SUPER
BRAIN-BOOSTING
SECRETS

Scientifically Proven Breakthroughs That Can Prevent Alzheimer's, Reverse Memory Loss and Keep Your Mind Sharp for Life

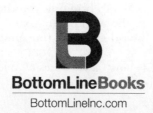

BottomLineBooks

BottomLineInc.com

10 9 8 7 6 5 4 3 2 1

ISBN 0-88723-764-9

Bottom Line Books® publishes the advice of expert authorities in many fields. These opinions may at times conflict as there are often different approaches to solving problems. The use of this material is no substitute for health, legal, accounting or other professional services. Consult competent professionals for answers to your specific questions.

Telephone numbers, addresses, prices, offers and websites listed in this book are accurate at the time of publication, but they are subject to frequent change.

Bottom Line Books® is a registered trademark of Bottom Line Inc., 3 Landmark Square, Suite 201, Stamford, CT 06901

BottomLineInc.com

Bottom Line Books® is an imprint of Bottom Line Inc., publisher of print periodicals, e-letters and books. We are dedicated to bringing you the best information from the most knowledgeable sources in the world. Our goal is to help you gain greater wealth, better health, more wisdom, extra time and increased happiness.

Printed in the United States of America

Contents

7 • STROKE RISKS, PREVENTION AND RECOVERY

Part 2: Make a Healthy Brain

8 • BRAIN FITNESS

9 • BRAIN FOOD AND SUPPLEMENTS

Part 3: Your Brain at Full Speed

12 • HOW YOUR BRAIN CAN HEAL YOUR BODY

13 • BRAIN TRICKS FOR A BETTER LIFE

PART 1

What Hurts Your Brain

CHAPTER 1

Alzheimer's and Dementia Prevention and Risks

Dr. Kosik's Alzheimer's Prevention Plan: 6 Powerful Secrets

If someone told you that there was a pill with no side effects and strong evidence showing that it helps prevent Alzheimer's disease, would you take it? Of course, you would!

The truth is, there's no such "magic bullet," but most adults do have the ability to dramatically decrease their risk for this dreaded disease.

A window of opportunity: According to the latest scientific evidence, slowing or blocking Alzheimer's plaques (buildups of dangerous protein fragments), which are now known to develop years before memory loss and other symptoms are noticeable, could be the key to stopping this disease.

Kenneth S. Kosik, MD, a renowned neuroscientist who has researched Alzheimer's for more than 25 years, shared the habits that he incorporates into his daily routine to help prevent Alzheimer's…

STEP 1: **Make exercise exciting.** You may know that frequent exercise—particularly aerobic exercise, which promotes blood flow to the brain—is the most effective Alzheimer's prevention strategy. Unfortunately, many people become bored and stop exercising.

Scientific evidence: Because exercise raises levels of brain-derived neurotrophic factor, it promotes the growth of new brain cells and may help prevent shrinkage of the hippocampus (a part of the brain involved in memory).

What I do: Most days, I spend 35 minutes on an elliptical trainer, followed by some weight training (increasing muscle mass helps

Kenneth S. Kosik, MD, the Harriman Professor of Neuroscience Research and codirector of the Neuroscience Research Institute at the University of California, Santa Barbara, where he specializes in the causes and treatments of neurodegeneration, particularly Alzheimer's disease. Dr. Kosik is coauthor of *Outsmarting Alzheimer's.* KennethSKosikMD.com prevent diabetes—an Alzheimer's risk factor). To break up the monotony, I go mountain biking on sunny days. I advise patients who have trouble sticking to an exercise regimen to try out the new virtual-reality equipment available in many gyms. While riding a stationary bike, for example, you can watch a monitor that puts you in the Tour de France!

Also helpful: To keep your exercise regimen exciting, go dancing. A recent 20-year study found that dancing reduced dementia risk more than any other type of exercise—perhaps because many types of dancing (such as tango, salsa and Zumba) involve learning new steps and aerobic activity. Do the type of dancing that appeals to you most.

STEP 2: **Keep your eating plan simple.** A nutritious diet is important for Alzheimer's prevention, but many people assume that they'll have to make massive changes, so they get overwhelmed and don't even try. To avoid this trap, keep it simple—all healthful diets have a few common elements, including an emphasis on antioxidant-rich foods (such as fruit and vegetables)…not too much red meat…and a limited amount of processed foods that are high in sugar, fat or additives.

Scientific evidence: Research has shown that people who consume more than four daily servings of vegetables have a 40% lower rate of cognitive decline than those who get less than one daily serving.

What I do: I try to eat more vegetables, particularly broccoli, cauliflower and other crucifers—there's strong evidence of their brain-protective effects.

Helpful: I'm not a veggie lover, so I roast vegetables with olive oil in the oven to make them more appetizing. Whenever possible, I use brain-healthy spices such as rosemary and turmeric.

STEP 3: **Guard your sleep.** During the day, harmful waste products accumulate in the brain. These wastes, including the amyloid protein that's linked to Alzheimer's, are mainly eliminated at night during deep (stages 3 and 4) sleep.

Scientific evidence: In a long-term Swedish study, men who reported poor sleep were

1.5 times more likely to develop Alzheimer's than those with better sleep.

Regardless of your age, you need a good night's sleep. While ideal sleep times vary depending on the person, sleeping less than six hours or more than nine hours nightly is linked to increased risk for cardiovascular disease—another Alzheimer's risk factor. If you don't feel rested when you wake up, talk to your doctor about your sleep quality.

What I do: I often take a 10-minute nap during the day. Brief naps (especially between 2 pm and 4 pm, which syncs with most people's circadian rhythms) can be restorative.

STEP 4: **Don't be a loner.** Having regular social interaction is strongly associated with healthy aging.

Scientific evidence: Older adults who frequently spend time with others—for example, sharing meals and volunteering—have about a 70% lower rate of cognitive decline than those who don't socialize much.

What I do: To stay socially active, I regularly Skype, attend conferences and stay in touch with other scientists and postdoc students.

If you're lonely, any form of social interaction is better than none. One study found that people who used computers regularly—to write e-mails, for example—were less lonely than those who didn't. If you can't connect in person, do a video chat or Facebook update at least once a day.

Also helpful: Having a pet. Pets are sometimes better listeners than spouses!

STEP 5: **Stay calm.** People who are often stressed are more likely to experience brain shrinkage.

Scientific evidence: In a three-year study of people with mild cognitive impairment (a condition that often precedes Alzheimer's), those with severe anxiety had a 135% increased risk for Alzheimer's, compared with those who were calmer.

What I do: I go for long walks.

Other great stress reducers: Having a positive mental attitude, deep breathing, yoga, tai chi, meditation—and even watching funny movies. Practice what works for you.

STEP 6: Push yourself intellectually. So-called "brain workouts" help prevent Alzheimer's—perhaps by increasing cognitive reserve (the stored memories/cognitive skills that you can draw on later in life)… and possibly by accelerating the growth of new brain cells.

Scientific evidence: In an important study, older adults (including those with a genetic risk factor for Alzheimer's) who frequently read, played board games or engaged in other mental activities were able to postpone the development of the disease by almost a decade.

But don't fool yourself—if you're an accomplished pianist, then banging out a tune won't help much even though a nonmusician is likely to benefit from learning to play. Push your mental abilities—do math problems in your head, memorize a poem, become a tutor, etc.

What I do: To challenge myself intellectually, I read novels and practice my foreign language skills—I do research in Latin America, so I work on my Spanish.

What You Don't Know About Preventing Alzheimer's

Dean Sherzai, MD, a neurologist and director of the Alzheimer's Disease Prevention Program at Cedars-Sinai Medical Center in Los Angeles.

Alzheimer's disease is hands down one of the most feared diseases. But simply worrying that you'll develop the illness doesn't do any good. A far better approach is to take action—now!

What's new: Around the country, respected medical centers and hospitals are now creating Alzheimer's prevention programs staffed by neurologists and researchers who help people do all that they can do to avoid this devastating condition.*

*To find an Alzheimer's prevention program near you, check with a local chapter of the Alzheimer's Association, ALZ.org, a local university or state or local agency for the aging.

Even if you're only in your 30s or 40s, it's wise to see a neurologist if you have a family history of Alzheimer's disease…or if, at any age, you're noticing mental changes (such as memory loss) that concern you. Everyone has momentary lapses—forgetting where you left your keys, for example—but those that impact your life, such as missing appointments, should be evaluated.

WHAT CAN YOU DO?

An increasing number of Alzheimer's experts now believe that preventive lifestyle approaches may help preserve memory and cognitive abilities. It's best to start before any disease-related changes occur in the brain. By the time symptoms are recognizable, the disease already has a foothold and the benefits of intervention will be nominal. While you may think that you already know the main Alzheimer's prevention strategies, key recommendations from Dean Sherzai, MD, director of the Alzheimer's Disease Prevention Program at Cedars-Sinai Medical Center in Los Angeles, include specifics that really make a difference. *Steps to take…*

• **Control your blood sugar.** Most Alzheimer's patients have higher-than-normal blood sugar levels or full-blown diabetes. In a study that tracked more than 2,000 patients for roughly seven years, those with a glucose reading of 115 mg/dL, on average, had an 18% higher risk for dementia than those with levels of 100 mg/dL or lower (normal range). The higher the blood sugar levels, the greater the Alzheimer's risk. It's not yet clear why elevated blood sugar increases cognitive risks, but it could be linked to the inflammation that accompanies blood glucose disorders.

Dr. Sherzai's advice: Avoid simple carbohydrates such as white bread and white rice that cause blood sugar to spike. Also, emerging evidence shows that eating a lot of sugar may cause Alzheimer's brain changes—so avoid sugar.

Recommended: No more than nine teaspoons of added sugars for men each day…six teaspoons for women. This may sound like a lot, but it's actually a lot less than many people get. Added sugars are in many foods—not

5

only in such things as sweetened yogurt and fruit drinks but also in pasta sauces, breads and salad dressings. Also, get screened for diabetes at three-year intervals, starting at age 45—sooner (and more frequently) if you have diabetes risk factors such as obesity and/or a family history.

• **Consume the "Big 3."** The Mediterranean diet, which includes fish, fruit, beans, vegetables, whole grains and monounsaturated fat (such as olive oil), has been widely promoted for brain health. But which specific foods are most likely to help keep you mentally sharp? *There's strong evidence for…*

• Fruit and vegetable juices, such as pomegranate, blueberry and grape. A nine-year study of 1,836 participants found that those who drank fruit or vegetable juices at least three times a week were 76% less likely to develop Alzheimer's than those who had them less than once a week. *Possible reason:* Juices have a high concentration of anti-inflammatory antioxidants—and this may help interrupt some of the brain changes (such as beta-amyloid deposits) that occur in Alzheimer's patients. A daily serving of a juiced mixture of fresh vegetables and low-sugar fruits, such as berries, lime or cantaloupe, is a good source of antioxidants and nutrients. Fruits high in sugar, such as bananas and mangoes, should be avoided, since as mentioned earlier, recent research has linked higher sugar levels with cognitive decline and dementia.

• Fatty fish. Researchers recently announced that people with high blood levels of omega-3 fatty acids had increased volume in the hippocampus, a part of the brain that's affected in those with cognitive decline. Other research has shown that there's less Alzheimer's in parts of the world where people eat the most fish.

One problem is that people often eat the wrong kind of fish. It must be omega-3–rich, fatty fish. *Best choices:* Salmon, herring, mackerel, sardines or tuna, eaten at least twice a week. If you don't like fish, you can take a daily supplement. Lovaza is the only fish oil supplement approved by the FDA. Because it's available by prescription, it may be covered by your insurance. Alternatively, you can take an over-the-counter fish oil supplement (check with your doctor first—fish oil can raise risk

for bleeding). Flaxseed, chia seeds and walnuts contain a plant-based omega-3.

• Vegetables—and more vegetables. With all the focus on brain-healthy fruits such as blueberries, vegetables are often forgotten. That's a mistake. In a study of more than 3,700 people, those who consumed the most vegetables (a median of 4.1 daily servings) had 38% less cognitive decline than those who ate the least. Good choices for those four or more daily servings are kale, spinach, brussels sprouts, broccoli and red bell peppers.

• **Give your mind the right kind of workout.** Crosswords and Sudoku help but less than you might think. They get easy with practice and target only some parts of the brain.

Better: Activities that challenge your brain on multiple levels—and stay challenging no matter how long you do them.

Examples: Playing a musical instrument, painting and even playing some challenging video or board games.

Also: Look for hobbies that use the hands and the mind—they require focus, memory, problem-solving, spatial visualization and other skills.

Dr. Sherzai's advice: List 10 activities that you enjoy, and try to do three or four of them daily. If one activity doesn't stimulate a part of your brain, another probably will.

• **Get more exercise—safely.** When it comes to preserving brain health, nothing beats exercise. It improves circulation and increases the amounts of glucose and oxygen that reach the brain.

Dr. Sherzai's advice: Be sure to exercise safely. An injury will deprive you of one of your strongest defenses against Alzheimer's. Outdoor exercise can increase risk for falls and other injuries. If you're not that sure-footed, go for indoor exercise using a machine such as a recumbent bicycle or elliptical trainer. Otherwise, take brisk walks outdoors. Aim for 30 minutes of moderate-to-vigorous exercise (breathing hard and fast with increased heart rate) on most days of the week, plus strength, flexibility and balance-improving activities. (Start with five-minute sessions if you're not used to it.)

A MEDICATION WORTH TRYING?

High blood pressure is widely known to increase Alzheimer's risk. What you may not realize is that the type of medicine used to control high blood pressure could also affect your Alzheimer's risk.

Interesting finding: When the medical records of more than five million patients were reviewed, those who took blood pressure drugs called angiotensin II receptor blockers (ARBs), such as *irbesartan* (Avapro), *losartan* (Cozaar) and *azilsartan* (Edarbi), had a 35% to 40% lower risk of developing Alzheimer's or other brain diseases than those prescribed other blood pressure drugs. What makes these drugs different? It's possible that blocking the renin-angiotensin system provides neurological benefits in addition to lowering blood pressure.

The research is not definitive, so your doctor won't prescribe an ARB just to prevent Alzheimer's disease. But if you're already taking blood pressure medication, you may want to ask about trying an ARB.

---

5 Surprising Ways to Prevent Alzheimer's . . . # 1: Check Your Tap Water

Marwan Sabbagh, MD, neurologist, and director of the Alzheimer's disease and memory disorders division at Barrow Neurological Institute at Dignity Health St. Joseph's Hospital and Medical Center, Phoenix, Arizona. He is author of *The Alzheimer's Prevention Cookbook: 100 Recipes to Boost Brain Health.* MarwanSabbaghMD.com

---

Every 68 seconds, another American develops Alzheimer's disease, the fatal brain disease that steals memory and personality. It's the fifth-leading cause of death among people age 65 and older.

You can lower your likelihood of getting Alzheimer's disease by reducing controllable and well-known risk factors. *But new scientific research reveals that there are also little-known "secret" risk factors that you can address...*

COPPER IN TAP WATER

A scientific paper published in *Journal of Trace Elements in Medicine and Biology* theorizes that inorganic copper found in nutritional supplements and in drinking water is an important factor in today's Alzheimer's epidemic.

Science has established that amyloid-beta plaques—inflammation-causing cellular debris found in the brains of people with Alzheimer's—contain high levels of copper. Animal research shows that small amounts of inorganic copper in drinking water worsen Alzheimer's. Studies on people have linked the combination of copper and a high-fat diet to memory loss and mental decline. It may be that copper sparks amyloid-beta plaques to generate more oxidation and inflammation, further injuring brain cells.

What to do: There is plenty of copper in our diets—no one needs additional copper from a multivitamin/mineral supplement. Look for a supplement with no copper or a minimal amount (500 micrograms).

I also recommend filtering water. Water-filter pitchers, such as ones by Brita, can reduce the presence of copper. I installed a reverse-osmosis water filter in my home a few years ago when the evidence for the role of copper in Alzheimer's became compelling.

VITAMIN D DEFICIENCY

Mounting evidence shows that a low blood level of vitamin D may increase Alzheimer's risk.

A study in *Journal of Alzheimer's Disease* analyzed 10 studies exploring the link between vitamin D and Alzheimer's. Researchers found that low blood levels of vitamin D were linked to a 40% increased risk for Alzheimer's.

The researchers from UCLA, also writing in *Journal of Alzheimer's Disease*, theorize that vitamin D may protect the brain by reducing amyloid-beta and inflammation.

What to do: The best way to make sure that your blood level of vitamin D is protective is to ask your doctor to test it—and then, if needed, to help you correct your level to greater than 60 nanograms per milliliter (ng/mL). That correction may require 1,000 IU to 2,000 IU of vitamin D daily...or another individualized supplementation strategy.

Important: When your level is tested, make sure that it is the 25-hydroxyvitamin D, or 25(OH)D, test and not the 1.25-dihydroxy-vitamin D test. The latter test does not accurately measure blood levels of vitamin D but is sometimes incorrectly ordered. Also, ask for your exact numerical results. Levels above 30 ng/mL are considered "normal," but in my view, the 60 ng/mL level is the minimum that is protective.

HORMONE REPLACEMENT THERAPY AFTER MENOPAUSE

Research shows that starting hormone-replacement therapy (HRT) within five years of entering menopause and using hormones for 10 or more years reduces the risk for Alzheimer's by 30%. But an 11-year study of 1,768 women, published in *Neurology*, shows that those who started a combination of estrogen-progestin therapy five years or more after the onset of menopause had a 93% higher risk for Alzheimer's.

What to do: If you are thinking about initiating hormone replacement therapy five years or more after the onset of menopause, talk to your doctor about the possible benefits and risks.

A CONCUSSION

A study published in *Neurology* showed that NFL football players had nearly four times higher risk for Alzheimer's than the general population—no doubt from repeated brain injuries incurred while playing football.

What most people don't realize: Your risk of developing Alzheimer's is doubled if you've ever had a serious concussion that resulted in loss of consciousness—this newer evidence shows that it is crucially important to prevent head injuries of any kind throughout your life.

What to do: Fall-proof your home, with commonsense measures such as adequate lighting, eliminating or securing throw rugs and keeping stairways clear. Wear shoes with firm soles and low heels, which also helps prevent falls.

If you've ever had a concussion, it's important to implement the full range of Alzheimer's-prevention strategies in this article.

NOT HAVING A PURPOSE IN LIFE

In a seven-year study published in *Archives of General Psychiatry*, researchers at the Rush Alzheimer's Disease Center in Chicago found that people who had a "purpose in life" were 2.4 times less likely to develop Alzheimer's.

What to do: The researchers found that the people who agreed with the following statements were less likely to develop Alzheimer's and mild cognitive impairment—"I feel good when I think of what I have done in the past and what I hope to do in the future" and "I have a sense of direction and purpose in life."

If you cannot genuinely agree with the above statements, there are things you can do to change that—in fact, you even can change the way you feel about your past. It takes a bit of resolve...some action...and perhaps help from a qualified mental health counselor.

One way to start: Think about and make a list of some activities that would make your life more meaningful. Ask yourself, Am I doing these?...and then write down small, realistic goals that will involve you more in those activities, such as volunteering one hour every week at a local hospital or signing up for a class at your community college next semester.

The following steps are crucial in the fight against Alzheimer's disease...

- **Lose weight if you're overweight.**

- **Control high blood pressure.**

- **Exercise regularly.**

- **Engage in activities that challenge your mind.**

- **Eat a diet rich in colorful fruits and vegetables and low in saturated fat,** such as the Mediterranean diet.

- **Take a daily supplement containing 2,000 milligrams of omega-3 fatty acids.**

More Than Half of Alzheimer's Cases Could Be Prevented with Lifestyle Changes

Many of the biggest risk factors for Alzheimer's disease are modifiable—lack of physical activity, depression, smoking, midlife hypertension, midlife obesity and diabetes. Changing or eliminating these risks could potentially prevent 2.9 million Alzheimer's cases in the US.

Deborah Barnes, PhD, MPH, associate professor of psychiatry, University of California, San Francisco, and leader of a comprehensive review published online in *The Lancet Neurology.*

How to Cut Your Risk for Alzheimer's…by Half

Majid Fotuhi, MD, PhD, neurologist, medical director of the NeuroGrow Brain Fitness Center in McLean, Virginia, and affiliate staff at Johns Hopkins Medicine, Baltimore. He is also author of *The Memory Cure* and coauthor of *The New York Times Crosswords to Keep Your Brain Young.*

The prevalence of memory and thinking problems—including Alzheimer's disease and other forms of dementia—declined in the US by nearly 30% during a recent nine-year period.

Why did this happen? Partly because many adults are doing a better job at controlling significant dementia risk factors, including blood pressure (below 120/80 mm Hg is optimal) and cholesterol (below 200 mg/dL is the target for most people's total cholesterol).

But there are other strategies to reduce dementia risk even further. Although some vulnerability to Alzheimer's and other forms of dementia can be genetic, an ever-increasing body of evidence shows that adopting a healthful lifestyle often can cut a person's risk by half. *What you need to know…*

OVERLOOKED RISK FACTORS

Dementia occurs when brain cells are progressively damaged by excessive accumulation of proteins, such as amyloid. These proteins trigger inflammation, causing more damage to nearby brain cells. But that's not the only trigger. The brain needs a constant supply of oxygen, hormones and nutrients such as blood sugar (glucose). Interruptions in the supply—due to narrowed and blocked blood vessels, multiple small strokes that may pass unnoticed and even heart failure, kidney disease and chronic lung disease—can kill brain cells.

Other dementia risk factors that are sometimes overlooked…

•**Belly fat.** Abdominal fat is strongly linked to an increased risk for heart disease, and two recent studies have shown an association between belly fat and dementia.

Evidence: A study of more than 6,500 men and women, published in *Neurology,* found that those with the most belly fat during their 40s were nearly three times as likely to develop dementia over the next 30 to 40 years, compared with those who had the least belly fat.

Alzheimer's prevention step: Regardless of your age, strive for a fit body. Your waist measurement in inches should be no more than half your height, in inches.

•**Diabetes.** Research supports a link between diabetes and dementia. One Swedish study of 2,269 men found that those whose secretion of the hormone insulin was low in response to glucose at age 50 (a sign of impaired glucose metabolism that is likely to progress to diabetes) were significantly more likely to develop dementia over the next 32 years.

Alzheimer's prevention step: Your blood glucose level after fasting overnight should be less than 100 mg/dL. People with levels of 100 mg/dL to 125 mg/dL may be at risk for diabetes and should be closely monitored by their physicians. Levels of 126 mg/dL and higher indicate diabetes. Follow your doctor's advice on the frequency of fasting blood-glucose testing.

•**Smoking and heavy drinking.** People with a history of smoking or heavy drinking appear to develop Alzheimer's sooner than others.

Evidence: In a Florida study of nearly 1,000 people diagnosed with Alzheimer's, those who smoked more than a pack per day developed Alzheimer's 2.3 years before those who were not heavy smokers. Those who drank more than two drinks per day developed it 4.8 years earlier than those who drank less.

Alzheimer's prevention step: If you smoke, quit now. If you drink, ask your doctor whether moderate drinking is beneficial for you. Moderate alcohol consumption has been shown in some studies to help prevent cognitive decline. Women should not exceed one drink (wine, beer or hard liquor) daily…men, no more than two drinks daily.

EXERCISE REALLY DOES HELP

Even if you're aware that exercise helps protect against dementia, few people realize just how important it is. Besides maintaining good circulation to ensure a steady supply of nutrients and oxygen to the brain, physical activity increases production of brain-derived neurotrophic factor—a protein that triggers brain cell growth.

Evidence: Sedentary retirees started walking three times a week. Six months later, their brains—as measured by magnetic resonance imaging (MRI) scans—had grown by 3%, on average, roughly the equivalent of taking three years off the age of their brains.

Alzheimer's prevention step: Get at least 30 minutes of moderate exercise (such as brisk walking) most days of the week. If you don't like walking, try dancing, cycling or golf. Any physical activity is better than nothing—and the more, the better.

GET THE RIGHT BRAIN FOODS

Foods that help protect your brain…

•**Omega-3 fatty** acids are the most abundant of the polyunsaturated fatty acids that comprise up to 20% of the brain's volume. Some people get their omega-3s from fish-oil capsules—which contain both eicosapentaenoic acid (EPA) and docosahexaenoic acid (DHA). DHA is the most important for brain health and is recommended (along with EPA)

for heart health by the American Heart Association.

Alzheimer's prevention step: Ask your doctor about taking an omega-3 supplement that contains at least 400 mg of DHA per daily dose. Or eat two to three servings of cold-water fish (such as wild salmon, mackerel and sardines) weekly.

•**Antioxidants** protect the brain against cumulative damage caused by highly reactive chemicals known as "free radicals." An eight-year study of 5,000 people identified vitamins E and C as particularly important for brain health.

Alzheimer's prevention step: Whenever possible, get your vitamins E and C from fruits and vegetables—this also will increase your intake of other powerful antioxidants. Kiwifruit, papaya and pomegranates are particularly good sources. Aim for four to five servings daily of fruits and vegetables. If you prefer a supplement, take 300 international units (IU) of vitamin E and 500 mg of vitamin C daily.

•**Curcumin** is the yellow pigment of turmeric, the primary ingredient in curry powder. Laboratory tests have shown that curcumin helps dissolve the abnormal amyloid formations of Alzheimer's disease.

Alzheimer's prevention step: Cook with curcumin (try it in curried chicken, soups and vegetables) or take a 200-mg supplement daily.

Also helpful: A regular regimen of "brain fitness" activities.

MEMORY SELF-TEST

Questions to ask yourself…

1. Have you ever gotten lost when you drive home?

2. Have you forgotten being at major appointments or events? Forgetting names of people you met at a recent party is not cause for concern, but forgetting that you attended the party could signal a possible memory problem.

3. Has anyone around you complained that you tend to repeat the same questions four or five times?

4. Have you stopped any of your hobbies or routines because of memory problems?

5. Have you reduced your work responsibilities or hours mainly due to poor memory? For example, did you take early retirement because you can't keep up with the same work you've done for years?

If you answered "yes" to any of these questions, speak to your doctor about getting a neurological evaluation.

Alzheimer's: Is It "Type 3" Diabetes?

Isaac Eliaz, MD, LAc, an integrative physician and medical director of the Amitabha Medical Clinic & Healing Center in Santa Rosa, California, an integrative health center specializing in chronic conditions. Dr. Eliaz is a licensed acupuncturist and homeopath and an expert in mind/body medicine. He has coauthored dozens of peer-reviewed scientific papers on natural healing. DrEliaz.org

---

For years, scientists from around the world have investigated various causes of Alzheimer's disease. Cardiovascular disease factors, such as hypertension, stroke and heart failure...other neurological diseases, such as Parkinson's disease...accumulated toxins and heavy metals, such as aluminum, lead and mercury...nutrient deficiencies, including vitamins B and E...infections, such as the herpes virus and the stomach bacterium H. pylori...and head injuries each have been considered at one time or another to be a possible contributor to the development of this mind-robbing disease.

However, as researchers continue to piece together the results of literally thousands of studies, one particular theory is now emerging as perhaps the most plausible and convincing of them all in explaining why some people—and not others—develop Alzheimer's disease.

A PATTERN EMERGES

An estimated 5.4 million Americans are now living with Alzheimer's, and the number is expected to increase with a rapidly aging population. Rates of obesity, diabetes and metabolic syndrome (a constellation of risk factors including elevated blood sugar, high blood pressure, abnormal cholesterol levels and abdominal fat) are also on the rise.

What's the potential link? Doctors have long suspected that diabetes increases risk for Alzheimer's. The exact mechanism is not known, but many experts believe that people with diabetes are more likely to develop Alzheimer's because their bodies don't properly use blood sugar (glucose) and the blood sugar–regulating hormone insulin.

Now research shows increased dementia risk in people with high blood sugar—even if they do not have diabetes. A problem with insulin appears to be the cause. How does insulin dysfunction affect the brain? Neurons are starved of energy, and there's an increase in brain cell death, DNA damage, inflammation and the formation of plaques in the brain—a main characteristic of Alzheimer's disease.

AN ALZHEIMER'S-FIGHTING REGIMEN

Even though experimental treatments with antidiabetes drugs that improve insulin function have been shown to reduce symptoms of early Alzheimer's disease, it is my belief, as an integrative physician, that targeted nondrug therapies are preferable in preventing the brain degeneration that leads to Alzheimer's and fuels its progression. These approaches won't necessarily reverse Alzheimer's, but they may help protect your brain if you are not currently fighting this disease...or help slow the progression of early-stage Alzheimer's.

My advice includes...

• **Follow a low-glycemic (low sugar) diet.** This is essential for maintaining healthy glucose and insulin function as well as supporting brain and overall health. An effective way to maintain a low-sugar diet is to use the glycemic index (GI), a scale that ranks foods according to how quickly they raise blood sugar levels.

Here's what happens: High-GI foods (such as white rice, white potatoes and refined sugars) are rapidly digested and absorbed. As a result, these foods cause dangerous spikes in blood sugar levels.

Low-GI foods (such as green vegetables…fiber-rich foods including whole grains…and plant proteins including legumes, nuts and seeds) are digested slowly, so they gradually raise blood sugar and insulin levels. This is critical for maintaining glucose and insulin function and controlling inflammation.

Helpful: GlycemicIndex.com gives glucose ratings of common foods and recipes.

• **Consider trying brain-supporting nutrients and herbs.*** These supplements, which help promote insulin function, can be used alone or taken together for better results (dosages may be lower if supplements are combined due to the ingredients' synergistic effects)…

• **Alpha-lipoic acid (ALA)** is an antioxidant shown to support insulin sensitivity and protect neurons from inflammation-related damage.

Typical dosage: 500 mg to 1,000 mg per day.

• **Chromium improves glucose regulation.**

Typical dosage: 350 micrograms (mcg) to 700 mcg per day.

• **Alginates from seaweed help reduce glucose spikes and crashes.**

Typical dosage: 250 mg to 1,000 mg before meals.

• **L-Taurine, an amino acid, helps maintain healthy glucose and lipid (blood fat) levels.**

Typical dosage: 1,000 mg to 2,000 mg per day.

KICK UP YOUR HEELS!

Regular exercise, such as walking, swimming and tennis, is known to improve insulin function and support cognitive health by increasing circulation to the brain. Dancing, however, may be the ultimate brain-protective exercise. Why might dancing be better than other brain-body coordination exercises, such

*Consult your doctor before trying these supplements, especially if you take any medications or have a chronic health condition, such as liver or kidney disease. If he/she is not well-versed in the use of these therapies, consider seeing an integrative physician. To find one near you, consult The Institute for Functional Medicine, FunctionalMedicine.org.

as tennis? Because dancing is mainly noncompetitive, there isn't the added stress of contending with an opponent, which increases risk for temporary cognitive impairment.

Best: Aerobic dances with a social component, such as Latin, swing or ballroom, performed at least three times weekly for 90 minutes each session. (Dancing for less time also provides some brain benefits.) If you don't like dancing, brisk walking for 30 minutes a day, five days a week, is also shown to help protect the brain against dementia.

Free courses: In addition to getting regular physical activity, it's helpful to learn challenging new material to "exercise" the brain. For 750 free online lectures provided by professors at top universities such as Stanford and Johns Hopkins, go to OpenCulture.com/freeonline courses. Subjects include art history, geography, international relations and biology.

System Predicts Dementia in People with Type 2 Diabetes

The diabetes-specific dementia risk score (DSDRS) is based on factors such as age, education, acute metabolic events, heart disease and depression. The system will make it easier for doctors to monitor patients at the highest risk for dementia.

Study of 29,961 patients by researchers from Kaiser Permanente Northern California Division of Research, Oakland, and University Medical Centre Utrecht, the Netherlands, published in *The Lancet Diabetes & Endocrinology.*

Even Slightly High Blood Sugar Hurts Memory

People with blood sugar at the high end of the normal range performed worse on a memory test than people with lower blood sugar levels.

Also: People with high blood sugar had a smaller hippocampus, the area of the brain that plays a crucial role in memory and spatial navigation.

Best: Get your blood sugar level checked regularly...monitor your diet...and exercise to keep your blood sugar levels low.

Study of 141 people, average age 63, by researchers at Charité-Medical University of Berlin, Germany, published in *Neurology*.

Alzheimer's in the Family

Lisa Mosconi, PhD, research assistant professor, department of psychiatry, New York University Langone Medical Center, Center for Cognitive Neurology, New York City, and leader of a study of 66 adults, presented at a recent Alzheimer's Association international conference.

People whose mothers have or had Alzheimer's have a heightened risk of getting the disease. (People whose fathers have or had Alzheimer's do not appear to be at increased risk.) But even if your mother had Alzheimer's, you can take special care of your health to lower controllable risk factors. The more factors you control, the less chance there is that you will develop the disease.

Get a thorough medical examination. Focus on reducing high blood pressure and cholesterol and preventing or controlling diabetes, all of which increase the risk for cardiovascular disease and, in turn, increase the risk for dementia. Exercise regularly...quit smoking...and eat a healthful diet rich in fruits and vegetables. Increase consumption of foods high in antioxidants (including vitamins C and E, beta-carotene and omega-3 fatty acids), such as oranges, grapefruit, salmon, nuts and broccoli. If you drink, have one glass of red wine a day.

Bad Vision Boosts Alzheimer's Risk

Mary A.M. Rogers, PhD, research associate professor, department of internal medicine, University of Michigan, and research director of the Patient Safety Enhancement Program, University of Michigan Health System, Ann Arbor.

Want to give yourself a better chance of evading Alzheimer's disease? Get your eyes checked. Recent research reveals that treating vision problems can actually reduce the risk for dementia, including Alzheimer's disease.

Seeds for this study were planted with information from the Aging, Demographics, and Memory Study, when University of Michigan researchers noticed that people with dementia tended to have had fewer eye procedures prior to their diagnoses than those without dementia. *This led the team to ask two questions...*

• **Does poor vision contribute to the development of dementia?**

• **Does treating visual disorders reduce the likelihood of developing dementia?**

CAN YOU SEE DEMENTIA IN YOUR FUTURE?

Using data from Medicare and the nationally representative Health and Retirement Study, the Michigan researchers followed 625 elderly Americans (none of whom had dementia at the outset) for an average of 10 years. Based on a scale that ranked vision from excellent (one) to totally blind (six), they found that the risk for dementia increased 52%, on average, with each step up the scale. Mary A.M. Rogers, PhD, a clinical epidemiologist and the study's lead author, said that the study results suggest that the problems with declining vision preceded the dementia. She said that this is the first epidemiologic study, to her knowledge, that points to treatment of vision problems as being protective against the development of late-life dementia.

Some of the connections between poor vision and dementia symptoms seem obvious, while others are not yet understood. For instance, Dr. Rogers pointed out that people with poor vision may be less likely to participate in the kinds of activities, such as reading, playing board games and engaging in physical activities, that can be protective against cognitive decline. She said that other research indicates that visual loss can lead to structural changes in the brain, but notes that more studies are needed to understand why.

SEE YOUR DOCTOR!

Good news came out of this study too. Dr. Rogers said that when elderly people received appropriate treatment for their visual difficulties—which can include procedures such as corneal transplant, cataract removal and lens insertion, and treatment for retinal detachment, lesions and other eye disorders—their probability of developing dementia decreased. Even one visit to an ophthalmologist was associated with a lower risk.

Unfortunately, at this point Medicare coverage of vision problems is spotty. While only about 13% of the Medicare population has Alzheimer's disease, this group accounts for 34% of Medicare spending—and, of course, Alzheimer's incidence is expected to increase, not decline. Dr. Rogers believes it would be very worthwhile to investigate whether expanding vision screenings and treatment to more elderly Americans would in fact save money for Medicare. In the meantime, it is wise to visit your doctor if you are having any vision problems—it may improve your health and your life in several important ways.

Better Brain Health

When researchers examined clinical records of 211 adults diagnosed with probable Alzheimer's disease, those who spoke multiple languages over their lifetimes showed initial Alzheimer's symptoms an average of five years later than those who spoke one language.

Theory: Bilingual people build concentration skills by focusing on the language they are speaking while minimizing interference from a second language.

If you are bilingual: It's not enough to hear or read a second language—contact libraries, universities and cultural centers to find groups that converse. If you are not bilingual, learning a second language can help promote brain health.

Fergus Craik, PhD, senior scientist, The Rotman Research Institute, Toronto, Canada.

What Really Causes Dementia

Peter V. Rabins, MD, MPH, Richman Family Professor for Alzheimer's and Related Diseases, vice-chair for academic affairs, department of psychiatry and behavioral sciences, Johns Hopkins University School of Medicine, Baltimore, and coauthor of *The 36 Hour Day*.

What really causes dementia? What a relief it would be to know the answer, since most people over 65 worry about whether the occasional "senior moment" or "brain fog" is a sign that something more serious is going on. Scientists are studying this issue from every possible angle, trying to learn what illnesses, lifestyle habits and environmental factors are at play—but, as yet, no one knows for sure.

Making this particular challenge even more difficult (or rewarding, depending on your perspective) is that dementia researchers seem to find new associations with every rock they turn over. Having a big head? Exposure to bright lights? Both may be protective. Living a sedentary lifestyle, smoking and having high cholesterol at midlife? Trouble lies ahead.

WHAT WE DO KNOW

Healthy habits that seem to protect against dementia...

•**Using your brain, living a full life.** A study of 951 older, dementia-free patients found that those who reported having a purpose in life at the study's start were half as likely to have Alzheimer's disease seven years later...while numerous studies showed that engaging in mentally stimulating activities, such as doing crossword puzzles, playing cards and attending movies and plays, holds back development of dementia.

• **Good nutrition—including drinking tea.** A four-year study of 2,258 dementia-free New Yorkers found 40% lower risk for Alzheimer's among those who followed the Mediterranean diet (lots of fruit, vegetables, fish, olive oil, legumes and cereals and moderate alcohol intake) than for those whose diets weren't as healthy. Studies have also found that drinking tea regularly is protective—for instance, one 14-year study found that tea drinkers were 37% less likely to develop dementia than those who don't drink tea.

• **Exercise.** A vast body of research finds regular exercise is protective. For instance, one study found that those who engage in active exercise, such as doing yard work or biking, had a 29% lower risk for dementia than people who got little or no exercise.

Meanwhile, signs that point to increased risk for other health problems are also associated with a higher risk for dementia...

• **Vitamin D deficiency.** An international group that assessed cognitive decline of 858 seniors over six years found that people deficient in vitamin D were more than 60% more likely to have experienced significant cognitive decline and 31% more likely to have problems with executive function (which includes thinking, learning and memory) than those with healthy levels of vitamin D.

• **Cardiovascular risk factors.** One large study that followed almost 10,000 people over age 40 found that even marginally high cholesterol (200 mg/dL to 239 mg/dL) at middle age increased risk for late-life dementia by about 50%, while other studies have correlated high blood pressure with dementia.

• **First- and secondhand smoking.** Beyond the countless studies linking smoking and cognitive impairment, a six-year study of almost 5,000 nonsmoking adults by researchers from the Universities of Cambridge and Michigan found that those who reported long-term exposure (30 years or more) to secondhand tobacco smoke were about 30% more likely to develop dementia than those who reported no regular exposure.

And if you already have certain diseases, odds are higher that you'll get dementia, too...

• **Diabetes.** Substantial research has found diabetes is a risk factor for dementia. For example, a recent study by London's Institute of Psychiatry found that participants with diabetes were nearly three times as likely as nondiabetics to develop dementia.

• **Depression.** Several studies find depression increases dementia risk. Of nearly 1,000 elderly participants from the Framingham Heart Study, those who were depressed when first examined had almost double the risk for dementia 17 years later.

IS THERE A THEME HERE?

It makes sense, in practical terms, to summarize risk factors for dementia as being pretty much inclusive of everything that we already know is bad for your heart. But when it comes to prevention—frustratingly—the massive amount of research has so far produced no strong evidence that we can "prevent" dementia by doing anything in particular.

A major problem is that most of the studies have some basic limitation or flaw in research design. For instance, most of the existing research compares people who develop dementia with those who don't...but recent research indicates that dementia may be present decades before symptoms are noticeable enough to make a diagnosis, so it may be that some of those patients weren't actually dementia-free.

Another flaw: Healthier people tend to take better care of themselves, so it's hard to tease out which factors or habits are responsible for cognitive health.

IN THE MEANTIME

What scientific advice can we offer, based on what we know at this point? When it comes to preventing dementia, the odds clearly favor those who live a healthy lifestyle. For instance, since 10% to 20% of dementia in the US is known to have vascular causes, we can infer that eating a healthy diet, exercising and managing stress are beneficial. The fact that only 30% to 60% of dementia risk is thought to be genetic means that there is plenty of reason to do all you can to reduce environmental risk—another argument for health-promoting habits and choices.

The search for the cause or cure will certainly continue, but reviewing what we already do know says quite a lot. Living well and with joy seems to boost the odds that you will remain cognitively intact, whereas all those things that are bad for you…are bad for you.

You Can Have a Much Younger Body and Mind— A Few Simple Changes Can Turn Back the Clock

Mike Moreno, MD, who practices family medicine in San Diego, where he is on the board of the San Diego Chapter of the American Academy of Family Physicians. He is also author of *The 17 Day Plan to Stop Aging.* Dr.MikeDiet.com

What is it that allows some people to remain robust and healthy well into their 80s and 90s while others become frail or virtually incapacitated? It's not just luck. Recent studies indicate that aging is largely determined by controllable factors.

Case in point: Millions of people have chronic inflammation, which has been linked to practically every "age-related" disease, including arthritis, heart disease and dementia.

Inflammation can usually be controlled with stress management, a healthful diet, weight loss (if needed) and other lifestyle changes, but there are other, even simpler, steps that can strengthen your body and brain so that they perform at the levels of a much younger person.

To turn back your biological clock…

• **Challenge your lungs.** You shouldn't be short of breath when you climb a flight of stairs or have sex, but many adults find that they have more trouble breathing as they age—even if they don't have asthma or other lung diseases.

Why: The lungs tend to lose elasticity over time, particularly if you smoke or live in an area with high air pollution. "Stiff" lungs cannot move air efficiently and cause breathing difficulty.

Simple thing you can do: Breathe slowly in and out through a drinking straw for two to three minutes, once or twice daily. Breathe only through your mouth, not your nose. This stretches the lungs, increases lung capacity and improves lung function.

Helpful: Start with an extra-wide straw, and go to a regular straw as you get used to breathing this way.

• **Drink thyme tea.** When the lungs do not expand and contract normally (see above), or when the tissues are unusually dry, you're more likely to get colds or other infections, including pneumonia. The herb thyme contains thymol, an antioxidant that may help prevent colds, bronchitis and pneumonia and soothe chronic respiratory problems such as asthma, allergies and emphysema.

Simple thing you can do: Add a cup of thyme tea to your daily routine. If you have a chronic or acute respiratory illness, drink two cups of thyme tea daily—one in the morning and one at night.

To make thyme tea: Steep one tablespoon of dried thyme (or two tablespoons of fresh thyme) in two cups of hot water for five minutes, or use thyme tea bags (available at most health-food stores).

If you take a blood thinner: Talk to your doctor before using thyme—it can increase risk for bleeding. Also, if you're allergic to oregano, you're probably allergic to thyme.

Another simple step: Drink at least six to eight eight-ounce glasses of water every day. This helps loosen lung mucus and flushes out irritants, such as bacteria and viruses.

• **Lower your heart rate.** Heart disease is the leading cause of death in the US. The average American would live at least a decade longer if his/her heart pumped blood more efficiently.

Simple thing you can do: Aim for a resting heart rate of 50 to 70 beats a minute—a good range for most adults. To do this, get 30 minutes of aerobic exercise, five days a week. Good aerobic workouts include fast walking, bicycling and swimming. Even if you're not in great shape, regular workouts will lower your resting heart rate.

To check your pulse: Put your index and middle fingers on the carotid artery in your neck, and count the beats for 15 seconds, then multiply by four. Check your pulse before, during and after exercise.

• **Walk just a little faster.** A study published in *The Journal of the American Medical Association* found that people who walked faster (at least 2.25 miles per hour) lived longer than those who walked more slowly.

Why: Faster walking not only lowers your heart rate and blood pressure but also improves cholesterol and inhibits blood clots, the cause of most heart attacks.

Simple thing you can do: You don't have to be a speed-walker, but every time you go for a walk, or even when you're walking during the normal course of your day, increase your speed and distance slightly.

• **Try this for better memory.** A study found that people who got even moderate amounts of exercise—either leisurely 30-minute workouts, five days a week, or more intense 20-minute workouts, three times a week—had better memories than those who exercised less. Aerobic exercise also lowers heart rate, which reduces risk of heart disease.

Why: Physical activity increases oxygen to the brain and boosts levels of neurotransmitters that improve mood as well as memory.

Simple thing you can do: Try an aerobic dance class, such as Zumba or salsa, or power yoga. These activities provide the physical activity needed to boost memory…and learning and remembering complicated routines will activate brain circuits and promote the growth of new brain cells for further brain benefit.

Bottom line: Just keep moving—even housecleaning and yard work count. *More on boosting brain function below…*

• **Shake up your mental routines.** In a study of about 3,000 older adults, those who performed mentally challenging tasks, such as memorizing a shopping list or surfing the Internet to research a complex topic, were found to have cognitive skills that were the typical equivalent of someone 10 years younger.

Why: These tasks trigger the development of new neurons in the brain, which boost cognitive function.

Simple thing you can do: Try to change your mental routines daily.

Fun ideas: If you're right-handed, use your left hand to write a note. Study the license number of the car in front of you, and see if you can remember it five minutes later. Overall, don't let your brain get into the rut of performing the same tasks over and over.

• **Fight brain inflammation.** You've probably heard that good oral hygiene can reduce the risk for heart disease. A recent study suggests that it also can promote brain health. Researchers found that men and women over age 60 who had the lowest levels of oral bacteria did better on cognitive tests involving memory and calculations than those who had more bacteria.

Why: Bacteria associated with gum disease also cause inflammation in the brain. This low-level inflammation can damage brain cells and affect cognitive function.

Simple thing you can do: Brush your teeth after every meal—and floss twice a day. I also recommend using an antiseptic mouthwash, which helps eliminate bacteria.

This Diabetes Drug May Be Good for Your Brain

Metformin encourages neuron growth in laboratory tests and enhances memory in mice. If further research confirms the findings, the drug may be used to help repair the brains of patients with neurological disorders.

Study by researchers at University of Toronto, published in *The Journal of the American Medical Association.*

BP Meds That Reduce Alzheimer's Risk 50%!

Patients who took medication for high blood pressure—specifically, diuretics, angiotensin receptor blockers (ARBs) or angiotensin-converting-enzyme (ACE) inhibitors—had 50% lower risk for Alzheimer's in a recent study. Patients who took other blood pressure medications did not show this benefit. Hypertension is a known risk factor for Alzheimer's, so talk to your doctor about the right medication for you.

Sevil Yasar, MD, PhD, assistant professor of medicine at The Johns Hopkins University School of Medicine, Baltimore, and leader of a study of 2,200 people, published in *Neurology.*

Having a Purpose in Life Prevents Dementia

Patricia A. Boyle, PhD, neuropsychologist, Rush Alzheimer's Disease Center, and associate professor, department of behavioral sciences, Rush University Medical Center, both in Chicago. Her study was published in *Archives of General Psychiatry.*

You already know that staying physically and mentally active may help stave off dementia, but researchers have found yet another protective trick—having a purpose in life.

The study analyzed 246 senior citizens who received annual cognitive testing for about 10 years. Each was asked questions to determine whether he or she had a strong purpose in life. When participants died, they underwent brain autopsies.

What the researchers found was that in participants who had a lot of plaques and tangles in their brains—abnormal structures in and around the brain's nerve cells that are hallmarks of Alzheimer's disease—the rate of cognitive decline had been about 30% slower for people who had a strong purpose in life compared with those who had had a weaker purpose or no purpose at all.

Here's a possible explanation: The stronger your purpose in life, the less likely you'll suffer cognitive decline as you age, even if your brain is affected by Alzheimer's signs. This might mean that you can preserve your cognitive ability by making sure that you have a purpose.

Of course, it could be the other way around—it could be that some people have a biological problem that makes them less able to cope with brain plaques and tangles and, also, less able to feel that their lives have purpose.

GO FOR IT ANYWAY

According to lead study author Patricia A. Boyle, PhD, a neuropsychologist in the Alzheimer's Disease Center at Rush University Medical Center in Chicago, her study doesn't prove whether purposefulness helps our brains work better or is simply a side effect of a brain that is already working better. Maybe research will determine that one day. But on the other hand, since having a sense of purpose seems to make people happier, she said, why not cultivate one?

Based on her work with the study subjects, Dr. Boyle defines a life purpose as "the sense that one's life has meaning and direction—that one is intentional and motivated to engage in activities that one finds important and fulfilling." In other words, it's what gets you out of bed each day and makes you feel that life is worth living.

A purpose doesn't have to be ambitious or complicated. In fact, many purposes are simple, said Dr. Boyle. It just can't have a definite end point—it has to last throughout your life. For example, some purposes include spending time every day with loved ones…helping other people (for example through long-term volunteer work)…learning something new every day…or passing down a certain set of knowledge or skills to a younger generation. If you love running marathons or writing novels, make sure that your goal is to continue pursuing those goals through life—and not just run one marathon or write one novel.

It's not so much what your purpose is, Dr. Boyle said—what's critical is how it makes you feel. If it stirs you up inside and makes you feel passionate, energetic and excited, then you've found it!

Fun Way to Boost Brain Health

Learn a new word every day! As people age, the brain relies on "cognitive reserve" (healthy neural networks) to compensate for loss of cognitive function such as memory. In a recent study of more than 300 people over age 50, healthy participants had a stronger vocabulary than those with mild cognitive impairment.

To keep your neural networks strong: Play daily word games, or sign up for Word of the Day apps.

Cristina Lojo Seoane, PhD, researcher, department of developmental psychology, University of Santiago de Compostela, Spain.

Good News for Grandmas!

Postmenopausal women who took care of their grandchildren one day a week had better memory and faster cognitive speed (im-portant for warding off dementia) than those who didn't.

Possible explanation: Active grandparenting includes positive interactions, ongoing learning and mental stimulation—all of which reduce risk for dementia.

Careful, though…women who cared for grandchildren five or more days a week had significantly lower cognitive scores, possibly because they felt exhausted.

Cassandra Szoeke, MD, PhD, associate professor of medicine, The University of Melbourne, Australia.

Don't Let Computer Use Harm Your Brain

Gary Small, MD, professor of psychiatry and director of the UCLA Longevity Center at the Semel Institue for Neuroscience & Human Behavior. He is author and coauthor of many books, including *2 Weeks to a Younger Brain*.

The average American uses the Internet for more than 80 hours each month—working, writing e-mails, searching for facts, streaming entertainment or simply shopping online. But does all this online activity help—or harm—our brains?

Gary Small, MD, a leading authority on brain function, explains that computer use has both positive and negative effects.

YOUR BRAIN ON THE INTERNET

"Use it or lose it" has long been the motto for brain health. And according to recent research, processing and responding to a shifting influx of information on the computer appears to dramatically increase mental activity.

Important recent finding: When 24 adults with and without computer experience had their brain activity measured while they searched the Internet for information, the experienced users' brains were twice as lively as the others'. The increased activity was most striking in the brain's prefrontal cortex—the area that weighs complex information and makes decisions.

But the newcomers caught up fast. After spending just an hour a day on Internet searching for five days, their brains were just as active, when retested, as their more experienced counterparts'.

ONLINE SOCIAL SKILLS

New technology means a world of new opportunities to socialize. For example, so-called social media outlets, such as Facebook (Facebook.com), MySpace (MySpace. com) and Twitter (Twitter.com), make it possible to easily communicate with friends and acquaintances, including many you've never actually met.

The more you socialize online, the more adept at it you become, as brain circuits engaged by the activity grow stronger. This type of social activity engages the "thinking center" of the brain, as well as areas involved in language and memory functions.

The potential cost: When you spend long hours in front of the computer screen, you have less time for face-to-face conversations, which communicate a far richer stream of information than digital messages can. Facial expression, eye contact, tone of voice and body language convey subtleties of thought and feeling that are otherwise lost.

In fact, face-to-face conversation activates the brain more broadly and deeply than does computer communication—speaking, listening and interpreting nonverbal cues engage neurons in areas such as the anterior cingulate, the insula and parts of the frontal cortex that can weaken from disuse.

Self-defense: Become aware of the hours you spend online and be ready to set limits. Spend more physical time with people you care about—for example, schedule family dinners to reconnect with each other. To engage your brain even more fully, make special note of nonverbal communication when you are with people. For example, what are people saying by the way they stand and gesture?

TOO MUCH AT ONCE?

Today's computer technology makes multitasking almost inevitable. Streams of information are constantly converging as e-mails and the lure of the Internet compete for our attention. Hopscotching back and forth grows easier with practice. Presumably it strengthens the part of the brain that lets us leave one task and focus on another—an area behind the forehead called the anterior prefrontal cortex.

The potential cost: Getting used to the staccato thinking style of dancing between tasks may make it more difficult to focus attention long enough to think through a problem. Some experts have suggested that symptoms of attention deficit hyperactivity disorder (ADHD) in adults—such as distractibility, impulsivity and inability to concentrate—may be due, in some cases, to brain shifts that occur in response to the continual bombardment of information delivered by technology.

You may think that you're getting more tasks done by multitasking, but in fact the brain is far more efficient when allowed to concentrate on one thing at a time. Studies have shown that mental efficiency declines during multitasking, and tasks take longer to complete than they do when done sequentially.

Self-defense: List your tasks in order of importance, and arrange your schedule accordingly. Set aside times when you focus on paying bills or returning phone calls—and turn off your e-mail if it distracts you.

Also helpful: When possible, take "power naps." A Harvard study found that a 30-minute nap renews the neural pathways depleted by multitasking and reduces overall fatigue.

ARE YOU ADDICTED TO YOUR COMPUTER?

Many people have gotten hooked on online shopping, computer games, Internet porn and/or Internet gambling. Even mundane Internet searching—just looking for interesting websites—may be seriously habit forming.

The potential cost: Whether they are true addictions—not all experts think so—such activities apparently activate the same "reward circuits" in the brain that drugs and alcohol do.

As with substance abuse, dependence on computer stimulation can become an unhealthy preoccupation that persists even to the point where it puts jobs and personal relationships in jeopardy—and efforts to stop may trigger withdrawal-like discomfort.

Self-defense: Each day, substitute offline diversions that you enjoy, such as hobbies and sports, for computer activities. If certain websites prove hard to resist, use a program that filters content. (Have a family member or friend set up the filter and keep the password.)

Helpful: If the lure of toxic technology is truly interfering with your life, seek professional help. Contact the Center for Internet Addiction (NetAddiction.com).

TRY BRAIN-BUILDING TECHNOLOGY

Research shows that regular mental stimulation can spur new connections between neurons and improve memory.

Solving crossword puzzles in the newspaper, for example, and learning new subjects may slow brain aging—or even lower the risk for Alzheimer's disease.

Used wisely, your computer also can help promote brain health. (See pages 253 and 254 to see how Google and Facebook helps your brain.) For example, there are websites that feature games and puzzles specifically designed to challenge the brain at varying levels of difficulty.

My favorite websites: BrainBashers.com (created by a math teacher in England, this free site offers puzzles, riddles, games and optical illusions)…and Braingle.com (this site will e-mail you a free brain teaser each day and allows you to chat online with other brain teaser enthusiasts).

Social Connections Prevent Memory Loss

A recent study of more than 16,000 people age 50 and older asked participants to take verbal memory tests over six years.

Findings: Those who had the fewest social connections with friends, family and in the community suffered decline in memory capacity at twice the rate as those with the most.

Conclusion: This is another example of how being socially engaged is beneficial for mental health.

Lisa F. Berkman, PhD, department of Sociology, Human Development and Health, Harvard School of Public Health, lead study author.

To Protect Your Brain: Hold Off on Retirement

Delaying retirement may protect your brain. For each additional year that a person worked before retiring, dementia risk dropped by 3% in a recent analysis. That means someone who retired at age 60 had a 15% greater chance of developing dementia, on average, than someone who retired at 65.

Theory: The mental stimulation and social connections at work may keep the brain healthy.

Analysis of the records of more than 400,000 retired workers in France by researchers at National Institute of Health and Medical Research, Paris, presented at the 2013 Alzheimer's Association International Conference.

Better Brain Health Found in Bookworms

Memory and thinking tests given to approximately 300 adults revealed that those who participated in reading, writing and similar activities throughout their lives had a 32% lower rate of memory decline than those who did not. Reading helps strengthen circuits in the cerebral cortex, making them more resilient. The brain needs exercise just like other body parts, so keep it in shape at any age with mentally challenging activities, such as reading and/or writing.

Robert Wilson, PhD, senior neuropsychologist, Rush Alzheimer's Disease Center, Chicago.

A Little Stress Can Actually Be Good for You

Rats under stress for three hours released fibroblast growth factor 2 (FGF2), which triggers the development of new nerve cells in the part of the brain needed for memory.

Caution: Too much stress can lead to obesity, depression, heart disease and brain-cell damage.

Animal study by researchers at Helen Wills Neuroscience Institute at University of California-Berkeley, published in *eLife*.

B-12 Deficiency May Be at the Root of Dementia

Andrew L. Rubman, ND, director, Southbury Clinic for Traditional Medicines, Southbury, Connecticut.

Many aging baby-boomers are deathly afraid that they will fall victim to the rising rates of Alzheimer's disease and dementia. The good news is that prevention may be as close as the vitamin aisle, thanks to research that suggests that vitamin B-12 (cobalamin) may help. Andrew L. Rubman, ND, director of the Southbury Clinic for Traditional Medicines, says that naturopathic physicians have long used B-12 as a treatment for dementia. While the mainstreamers are just catching on, once again naturopaths have been aware of its benefits for many years.

B-12 DEFICIENCY: MORE COMMON AS WE AGE

Vitamin B-12 is a central player in brain and nervous system processes, observes Dr. Rubman. In addition, a B-12 deficiency can lead to a wide variety of neurological problems. In mild cases, these might pass unnoticed—subtle changes in memory, depression, irritability and the like. But in extreme cases, B-12 deficiency may contribute to more serious disorders such as dementia.

Unfortunately, B-12 deficiency is very common among older adults, especially those over 60. Americans get plenty of B-12 in their diet through foods such as shellfish and beef. Yet older people have problems digesting B-12-rich foods and absorbing B-12, so its deficiency commonly increases as we age, explains Dr. Rubman. Given how important B-12 is to brain and nervous system function, along with the body's reduced digesting ability, it is easy to see why dementia may result.

WHAT YOU CAN DO

Even though we have broad government guidelines as to how much B-12 we should take in, Dr. Rubman points out that we must also take into account individual differences in how it is absorbed and utilized. Dr. Rubman encourages people to get a serum B-12 blood test through their doctor to assess their level of B-12. If there is a deficiency—contrary to the emphasis on B-12 shots in conventional medical practice—he says that certain oral forms work equally well. In particular, Dr. Rubman often prescribes sublingual B-12 pills, either hydroxycobalamin or methylcobalamin, which dissolve under the tongue. (Avoid cyanocobalamin, which may be poorly absorbed.) B-12 should be taken under a doctor's supervision. In order for it to function properly, other B vitamins are also required. One B-50 multi, taken twice daily, is quite often prescribed along with the B-12, as they do not last 24 hours in circulation. If you're taking in sufficient B vitamins, urine should remain yellow.

Dr. Rubman adds that B-12 works best as a catalyst with other nutrients. In addition, if you have a poor diet or have digestive challenges that inhibit proper absorption and utilization of nutrients, B-12 can't function efficiently. He also warns that when you take acid-reducing or acid-suppressing drugs, the level of B-12 absorption can drop. To properly absorb nutrients, you need to work on digestion. In most cases, a naturopathic physician can get impaired digestion back on track within just a few weeks.

Common Vitamin May Slow Alzheimer's Symptoms

When people with mild-to-moderate Alzheimer's took a high dose of vitamin E—2,000 international units (IU) daily—they had slower declines in activities of daily living, such as dressing and bathing without help, than people who didn't take the vitamin or took the Alzheimer's drug *memantine* (Namenda). Vitamin E provided just over a six-month delay in the disease's progression over a two-year period.

Note: A doctor should be consulted before this therapy is tried—vitamin E may increase risk for bleeding and/or interact with medications.

Maurice Dysken, MD, geriatric psychiatrist, Minneapolis VA Health Care System, Minnesota.

Stay Away from Artificial Butter

Artifical butter flavorings harm brain cells. Many contain the chemical diacetyl, which promotes the protein clumps associated with Alzheimer's disease. Make unbuttered popcorn and add salt, herbs or real butter. At the movies, order popcorn without the buttery topping.

Study by researchers at University of Minnesota, Minneapolis, published in *Chemical Research in Toxicology*.

Get These Minerals Out of Your Brain!

Neal D. Barnard, MD, president of the nonprofit Physicians Committee for Responsible Medicine. He is author of *Power Foods for the Brain: An Effective 3-Step Plan to Protect Your Mind and Strengthen Your Memory.* PCRM.org

Chances are you're doing everything that you can to eat plenty of "superfoods"—blueberries, walnuts and other nutritious and antioxidant-rich wonders—that many scientists believe help reduce risk for a variety of chronic health problems, including Alzheimer's disease.

The missing part of the story: What you may not know is that most people get too much of certain nutrients—even those found in some superfoods—that have long been considered an important part of a nutritious diet.

Iron, copper and zinc, which are widely recognized as key nutrients, actually are metallic minerals. They are common in many of the foods you may be eating, the water you drink—and even in some of the supplements you may be taking to improve your health.

What researchers are now discovering: Excessive amounts of iron, copper and zinc can produce free radicals that impair memory.

In fact, scientists have discovered that these metals are more prevalent in the brains of Alzheimer's patients than in people without the disease. Even in healthy adults, high levels appear to interfere with normal brain functions.

3 NEWLY DISCOVERED DANGERS

Your body does need iron, copper and zinc, but only in miniscule amounts. If you exceed these levels, your brain is at risk. *What to watch out for…*

•**Iron.** Unless you have been diagnosed with a condition that requires supplemental iron, such as anemia, you probably don't need more than you're already getting from your diet—and even that might be too much.

Compelling evidence: In a study of 793 adults, those who had the most iron in their

23

blood did worse on cognitive tests than those with normal levels.

In a study of 881 adults, those with high hemoglobin levels (a measure of iron in the blood) were three times more likely to develop Alzheimer's disease than those with normal levels. Hemoglobin levels above 13.7 g/dL were associated with increased Alzheimer's risk. Those whose iron levels are too low are also at risk for Alzheimer's.

My advice: Emphasize plant-based foods in your diet. These foods can contain as much iron as what's found in meat—but our bodies are better able to regulate our intake of the type of iron found in plant-based foods, such as spinach, dried apricots, lima beans and wheat germ. Your body absorbs more of this nonheme iron when you need it and absorbs less when you don't.

In contrast, the heme iron in meats, poultry, fish and shellfish (particularly oysters) is absorbed whether you need it or not. Because of this, a high-meat diet is a main cause of iron overload, which potentially damages not only your brain but also your heart.

Other smart steps…

•**Don't use iron cookware.** A significant amount of iron leaches from uncoated cast-iron pots, pans and skillets into foods—particularly acidic foods, such as tomatoes.

•**Choose an iron-free product if you take a daily multisupplement.**

•**Read cereal labels.** Many breakfast cereals are fortified with iron. You don't need it.

Amount of iron you need in your diet: 8 mg per day for men age 19 and older and women age 51 and older. Women age 19 to 50 need 18 mg per day. (In general, women should get the lower amount of iron when they stop menstruating.)

•**Copper.** At proper levels, copper is essential for enzyme function and helps promote heart health and bone strength. At excess levels, copper—like iron—triggers the production of free radicals that can damage brain cells.

Important finding: A study of 1,451 people in southern California found that those who had the least copper in their blood were

mentally sharper and had fewer problems with long- and short-term memory than those whose levels were high.

How copper may promote almost 20 years of aging: When high copper levels are combined with excess saturated fat in the diet—another risk factor for brain problems—the effect is particularly detrimental. Data from the Chicago Health and Aging Project found that high copper/saturated fat caused a loss of mental function that was the equivalent of 19 years of aging.

My advice: Don't take any supplement that contains copper. If you have copper plumbing, it's fine to use tap water for doing dishes and washing but not for cooking or drinking. It is better to use bottled water or water filtered with an activated carbon filter (such as those found in Brita pitchers).

You are unlikely to get too much copper from plant foods that are rich in the mineral such as whole grains, nuts and beans because they also contain natural compounds called phytates that limit copper absorption.

Amount of copper you need: 0.9 mg daily.

•**Zinc.** Our bodies need adequate zinc levels for key functions such as immunity, skin health and sexual function. Excessive amounts, however, are thought to promote the clumping of beta-amyloid proteins in the brain—the hallmark of Alzheimer's disease.

Much of the excess zinc in the American diet comes from supplements. If you take a multivitamin-mineral supplement and also eat fortified cereals or other foods that include zinc, such as oysters, pumpkin seeds or cocoa, you could be getting too much.

Amount of zinc you need: 11 mg daily for men and 8 mg for women.

TAKEAWAY ON MINERALS

Testing is not needed to check levels of iron, copper and zinc in your blood. It is wise to simply avoid the mineral sources in this article. If you are getting too much of these minerals, your levels will gradually decline when you avoid excessive intakes.

Important: Avoid multivitamin-mineral supplements.

Better choices: "Vitamin only" supplements such as No Minerals Multi-Vitamin by Nature's Blend or Vitamins Only by Solgar.

More from Dr. Barnard...

What About Aluminum?

This ubiquitous metal has never been considered a nutrient—it plays no role in the body. While questions have persisted for several years about whether aluminum interferes with brain health, recent studies suggest that the risk is real.

In the UK, researchers found that Alzheimer's cases occurred 50% more often in counties with high aluminum levels in the water. Other studies have had similar results.

My advice: While researchers search for definitive findings on aluminum, err on the side of caution...

• **Don't buy foods that contain aluminum.** Check food labels. Cheese products (such as the cheese on frozen pizza) often contain aluminum. So do baking powders and the baked goods that include them. You can buy an aluminum-free baking powder, such as the Rumford brand.

• **Don't take aluminum antacids.** Use an aluminum-free product, such as Tums. Other drugs, such as buffered aspirin, may also contain aluminum. Check the label.

• **Cook with steel-clad or porcelain-coated pots**...use wax paper instead of aluminum foil...and don't consume foods or beverages that come in aluminum cans.

• **Check your tap water.** If it's high in aluminum or other metals, use bottled water or a reverse osmosis filter. You can use the EPA website, cfpub.EPA.gov/safewater/ccr, to get information about the water sources in your area.

• **Avoid antiperspirants with aluminum.** Labels may say aluminum or alum to indicate an aluminum-containing ingredient.

Chemical Caution

The brain may never recover from chemical fumes. In a study of more than 2,000 retired industrial workers, those who had high exposure to benzene, petroleum, paint, glue, chlorinated solvents and other chemicals scored worse on tests for cognitive functioning—and impairment was detected in people whose exposure dated back 50 years.

Explanation: Industrial solvents may permanently damage brain cells, so if you're around them, be sure to wear a face mask and keep the area ventilated.

Erika Sabbath, ScD, assistant professor, Boston College Graduate School of Social Work, Chestnut Hill, Massachusetts.

"Dirty Drugs": Common Medications with Really Bad Side Effects

James Rudolph, MD, geriatrician and palliative care physician, director, VA Boston Geriatric Research, Education, and Clinical Center, and acting clinical director, division of aging, Brigham and Women's Hospital, and associate professor of medicine, Harvard Medical School, all in Boston.

Shannon Risacher, PhD, assistant professor of radiology and imaging sciences at Indiana Alzheimer Disease Center, Indiana University School of Medicine, Indianapolis, and leader of a study of 451 older adults, average age 73, published in *JAMA Neurology*.

If you're like most Americans, you have probably taken—or may currently take—an over-the-counter (OTC) allergy or cold drug, pain reliever or sleep aid containing *diphenhydramine*. This generic medication has become widely available without prescription in such products as Benadryl, Excedrin PM and Tylenol PM.

What you may not know: These drugs, as well as dozens of others that are used by millions of Americans, block the action of acetylcholine, a neurotransmitter that controls several critical functions in the body ranging from body secretions to cognitive function.

Why is this a potential problem? Cells in virtually every part of the body have molecular openings (receptors) that respond to acetylcholine. A drug that's used to treat a condition in one part of the body invariably affects receptors somewhere else.

Result: A high incidence of unintended effects. In some cases, people who use these so-called anticholinergic drugs suffer side effects such as constipation, urinary retention, blurred vision and dry mouth, and now researchers say use of these drugs increases risk of Alzheimer's disease.

"DIRTY" DRUGS

Medications that cause a high rate of unintended effects are known in the health-care community as "dirty" drugs. The same active ingredient that reduces bladder spasms, for example, might also cause constipation by reducing intestinal contractions or eye dryness by blocking acetylcholine at the receptors that control body secretions.

Important finding: A study published in *JAMA Internal Medicine* tracked health outcomes and anticholinergic drug use for 3,434 people age 65 years or older for more than seven years. None of the study participants had dementia at the beginning of the study, but nearly one-quarter developed it during the study period—most in the form of Alzheimer's disease. Alarmingly, the researchers discovered that the higher the dose of an anticholinergic drug and the longer a person was on it, the higher that person's risk of dementia. In fact, risk was 54% greater for those taking high doses of anticholinergic drugs for more than three years than for those who did not take such drugs. Specifically, those at risk included people taking at least 10 mg per day of *doxepin* (Silenor), 4 mg per day of *diphenhydramine* (Nytol, Benadryl) or 5 mg per day of *oxybutynin* (Ditropan).

Additional research: Older people who regularly took an AC drug had brain cavities up to 32% larger than other seniors. Increased cavity size reflects brain atrophy. AC-medication users also did worse on tests of brain function including short-term memory, verbal reasoning, planning and problem solving.

COMMON USES AND ALTERNATIVES

Popular anticholinergic drugs…

• **Allergies.** Many of the older allergy drugs, including Benadryl and Dimetapp, are effective at relieving irritated eyes, sneezing and runny nose. That's not surprising, since one of the main anticholinergic effects is to reduce mucus and other secretions. But the side effects, such as drowsiness and a dry mouth and eyes, are pronounced. Few can take these drugs and function well the next day.

My advice: Avoid diphenhydramine or brompheniramine.

Better: Avoid allergens in the first place. If this is not possible, take a nonsedating antihistamine, such as *fexofenadine* (Allegra) or *loratadine* (Claritin). These drugs have relatively mild anticholinergic effects—most people can take them without experiencing side effects. The researchers advised that, whenever possible, nonanticholinergic medications should be substituted for these drugs.

• **Urinary incontinence.** People who suffer from an unusually intense and frequent need to urinate, known as urge incontinence, are often treated with overactive bladder medications such as *oxybutynin* (Ditropan) or *tolterodine* (Detrol). These drugs may cause dry mouth, blurred vision, constipation and/or cognitive impairments. Adults age 65 and older have the highest risk for side effects. This is partly because the blood-brain barrier becomes more porous with age. These drugs are not supposed to enter the brain—but often do.

My advice: After discussing dosages and potential side effects with your physician, you may want to consider taking one of these drugs if incontinence is preventing you from living a normal life. It may be better to cope with drug side effects than to become housebound due to fear of having an "accident."

Even better: Bladder training, in which a doctor or therapist teaches you to gradually increase the intervals between urinating by waiting longer than you think you can. Most people can gradually increase their "holding" time by several minutes to several hours.

If urgency/frequency occurs during the night, see your doctor. Nighttime urination may especially be a problem for men with enlarged prostates, but incontinence drugs are unlikely to help—and may even be harmful.

• **Depression.** Before selective serotonin reuptake inhibitor (SSRI) antidepressants were developed, doctors often prescribed *amitriptyline* (Elavil) for depression. This drug has fallen out of favor because it tends to cause strong anticholinergic side effects. But some of the newer drugs, such as *paroxetine* (Paxil), the most anticholinergic of the SSRIs, have similar effects.

My advice: If your doctor is going to prescribe an antidepressant, ask him/her about SSRI antidepressants with the least anticholinergic effects, particularly those with a shorter "half-life," such as *sertraline* (Zoloft). These drugs are eliminated from the body more quickly, so they're less likely to cause side effects. This is particularly important for older adults, who metabolize drugs more slowly.

• **Insomnia.** Most OTC drugs taken for insomnia, including the allergy medication Benadryl and sleep aid Sominex, contain diphenhydramine. It can cause constipation, difficulty concentrating, urinary retention and trouble with eye focus—and stays active in the body for 12 to 18 hours, which can lead to next-day grogginess.

My advice: Avoid taking diphenhydramine for insomnia.

Better: Practice good sleep habits. *Examples:* Go to bed at a reasonable hour, and maintain the same schedule every night. Exercise regularly but not within two hours of your bedtime—it will make falling asleep more difficult. Take a warm bath before bed to help you relax.

Important: Make the bedroom a peaceful place—no TV, computer, etc. If you don't fall asleep within a half hour, get up and do something else until you're ready to try to sleep again. Avoid the computer and all electronics—their glow delays release of the sleep-inducing hormone melatonin.

• **Motion sickness.** Many anticholinergic drugs prevent and/or relieve motion sickness. However, the doses needed to reduce motion sickness can also cause drowsiness or confusion as a side effect.

My advice: Avoid motion sickness drugs such as *dimenhydrinate* (Dramamine).

Better: Use a prescription *scopolamine* patch (such as Transderm Scop). The active ingredient enters the body slowly and is less likely to cause side effects than oral dimenhydrine. The patches deliver about 1.5 mg of scopolamine over three days. Apply the patch to a hairless area at least four hours before traveling/sailing. Remove the patch if you notice any of the anticholinergic side effects described above.

PROTECT YOURSELF

Older people who use an AC drug for a chronic condition should ask their physicians whether non-AC alternatives are available. A list of medications that have possible or definitive AC properties can be found by putting "Anticholinergic Burden (ACB) Scale" into any search engine. Drugs with an ACB score of 3 (found in the right-most column) are the most problematic.

Heartburn Drug Danger

Regular use of a proton-pump inhibitor (PPI), such as *omeprazole* (Prilosec) or *esomeprazole* (Nexium), increased risk for dementia by up to 44% in a recent seven-year study of adults age 75 and older. Further research is needed on long-term use of PPIs and the possible effects on cognition in the elderly.

If you take a PPI: Follow your doctor's guidance.

Britta Haenisch, PhD, group leader, German Center for Neurodegenerative Diseases, Bonn, Germany.

Statin Curbs Dementia Risk

Researchers who analyzed medical data on more than 700,000 users of *simvastatin* (Zocor) found that the cholesterol-lowering drug reduced the incidence of Alzheimer's disease and Parkinson's disease by nearly 50% in people age 65 or older who had taken statins for at least seven months. No similar results were found in study subjects taking the statins *lovastatin* (Mevacor) or *atorvastatin* (Lipitor).

Theory: Simvastatin's beneficial effect may be due to its ability to enter the brain and reduce both inflammation and cholesterol. More research is needed, but if you take simvastatin to lower cholesterol, a brain-protective effect may be an added benefit.

Benjamin Wolozin, MD, PhD, professor of pharmacology, Boston University School of Medicine.

Cholesterol Affects Future Dementia Risk

Much of the recent news about dementia prevention has been discouraging. But a recent large-scale, long-term study lends support to one risk-reduction strategy over which we do have significant control—cholesterol levels.

What this study found: Compared to people with normal cholesterol levels, those who had borderline-high cholesterol (200 mg/dL to 239 mg/dL) at age 40 to 45 were 52% more likely to develop dementia within 40 years. For those who had high cholesterol (240 mg/dL or above) at midlife, dementia risk was elevated 66%.

Lesson: What's good for the heart is good for the brain—so no matter what your age, if you have high cholesterol, talk to your doctor about cholesterol-reducing strategies, such as dietary changes, exercise and, if necessary, medication.

Rachel Whitmer, PhD, research scientist and epidemiologist in the division of research at Kaiser Permanente in Oakland, California, and senior author of a study of 9,844 people.

HRT May Reduce Alzheimer's Risk

Women who take hormones within five years of menopause have a 30% lower risk

for Alzheimer's, compared with women who never take them. The issue of HRT remains complex and controversial—discuss your personal situation with your doctor.

Study of 1,768 women by researchers at Johns Hopkins Bloomberg School of Public Health, Baltimore, published in *Neurology*.

Dementia Linked to Common Heart Condition

Atrial fibrillation alone is associated with higher dementia risk, and it often is treated with *warfarin*—but when warfarin doses must be adjusted frequently because the blood levels of the medicine are too high or low, dementia risk also rises. Patients may do better on newer forms of blood thinners such as *dabigatran*, *apixaban* or *rivaroxaban*. And there is a new, implantable device—the Watchman left atrial appendage closure device—for some A-fib patients who cannot take warfarin.

T. Jared Bunch, MD, medical director of heart rhythm services for Intermountain Medical Center, Salt Lake City, Utah.

Say No to Benzodiazepines

Sedatives increase the risk for Alzheimer's, warns Malaz Boustani, MD, MPH. Older adults who used benzodiazepine sedatives, such as *lorazepam* (Ativan), *diazepam* (Valium) and *alprazolam* (Xanax), for more than three months within a five-year period had a 51% increased risk for Alzheimer's. These drugs often are prescribed for insomnia or anxiety, but they should not be used long term.

Better approach: The underlying cause of the anxiety or insomnia should be identified and treated without using medicines—for example, with talk therapy.

Malaz Boustani, MD, MPH, chief innovation and implementation officer at Indiana University Health and Richard M. Fairbanks Professor of Aging Research at Indiana University School of Medicine, both in Indianapolis.

Watch for Anemia to Avoid Dementia

Study titled "Anemia and risk of dementia in older adults: Findings from the Health ABC study," published in *Neurology*.

Anemia—a shortage of oxygen-carrying red blood cells—is fairly common in older adults, affecting up to 24% of people age 65 and older. Meanwhile, Alzheimer's disease, the most common form of dementia, affects 15% of people age 65 to 74 and 44% of people age 75 to 84. And now studies have shown a link between the two disorders, and that's good news. Looking out for and addressing one (anemia) may have a strong impact on avoiding the other (dementia).

In one small study, the risk of dementia doubled within three years of an anemia diagnosis and, in another, anemia was associated with a 60% increased risk of Alzheimer's disease within 3.3 years. But while small studies are all well and fine to get a glimpse into new ways of seeing health problems, larger studies are needed to really make a strong case. And that's what an international team of researchers has done.

The team followed 2,552 people, age 70 to 79, who participated in an 11-year study called *Health, Aging and Body Composition*. Over the course of the study period, all of the participants were given memory tests to check for signs of dementia and blood tests for anemia. None of them had dementia at the start of the study, and 15% of them had anemia. By the end of the study, 18% of participants had Alzheimer's or another form of dementia. When the researchers compared rates of dementia between people who had or didn't have anemia, they discovered that having anemia was associated with a 41% higher risk for Alzheimer's or another form of dementia.

WHAT TO DO

How anemia is linked to dementia is not completely understood. Possible factors include simply being in poor health, not getting enough oxygen to the brain (those red blood cells!) or having an iron or vitamin B-12 deficiency. Whatever the connection, in case it is anemia that is actually causing dementia, you'll want to do whatever you can to recognize and treat the symptoms of anemia—and, of course, prevent anemia from ever happening in the first place.

Signs of anemia can be subtle at first and include fatigue, weakness, pale skin, fast or irregular heartbeat, trouble breathing, chest pain, trouble with memory and concentration, cold hands and feet and headache. So if you've been feeling fatigued and don't know why or have other symptoms just mentioned, make an appointment with your doctor, who will order a blood test to check for anemia.

If anemia is found, additional tests will be done to find the exact cause, and the results will determine treatment.

Although rare or hereditary forms of anemia require blood transfusions, others are corrected by treating the underlying cause, whether it be loss of blood from a bleeding ulcer or complications from an infection or a medication side effect. Fortunately, the most common form of anemia—that caused by an iron or B-12 deficiency—is managed with good nutrition and vitamin and mineral supplements. It might be a simple correction that lets you avoid a horrific outcome.

PREVENTING ANEMIA

Since prevention is best, keep your diet rich in iron, folate, vitamin B-12, and vitamin C (which is essential for iron absorption). Foods that will give you the iron you need include red meat, beans, dried fruit, and green leafy vegetables, such as spinach. Besides vitamin C, citrus fruits provide folate. Other good sources of folate include green leafy veggies, beans and bananas. As for vitamin B-12, rely on salmon, shellfish, beef and dairy. And if you are vegan or vegetarian (or have a large B-12 deficiency), you likely already know that you need to get B-12 from supplementation.

General Anesthesia Linked to Dementia... Even Years Later

A study, "Exposure to general anaesthesia could increase the risk of dementia in elderly," from researchers at the University of Bordeaux, France, presented at Euroanaesthesia, the annual meeting of the European Society of Anaesthesiology.

G iven a choice, many people would prefer to have general anesthesia and sleep through surgery rather than have local anesthesia and be awake for the procedure. But this may change their minds—there's worrisome scientific evidence that general anesthesia significantly increases a person's risk of developing dementia. Scarier still, this risk may remain elevated even years after the surgery is over, a recent French study suggests.

The participants, all of whom were 65 or older, were interviewed and examined at the beginning of the study...and then again two, four, seven and 10 years later. Each exam included a cognitive evaluation to screen for dementia. From the two-year follow-up onward, 7,008 nondemented participants were asked at each follow-up whether they had had anesthesia since the last follow-up and, if so, what type they'd received.

Analysis: Over the next eight years, 9% of the study participants were diagnosed with some type of dementia, most often Alzheimer's disease. After adjusting for other health problems that might have influenced the results, the researchers calculated that receiving general anesthesia at least once during the study increased the seniors' risk of developing dementia by a startling 35%, compared with participants who did not receive anesthesia.

Caveats: It's too early to say whether or not general anesthesia actually causes dementia, but this study does show a worrisome association. What could be behind this link? Researchers suspect that certain anesthetizing drugs promote inflammation of parts of the nervous system and/or trigger formation of beta-amyloid plaques and other precursors to Alzheimer's disease. As for whether the same long-term risk applies to younger people who receive general anesthesia, only additional research can answer that question.

Exploring safer options: Are you facing surgery or some other medical procedure for which general anesthesia may be used? If the procedure isn't truly necessary, it's worthwhile to consider all your nonsurgical options before you agree to go under the knife. If you do need the procedure, ask your doctor whether local anesthesia, a sedative or a relatively new technique called ultrasound-guided nerve block might be an appropriate alternative to general anesthesia. If general anesthesia is unavoidable—or if you received general anesthesia in the past, particularly if you had it repeatedly—it would be wise to talk with your doctor about how the two of you can be on the lookout for early warning signs of dementia in the coming years. For dementia patients, early detection offers the best chance for optimal management of the condition.

Delirium Danger

Malaz Boustani, MD, MPH, professor of medicine at the Indiana University School of Medicine and scientist at the Indiana University Center for Aging Research. He is also research director of the university's Healthy Aging Brain Center and a research scientist at the Regenstrief Institute, Inc. Regenstrief.org

I f you are admitted to a hospital, you're at greater risk for a disorder that very few doctors recognize and treat appropriately...delirium.

Frightening statistic: Delirium—a condition characterized by confusion and changes in memory and emotion—affects 60% of patients age 65 and older recovering from major orthopedic surgery and 80% of intensive care unit (ICU) patients.

What's more, research now shows that the brain trauma associated with delirium also can have significant negative effects on long-term mental and physical health.

Important finding: A meta-analysis published in *The Journal of the American Medi-*

cal Association found that older patients with delirium were, on average, more likely to die within 22 months…at increased risk of entering a nursing home within 14 months…and more likely to develop dementia within four years. These patients also are more likely to suffer a serious physical disability.

Equally disturbing: Up to about 60% of delirium cases go unrecognized by the patients' doctors.

The good news: Protocols now exist to help doctors and patients' families prevent delirium in people who are at highest risk and to detect the condition when it occurs. Various approaches to treating and reversing delirium also are now being studied.

WHAT IS DELIRIUM?

Delirium is an acute mental state that is typically characterized by confusion, inattention and disorientation. Delusions (false beliefs) or hallucinations (perceiving something that is not there) also may occur with delirium.

ARE YOU AT RISK?

Delirium is most prevalent among adults age 65 and older. At particular risk are older adults with existing mild cognitive impairment, such as early-stage Alzheimer's disease or some other form of dementia, who are undergoing major vascular surgery, such as abdominal aneurysm repair, or orthopedic surgery. Hearing or vision loss is another risk factor since this can result in diminished sensory input (a trigger for delirium).

Also at risk are people who take anticholinergic medications, such as *diphenhydramine* (Benadryl), *paroxetine* (Paxil) and *amitriptyline*, on a regular basis. These drugs inhibit the neurotransmitter acetylcholine, which is crucial for memory and coherent thought. Disruption of acetylcholine production, which is already reduced in older people, is what causes delirium.

Particularly troublesome are drugs called benzodiazepines, which act on the central nervous system and are used as sedatives. These include *lorazepam* (Ativan), *alprazolam* (Xanax), *chlordiazepoxide* (Librium), *clorazepate dipotassium* (Tranxene), *diazepam* (Valium) and *oxazepam*. It's now believed that such sedatives—which are widely used for ICU patients on ventilators to keep them from "fighting" the machine—play a major role in triggering or exacerbating delirium.

PREVENTING DELIRIUM

For at-risk patients, a variety of stressors can nudge them into delirium. These include pain, infection, disturbed sleep patterns, dehydration or a fall. Starting a new anticholinergic drug also can trigger delirium.

Prevention focuses on doing everything possible to avoid such triggers. *Steps typically include…*

• **Not disturbing the patient's sleep unnecessarily.**

• **Preserving normal body rhythms.**

How: Turn lights on at 7 am and dim them at 7 pm.

• **Managing pain effectively.**

• **Keeping the patient well-hydrated.**

• **Making sure that the patient's hearing and vision aids are being used.**

• **Keeping the patient oriented to the time of day.**

• **Reducing the use of ventilators.**

Also: Minimizing the use of sedatives when a patient is on a ventilator.

Implementing these measures has been shown to reduce hospital-wide incidence of delirium by 60%.

DETECTING DELIRIUM

Even when preventive steps are taken, delirium remains a risk. That's why hospital staff and patients' families need to be alert to its symptoms, which can arise over a period of just a few hours. *Symptoms include…*

• **Sudden confusion, change in personality, disorientation and/or memory problems.**

• **Difficulty sleeping.**

• **Speech disturbances.**

• **Delusions (false beliefs).**

• **Visual and/or auditory hallucinations.**

These symptoms tend to come and go, so even a brief occurrence is cause for alarm.

Important: While patients with delirium may be agitated, they also can be very quiet and still be suffering from these symptoms.

31

Many hospitals now use a structured interview called Confusion Assessment Method (CAM) to evaluate at-risk patients. It takes only a few minutes to administer and has proven highly effective at identifying delirium when it occurs. If you think a loved one might have delirium, ask a nurse or doctor to administer the CAM interview.

TREATING DELIRIUM

If delirium is suspected, the goal is to identify and treat the medical condition, such as infection, that triggered the delirious state as soon as possible. Any agitation that may be induced by the delirium also is treated.

Recent research: Studies that involve immediately stopping all use of benzodiazepines or anti-cholinergic drugs and administering a very low dose of the antipsychotic medication *haloperidol* (Haldol) are ongoing.

In addition, researchers are looking at ways to reduce the use of ventilators in ICUs. In one study, patients were taken off sedatives briefly and encouraged to breathe on their own each day to wean them off the ventilator—an approach shown to shorten time in the ICU by four days, on average, and reduce one-year risk for death by 32%.

Important to remember: Some doctors tend to focus too much on medicating the body without taking into account a drug's effects on the brain. When it comes to delirium, the less medication, the better.

Going to the Hospital for Surgery? Vitamin D May Protect Your Mind

Study titled "Association between pre-hospital vitamin D status and hospital-acquired new-onset delirium" by researchers in the department of medicine, Harvard Medical School, and Brigham and Women's Hospital, both in Boston, published in *British Journal of Nutrition*.

I t's terrible what hospitals can do to you. We all know someone who checked into the hospital with his/her mind completely intact, but then quickly (especially if there was surgery) became confused and disoriented in a most disturbing way.

It's called hospital-acquired delirium. And, yeah, it's scary.

Delirium in the hospital is more common—and more dangerous—than you may think. It's a severe condition that mostly affects older patients (although not only older patients) and is often missed by hospital staff, especially in emergency rooms. If it's not treated promptly, it can lead to longer hospital stays and poor health outcomes, including permanent cognitive problems and even a higher risk for mortality. It's more common if there's already some cognitive impairment, but research shows that between 3% and 29% of "low risk" patients without any existing cognitive problems succumb to delirium after a hospital stay. A combination of surgery, infection, social isolation, dehydration, poor nutrition and mind-affecting pharmaceuticals such as painkillers, sedatives and sleeping pills can bring it on…quickly.

You can't control all of these factors, especially in the heat of the moment during emergency treatment. But researchers have discovered a nutritional factor that may protect against hospital-induced delirium…vitamin D.

D IS FOR…NO DELIRIUM

Researchers examined records of about 4,500 men and women (average age 59) who were admitted to one of two large teaching hospitals in Boston from 1993 to 2006. They included patients who had been tested before their hospitalization for blood levels of vitamin D and excluded those who had a history of delirium or dementia. Of all the patients, 198 (4%) were ultimately diagnosed with hospital-acquired new-onset delirium.

Their vitamin D levels told a story. Even after adjusting for age, sex, race, other illnesses and reason for hospitalization (medical or surgical), low preadmission vitamin D status was strongly associated with risk for hospital-acquired delirium.

Among all the patients studied, the average blood level of vitamin D was 22 nanograms per milliliter (ng/mL), which is on the low end of normal (20 ng/mL to 40 ng/mL). (A blood level of 35 ng/mL to 40 ng/mL is probably ideal, experts believe.) But those with the lowest vitamin D levels were most prone to delirium. Compared with patients who had blood levels 30 ng/mL and over, patients with levels from 10 ng/mL to 20 ng/mL were 50% more likely to develop delirium—and those with levels under 10 ng/mL faced double the risk. And that wasn't just a handful—about one in six (16%) of all the patients studied had levels under 10 ng/mL. Adjusting for other possible factors, including history of depression, calcium level and season of vitamin D testing, didn't change the results.

A NO-BRAINER APPROACH TO PROTECTING THE BRAIN

It's an observational study, which means it can't prove (or disprove) that a lack of vitamin D caused delirium, so it's possible that whatever caused delirium in these patients also made their vitamin D levels plummet. Nor does this study show that bringing vitamin D levels up to speed proactively prevents delirium. More studies will be needed to explore that hypothesis.

But it's a reasonable hypothesis, and there is good reason to believe that vitamin D may play a specific role in protecting the brain and the mind. The brain has vitamin D receptors throughout, and there is evidence that the active form of vitamin D may remove plaque, a hallmark of Alzheimer's, from brain cells, scientists have recently discovered. Research has shown that low blood levels of vitamin D are linked with dementia, Alzheimer's disease and depression.

In a way, though, the exact question is beside the point. Medicine is about balancing benefit and harm, and in this case, if you're vitamin D–deficient, there's no harm, and potentially much benefit, in bringing your body's vitamin D level up to normal! According to the National Institutes of Health, 77% of Americans are deficient in vitamin D, with blood levels under 30 ng/mL, and 6% have levels under 10 ng/mL. Even if you don't know your level, taking a daily supplement that contains up to 2,000 IU or 3,000 IU is considered safe.

An even better idea: Get a blood test. It's simple, quick and inexpensive. If your level is low, your health-care provider may prescribe a higher dosage for a while or even recommend vitamin D injections to get your level up to normal quickly.

If you are going into the hospital or know someone who is, the idea of getting tested for vitamin D beforehand…and reaching a normal level with a supplement if need be…is a no-brainer. It may prevent a scary form of delirium that can take hold in the hospital and lead to a downward health spiral. Even if it doesn't, it's a healthy thing to do.

MORE WAYS TO PREVENT HOSPITAL DELIRIUM

Ensuring you get enough vitamin D is something you can do before hospitalization. Once there, there are additional steps you can take to avoid delirium…or arrest it before it gets too bad. Whether it's you or a loved one, make sure that items such as eyeglasses or hearing aids are readily available, books and other familiar objects are nearby, and that the patient walks around if possible, stays hydrated, and gets as much sleep as possible in the sleep-depriving hospital environment. Regular visits from friends and family are key, since being (and feeling) isolated can lead to loneliness and fear that in turn can be a factor in delirium. Monitor medications carefully, especially pain and sleep drugs, which can contribute to confusion and push a patient toward delirium. If you're caring for a loved one who does become agitated, confused or disoriented while in the hospital—even if it comes and goes, a common feature of hospital-induced delirium—alert the staff and ask specifically for a delirium evaluation from a mental health care provider. Basic treatment, including making sure the patient is well hydrated and nourished…stops taking dangerous medications if possible…gets daily exercise…is surrounded by familiar objects…and stays connected to family and friends, can often turn incipient delirium around before it gets too bad.

The Truth About Weight and Dementia

Deborah Gustafson, PhD, professor of neurology, SUNY Downstate Medical Center, Brooklyn, New York. Her review, titled "2003-2013: a decade of body mass index, Alzheimer's disease, and dementia," was published in *Journal of Alzheimer's Disease.*

A ttention skinny people—you may get dementia. That's the finding from a study of more than two million people that looked at the relationship between body mass index (BMI) in middle age and dementia later in life. This study has gotten a lot of press because it found, essentially, that the thinner you are, the greater your dementia risk…which goes against what most people might think and implies that there's no need to worry about staying trim.

Before you break out the cheesecake to celebrate, though, let's take a closer look.

"CONTRADICTING EVERYTHING WE THOUGHT WE KNEW"

The researchers used a health-care database from a network of primary-care practices in the United Kingdom to find height/weight measurements on people aged 40 and older. They followed these people until they either left the network, were diagnosed with any form of dementia or died.

The result was more than a little surprising: Dementia risk decreased with each bump up in BMI. People who were underweight (BMI 20 or lower in this study, or under 139 pounds for a 5'10" tall person) had a 34% higher risk than average of developing dementia over 20 years than average—maybe not so surprising, since being underweight is obviously not a healthy thing to be. But then the higher that people went up on the weight spectrum, the lower their risk for dementia became, and that seemed downright odd. At the far end of the weight scale, those who were morbidly obese in midlife, with a BMI of 40 or higher (279 pounds for a 5'10" person) had a 29% lower risk for dementia than average. Crazy, huh? As one headline put it, "Being Fat Lowers Dementia Risk In Middle And Old Age, Contradicting Everything We Thought We Knew."

Deborah Gustafson, PhD, a professor of neurology at SUNY Downstate Medical Center in Brooklyn, New York and the University of Gothenburg in Sweden, was not involved with the UK study, but has done extensive research on the risk factors for cognitive decline and was among the first to study the relationship between body weight and dementia.

Regarding the recent study, she was somewhat skeptical.

OOPS, DID WE MEASURE RIGHT?

Like all observational studies, the UK weight study has some inherent limitations. While these kinds of studies are valuable for pointing researchers toward associations, they can't show cause and effect. *Beyond this general limitation, there are specific concerns about this particular study's methods…*

• **It included mixed age groups.** You had to be 40 or older to be included, but there was no upper limit. Some people were 80 years old when their baseline info was recorded. (No matter how you slice it, being 80 isn't middle-aged.) So it's hard to draw conclusions from this data about how weight in middle age affects dementia risk when you're older. During midlife, a person normally gains weight. At around 65 or 70 years old, a person typically loses skeletal muscle and gains fat, but overall, BMI tends to decrease. Mixing up data from these two very different stages of life, means the study is not going to work.

• **It likely missed many cases of dementia.** Patients with dementia were identified only through a review of medical records in this study, but people may come into the health-care system with more acute illnesses that mask dementia, so this approach misses many late-onset cases of dementia. A better approach would be to conduct thorough evaluations among a representative sample, which can take hours, followed by discussion among more than one expert to confirm the diagnoses. That's what Dr. Gustafson has done in her studies. "It's expensive to conduct a study with time-consuming evaluations, which is why it can't be done on two million people. But it's more accurate," she said.

• **It didn't distinguish between different types of dementia.** Certain hereditary forms of dementia tend to strike earlier in life. Early-onset dementia is a different beast, so it would have helped if the researchers had separated dementias diagnosed before age 65 from those diagnosed after age 65. Late-onset dementia may be influenced by being overweight, while early-onset dementia is more likely to be hereditary and influenced by specific genes.

WHAT DO WE REALLY KNOW ABOUT WEIGHT AND DEMENTIA?

• **Watch your weight in midlife.** Studies investigating the association between midlife BMI and risk for dementia demonstrated generally an increased risk among overweight and obese adults. One reason may be that excess weight increases your risk for high blood pressure, high cholesterol levels and diabetes. All of these factors have been shown to increase the risk for dementia.

• **Being too skinny over the age of 70 increases your risk.** Being underweight (BMI 18.5 or lower) is associated with increased dementia risk. That's quite thin, such as 5' 4" and 107 pounds. No one is sure why, but there may be metabolic abnormalities that keep people underweight that also contribute to dementia risk. In some cases, the dementia process may begin decades before clinical symptoms and lead to a lower body weight.

• **A little extra weight in later life may be protective.** There is a consistent finding in the medical literature that over age 70, having a BMI in the "overweight" range (25 to 29.9) is protective. Some but not all studies find that even being obese (BMI 30 to 34.9) protects, too. If you're a little heavier going into late life, you may be less likely to develop dementia. While no one is sure why, it may be that fat tissue produces hormones that are protective for the brain.

It's not quite as much fun as a headline that says being fat is a good thing for your brain and memory. That would be nice for people who are heavy. But the real story appears to be that a healthy lifestyle that helps keep weight in the normal range throughout your middle years and into your 70s is good for your brain, too. Once you get into your 70s, a little extra weight may be fine.

At any age, however, a healthy diet and exercise is important for body—and mind. All of the things that we have been promoting for a long time—eating right and getting physical exercise—are actually relevant for dementia, too.

Trans Fats Linked to Poor Memory

M en age 45 and younger who ate the highest amounts of trans fats daily performed poorly on a word-memory test. Men with high daily intake of 16 to 28 grams of trans fats recalled, on average, 12 to 21 fewer words than men with a lower intake of trans fats. Trans fats are commonly found in french fries, cakes, cookies, taco shells and microwave popcorn. The US Food and Drug Administration has announced a three-year phaseout of partially hydrogenated oils, a primary source of trans fats, from the American food supply.

Study of 645 men by researchers at University of California, San Diego School of Medicine, published in *PLOS ONE*.

Smoking and Heavy Drinking: Path to Alzheimer's

S moking and drinking are among the most important preventable risk factors for Alzheimer's disease.

Recent findings: People who smoke a pack or more of cigarettes daily develop Alzheimer's more than two years earlier than those who do not smoke. People who have more than two alcoholic drinks a day develop the disease almost five years sooner than people who drink more moderately.

Study of 938 people by researchers at Wien Center for Alzheimer's Disease at Mount Sinai Medical Center, Miami Beach, published in *Neuropsychiatry Reviews*.

The Scary Link Between Binge Drinking and Dementia

Iain A. Lang, PhD, consultant and senior lecturer in public health, National Institute for Health Research Collaboration for Leadership in Applied Health Research and Care for the South West Peninsula (NIHR PenCLAHRC), University of Exeter Medical School, Exeter, UK.

Astonishingly, senior citizens (ages 65+)—not college students or 20 somethings—binge drink most frequently, according to the Centers for Disease Control and Prevention (CDC).

Binge drinking is defined as consuming four or more servings of alcohol on one occasion. That kind of drinking isn't healthy for anyone…but for seniors, it's particularly risky.

Reason: Binge drinking can greatly increase the risk for cognitive decline, recent research reveals—and there's a proven link between cognitive decline and dementia.

BRAIN STRAIN

The brain study looked at American men and women age 65 and older. For eight years, participants reported their drinking patterns. Also, at the start and end of the study period, they took standardized tests (such as doing arithmetic and recalling lists of common words) to assess their cognitive function, including memory.

Then researchers analyzed the data to identify the 10% of people who experienced the worst decline in cognition…and the 10% who suffered the worst decline in memory.

Findings: Compared with seniors who did not binge drink…

• **Those who reported binge drinking at least twice a month** were 2.5 times more likely to be in the groups that experienced the worst declines in cognitive function and/or in memory.

• **Even participants who reported bingeing only once a month or more** were 62% more likely to be among those who had the worst cognitive decline…and 27% more likely to be among those who had the worst memory decline.

Gender bender: Frequent bingeing was mostly a "guy thing"—4.3% of men in the study reported binge drinking twice a month or more, while 8.3% did so at least once a month. Women weren't entirely immune, though—0.5% binged twice or more per month and 1.5% did so at least monthly. And the damaging effects of binge drinking on cognition and memory were about the same for both genders.

SIZE DOES MATTER

It can be tricky to gauge how much alcohol you're actually consuming on any given occasion—in part because today's beverage glasses tend to be oversized. For instance, you might think that you had "just two glasses of wine" with dinner. But if your goblet held 10 ounces—rather than the standard five ounces—you really drank the equivalent of four glasses. In other words, you had a binge.

Reality check: The standard US definition of one drink is 12 ounces of beer…eight to nine ounces of malt liquor…five ounces of table wine…three to four ounces of fortified wine, such as sherry or port…two to three ounces of cordial, liqueur or aperitif…or 1.5 ounces of hard liquor or brandy. Recognize, too, that a single mixed drink may contain up to three times the amount of alcohol in a single serving of a plain drink, depending on what spirits are combined in the recipe.

Moderate drinking means no more than two drinks per day for men or one drink per day for women. But don't fool yourself into believing that it's OK to "save up" some of those drinks and consume them all at once. Having four drinks over the course of four days is fine for many adults—but abstaining for three days and then having four drinks on the fourth day is most definitely not fine.

Best: If you're having trouble limiting your alcohol intake—even if you drink only occasionally—confide in your doctor. With help, you can overcome binge drinking…and safeguard your memory and your mind.

Living Alone Raises Dementia Risk

In a study of 1,449 men and women, researchers found that those who were single or divorced during middle age had twice the risk for dementia later in life as those who were married or living with partners. The risk was seven times higher for those who were widowed during middle age and still lived without a partner 21 years later.

Theory: Social engagement promotes healthy brain function.

If you live alone: Aim to stay engaged by participating in social, cultural and recreational activities.

Krister Hakansson, research fellow, Aging Research Center, Karolinska Institute, Stockholm, Sweden.

Loneliness Doubles Alzheimer's Risk

Robert S. Wilson, PhD, senior neuropsychologist of the Rush Alzheimer's Disease Center, Rush University Medical Center, Chicago.

For some time we've known that social isolation is a risk factor for dementia. A recent study goes far deeper, with findings offering fascinating insight. Researchers at Rush University in Chicago and the University of Pennsylvania followed 823 people older than 70 for four years, using questionnaires administered by researchers to assess social isolation and conducting tests of cognitive functioning. They discovered that people who scored highest on the loneliness scale—regardless of whether or not they actually spent much time with people—were more than twice as likely to develop AD during the follow-up period as people whose score was the lowest.

WHO GETS ALZHEIMER'S... AND WHO DOESN'T

Robert S. Wilson, PhD, senior neuropsychologist of the Rush Alzheimer's Disease Center, was the lead author of the study. He said that loneliness is sometimes considered an early sign of AD, but these findings show it is associated with increased risk and not an early symptom of its pathology.

Culturally, we've been inclined to regard problems of age to be inevitable with the passing of years, says Dr. Wilson. This study shows it's time to correct that assumption and more closely investigate ways to prevent the debilitation of old-age diseases including dementia. The kind of loneliness this study talks about is more like a trait than an emotional state—it's not the type of loneliness you might experience being away from home for an extended period, which is loneliness as a state, but rather the type that you feel all or most of the time, loneliness as a trait, that follows you everywhere. Even so, there are still many ways to address and modify it. Medicine helps treat depression, which is usually part of loneliness, but non-drug therapies including regular exercise, joining like-minded groups for activities and expanding your circle of friends and acquaintances in general can be hugely beneficial—most especially when you've got strong networks already in place. If you live alone, you may want to consider moving to a retirement community, where even shy people can make connections, since most residents are looking to do so. Not only will being with others possibly help people avoid Alzheimer's in years to come, it will make for happier years right now.

Caregiver Dementia: It's Real

Brenda Avadian, founder of The Caregiver's Voice, an organization that provides information and support to family caregivers, Los Angeles. She is author of the *Finding the Joy in Alzheimer's* series of books. She previously served as a caregiver for her father, who lived with Alzheimer's. TheCaregiversVoice.com

People who provide prolonged care to family members living with dementia often develop dementia symptoms themselves, including memory loss and disorientation.

This "caregiver dementia" usually is not the result of a degenerative brain condition—it stems from stress and lack of sleep. People who experience it typically recover after their caregiving duties end. But not all do—some face elevated risk for permanent dementia. A study published in *Journal of the American Geriatrics Society* found that people who care for spouses who have dementia are six times more likely to later develop permanent dementia than people whose spouses are dementia-free. The study's authors concluded that the "chronic and often severe stresses associated with dementia caregiving" might be responsible.

Four things caregivers can do…

• **Learn as much as possible about the specific disease affecting the person you care for.** Increasing your knowledge can decrease your frustration.

• **Find moments of joy with your loved one.** Give silent thanks for a quiet moment sitting together. Share a laugh when you can.

• **Take respites.** Caregivers need time off. Sometimes this can be accomplished through assistance from professional caregivers, friends and other family members. When that isn't possible, at least grant yourself five-minute respites. Step outside to take a deep breath. Walk into another room. Pet your cat or dog—research shows this is calming.

• **Replace obligation with empathy.** Reflect on how much your loved one is trying to make sense of his/her world…and how you would feel if the roles were reversed. This can help you provide care out of a sense of love rather than duty.

Distrust Harms the Brain

People who habitually distrust others, believing that others act mainly in their own self-interest, are three times more likely to develop dementia than those who do not. That

was the finding of a recent eight-year study of older adults (average age 71).

Why: Chronic negative emotions can impair cognitive function.

Anna-Maija Tolppanen, PhD, development director of neurology, University of Eastern Finland, Kuopio.

Boost the Good Stuff

Memory loss is associated with low levels of "good" (HDL) cholesterol.

Recent study: People whose HDL was below 40 mg/dL at age 55 were 27% more likely to have a memory deficit than people whose HDL was above 60 mg/dL. At age 61, those with low HDL levels were 53% more likely to suffer memory problems.

To boost HDL: Get regular aerobic exercise…maintain a healthy weight…limit intake of saturated fat…don't smoke.

Archana Singh-Manoux, PhD, senior research fellow in epidemiology and public health, University College London, England, and lead author of a study of 3,673 people, published in *Arteriosclerosis, Thrombosis and Vascular Biology*.

Another Reason to Lower Your Blood Pressure

High blood pressure may raise Alzheimer's risk. High blood pressure reduces blood flow to the part of the brain that controls memory and learning.

Self-defense: Exercise and proper diet are very effective at keeping blood pressure down. Ask your doctor what is best for you.

Cyrus Raji, an MD/PhD candidate at University of Pittsburgh School of Medicine and coauthor of a study of blood flow in the brains of older adults, presented at a recent meeting of the Radiological Society of North America.

How BP Changes Affect Memory

Blood pressure fluctuations may lead to memory loss. In a study of 5,400 adults over age 70, those with the greatest fluctuations in blood pressure performed worse on tests of memory, attention and reaction time than those with more stable levels, even if blood pressure was high. Extreme swings in blood pressure are also associated with brain microbleeds, which may contribute to cognitive decline.

Possible explanation: Unstable blood pressure can disrupt blood flow to the brain, which could lead to dementia over time.

Simon Mooijaart, MD, PhD, director, Institute for Evidence-Based Medicine in Old Age, Leiden University Medical Center, the Netherlands.

Low Blood Pressure May Harm the Brain

It's long been known that high blood pressure in middle age may cause brain shrinkage, or atrophy, later in life. But when 663 middle-aged patients with coronary artery disease or other vascular conditions were followed for about four years, those with low diastolic (bottom number) blood pressure readings (under 60 mm/Hg) also showed signs of atrophy.

Theory: Low blood pressure may be inadequate for healthy blood flow to the brain, which can lead to brain tissue loss. More research is needed to determine if low pressure should be treated to minimize risk for brain atrophy.

Majon Muller, MD, PhD, geriatrician, VU University Medical Center Amsterdam, the Netherlands.

Easy Way to Keep Alzheimer's Away

Walking six miles weekly may prevent Alzheimer's.

Recent finding: In a study of 426 adults with or without cognitive decline, those who walked at least six miles weekly were half as likely to develop Alzheimer's disease over 13 years as nonwalkers. Among those with cognitive impairment, walking five miles a week reduced cognitive decline by more than half.

Theory: Exercise improves blood flow to the brain, which helps keep neurons healthy.

To help preserve brain health: Aim to walk at least three-quarters of a mile daily.

Cyrus Raji, MD, PhD, physician-scientist, department of radiology, University of Pittsburgh.

Don't Let Stress Wreck Your Memory

Irene Louise Dejak, MD, an internal medicine specialist who focuses on preventive health, including counseling patients on the dangers of chronic stress.

It's widely known that acute stress can damage the heart. But even low-level, ongoing stress, such as that from a demanding job, marriage or other family conflicts, financial worries or chronic health problems, not only increases inflammation in the arteries, it can also harm your brain…

What it does: After just a few weeks of stress, nerves in the part of the brain associated with memory shrink and lose connections with other nerve cells, according to laboratory studies.

Result: You might find that you're forgetting names or where you put things. These lapses are often due to distraction—people who are stressed and always busy find it difficult to store new information in the brain. This type of memory loss is rarely a sign of dementia unless it's getting progressively worse.

39

What helps: Use memory tools to make your life easier. When you meet someone, say that person's name out loud to embed it in your memory. Put your keys in the same place every day.

Also: Make a conscious effort to pay attention. It's the only way to ensure that new information is stored. Sometimes the guidance of a counselor is necessary to help you learn how to manage stress. Self-help materials, such as tapes and books, may also be good tools.

STRESS-FIGHTING PLAN

There are a number of ways to determine whether you are chronically stressed—you may feel short-tempered, anxious most of the time, have heart palpitations or suffer from insomnia.

However, I've found that many of my patients don't even realize how much stress they have in their lives until a friend, family member, coworker or doctor points it out to them. Once they understand the degree to which stress is affecting their health, they can explore ways to unwind and relax.

In general, it helps to...

•**Get organized.** Much of the stress that we experience comes from feeling overwhelmed. You can overcome this by organizing your life.

Examples: Use a day calendar to keep your activities and responsibilities on-track, and put reminder notes on the refrigerator.

•**Ask for help.** You don't have to become overwhelmed. If you're struggling at work, ask a mentor for advice. Tell your partner/spouse that you need help with the shopping or housework.

Taking charge of your life is among the best ways to reduce stress—and asking for help is one of the smartest ways to do this.

•**Write about your worries.** The anxieties and stresses floating around in our heads often dissipate, or at least seem more manageable, once we write them down.

•**Sleep for eight hours.** No one who is sleep-deprived can cope with stress effectively.

Don't Forget to Tell Your Doctor!

Older adults tend not to discuss memory problems with doctors, and doctors often don't raise the subject. Only 25% of adults age 45 or older with memory problems talked about their problems with health-care professionals during routine checkups—and the likelihood of discussing memory concerns declined with advancing age.

Likely reason: Denial and avoidance on the part of both patient and doctor.

Self-defense: Bring up any memory concerns at your annual physical. Memory issues often are not the start of dementia but result from a different, highly treatable cause, such as depression. And memory trouble that is linked to dementia needs to be caught early for treatment to be effective.

Analysis of government data from 2011 on more than 10,000 people by researchers at On Target Health Data, West Suffield, Connecticut, published in *Preventing Chronic Disease*.

Hearing Loss Is Linked to Memory Loss

Older adults with even mild-to-moderate hearing loss may experience a decline in brain function up to 41% faster—or three years sooner—than those who have not become hearing impaired.

Reasons: When people are faced with hearing loss, the brain works harder to process sounds rather than dedicating energy to memory and thinking. And the social isolation that occurs among people with poor hearing may result in cognitive decline.

Study of 1,984 people, ages 75 to 84, by researchers at The Johns Hopkins University School of Medicine, Baltimore, published in *JAMA Internal Medicine*.

Signs of Dementia and Alzheimer's: Symptoms and Diagnosis

Worried About Dementia?

Chances are you notice every little blip in your memory if you're over age 40. That's because most people who are middle-aged or beyond fear that any sign of memory loss is a red flag for Alzheimer's disease.

What you may not realize: While memory loss does occur with Alzheimer's disease, there are other symptoms that often get overlooked by patients and their doctors. These symptoms can also be the key to identifying other causes of dementia that are less well-known than Alzheimer's disease.

Important: Dementia-like symptoms are sometimes due to medical conditions, including depression…traumatic brain injury…diabetes…tumors…thyroid disease…vitamin B-12 deficiency…and kidney disease. Certain medications can also be to blame—including drugs that block the neurotransmitter acetylcholine,

such as those for overactive bladder, allergies, anxiety and depression.

If you or a loved one is showing any of the symptoms described in this article, consult your primary care provider. He/she can perform simple memory tests or refer you to a specialist, such as a neurologist, psychiatrist, neuropsychologist or geriatrician, for a more comprehensive evaluation, which may include an imaging test of the brain, such as an MRI or a CT scan.

James E. Galvin, MD, a renowned authority on dementia, explained more about the complex interplay between memory and dementia…

James E. Galvin, MD, MPH, professor and associate dean for clinical research at the Charles E. Schmidt College of Medicine and professor in the Christine E. Lynn College of Nursing, both at Florida Atlantic University (FAU) in Boca Raton, Florida. He also has developed a number of dementia-screening tools, including the "Lewy Body Composite Risk Score" and the "Quick Dementia Rating System." You can find these tests by searching at FAU.edu.

4 MAIN CAUSES OF DEMENTIA

Of all the possible causes of dementia, the majority of cases are due to one of the following disorders—and many people have a combination of two or more disorders…

•**Alzheimer's disease.** It's true that memory (problems with learning new things and recalling past information) is significantly affected by this disease. But memory problems aren't the only warning signs.

Non-memory symptoms include: Changes in mood (including the onset of depression, anxiety or paranoia)…behavior (such as withdrawing from hobbies and social activities)…language ability (such as difficulty finding the right word)…and problem-solving skills and concentration (such as finding it hard to keep track of monthly bills).

When Alzheimer's typically strikes: It mainly hits people in their mid-60s to mid-80s. Early-onset Alzheimer's disease can appear in one's 40s or 50s.

•**Lewy body dementia.** Lewy body dementia and a related form of dementia that accompanies Parkinson's are caused by clumps (called Lewy bodies) of a protein that forms in cells throughout the brain. With Lewy body dementia, the protein clumps start in the cerebral cortex, which can lead to memory loss.

Non-memory symptoms that may occur with Lewy body dementia: Visual hallucinations…perceptual difficulties (for example, bumping into doors)…frequent staring spells…and/or sleep disruptions that cause one to act out dreams.

When dementia accompanies Parkinson's, similar cognitive symptoms develop a year or more after the onset of the movement changes that characterize Parkinson's, including slow movement, muscle rigidity and tremors. The movement problems occur when abnormal protein clumps form in the brain stem and later spread to other brain regions.

When Lewy body dementia and Parkinson's disease with dementia usually strike: In one's 60s to late 70s, but early-onset Parkinson's with dementia can occur under age 50. (See the following article for more information and how not to be misdiagnosed.)

•**Vascular dementia.** In people with vascular dementia, brain cells become damaged by "mini" strokes that are often so small that they may go unnoticed. Memory problems may occur but sometimes after the other symptoms described below.

Non-memory symptoms may include: Changes in one's ability to plan, organize and make decisions (such as those required for daily activities)…and mood (such as depression and lack of motivation).

When vascular dementia strikes: Risk is highest after age 65, but it can occur at any age.

•**Frontotemporal dementia (FTD).** This degenerative disorder mainly affects brain cells in two parts of the brain—the frontal lobe (responsible for behavior and emotions) and temporal lobe (involved in language and memory skills).

Memory problems are more prominent at a later stage than with Alzheimer's disease. Language is frequently affected, either with difficulty producing words or in understanding the meaning of words. For more on frontotemporal dementia, see page 52.

Non-memory symptoms that may occur: Changes in personality (a shy person becoming boisterous, for example) and/or trouble with problem solving and other executive functions (such as the ability to handle everyday situations, including driving a car and shopping for groceries) develop when the frontal lobe is mainly affected.

When FTD strikes: Typically in one's 50s or 60s.

TREATMENT OPTIONS

Regardless of the cause of dementia, an early diagnosis helps…

For Alzheimer's disease, medications are available to help slow the progression, and doctors may use the same medications to help treat the symptoms of other causes of dementia.

For vascular dementia, you can work with a doctor to control risk factors, such as high blood pressure or high cholesterol. For Lewy body dementia and frontotemporal dementia, there are no treatments for the diseases themselves, but research is ongoing to change that.

There is also accumulating evidence that certain lifestyle factors may reduce risk of developing dementia and slow symptoms of disease. These include daily exercise (aerobic, resistance training, flexibility)…mental stimulation (games, lectures)…social engagement… and a healthful diet (fruits, vegetables, whole grains, lean meats).

Parkinson's, Alzheimer's or Lewy Body Dementia— Don't Be Misdiagnosed Like Robin Williams

Susan M. Maixner, MD, associate professor of psychiatry, director of the geriatric psychiatry clinic at the University of Michigan Health System, Ann Arbor.

The world was shocked and grieved when beloved comedian Robin Williams took his own life in 2014. The media went on about how he had been battling depression. Then news came out that he had Parkinson's disease, so the media conjectured whether that diagnosis played a role in him deciding to end it all. But as it turns out, Robin Williams may have had Parkinson's—or a common type of dementia that is often mistaken for Parkinson's disease or Alzheimer's. In fact, medication that Williams was taking for Parkinson's may have worsened his dementia symptoms, possibly even driving him to suicide!

The disease that Williams's doctors apparently never detected is called Lewy body dementia. Because doctors and other medical professionals are just learning about how to distinguish this dementia from other types, it can take longer—up to 18 months—to get a correct diagnosis. This can have tragic consequences, as Robin Williams's sad story seems to show. So arm yourself with information about this kind of dementia.

WHY IT'S A TRICKY DIAGNOSIS

Lewy body dementia (also called dementia with Lewy bodies) is a condition in which

small, orblike proteins called Lewy bodies begin to form in brain cells, ultimately crowding out the normal structures of those cells. The exact diagnosis can be made only at autopsy, and that is, in fact, when Robin Williams's diagnosis was made. But the clinical knowledge to distinguish Lewy body dementia from Alzheimer's or Parkinson's in the living has greatly improved in the past 10 years—and now this information needs to get out there.

"The early symptoms of Lewy body dementia usually involve cognitive and psychiatric problems, whereas early symptoms of Parkinson's disease are usually related to problems with movement," said Susan Maixner, MD, an associate professor of psychiatry and director of the Geriatric Psychiatry Clinic at the University of Michigan Health System. As the two different but related diseases progress, they look more and more alike because a degree of Lewy body–protein buildup also occurs in Parkinson's disease.

Lewy body dementia also can be difficult to distinguish from Alzheimer's disease because the symptoms of cognitive decline are similar. But, unlike with Alzheimer's disease, short-term memory loss is usually not the first symptom, said Dr. Maixner. "In contrast to Alzheimer's, people with Lewy body dementia have early challenges with problem-solving. They can fluctuate between having normal and very confused days, and often see things that aren't there—most commonly little people or animals. Depth perception can be off, and they are more sensitive to medications given to treat hallucinations," she explained. REM sleep disorder, a condition in which you physically act out dreams because the brain chemistry that keeps your body still while asleep does not kick in, is also more common with Lewy body dementia. There's also a higher risk of dizziness and falls in people with Lewy body dementia because one of the symptoms is a sudden drop in blood pressure.

If you notice signs of dementia in yourself or someone you know, the diagnostic process starts by getting a good medical exam to rule out other possible causes of cognitive decline, such as a vitamin deficiency or thyroid disease. Although brain scans can't diagnose Lewy body dementia, an MRI or CT scan can help rule out mini-strokes or brain tumors. In fact, the process of diagnosis is similar to that for Alzheimer's disease.

TREATING IT

Like Alzheimer's and Parkinson's, Lewy body dementia is progressive (symptoms can be expected to worsen over time) although medication, complementary therapies and lifestyle modification can slow down the disease symptoms. Still, those affected will ultimately need to be in the care of another person or placed in a long-term-care facility.

Drugs called cholinesterase inhibitors (such as *rivastigmine* (Exelon) and *donepezil* (Aricept), which are used to slow the worsening of dementia symptoms in Alzheimer's, are also used to treat Lewy body dementia, and some studies suggest that they are more effective in treating Lewy body dementia than Alzheimer's. Levodopa, the key medication to control movement in Parkinson's disease, is also used in patients with Lewy body dementia who have Parkinson's symptoms, such as rigid muscles and slow movements, but it can intensify symptoms of confusion, delusions and hallucinations in some people. "Antipsychotic drugs, which are given for hallucinations, can worsen walking problems, other Parkinson-like symptoms and confusion," said Dr. Maixner.

Having a safe, uncluttered, comfortable environment prepared for you or an affected loved one is preferable to medications, she said, adding that physical, social and mental activity can slow down symptoms. In addition, establishing routines and predictability to provide the affected person with a sense of structure is important. "However, due to the severity of some Lewy body symptoms, a person's quality of life can be improved through careful use of medications if the above strategies are not enough," she said.

Complementary nondrug treatments of benefit include physical therapy to fortify cardiovascular and muscular health and gait… speech therapy to help improve enunciation… occupational therapy to help maintain skills and promote independence…and treatments, such as music therapy or aromatherapy, to reduce anxiety and improve mood.

More information on Lewy body dementia, including information on support groups for patients, families and caregivers, can be found on the website of the Lewy Body Dementia Association, LBDA.org.

What Do "Senior Moments" Really Mean?

Barry Reisberg, MD, leader of the Clinical Core of the Alzheimer's Disease Center of the New York University (NYU) School of Medicine and clinical director of the school's Aging and Dementia Research Center, both in New York City. He is also director of the university's Zachary and Elizabeth M. Fisher Alzheimer's Disease Education and Resources Program.

Until recently, most physicians have reassured older adults that so-called "senior moments" are usually a normal part of aging.

Now, recent research shows that complaints of subtle memory loss—for example, not remembering the name of a longtime acquaintance as easily as you might have five to 10 years earlier—may mean more than doctors once thought.

What's new: Researchers at New York University (NYU) School of Medicine have found that people who are concerned about episodes of memory loss may, in fact, be absolutely right, and they are at increased risk of developing Alzheimer's disease years later.

Barry Reisberg, MD, a renowned Alzheimer's researcher who led this important recent research, explained more about the recent research…

WHEN DOES ALZHEIMER'S BEGIN?

The warning signs of Alzheimer's disease are now well-known and include a gradual decline of memory and reasoning skills. However, the stages that precede Alzheimer's now are a great focus of investigation.

In the 1980s, my associates and I first identified a condition that we termed mild cognitive impairment (MCI), which is generally characterized by measurable memory loss beyond the personal experiences of forgetfulness that can be associated with normal aging. With MCI, memory problems, such as forgetting recent events and frequently repeating yourself in conversations, usually are noticeable to family members and/or friends.

Research findings are mixed, but most evidence shows that about half of people who experience MCI go on to develop overt Alzheimer's disease within about four years.

Important recent research: NYU investigators have found that a condition they've termed subjective cognitive impairment may be evident up to 22 years before noticeable Alzheimer's symptoms manifest—many, many years before MCI.

What's the implication of this recent finding?

It means that scientists can refocus their research to try to find ways to prevent Alzheimer's by addressing it a decade or two before it surfaces—and individuals may have a crucial new clue that signals the importance of seriously following the lifestyle habits that promote brain health.

A NEW—EVEN EARLIER—SIGN

Subjective cognitive impairment is so subtle that it usually is not recognized by a patient's doctor or his/her family. In fact, the condition is generally apparent only to the individual, although he may confide in a spouse or close friend about the self-perceived problem.

Interestingly, when people with subjective cognitive impairment are tested, they continue to perform within normal ranges on mental and psychological tests.

So, how can subjective cognitive impairment be detected—and is it important to even do so?

What researchers currently know: Up to 56% of adults ages 65 and older experience subjective cognitive impairment. Its key known characteristic is that the person believes his memory is not as good as it was five to 10 years before. Specifically, a person with the condition may complain—or simply note—that he can't remember, say, names or where he has placed things as well as he did in previous years.

Compared with people who don't have subjective cognitive impairment, those who have the condition are 4.5 times more likely to develop MCI or full-blown Alzheimer's within seven years. In a recent study, more than half of people advanced to these more evident and more serious conditions after seven years.

What's more, research shows that those with subjective cognitive impairment who progress to MCI or Alzheimer's do so about 3.5 years sooner, on average, than those who didn't have subjective cognitive impairment.

IS THIS JUST NORMAL AGING?

Since studies show that as many as 56% of people ages 65 and older have subjective cognitive impairment, it can be technically considered part of the normal aging process. Advanced age is, after all, the single biggest risk for dementia.

However, there are unique psychological and physiological characteristics that accompany subjective cognitive impairment.

For example, research conducted at the NYU School of Medicine found that people with subjective cognitive impairment have increased urinary levels of the stress hormone cortisol and decreased brain activity in the memory and other brain regions, compared with people who don't have the condition. Increased cortisol levels have been shown in some studies to damage the brain.

In addition, European researchers have found that people with subjective cognitive impairment have significantly higher levels of spinal fluid markers that often accompany Alzheimer's, compared with people who don't have subjective cognitive impairment.

THREE IMPORTANT QUESTIONS

Here are a few of the questions that were used by the NYU researchers to help identify subjective cognitive impairment. *If you answer "yes" to one or more of the following, discuss this with your physician…*

1. Am I having trouble recalling names (especially names of people) more than I did five to 10 years ago?

2. Am I having trouble recalling where I placed things more than I did five to 10 years ago?

3. Has my ability to concentrate decreased compared with five to 10 years ago?

WHAT YOU CAN DO

If you suspect that you have subjective cognitive impairment or MCI, your doctor can determine whether a treatable factor—such as depression…anxiety…a thyroid disorder…a nutritional deficiency (such as too little vitamin B-12)…or medication (such as anticholinergic drugs taken for conditions including allergies or overactive bladder…and painkillers)—is causing memory loss. Chronic stress also may affect memory.

If your doctor rules out a treatable cause for your impairment difficulty, it's crucial to adopt lifestyle habits, such as regular exercise, that promote brain health.

This includes eating a heart-healthy diet. A diet that emphasizes vegetables and fruit, lean protein and whole grains…avoids saturated and trans fats…and includes healthful fats, such as olive oil, promotes cardiovascular health and, in turn, the health of your brain.

There is no medication that is prescribed at the present time for people with subjective cognitive impairment. There are also no medications that have been approved specifically for MCI. However, medications such as *donepezil* (Aricept) or *rivastigmine* (Exelon), which are approved for the treatment of Alzheimer's symptoms, have been studied in MCI patients. But these medications have not shown sufficient benefit to win FDA approval as a treatment for MCI.

How to Avoid the Memory Hiccups That Cause Panic

Aaron P. Nelson, PhD, chief of neuropsychology in the division of cognitive and behavioral neurology at Brigham and Women's Hospital and an assistant professor of psychology at Harvard Medical School, both in Boston. He is coauthor, with Susan Gilbert, of *The Harvard Medical School Guide to Achieving Optimal Memory.*

With all the media coverage of Alzheimer's disease and other forms of dementia, it's easy to imagine the worst every time you can't summon the name of a good friend or struggle to remember the details of a novel that you put down just a few days ago.

Reassuring: The minor memory hiccups that bedevil adults in middle age and beyond usually are due to normal changes in the brain and nervous system that affect concentration or the processing and storing of information. In fact, common memory "problems" typically are nothing more than memory errors. Forgetting is just one kind of error.

Important: Memory problems that are frequent or severe (such as forgetting how to drive home from work or how to operate a simple appliance in your home) could be a sign of Alzheimer's disease or some other form of dementia. Such memory lapses also can be due to treatable, but potentially serious, conditions, including depression, a nutritional deficiency or even sleep apnea. See your doctor if you have memory problems that interfere with daily life—or the frequency and/or severity seems to be increasing. *Five types of harmless memory errors that tend to get more common with age…*

MEMORY ERROR #1: **Absentmindedness.** How many times have you had to search for the car keys because you put them in an entirely unexpected place? Or gone to the grocery store to buy three items but come home with only two? This type of forgetfulness describes what happens when a new piece of information (where you put the keys or what to buy at the store) never even enters your memory because you weren't paying attention.

My advice: Since distraction is the main cause of absentmindedness, try to do just one thing at a time.

Otherwise, here's what can happen: You start to do something, and then something else grabs your attention—and you completely forget about the first thing.

We live in a world in which information routinely comes at us from all directions, so you'll want to develop your own systems for getting things done. There's no good reason to use brain space for superfluous or transitory information. Use lists, sticky notes, e-mail reminders, etc., for tasks, names of books you want to read, grocery lists, etc. There's truth to the Chinese proverb that says, "The palest ink is better than the best memory."

Helpful: Don't write a to-do list and put it aside. While just the act of writing down tasks can help you remember them, you should consult your list several times a day for it to be effective.

MEMORY ERROR #2: Blocking. When a word or the answer to a question is "on the tip of your tongue," you're blocking the information that you need. A similar situation happens when you accidentally call one of your children by the name of another. Some patients are convinced that temporarily "forgetting" an acquaintance's name means that they're developing Alzheimer's disease, but that's usually not true.

Blocking occurs when the information that you need is properly stored in memory, but another piece of information is getting in the way. Often, this second piece of information has similar qualities (names of children, closely related words, etc.) to the first. The similarity may cause the wrong brain area to activate and make it harder to access the information that you want.

My advice: Don't get frustrated when a word or name is on the tip of your tongue. Relax and think about something else. In about 50% of cases, the right answer will come to you within one minute.

MEMORY ERROR #3: Misattribution. This is what happens when you make a mistake in the source of a memory.

More than a few writers have been embarrassed when they wrote something that they thought was original but later learned that it was identical to something they had heard or read. You might tell a story to friends that you know is true because you read about it in the newspaper—except that you may have only heard people talking about it and misattributed the source.

Misattribution happens more frequently with age because older people have older memories. These memories are more likely to contain mistakes because they happened long ago and don't get recalled often.

My advice: Concentrate on details when you want to remember the source of information.

Focus on the five Ws: Who told you…what the content was…when it happened…where you were when you learned it…and why it's important. Asking these questions will help to strengthen the context of the information.

MEMORY ERROR #4: Suggestibility. Most individuals think of memory as a mental videotape—a recording of what took place. But what feels like memories to you could be things that never really happened. Memories can be affected or even created by the power of suggestion.

In a landmark study, researchers privately asked the relatives of participants to describe three childhood events that actually happened. They were also asked to provide plausible details about a fourth scenario (getting lost in a shopping mall) that could have happened, but didn't.

A few weeks later, the participants were given a written description of the four stories and asked to recall them in as much detail as possible. They weren't told that one of the stories was fictional.

What happened: About 20% of the participants believed that they really had been lost in a shopping mall. They "remembered" the event and provided details about what happened. This and other studies show that memories can be influenced—and even created—from thin air.

My advice: Keep an open mind if your memory of an event isn't the same as someone else's. It's unlikely that either of you will have perfect recall. Memories get modified over time by new information as well as by individual perspectives, personality traits, etc.

MEMORY ERROR #5: Transience. You watched a great movie but can't remember the lead actor two hours later. You earned an advanced degree in engineering, but now you can hardly remember the basic equations.

These are all examples of transience, the tendency of memories to fade over time. Short-term memory is highly susceptible to transience because information that you've just acquired hasn't been embedded in long-term storage, where memories can be more stable and enduring.

This is why you're more likely to forget the name of someone you just met than the details of a meaningful book that you read in college—although even long-term memories will fade if you do not recall them now and then.

My advice: You need to rehearse and revisit information in order to retain it. Repeating a name several times after you've met someone is a form of rehearsal. So is talking about a movie you just watched or jotting notes about an event in a diary.

Revisiting information simply means recalling and using it. Suppose that you wrote down your thoughts about an important conversation in your journal. You can review the notes a few weeks later to strengthen the memory and anchor it in your mind. The same technique will help you remember names, telephone numbers, etc.

Is the Way You Walk Giving You a Warning?

Mary Harward, MD, a geriatrician in private practice in Orange, California. She specializes in the diagnosis and treatment of gait disorders and other diseases affecting older adults. She is editor of *Medical Secrets*.

Have you surprised yourself recently with a stumble or a fall? If you blamed it on your shoes...your eyesight...or an obstacle, such as a throw rug, you may not be getting at the root cause of why you stumbled or fell. The fact is, the real reason many people fall (and sometimes die from it) is the way that they walk.

A problem that goes undetected: Most people who have treatable abnormalities in their gait (the way in which a person walks) never even discuss it with their doctors.

Here's why: When you go to the doctor, odds are that you are taken to an exam room and asked to "have a seat" until the doctor arrives. The problem is, you'll probably stay

seated during the entire visit, and your doctor may miss a symptom—a dangerous gait—that's just as important as abnormal X-rays or blood tests.

TAKE IT SERIOUSLY

It's never normal to shuffle, be off-balance or have an unusual posture. A gait disorder always means that something—or, in most cases, a combination of factors—is awry.

Problems with gait affect about 15% of adults age 60 and older and more than 80% of those age 85 and older. Gait disorders, which interfere with stability and balance, are not only among the most common causes of falls and subsequent hospitalizations, but also can be one of the first health problems that eventually leads to nursing home care.

My advice: Doctors should ask every patient if he/she has fallen in the last year. In addition, if you're age 65 or older, you should ask your doctor to check your gait at least once a year.

WHAT'S BEHIND IT?

Patients often assume that problems with one's gait are due to neurological disorders, such as Parkinson's disease or multiple sclerosis (MS). With Parkinson's disease, patients also experience a resting tremor or shaking of one hand, muscle rigidity and slow movements, while MS typically is accompanied by vision problems, dizziness and trouble speaking. *But there are other possible causes of gait problems...*

•**Arthritis.** Gait problems are common in patients with arthritis, particularly osteoarthritis of the knee or hip. If you have knee or hip pain, you may favor that side and use other muscles to compensate. This throws off your posture and body mechanics, which may cause you to limp or take tentative steps.

Helpful: Ask your doctor if it's appropriate to see a physical therapist for advice on exercises to strengthen the muscles around the arthritic joint—this will help you walk normally and with less pain.

Pain control is also very important. Apart from making you more comfortable, it will help you do the exercises that you need for a better gait. If you don't get adequate relief from over-the-counter pain relievers, talk to your doctor about stronger forms of pain control. Stretching, massage, heating pads, cold packs and/or acupuncture are helpful to some people.

• **Back problems.** A gait problem often is due to a painful back. Patients with lumbar stenosis, for example, will frequently experience nerve pressure from damaged vertebrae in the spine, affecting their ability to walk. Patients with sciatica (nerve pain that often accompanies lower-back problems) will have difficulty walking or standing. Suspect nerve problems if you have back or leg pain that gets worse when you walk or stand for more than a few minutes and gets better when you're off your feet. See your doctor for treatment advice.

• **Balance disorders.** If you sometimes feel as though you're about to fall (even when you're not), see a doctor right away. Problems with balance—often accompanied by dizziness, spinning sensations, etc.—are a major cause of falls. Potential causes include ear infections, inner-ear disorders, neuropathy (nerve damage) and circulatory problems.

Also: Ask your doctor to test your vitamin B-12 level. Older adults often have low levels of intrinsic factor, a protein that's needed for B-12 absorption. It's also common for vegetarians to be deficient in this vitamin because meat is a major source of B-12. Low B-12 can make you feel light-headed, cause numbness and/or tingling in the feet and make it difficult to walk.

Similar foot and leg symptoms are caused by diabetic neuropathy, nerve damage that may occur in patients with poorly managed (or undiagnosed) diabetes. Bunions and other foot conditions also can contribute to gait disorders.

• **Drug side effects.** It's not surprising that sedating medications such as *diazepam* (Valium) can increase fall risk. What many people don't realize is that nonsedating medications also can be an issue.

Example: Medications that lower blood pressure, such as diuretics, can cause orthostatic hypotension, a sudden drop in blood pressure that can make you dizzy or light-headed. Some blood pressure drugs also decrease magnesium, which can cause leg weakness or cramps. Your doctor might advise changing medications. Alcohol or drugs that lower blood sugar or affect mood or sleep also can change one's gait.

Important: Be especially careful after eating. Studies have shown that dizziness and gait problems tend to get worse about 30 minutes after meals—blood travels to the digestive tract after meals, sometimes lowering blood pressure.

• **Reduced brain circulation.** Gait disorders are often the first sign of infarcts, areas of brain damage caused by impaired circulation. Infarcts occur in patients who have had a stroke or other problems that affect blood vessels in the brain, such as hypertension or high cholesterol.

A patient who has multiple infarcts might walk very slowly...take short steps...stand with his feet wider apart than usual...and/or hesitate when starting to walk or have trouble slowing momentum when stopping.

HOW'S YOUR GAIT?

If you've noticed changes in the ways in which you move, see your doctor for an evaluation. *He/she will give you tests that may include...*

• **The timed get-up-and-go test.** This measures the time it takes you to get up from a chair (without using your hands to push off from the armrests), walk 10 feet, turn around and walk back to the chair. You should be able to complete the sequence safely in 14 seconds or less. If it takes longer than 20 seconds, your gait is seriously impaired.

Sleep Disorder Predicts Brain Disease

John Peever, PhD, associate professor of cell & systems biology, University of Toronto, Canada.

Up to 90% of people with rapid-eye-movement sleep behavior disorder (RBD) will develop a brain disease, such as Parkinson's, up to 15 years later. RBD causes people to act out their dreams, often hurting themselves or their bed partners. In healthy brains, the muscles are paralyzed during sleep to prevent this. See your doctor if you or your bed partner experiences restless dreaming during sleep.

If it turns out that the neurologist says, yes, you have REM sleep behavior disorder, he or she may suggest a treatment that will reduce the symptoms, such as the antiseizure medication *clonazepam* or the sleep aid melatonin. If your neurologist doesn't bring up the link between this sleep disorder and the very high risk of neurodegenerative disease down the road, you must bring up this link and make a plan with this neurologist—or another one you have confidence in, if necessary—for monitoring and staving off symptoms of neurodegeneration.

Trouble Smelling? It May Signal Serious Illness

Richard L. Doty, PhD, professor of otorhinolaryngology (ear, nose and throat disorders) at the University of Pennsylvania School of Medicine and director of the school's Smell and Taste Center, both in Philadelphia. He is author of *The Neurology of Olfaction*.

M ost of us take our sense of smell for granted. But for the surprising number of people for whom this vital sense is dulled, the consequences can be more serious than you might imagine. Smell disorders affect half of people age 65 and older, with more cases occurring in men than in women.

Danger: When a person's sense of smell is not functioning properly, it can lead to related health problems, such as loss of appetite, high blood pressure (due to the use of too much salt) and/or weight gain (due to excessive sugar intake). Gas leaks and fires also may endanger people with an impaired sense of smell.

Why your sense of smell is so important…

WHEN OUR SENSE OF SMELL FALTERS

We all know that allergies, colds and nasal congestion interfere with our sense of smell. These conditions cause nasal obstruction that prevents odors from reaching olfactory receptors (sensory nerve cells) in the nasal lining.

A blunted sense of smell is common with this type of obstruction, but the sense usually returns within a few days or weeks. When the damage is severe or repeated enough times, the cells can be permanently disabled. The persistent state of inflammation that occurs with chronic sinusitis also can permanently impair olfactory cells.

Other causes of impaired smell…

•**Aging.** As we grow older, the nerves involved in smell weaken, and membranes lining the nose become thin and dry.

•**Head injury.** When the brain is jarred within the skull, olfactory nerve fibers may be damaged. Smell loss from traumatic head injury is usually more severe than that caused by infection. Even a relatively mild impact—not enough to cause a concussion—can lead to permanent loss of smell.

•**Medications.** Heart drugs, such as the cholesterol-lowering medication *atorvastatin* (Lipitor), the calcium channel blocker *verapamil* (Covera) and the blood pressure–lowering agent *doxazosin* (Cardura), are among the medications most likely to impair one's sense of smell or taste. Other blood pressure drugs, such as angiotensin-converting enzyme (ACE) inhibitors, including *enalapril* (Vasotec) and *enalapril maleate-hydrochlorothiazide* (Vaseretic), also may lead to loss of smell or taste.

•**Environmental toxins.** The precise effect of environmental toxins, such as pesticides, is uncertain, but they can clearly damage one's sense of smell. In a study published in *Experimental and Toxicologic Pathology*, a group of residents of Mexico City—notorious for its air pollution—scored significantly lower on a smell identification test than residents of cleaner environments. Upon closer examination, signs of damage in the nasal lining and in the olfactory bulb (which processes smell signals) within the brain were found in the study subjects.

A WARNING SIGN

The olfactory system is highly vulnerable to brain disorders, and a noticeable decline in the sense of smell occurs in 85% to 90%

of people in the early stages of Alzheimer's and Parkinson's disease. In fact, the American Academy of Neurology recommends the use of smell tests as an aid to help diagnose Parkinson's disease.

There's even increasing evidence that smell loss begins in the so-called "preclinical" period—preceding classic symptoms of Alzheimer's (such as memory loss) and Parkinson's (such as movement problems) by several years.

Low thyroid function (hypothyroidism) also can lead to loss of smell. Distorted or phantom smells (smelling an odor, such as a chemical or floral scent, that is not present) may point to epilepsy or a brain tumor or Alzheimer's disease.

HOW WELL DO YOU SMELL?

If you think that your ability to distinguish odors has gotten significantly worse, it may be worth having it tested by your doctor. Few physicians routinely provide smell testing, so you will probably need to ask for it.

Or you can take a self-administered smell test that was developed by myself and other researchers at the University of Pennsylvania. Known as the Smell Identification Test (SIT), it is a scratch-and-sniff–type test and is available from the manufacturer (800-547-8838, Sensonics.com).

Cost: $27 for the test and $3.50 for the scoring key. For the most accurate results, take the test in your doctor's office and ask him/her to help you interpret the results.

PROTECT YOUR SENSE OF SMELL

Once seriously damaged, one's sense of smell may improve but is unlikely to recover fully.

Smell loss due to nasal inflammation can be treated with steroid drugs, such as *prednisolone* (Prelone), in nasal spray or pill form. But long-term use of the pill form of prednisolone and overuse of the nasal spray are not recommended because damage to the liver, kidney or bones may result.

Meanwhile, research using stem cells is under way at several universities to explore whether damaged olfactory receptor cells could be replaced with healthy cells in the future.

Prevention is the best defense against loss of smell. Exposure to tobacco smoke—both through smoking and exposure to secondhand smoke—dulls the sense of smell but is generally less devastating than one might expect. If you smoke, quitting cigarettes generally will restore any loss of your sense of smell—but that recovery can take years.

Other prevention strategies…

•**Avoid infection.** While occasional colds and the flu are inescapable, good hygiene practices (including frequent hand-washing) will make them less frequent.

•**Protect your head.** Wear seat belts in the car and a helmet when riding a bike, rollerblading, skiing or participating in any sport or activity that could lead to a head injury. Don't participate in sports, such as boxing or football, that may involve frequent blows to the head.

•**Breathe clean.** Take precautions around toxic chemicals at work, and herbicides and pesticides at home. Use these substances only in well-ventilated areas and wear a mask. Instead of using toxic household cleansers, detergents and other such products, choose safer alternatives, such as vinegar and baking soda.

Inability to Spot Lies May Warn of Dementia

Katherine P. Rankin, PhD, a neuropsychologist and associate professor of neurology at the University of California, San Francisco, Memory and Aging Center and coauthor of a study presented at a meeting of the American Academy of Neurology.

Does someone you love seem increasingly gullible? Don't be too quick to dismiss this as a normal sign of aging. *Here's why…*

A recent study included 175 people ages 45 to 88, more than half of whom were in the early stages of some type of neurodegenerative disease that causes certain parts of the brain to deteriorate. Participants watched videos of two people talking. In addition to truthful statements, the video dialogue included sarcasm and lies, plus verbal and nonverbal clues to help participants pinpoint the false or insincere statements. Participants then answered yes/no questions about the video… and researchers compared their scores with results of MRI scans that measured the volume of different brain regions.

Results: Cognitively healthy people easily picked out the lies and sarcasm in the video, as did most participants with certain neurodegenerative diseases, including Alzheimer's. However, participants whose brain scans showed degeneration of the frontal and temporal lobes, a condition called frontotemporal dementia—which is as common as Alzheimer's disease among people under age 65—found it very difficult to distinguish factual statements from untruthful or sarcastic ones.

Bottom line: Increasing inability to recognize deception or sarcasm merits a consultation with a neurologist, especially if accompanied by other possible symptoms of frontotemporal dementia, such as severe changes in behavior and/or personality—yet often these are mistaken for signs of depression, a midlife crisis or normal aging. Early diagnosis of frontotemporal dementia may maximize treatment options and help protect patients vulnerable to being scammed due to their blind trust.

Frontotemporal Degeneration: The Dementia Doctors Mistake for a Midlife Crisis

Bradford C. Dickerson, MD, associate professor of neurology, Harvard Medical School, and director of the Frontotemporal Disorders Unit, Massachusetts General Hospital, both in Boston. Dr. Dickerson conducts research on memory disorders, including frontotemporal dementia, and treats patients with the condition.

A loved one turns 50 (or so), impulsively buys a flashy sports car that he can't afford, aggressively propositions women in restaurants, swears at his boss, then lobs insults at you when you suggest that he settle down. You might think that he's having a somewhat tardy midlife crisis…but he's not.

The real problem may be a type of dementia called frontotemporal degeneration (FTD) that leaves memory intact while causing disturbing changes in behavior, personality and/or language. FTD occurs equally in men and women. People with this progressive brain disorder often alienate friends and family, jeopardize their jobs, maybe even get into legal trouble—yet often they're completely unable to recognize that they have a problem. And even if they do see their doctors, they're likely to be misdiagnosed with depression or some other psychiatric problem, at least in the early stages.

That's why it's important to be aware of the warning signs…so patients can get the help they need and appropriate plans can be made for their future. *Here's what you should know about FTD…*

RECOGNIZING AN UNRECOGNIZED DISORDER

One reason why FTD often goes undiagnosed is that it tends to strike earlier than other forms of dementia, typically developing in a person's 50s or 60s—which people may think of as "too young" for dementia. Alzheimer's disease, in comparison, appears 10 to 13 years later, on average. Another source of confusion is the fact that FTD patients usually ace memory tests used to detect Alzheimer's—for instance, they often have no trouble keeping track of day-to-day events and staying oriented to space and time. Also, many people have never heard of FTD (also called frontotemporal dementia or Pick's disease) even though it accounts for up to 20% of all dementia cases.

The term FTD actually encompasses several related disorders, all of which are characterized by progressive damage to the frontal lobe, a brain area associated with decision-making and behavior control…and/or the temporal lobe, which is associated with emotion and language.

Though genetics plays a role in about 15% to 20% of FTD cases, the majority of cases do not appear to be inherited. Doctors aren't sure what triggers FTD, though they do know that in some cases the disorder occurs when a protein called *tau* degenerates and is no longer able to perform its main function, which is to stabilize the structure of brain cells, said

Bradford C. Dickerson, MD, an associate professor of neurology at Harvard Medical School and director of the Frontotemporal Disorders Unit at Massachusetts General Hospital. Other cases result from changes in other proteins, he added. As a result, neurons die or become shrunken and misshapen…scar tissue forms…and there is an accumulation of abnormal protein within brain cells.

As a consequence of the brain degeneration, patients experience progressive changes in behavior, language and/or motor skills. Symptoms may include any or all of the following…

•**Personality changes**—including loss of empathy…heightened aggression…and increasingly inappropriate social behavior (hypersexuality, excessive swearing, laughing at others' misfortunes, etc.).

•**Impulsivity, distractibility, poor judgment and impaired decision-making skills.**

Examples: Impulsive spending or financial risk-taking…inability to plan and prepare a meal…inattention to personal hygiene…driving like a reckless teenager.

•**Compulsive behaviors,** such as repetitive hand clapping, incessant humming or shoplifting…and intense cravings for sweets or other carbohydrates.

•**Apathy, lack of motivation, listlessness, irritability**—symptoms easily mistaken for depression.

•**Increasing problems with language,** such as difficulty naming familiar objects, expressing thoughts and comprehending words. Ultimately, some patients are rendered incapable of speaking…and some lose the ability to comprehend the speech of others.

•**Muscle rigidity, weakness and tremors, which can lead to trouble balancing and walking.** Early on, such symptoms often are misconstrued as signs of Parkinson's disease. Eventually patients become unable to perform daily activities.

Sadly, FTD is ultimately fatal, with the duration of the disease ranging from two years to more than 10 years.

It's tragic to think that, during the early stages, an undiagnosed patient might so alienate his/her family and friends—who are understandably bewildered and upset by the person's disturbing behavior—that he winds up alone during the later stages, with no loved ones to help him. That's one reason why a diagnosis is so crucial.

GETTING HELP

"In many people with FTD, the changes in the brain reduce insight and self-awareness to a degree that the patient is not able to recognize his impairments," Dr. Dickerson said. So if you suspect that a loved one has FTD, insist on accompanying him to see his doctor and request a referral to a neurologist with expertise in the disorder. No single diagnostic test exists to confirm or rule out FTD. Diagnosis is based on a detailed cognitive and neurological exam…a neuropsychological exam to assess behavior, language and decision-making functions…and neuroimaging tests such as MRI or PET scans to check for atrophy in various areas of the brain.

There is no known way to cure FTD or stop the progression of the disease, but there are treatments that can help ease some of the symptoms. *For instance…*

•**Antidepressant selective serotonin reuptake inhibitors** may be able to help control aggressive behaviors, impulsivity and carbohydrate cravings.

•**Antipsychotic or mood-stabilizing medications** may be able to help manage irrational or compulsive behaviors and ease agitation. However, these drugs can have serious side effects, including accelerating heart disease, so the benefits need to be carefully weighed against the risks, Dr. Dickerson said.

•**Speech and language therapy** can help a patient learn alternative ways to communicate (such as with gestures or by pointing to pictures), reducing frustration and improving quality of life.

•**Occupational therapy** makes it easier for a patient to perform basic activities of daily living and to avoid falls.

Counseling or psychotherapy rarely helps FTD patients, Dr. Dickerson noted—but it almost always helps their families.

FTD eventually progresses to the point that patients need 24-hour care. The sooner a patient is properly diagnosed, the sooner plans can be put in place to make his life as secure and comfortable as possible.

For additional information: Visit the website of The Association for Frontotemporal Degeneration (AFTD), TheAFTD.org. This organization can also help you find doctors with expertise in FTD…as well as programs that provide FTD caregivers with invaluable support.

Apathy May Mean Your Brain Is Changing

Older adults who show a lack of interest, energy and emotion and drop activities to stay at home have less brain volume than their active peers. That was the finding in a recent study of more than 4,000 healthy adults (average age 76) who underwent MRI brain scans.

The upshot: It's normal to lose some brain volume as you age, but the larger losses found in this study could be a sign of a brain disorder, such as dementia. If you frequently feel apathetic, discuss this with your doctor.

Lenore Launer, PhD, chief of neuroepidemiology, National Institute on Aging, Bethesda, Maryland.

Is It an Illness or Are You Just Getting Old?

John Whyte, MD, MPH, an internist and former chief medical expert and vice president, health and medical education, at the Discovery Channel. He is the author of *Is This Normal?: The Essential Guide to Middle Age and Beyond.*

With all the physical changes that occur as we grow older, it's tempting to chalk up all our infirmities to the effects of aging.

But that's a mistake. In some cases, physical changes that appear to be a normal part of aging signal the onset of a treatable condi-tion. To protect yourself—and feel as good as possible!—it's crucial to know what's normal and what's not as we grow older. *For example…*

STOOPED POSTURE

The vertebrae in the spine are separated by intervertebral discs, which act like shock absorbers. It's normal for the discs to dehydrate and flatten with age. This is why the average person loses about half an inch in height every decade after about age 40. The same changes can alter the curve of the spine and cause a slight stoop.

What isn't normal: Extreme curvature of the upper spine. In general, aging should cause no more than a 20-degree curvature of the spine. An extreme curvature is typically due to a condition known as "dowager's hump" (kyphosis), which is usually caused by osteoporosis. Weak bones in the spine eventually crumble, changing the alignment of the spine and causing a stooped posture. Osteoporosis that has advanced this far can't be reversed.

That's why prevention is critical. Perform weight-bearing exercises, preferably before the bones have weakened. Walking and even dancing promote the development of new bone and protect your posture later in life. Weight-bearing exercise also can help even after bones are weakened—just be sure not to overdo it since you don't want to cause more damage. Depending on the condition of your bones, you may need to switch to non–weight-bearing exercise, such as swimming.

Important: Make sure you're getting enough vitamin D. Depending on where you live, it's possible to get more than 90% of the vitamin D that you need just from sun exposure—the rest can come from D-fortified foods and/or supplements. Vitamin D enables the movement of calcium from the bloodstream into the bones. Ask a doctor for a blood test to check your vitamin D level. If it's low, he/she can suggest the best ways for you to get more of this crucial vitamin.

PAIN

We all notice more aches and pains as we get older, often due to back problems, arthritis or other common conditions. These aches are normal if they are occasional.

What isn't normal: Pain that's severe or chronic.

Good rule of thumb: See a doctor if you have severe pain and don't know why—or if chronic pain interferes with your ability to live a normal life.

Important: Consider your mental health as well as your physical health. Pain and depression frequently go together—they actually share some of the same biochemical pathways.

That's why drugs called tricyclic antidepressants, such as *imipramine* (Tofranil), are sometimes used to relieve chronic pain—even in patients who aren't depressed. When pain is due to a physical problem, such as arthritis, depression also is common.

Get help right away, either from a doctor or a mental health professional (or both). Otherwise, you could be setting yourself up for a difficult cycle—ongoing pain increases depression, and the more depressed you are, the more pain you'll experience.

Helpful: I strongly advise pain patients to do some kind of exercise, even if it's just gentle stretches. Exercise increases endorphins, the body's natural painkillers.

LESS SLEEP

After about age 50, most people tend to sleep less soundly, and they may sleep fewer total hours than younger people. The reasons for these differences in sleep habits are varied but may include more pain, medication use and nighttime urination in older adults.

What isn't normal: Taking more than 10 to 15 minutes to fall asleep. See your doctor if you have trouble falling asleep more than, say, two nights a week. This delay in sleep onset might be due to stress. Or you could be having side effects from medications. Offenders include decongestants, beta-blockers and some asthma drugs. Don't ignore sleep problems—over time, they can increase one's risk for heart disease, diabetes and other serious conditions.

SLEEPWALKING

We still don't know why people sleepwalk, but it's been shown that sleepwalkers can engage in surprisingly complex activities, such as going to the refrigerator, then preparing—and consuming—a complete meal.

Sleepwalking is more common in children but also occurs in older adults. It's usually not cause for concern unless you are putting yourself in dangerous situations, such as leaving the house or walking outside onto an unprotected balcony.

What isn't normal: A condition known as sun-downing, which can mimic sleepwalking. With sun-downing, older adults sometimes are awake late at night and wander around the house. They're partly conscious but confused and often combative. You can distinguish sun-downing from sleepwalking by the person's degree of engagement. Sun-downers can interact with other people—sleepwalkers usually don't.

If you suspect that you or a loved one may be suffering from sun-downing, see a doctor. It could be a sign of early-stage dementia. Sun-downing can also be a side effect (or wearing off) of medications, such as antidepressants, sleeping pills or antipsychotic drugs. In addition, it can be caused by narcotic painkillers, such as *meperidine* (Demerol). Once a physician changes the person's medications—or adjusts the dosages—the nighttime wandering may stop.

What a Good Physical Tells About Your Brain

Richard Carmona, MD, FACS, MPH, president of the Tucson, Arizona–based Canyon Ranch Institute and vice chairman of Canyon Ranch, a health resort, spa and wellness retreat. He served as US Surgeon General from 2002 to 2006 and is author of *Canyon Ranch 30 Days to a Better Brain*.

Put yourself on a weight-loss diet, and you can measure your success with a bathroom scale. If fitness is your goal, you can track your improvement by charting how fast you can run or walk a mile.

But how can you tell if your brain is as fit as the rest of you?

If you're having memory problems, that's an obvious red flag. But even if you're basically healthy (or are being treated for a chronic condition such as high blood pressure), a routine medical exam can tell a lot about your brain health—if you know what the seemingly basic tests may mean, according to former US Surgeon General Richard Carmona, MD. *What a physical checkup reveals about your brain— and the additional tests you may need…*

LAY IT ALL OUT

Doctors aren't mind readers—they don't know what you're worried about unless you tell them. At your physical, tell your doctor about any changes in your health (even if you think they sound trivial).

Where most people get tripped up: There's always that routine question about medications you're taking. Don't assume that your doctor knows everything he/she has prescribed—include every medication and supplement you're taking.

Many common prescription or over-the-counter drugs—alone or in combination—can affect your brain. The following types of drugs are among the most commonly associated with dizziness, fuzzy thinking and/or memory problems. *All drugs within each class can addle a person's brain—not only the specific drug examples given…*

•**Allergy medications,** including antihistamines (such as Benadryl and Claritin).

•**Antianxiety medications** (such as Valium and Xanax).

•**Antibiotics** (such as Cipro and Levaquin).

•**Antidepressants** (such as Prozac and Lexapro).

•**Blood pressure medications** (such as Zestril and Procardia).

•**Sleep aids** (such as Ambien).

If you are taking one of these types of medications and are experiencing cognitive problems, ask your physician about switching to a different drug.

Fortunately, the fuzzy thinking and/or problems with memory usually go away when the drug is discontinued. And because everyone responds differently to individual medications, you may be able to safely take a different drug that's within the same class.

CLUES FROM YOUR PHYSICAL

Even if you're not having cognitive problems, your physical can give you a measure of key markers of brain health. For example, most people know that high blood pressure is linked to increased risk for certain types of dementia (normal blood pressure is 120/80 or below). But low blood pressure (lower than 90/60) may make you dizzy, fatigued and unable to think clearly. *Other important brain-health markers…*

•**Eyes.** When your doctor shines that bright light in your eyes, he is looking at the retina, the light-sensitive tissue at the back of the eye that is connected directly to the optic nerve leading to the brain. Blood vessels in the retina reflect vascular health in the whole body—including the brain.

•**Hearing, balance and coordination.** While many diseases can cause problems with hearing, balance or coordination, one possibility is dysfunction of the eighth cranial nerve, which connects directly to the brain. Ears have fluid-filled canals that relay information to the brain via the eighth cranial nerve and act as a kind of gyroscope, giving us our sense of orientation in space. When we change position, the fluid moves, and the brain adjusts our balance and coordination. With some inner-ear disorders, such as Ménière's disease or labyrinthitis, people are dizzy, lose hearing or fall frequently due to loss of balance and coordination.

•**Reflexes.** A tap on your knee with a tiny hammer sends an electrical impulse to the spinal cord, which then sends a signal back to the foot, triggering a kick. A weak or delayed response could indicate a problem with the nervous system or brain.

•**Sensation.** All of the senses are housed in the brain, including the sense of touch. Any change in sensation—tingling hands or feet…

weak hands…and/or numbness anywhere in the body—could signal a problem in the brain.

DIGGING DEEPER

If your memory is failing or you're having other cognitive problems, such as difficulty making decisions or planning activities, your doctor may want to run tests for…

• **Inflammation.** A blood test for C-reactive protein (CRP) measures general levels of inflammation in the body. High levels of CRP (above 3.0 mg/L) could be due to a simple infection…cardiovascular disease that may also be putting your brain at risk…or an autoimmune disease, such as lupus or multiple sclerosis, which can cause problems with memory and thinking as well as physical symptoms.

• **Vitamin deficiencies.** A vitamin B-12 deficiency can lead to memory loss, fatigue and light-headedness. Other common nutrient deficiencies that can affect thinking include vitamin D and omega-3 fatty acids—there are tests for both.

• **Diabetes and glucose tolerance.** Left untreated, diabetes can dramatically increase one's risk for dementia. If your doctor suspects you have diabetes (or it runs in your family), get your blood glucose level tested (following an overnight fast).

Useful: An HbA1C test, which gives a broader picture of your glucose level over the previous six to 12 weeks. While most people, especially after age 45, should get glucose testing at least every three years, it's particularly important for those having cognitive symptoms.

• **Tick-borne illness.** Lyme disease and Rocky Mountain spotted fever can cause mental fuzziness.

Also helpful: Liver function tests, including new genomic tests, also may be ordered to assess your liver's ability to remove toxins. If the body doesn't clear toxins, this can alter brain metabolism, possibly leading to cognitive decline.

Memory Trouble? A Neurological Exam Has the Answers

Majid Fotuhi, MD, PhD, neurologist, medical director of the NeuroGrow Brain Fitness Center in McLean, Virginia, and affiliate staff at Johns Hopkins Medicine, Baltimore. He is also author of *The Memory Cure* and co-author of *The New York Times Crosswords to Keep Your Brain Young.*

If you or members of your family are concerned about your memory, a thorough neurological exam can determine with 90% to 95% accuracy whether you have normal age-related memory loss or some form of dementia.

Good news: People who are alert enough to worry about their memories are less likely to have significant problems. Declines in memory or cognition that are apparent to others—but not to the patient—are usually more serious.

Key parts of a neurological exam…

YOUR MEDICAL HISTORY

Neurologists who specialize in memory loss usually can identify underlying problems from a person's medical history alone.*

Important: A friend or family member should accompany the patient to a neurological exam to help provide information regarding the patient's memory and/or lifestyle.

Questions typically asked…

• **Does the memory loss occur often?** People who repeat themselves frequently or repeatedly ask the same question during conversations are more likely to have a significant memory impairment than those who forget only occasionally.

• **Are there recent triggers?** A patient who recently had surgery might be taking a prescription painkiller or sedative that impairs memory. A head injury—even one that occurred years ago—also can result in memory loss, particularly if the patient also has high

*Ask your doctor to refer you, if possible, to a neurologist affiliated with an academic medical center. He/she will be more likely to be up-to-date on the latest research.

blood pressure, diabetes or other health problems. These factors—in combination with an old head injury—can have additive effects on the brain that can result in dementia.

• **Is the patient depressed?** Depression can cause trouble with attention and focus, both of which can lead to memory problems.

• **Is the problem progressing?** Memory loss that keeps getting worse or occurs with confusion—such as getting lost in a familiar area—usually indicates an underlying problem, such as dementia.

MENTAL STATE EXAM

The Mini-Mental State Exam (MMSE), which is commonly used to assess memory, evaluates…

• **Recent versus long-term memory.** The doctor may name three common objects, such as an apricot, a flag and a tree, and ask the patient to repeat the objects three minutes later.

What the results may mean: In the early stages of Alzheimer's, a patient might not remember the three objects that were named just minutes earlier, but is probably able to recall details, such as a favorite childhood song or beloved pet, from the distant past.

• **Orientation.** The patient will be asked to state his/her name, the year, season, day of the week and the date. Such questions test a patient's general awareness.

What the results may mean: Orientation can be impaired by medication side effects or substance abuse as well as different types of dementia, such as Alzheimer's. A patient is more likely to have dementia if he can't remember major details such as the name of the city where he lives.

• **Attention span.** The patient will be asked to count backward (by sevens) from, say, 100…or to spell a short word, such as "holiday" or "pitcher," backward.

What the results may mean: These tests measure alertness and mental focus. A poor score indicates that a patient might have delirium (a usually temporary decline in mental function due to an acute problem, such as a urinary tract infection) rather than, or in addition to, dementia.

Example: I recently saw in my practice a 102-year-old patient who didn't know where she was. I ordered a urine test, and it turned out that she had a urinary tract infection. I gave her antibiotics, and two days later she was back to normal.

PHYSICAL EXAM

The neurologist also will perform a physical examination that tests, among other things, reflexes and muscle movements to determine whether the patient has had a stroke or has thyroid problems, heart problems, Parkinson's disease or other conditions that can contribute to dementia.

DIAGNOSTIC TESTS

Depending on the results of the medical history and clinical exam, other tests, including the following, may be performed…

• **Imaging tests.** A magnetic resonance imaging (MRI) scan can show evidence of a stroke, bleeding in the brain, a brain tumor or brain shrinkage.

• **Blood tests.** Low levels of thyroid hormone and vitamin B-12 (both are detected by blood tests) may contribute to dementia.

Next Steps If You Suspect Early-Onset Alzheimer's Disease

Susan M. Maixner, MD, associate professor of psychiatry, director of the Geropsychiatry Program, director of the geriatric psychiatry clinic at the University of Michigan Health System, and psychiatric consultant at Arbor Hospice, Ann Arbor.

If you haven't seen the acclaimed movie *Still Alice*, starring Julianne Moore, who won an Academy Award for her performance, all we can say, without being "spoilers," is that the movie provides powerful food for thought for anyone concerned that dementia is setting in—and happening way too soon. The movie is about a linguistics professor and mother of three who is diagnosed with Alzheimer's disease at the tender age of 50.

For those of you who are middle-aged and feeling more distracted and forgetful—or more easily agitated than you once were—the movie will shake you up. It's not always easy to tell whether these symptoms are simply due to stress and multitasking or the beginnings of true cognitive decline. So how can you tell?

SUSPICIOUS SIGNS

The key symptom to look out for is trouble managing "bills and pills," said Susan Maixner, MD, an associate professor of psychiatry and director of the Geropsychiatry Clinic at the University of Michigan Health System. If you are younger than 65 and bill-paying becomes increasingly difficult to keep track of and if you find yourself forgetting to take medications or doubling up on doses (a danger in and of itself), you may be in the danger zone for early-onset Alzheimer's disease. For those still working, being unable to retain information for work, such as frequently used computer passwords, may be a very early sign of cognitive difficulties, said Dr. Maixner.

A decline in short-term memory, such as too often forgetting whether or not you paid that bill or took that med, usually comes first when early-onset Alzheimer's sets in, said Dr. Maixner. Other telltale signs are the same as those for Alzheimer's in older age groups—getting lost while driving, repeating yourself, inability to plan or to solve problems, confusion with time or place, the inability to comprehend visual images (for example, not recognizing acquaintances), difficulty writing or speaking, often misplacing things, failing judgment, social withdrawal and change in mood or personality, such as feeling more short-tempered or frustrated.

GETTING DIAGNOSED

The first step to getting a diagnosis is scheduling a thorough medical exam that your family doctor can perform, said Dr. Maixner. "Make sure that you tell your primary care doctor, up front, that you are scheduling the physical exam because you are experiencing memory problems and are concerned about early-onset Alzheimer's," said Dr. Maixner. The exam will be tailored to rule out physical as well as psychological ailments that may be causing the cognitive decline. And, because approximately 20% of early-onset Alzheimer's disease is inherited (genetic), tell your family doctor if you have a family history of dementia. Many primary care physicians won't think to ask this question—so be sure to bring it up, said Dr. Maixner.

Make sure blood work is done to rule out thyroid problems or vitamin deficiencies that can cause memory issues, advised Dr. Maixner. Medications and the use of drugs and alcohol also should be considered. The primary care doctor should then perform in-office cognitive tests, such as the Mini-Mental State Exam or Montreal Cognitive Assessment, which evaluate mental sharpness and short- and long-term memory. If the test results reveal signs of cognitive decline, your doctor should refer you to a geriatric psychiatrist or a neurologist with expertise in managing cognitive disorders such as dementia. The specialist may order an MRI or a CT scan of the brain to rule out whether a stroke, brain injury lesion or tumor may be causing the symptoms. A geriatric psychiatrist also has special training in differentiating dementia from depression, anxiety and other conditions that can accompany memory problems, said Dr. Maixner.

COPING WITH EARLY-ONSET ALZHEIMER'S

So far, there is no cure for Alzheimer's disease. Although progressive worsening of the disease is inevitable, the clock can be turned back on symptoms with lifestyle interventions and medications. It is crucial to keep up physical activity, social interactions and mental stimulation, according to Dr. Maixner. Also, routines, predictability and structure are essential coping tools that will help you or a loved one with early-onset Alzheimer's function better.

Planning about who will manage financial affairs and health decisions is important because if it is Alzheimer's, a time will come when you or your loved one will no longer be able to make those decisions, said Dr. Maixner. Support groups and a 24/7 information hotline that can help with finding a dementia specialist, coping, staying active and legal issues are available through the Alzheimer's Association.

Forgetting a Famous Face Could Mean Dementia

Rec *ecent research*: Nearly 60 adults ages 40 to 65 (half of whom had a form of early-onset dementia) were asked to identify pictures of 20 famous people, including John F. Kennedy, Bill Gates and Elvis Presley.

Result: Only 46% of those with dementia could name all the faces (although nearly 80% recognized them). In participants with normal brain function, more than 90% could name the faces.

Explanation: Naming and recognition abilities decline with loss of brain tissue.

If you're having trouble identifying people you once knew: See a neurologist for an evaluation.

Emily J. Rogalski, PhD, research assistant professor, Northwestern University Feinberg School of Medicine, Chicago.

Worried That a Loved One Might Have Dementia? How to Tell

John C. Morris, MD, director, Charles F. and Joanne Knight Alzheimer's Disease Research Center, Washington University School of Medicine, St. Louis.

I t's an increasingly common problem—someone you care about seems to be showing signs of cognitive slippage, but you're not sure whether it's serious enough to merit testing or not. Should you schedule an appointment to see what the doctor thinks?

Not so fast. It turns out that the best person to judge whether or not there's a real reason to worry may not be a medical professional but a family member or close friend, a recent study shows. If this doesn't seem particularly surprising to you (after all, who better to evaluate changes in cognitive function than those who know a person best?), you may still find the study results startling—because a standard screening test used by health professionals to detect dementia was so much less effective in recognizing serious situations than the observations of family and friends.

Researchers at the Washington University School of Medicine in St. Louis wanted to see which of two tools to identify early-stage dementia worked better. One, called the Ascertain Dementia 8 (AD8) questionnaire, consists of an eight-question survey that is completed by a family member (usually the spouse or an adult child) or a friend of the person whose cognitive function is in question. The other is the commonly used Mini Mental State Exam (MMSE), a more detailed dementia screening test that is administered to the patient by a health-care professional. Researchers compared the results when both tests were used to evaluate 257 individuals (average age 75.4 years), some of whom were cognitively normal while others had mild Alzheimer's symptoms. Then they examined these people using imaging and spinal fluid tests that identify Alzheimer's changes in the brain, such as amyloid plaque. Although there were some "false positive" results, the AD8 questionnaire (the one done without using a doctor) picked up all but five of 101 individuals with dementia… while the MMSE test missed 74 of these mildly affected individuals!

Moreover, the AD8 is free, noninvasive and easy to complete in just a few minutes.

John C. Morris, MD, director of The Charles F. and Joanne Knight Alzheimer's Disease Research Center at Washington University School of Medicine, who was involved in the research, said that the AD8 questionnaire itself is not a diagnostic instrument but a reliably sensitive screening tool to determine the need to seek definitive diagnostic evaluation for Alzheimer's. "Instead of just saying, 'Dad's not really remembering to pay the bills like he used to,' this questionnaire can give you a way to structure your concerns and then present them to your physician," he said.

HERE'S THE TEST

To administer the questionnaire, answer the following yes-or-no questions regarding the loved one you're concerned about. Two or more "yes" answers may mean that further diagnostic testing is in order.

Over the last several years, have you noticed a change in cognitive abilities for your loved one in regard to...

•**Having problems with judgment** (e.g., problems making decisions, bad financial decisions, problems with thinking).

•**Showing less interest in hobbies/activities.**

•**Repeating the same things over and over** (questions, stories or statements).

•**Having trouble learning how to use a tool, appliance or gadget** (e.g., computer, microwave, remote control).

•**Forgetting the correct month or year.**

•**Having trouble handling financial affairs** (e.g., balancing a checkbook, income taxes, paying bills).

•**Having trouble remembering appointments.**

•**Having daily problems with thinking and/or memory.**

If you answered yes to two or more questions, don't panic—Dr. Morris stresses that the AD8 isn't a diagnostic tool, but one that is meant to determine whether more testing should be done. To families facing uncertainty about what to do about a loved one who seems to be declining, this looks like a safe, wise and supportive first step to take.

Surprising Early Symptoms of Alzheimer's

Patricia A. Boyle, PhD, associate professor, department of psychology, Rush University Medical Center, Chicago.

For obvious reasons, testing for Alzheimer's disease focuses on cognitive symptoms. But the disease does more damage than that—it often causes impaired motor functions, such as changed gait and weakened grip strength. Recently, researchers at Rush University Medical Center in Chicago studied 970 adults, average age 80.3, who had no signs of dementia. Participants were tested annually for cognitive and neurological function and for muscle strength in 11 different muscle groups. Three and a half years later (on average), 138 participants had developed Alzheimer's—and, most intriguingly, it turned out that participants who had been the strongest when the study started (the ones in the top 10%) were 61% less likely to have developed the disease than those who had been the weakest (bottom 10%).

ANOTHER EARLY SIGN?

Study author Patricia A. Boyle, PhD, explained that the value of the study is that it gives doctors another clue for early identification of Alzheimer's. But she said that there's no evidence that having weak muscles can cause the disease, or that you can prevent it by working out. Dr. Boyle explains that the study controlled for current physical activity, body mass index (which she calls "a valuable indicator of health across lifespan"), vascular function and genetic markers associated with Alzheimer's—and the link with weaker muscle strength held in spite of these.

Dr. Boyle said that the probable explanation is that in people with early Alzheimer's several pathological processes are taking place in the brain that reduce cognition and muscle strength. These could include vascular issues or inflammation or they might even be very early symptoms of the disease itself. Another theory concerns aging of the mitochondria (the energy producing parts of cells), which a few animal studies have suggested can cause impaired cognition, muscle strength and motor function.

While the specific connection remains unknown, Dr. Boyle said that we do know that "what's good for the body is good for the brain." Staying physically strong is always a good idea.

Alzheimer's Imaging Drugs Improve Detection

Norman Foster, MD, professor of neurology and director of Center for Alzheimer's Care, Imaging and Research at the University of Utah.

Know thy enemy! The Food and Drug Administration recently approved three diagnostic drugs (*florbetapir* [Amyvid], *flutemetamol* [Vizamyl] and *florbetaben* [Neuraceq]) that may make it possible for people to find out their risk for Alzheimer's disease (AD). These drugs are used with positron emission tomography (PET) imaging of the brain to detect amyloid plaque density in adults with cognitive impairment. Besides being a powerful tool for managing risk, this test helps to reduce diagnostic errors when symptoms such as memory loss or confusion in a particular patient are mistakenly attributed to Alzheimer's—a sad situation that happens 20% of the time or more, by some estimates.

Even though there is no effective cure for Alzheimer's (and few promising ones on the horizon), this diagnostic test is a great advance, says Norman L. Foster, MD, professor of neurology and director of the Center for Alzheimer's Care, Imaging and Research (CACIR) at the University of Utah. Apart from the PET imaging, the only way to know, absolutely and for sure, that a person has Alzheimer's is to wait until he/she dies and examine the brain via autopsy—which clearly is not helpful. *Dr. Foster spoke about what this new test will mean for diagnosis and treatment of patients with Alzheimer's disease…*

NEARLY 100% RELIABLE

Dr. Foster explained that a radioactive contrast dye (or "imaging tracer") is injected into people suspected of having AD. The dye travels to the brain. Doctors can then use a PET scanner to detect whether there are any amyloid plaques in the brain—along with other symptoms, the presence of these plaques can confirm that a person has AD. This test is considered quite safe, because the dye is similar to other agents already widely in use.

Confirmation that it works: Recent studies on living AD patients have demonstrated a near perfect (96%) correspondence between what the scans showed and what subsequent autopsies of those patients revealed, Dr. Foster notes.

WHAT THE TEST CAN'T TELL YOU

It's important to keep in mind, however, that while amyloid PET scanning reliably detects plaques in the brain, it does not on its own provide a definitive diagnosis—doctors still must use their clinical judgment to interpret the results in the context of a person's medical history and symptoms. It is possible to have plaques but not have the typical problems associated with AD, Dr. Foster explained. Indeed, 30% of people who have amyloid plaques do not experience memory problems. But, importantly, without amyloid plaques a person does not have AD.

What the test can tell you is the probability of Alzheimer's…

• **A low level of amyloid plaques in the brain indicates a low risk for AD.**

• **A high level suggests that a person has or is likely to develop the disease.**

If there are symptoms (such as memory loss or dementia) and there are no amyloid plaques in the brain, Alzheimer's can be ruled out—so doctors know to look for other causes of the symptoms (e.g., minor strokes, medication side effects or malnutrition).

THIS TEST CAN BE USED FOR SCREENING

Dr. Foster compares detecting amyloid plaques in your brain with detecting atherosclerosis in your coronary arteries. If you have plaque buildup and hardening in your coronary arteries, you are at a higher risk for heart attack and/or stroke—but that does not necessarily mean you will have one. Likewise, amyloid plaques in your brain predict a higher risk for problems due to AD—but you will not necessarily develop it. This leads Dr. Foster to predict that it may become commonplace within the next decade to use amyloid PET scanning to screen for AD in people who are exhibiting symptoms. He said that research is currently evaluating how accurate a predictor of the disease it truly is.

Dr. Foster believes that the scans are particularly useful when there are doubts about diagnosis. Even if the diagnosis is AD, knowing can help you plan for what lies ahead. There are medications that improve Alzheimer's symptoms, as well as drugs to avoid if you have the disease. And it is never too late to improve your quality of life—even as the disease progresses—by taking active steps to stay mentally engaged… physically active… and socially connected. You also can look into community health and support services to help you cope with further challenges down the road.

Grappling with the uncertainty of AD can be a harrowing experience. Dr. Foster sees the amyloid PET scan as a major step forward in helping families plan for the future and avoid unnecessary delays in getting treatment.

Important Alzheimer's Scan

People at high risk for Alzheimer's should have a scan to detect leakage in the barrier between blood vessels and the brain. This barrier can become leaky with age, beginning in the hippocampus—an important learning and memory center. Identifying the leaks before Alzheimer's develops would allow treatment to start earlier and possibly slow development of the disease. Brain scans could be useful for people with symptoms of mild dementia on neuropsychological tests and people with genetic risks for Alzheimer's.

Berislav V. Zlokovic, MD, PhD, professor and chair, department of physiology and biophysics, Keck School of Medicine, University of Southern California, Los Angeles, and leader of a study published in *Neuron*.

An MRI May Reveal Alzheimer's Risk

By using arterial spin labeling (ASL), which can be done by all modern MRI scanning machines, it may be possible to detect very subtle blood flow changes in parts of the brain linked to memory. Early detection could make it possible to start medicines to slow decline.

Sven Haller, MD, a senior physician in clinical neuroradiology at Geneva University Hospital, Switzerland, and leader of a study published online in *Radiology*.

CHAPTER 3

Alzheimer's Imposters

Memory Robbers That Are Often Overlooked

Alzheimer's disease is such a dreaded diagnosis that you may be filled with panic if you experience occasional memory loss. But these worries may be unnecessary.

As people age, the brain undergoes changes that may lead to some decline in short-term memory. This is normal.

Of course memory loss that truly concerns you is another matter. *Ask your primary care physician to refer you to a neurologist or geriatrician for an evaluation if...*

• **You have noticed a significant change in your everyday memory over the past six months.**

• **Friends or family members have expressed concern about your memory.**

• **You have begun forgetting recent conversations.**

In the meantime, consider whether your occasional forgetfulness may be due to one of the following causes, all of which can be easily corrected...

NOT ENOUGH SLEEP

Poor sleep is probably the most common cause of occasional memory lapses. The ability to concentrate suffers with insufficient rest. Sleep also appears to be essential for consolidating memory—whatever information you learn during the day, whether it's the name of a colleague or the street where a new restaurant opened, you need sleep to make it stick in your mind.

Self-defense: If you're not sleeping seven to eight hours nightly, make it a priority to get more sleep. If you are unable to improve your sleep on your own, talk to your doctor.

Cynthia R. Green, PhD, assistant clinical professor of psychiatry at Mount Sinai School of Medicine in New York City and president of Memory Arts, LLC. Memory Arts.com. She is author of *Total Memory Workout.*

WIDELY USED DRUGS

Impaired memory is a potential side effect of many medications. Obvious suspects include prescription sleeping pills…opiate pain-killers, such as *meperidine* (Demerol)…and antianxiety drugs, such as *diazepam* (Valium) and *alprazolam* (Xanax).

Certain blood pressure–lowering medications, such as beta-blockers, and antidepressants also cause memory problems in some people. Even over-the-counter antihistamines, such as *diphenhydramine* (Benadryl), can have this effect.

If you're taking multiple medications, more than one may cause impaired memory, making it even more difficult to identify the culprit.

Timing is often a tip-off: When impaired memory is an adverse drug effect, it's most likely to appear when you start taking a new medication or increase the dose. But not always.

As we grow older, our bodies become less efficient at clearing medications from the body, so the same dose you've been taking safely for years may cause problems you never had before.

Self-defense: If you think medication might be affecting your memory, do not stop taking the drug or reduce the dosage on your own. Talk to your doctor or pharmacist for advice.

EMOTIONAL UPSET

When you're anxious, stressed or depressed, your ability to concentrate suffers. Whatever it is that worries or preoccupies you keeps your mind from focusing on facts, names, faces and places, so they aren't absorbed into memory.

Self-defense: To keep everyday tensions from undercutting your memory, practice some form of relaxation or stress reduction. Yoga, meditation, deep breathing—or something as simple as allowing yourself a soothing time-out to walk or chat with a friend—can relieve accumulated stress and bolster your recall.

True depression is something else: Even mild-to-moderate depression can sap your energy, take pleasure out of life and affect your memory. If you suspect that you may be depressed, be alert for other symptoms—such as difficulty sleeping, sadness, apathy and a negative outlook—and see your doctor or a mental-health professional.

TOO MUCH ALCOHOL

Moderate red wine consumption has been shown to promote the health of your heart and arteries. Because of this cardiovascular health benefit, red wine also may reduce risk for dementia.

Excessive drinking, on the other hand, is harmful to the brain. Among its devastating toxic effects is a severe and often irreversible form of memory loss called Korsakoff's syndrome, a condition that occurs in alcoholics.

Alcohol's effect on memory can be subtle. Some people find that even a glass or two of wine daily is enough to interfere with learning facts and recalling information. Pay attention to how mentally sharp you feel after having a drink. If you think your alcohol intake may be causing forgetfulness, cut back. Remember, tolerance for alcohol generally declines with age, giving the same drink more impact.

Self-defense: There is more scientific evidence supporting red wine's brain-protective effect than for any other form of alcohol. If you are a man, do not exceed two glasses of red wine daily, and if you are a woman, limit yourself to one glass daily.

ILLNESS

A simple cold or headache is enough to interfere with your concentration and recall.

Illnesses that commonly go undiagnosed also may play a role. For example, when the thyroid gland (which regulates metabolism) is underactive, the mind slows down along with the body. (Other signs of an underactive thyroid include weight gain, constipation, thin or brittle hair and depression.) An overactive thyroid can affect your memory by making you anxious, "wired" and easily distracted.

Memory impairment also may be a symptom of other disorders, such as Parkinson's disease, multiple sclerosis or Lyme disease.

NUTRITIONAL DEFICIENCY

An easily overlooked memory robber is a vitamin B-12 deficiency, often marked by general fatigue and slowed thinking. Older people are especially at risk—as we age, our ability to absorb vitamin B-12 from foods diminishes.

Self-defense: If you have occasional memory lapses, ask your doctor for a blood test to check your vitamin B-12 level.

SAFEGUARDING YOUR MEMORY

Even if you've identified a relatively harmless cause for occasional forgetfulness, it's still wise to take steps to guard against cognitive decline in the future. *My advice…*

•**Get enough exercise.** Exercise helps prevent a wide range of serious health problems, including heart disease, diabetes and some types of cancer. The evidence also is strong that exercise protects against dementia—and enhances everyday memory performance by improving overall circulation and lowering risk for disorders that can affect memory, such as high blood pressure and obesity.

Self-defense: A leisurely stroll around the block may be relaxing, but you must get 30 minutes of moderate exertion (such as brisk walking or swimming), three to four days a week, to keep your memory intact.

•**Stay on top of chronic health problems.** Studies have shown repeatedly that people with high blood pressure, atherosclerosis (fatty buildup in the arteries), obesity and/or diabetes are at dramatically increased risk of developing dementia in their later years.

The effect of these chronic medical conditions on day-to-day memory is less clear. Research shows that memory declines when blood sugar rises in people with diabetes and improves when they take dietary steps to stabilize it.

Self-defense: If you have a chronic health problem, work with your doctor to keep your symptoms under control.

•**Give your brain a timed workout.** A growing body of research shows that mental exercise helps fend off everyday age-related cognitive changes that contribute to occasional forgetfulness.

Self-defense: Crossword puzzles and the number game Sudoku have gotten a lot of attention as "brain" workouts, but I prefer timed games, such as the word game Boggle or the card game Set (both available online or at dis-

count stores). Racing against the clock gives your mental muscles a real workout by challenging such intellectual skills as attention, speed and multitasking.

It Might Not Be Alzheimer's

Jacob Teitelbaum, MD, board-certified internist and founder of Practitioners Alliance Network. He is the primary investigator on a nationwide study using MIND to treat Alzheimer's and dementia and creator of the popular Cures A-Z app. Based in Kona, Hawaii, he is author, with Bill Gottlieb, of *Real Cause, Real Cure.*

If a doctor says that you or a loved one has Alzheimer's disease, take a deep breath and get a second opinion. Studies have shown that between 30% and 50% of people diagnosed with Alzheimer's turn out not to have it.

Bottom line: The symptoms common to Alzheimer's can be caused by other reversible conditions. Problems with memory and other cognitive functions often are linked to what I call MIND—metabolism, infection or inflammation, nutrition or drug side effects— or a combination of these factors. Addressing these can markedly improve cognitive function. Even people who do have Alzheimer's will see improvements.

METABOLISM

Anyone who is experiencing confusion, memory loss or other cognitive problems should have tests that look at the hormones that affect metabolism. *In particular…*

•**Thyroid hormone.** A low level of thyroid hormone often causes confusion and memory loss. It also increases the risk for Alzheimer's disease. In recent studies, thyroid levels on the low side in the normal range are associated with a 240% higher risk for dementia in women. Borderline low thyroid hormone is associated with as much as an 800% higher risk in men.

My advice: For most people with unexplained chronic confusion and memory loss, I recommend a three-month trial of desiccated thyroid (30 mg to 60 mg) to see if it helps. It is a thyroid extract containing the two key thyroid hormones. (The commonly prescribed medication Synthroid has just one of the two.) If you have risk factors for heart disease—such as high LDL cholesterol and high blood pressure—your doctor should start you with a low dose and increase it gradually.

• **Testosterone.** This hormone normally declines by about 1% a year after the age of 30. But in one study, men who went on to develop Alzheimer's disease had about half as much testosterone in their bloodstreams as men who did not.

Every 50% increase in testosterone is associated with a 26% decrease in the risk for Alzheimer's.

My advice: Men should ask their doctors about using a testosterone cream if their testosterone tests low—or even if it's at the lower quarter of the normal range. Limit the dose to 25 mg to 50 mg/day. More than that has been linked to heart attack and stroke.

INFECTIONS & INFLAMMATION

You naturally will get large amounts of protective anti-inflammatory chemical compounds just by eating a healthy diet and using supplements such as fish oil and curcumin (see next column). For extra protection, take aspirin. In addition to reducing inflammation, it's among the best ways to prevent blood clots and vascular dementia, which is as common as Alzheimer's disease. In addition, infections leave us feeling mentally foggy. Have your doctor look for and treat any bladder and sinus infections.

My advice: Talk to your doctor about taking one enteric-coated low-dose (81-mg) aspirin daily to improve circulation and reduce the risk for ministrokes in the brain. Even people with Alzheimer's may have had a series of ministrokes, adding to their cognitive decline. This is especially important when mental worsening occurs in small distinct steps instead of gradually.

NUTRITION

The typical American diet is just as bad for your brain and memory as it is for your heart. Too much fat, sugar and processed food increase cell-damaging inflammation throughout the body, including in the brain.

In one study, Columbia University researchers studied more than 2,100 people over the age of 65 who consumed healthy foods such as nuts, fruits, fish, chicken and leafy, dark green vegetables and who limited their consumption of meat and dairy. They were 48% less likely to be diagnosed with Alzheimer's over a four-year period. *Especially important…*

• **B-12.** Millions of older adults don't get or absorb enough vitamin B-12, a nutrient that is critical for memory and other brain functions. You might be deficient even if you eat a healthful diet due to the age-related decline in stomach acid and intrinsic factor, a protein needed for B-12 absorption.

My advice: Take a multivitamin that contains 500 micrograms (mcg) of B-12 and at least 400 mcg of folic acid and 50 mg of the other B vitamins. If you test low-normal for B-12 (less than 400 ng/ml), also ask your doctor about getting a series of 10 B-12 shots.

Helpful: Have one teaspoon of apple cider vinegar with every meal. Use it in salad dressing, or mix it into eight ounces of vegetable juice or water. It will increase B-12 absorption.

Caution: Vinegar is highly caustic if you drink it straight.

• **Fish oil.** The American Heart Association advises everyone to eat fish at least twice a week. That's enough for the heart, but it won't provide all of the omega-3 fatty acids that you need for optimal brain health. Fish-oil supplements can ensure that you get enough.

My advice: I recommend three to four servings a week of fatty fish, such as salmon, tuna, herring or sardines. Or take 1,000 mg of fish oil daily. You will need more if you're already having memory/cognitive problems. Ask your doctor how much to take.

• **Curcumin.** Alzheimer's is 70% less common in India than in the US, possibly because of the large amounts of turmeric that are used in curries and other Indian dishes.

Curcumin, which gives turmeric its yellow color, reduces inflammation and improves blood flow to the brain. Animal studies show that it dissolves the amyloid plaques that are found in the brains of Alzheimer's patients.

My advice: Unless you live in India, you're not likely to get enough curcumin in your diet to help, because it is poorly absorbed. Use a special highly absorbed form of curcumin (such as BCM-95 found in CuraMed 750 mg), and take one to two capsules twice a day.

Caution: Taking curcumin with blood thinners can increase the risk for bleeding.

When It's More Than a "Senior Moment"— The Mild Memory Disorder You Can Fight

Scott Roberts, PhD, associate professor in the department of health behavior and health education at University of Michigan School of Public Health, in Ann Arbor. He is co-principal investigator of the REVEAL Study, an NIH-funded clinical trial of a genetic risk-assessment program for people with mild cognitive impairment.

We all know the embarrassment of losing our train of thought in the middle of a sentence or forgetting the name of a friend. For most of us, these so-called "senior moments" are just a normal part of getting older—and you don't even have to be a senior to experience them.

But what if you're more forgetful than most of your friends? What if you're forgetting important things that you shouldn't forget, such as making a mortgage payment or the best route to get home? What if you're forgetting appointments or whether your favorite team won a recent game?

These could be signs of mild cognitive impairment (MCI), a subtle memory disorder that is more pronounced than normal memory lapses but not serious enough to significantly interfere with daily life. *If you have it, you can take steps that might keep it from progressing…*

A NEW DIAGNOSIS

MCI was first described by researchers at the Mayo Clinic in 1999. Only in the last few years has it become an official diagnosis that is recognized by physicians and insurance companies. The disorder is characterized by memory lapses serious or frequent enough that other people notice but that are not accompanied by problems with basic thinking or reasoning skills. The affected individual typically is able to carry out his/her usual activities. Because it's a new diagnosis, there's a lot that doctors still don't know, including how many Americans have it…how it will progress over time…and what can be done to treat it.

The risk: Preliminary research suggests that about 40% to 50% of people diagnosed with MCI will go on to develop Alzheimer's disease within three to four years. It's possible that many cases of MCI are an early form of dementia, although some patients never get worse and live normal lives.

HOW IT'S DETECTED

Because MCI's symptoms are subtle, it is difficult to distinguish it from normal, age-related changes. A physician with expertise in cognitive disorders and aging, such as a neurologist or geriatrician, is best qualified to make an MCI diagnosis.

To make a diagnosis, he/she can do the following…

• **Standard memory tests** can determine whether your mental capacities are normal for a person of your age. These tests usually are performed by a neurologist or a neurological testing service.

• **Hippocampus measurement.** Your doctor might recommend tests that measure the size and metabolism of the hippocampus, the part of the brain associated with memory. Studies have shown that patients with MCI have lower glucose metabolism in this part of the brain and possibly atrophy (shrinking) of the tissues.

• **Medical history and testing.** Many physical problems can cause symptoms that mimic MCI. These include a deficiency of vitamin B-12…depression…and an underactive thyroid gland. The side effects of certain medications can cause memory problems as well. These medications include antispasmotics, antihistamines and antidepressants.

WHAT CAN YOU DO?

There are no FDA-approved treatments for MCI. However, drugs that are used to treat Alzheimer's disease might be helpful.

Example: A three-year study that looked at more than 750 adults with MCI, published in *The New England Journal of Medicine*, found that those who were given *donepezil* (Aricept) were less likely to develop Alzheimer's disease within one year than those who didn't take it. Unfortunately, the same study found that the benefits did not last. After three years, the Alzheimer's risk was the same in people who took the drug and those who didn't.

What you can do now that might help…

• **Exercise.** People who exercise regularly do better on neuropsychological tests than those who don't exercise. Exercise increases levels of nerve growth factor, a substance used by brain cells. It also improves circulation to the brain, which is helpful for memory and mood.

We don't know what effects, if any, exercise will have on the progression of MCI, but anything that improves memory, mood and cognitive functions might be helpful.

Recommended: Some form of aerobic exercise, such as walking, for 30 minutes most days.

• **Maintain a healthy weight.** Recent research from the Mayo Clinic suggests that consuming between 2,100 and 6,000 calories per day may double the risk for MCI among people age 70 and older. The higher the amount of calories consumed, the higher the risk. Also, people who are obese in middle age are about four times more likely to develop Alzheimer's or other forms of dementia in later life than those who are leaner. It's possible that inflammatory substances produced by fat increase brain damage that can lead to dementia.

• **Stay mentally active.** The brain continues to form neurons and connections between neurons throughout life. Patients who are mentally active form the most connections and develop reserves that can slow the onset of Alzheimer's symptoms.

There's no evidence that mental workouts can reverse MCI, but people who keep their minds challenged—by working, taking classes, volunteering, doing puzzles, etc.—will have better cognitive function.

Time for Your Cognitive Exam: Is It Serious Memory Loss?

Malaz A. Boustani, MD, the Richard M. Fairbanks professor in aging research at the Indiana University Center for Aging Research and founding director and chief innovation and implementation officer at the Sandra Eskenazi Center for Brain Care Innovation, both in Indianapolis. AgingBrainCare.org.

One of your favorite actors appears on the screen, but you can't put a name to the face. Or you walk into the kitchen for—well, you walked in there for something, but you can't remember what.

Sound familiar? If so, you are probably at least middle-aged. These and other memory hiccups usually reflect nothing more than normal brain changes, but how can you be sure? It's a legitimate concern because up to 76% of cases of cognitive impairment aren't spotted by primary care physicians during the mild-to-moderate phases.

Recent development: You may have heard about the "annual wellness visit" that the Affordable Care Act has added as a new Medicare/Medicaid benefit. As you might imagine, this free checkup includes standard tests (such as blood pressure), a review of screening tests, etc. But this exam also includes a thorough assessment to detect memory problems or other cognitive impairments. Some private insurance policies may also cover this type of exam.

Why it's important: People with Alzheimer's or other forms of dementia are typically diagnosed three to five years *after* they've developed impairments. The cognitive checkup offers the chance for earlier detection of a problem and the opportunity to develop an effective plan for coping with symptoms of cognitive impairment.

WHAT THE EXAM INCLUDES

During the annual wellness visit, your doctor will start with a general health assessment. If you're like most adults, you probably have one or more health issues—such as high blood pressure or diabetes—that increase the risk for cognitive impairments. Certain medications can also cause cognitive problems.

The exam (combined with subsequent tests) can also help identify reversible causes of cognitive declines, such as thyroid problems, low vitamin B-12 and depression.

After that, the exam will include…

•**Personal stories.** Your doctor will ask how your life is going. This is your chance to discuss any changes you might have noticed—maybe it's getting harder to balance your checkbook…perhaps you're forgetting to take medications (or you're taking them at the wrong times). Such self-reported observations can raise important red flags.

•**A conversation with a family member/ close friend.** It's common for patients with cognitive changes to be unaware (or only partly aware) of how much they're affected. You may think that you're on top of daily details, but someone else in your life might notice that you keep missing appointments or taking wrong turns on your drive home. A different perspective is helpful.

My advice: I strongly encourage patients to bring someone with them to their wellness visits whether they suspect cognitive problems or not. The doctor or a member of the medical team may interview the person separately so that he/she can speak freely. If you and your companion say that your memory is good, there's a strong likelihood that everything's fine…and that you won't need further testing for another year.

POSSIBLE PROBLEM AREAS

If you have noticed changes in your memory or daily routines, your doctor will ask focused questions.

Examples: "During the last 12 months, have you noticed that confusion/memory loss is happening more often or getting worse?" "Did you need help from others during the last week in performing daily activities, such as grooming, walking or getting dressed?"

Problems in any of these areas could mean that you need…

•**Cognitive testing.** If your doctor suspects (based on the above discussions) that you might have some degree of cognitive impairment, commonly used tests include the Memory Impairment Screen (MIS)…the General Practitioner assessment of Cognition (GPCOG)…or the Mini-Cog. Each can be administered by a medical staff member in less than five minutes.

Example: The MIS is a verbally administered word-recall test. You may also be asked to spell a word (such as "world") backward… or count back from 100 by sevens.

Patients who "fail" a test may have cognitive impairments—or they could simply be having an off day. Further evaluation by a neurologist, geriatrician or other specialist will be recommended.

WHAT'S NEXT?

If the wellness visit and subsequent testing point to a cognitive decline, you'll need appropriate follow-up.

Recent research: The collaborative care model (a team approach to care) has been shown to be more effective than the standard one-doctor/one-patient approach. With the collaborative approach, a team of clinicians (which may include a primary care doctor and memory care doctor) led by a care coordinator (a registered nurse or a social worker) works with the patient and family to improve quality of care.

In a study of 153 patients with mild-to-moderate Alzheimer's, patients who received collaborative care had fewer behavioral/psychological problems and were more likely to be given effective drug treatments than patients receiving "standard" care with one doctor.

Many patients can live a relatively normal life with cognitive decline, but they'll need a lot of help along the way. A collaborative program is the best way to provide it.

Note: All aspects of this care may not be covered by insurance.

Alzheimer's Could Be This Dangerous Deficiency

Irwin Rosenberg, MD, senior scientist and former director, Nutrition and Neurocognition Laboratory, Tufts University, Boston.

It may seem like an extreme form of wishful thinking to suggest that symptoms believed to signal the onset of Alzheimer's disease could instead be due to a lack of one particular vitamin—and yet studies over the years have been telling us just that. Some people 50 and older who are suffering from memory problems, confusion, irritability, depression and/or paranoia could see those symptoms dramatically diminish simply by taking vitamin B-12.

Frighteningly, recent research shows that up to 30% of adults may be B-12 deficient—making them vulnerable to misdiagnosis of Alzheimer's. For years, doctors had believed that B-12 deficiency showed itself most significantly as the cause of anemia (pernicious anemia), but they now realize the lack of B-12 may even more dramatically be causing neurological symptoms, some of which are similar to Alzheimer's.

OTHERS AT RISK...

Age is not the only risk factor for having a B-12 deficiency—other at-risk groups include vegetarians (dietary B-12 comes predominantly from meat and dairy products) and people who have celiac disease, Crohn's disease or other nutrient malabsorption problems. Evidence accumulating over the past few decades shows that regular use of certain medications also can contribute to vitamin B-12 deficiency. These include antacids, in particular proton pump inhibitors (PPIs) such as *esomeprazole* (Nexium), *lansoprazole* (Prevacid) and many others which reduce stomach acid levels, making it difficult for B-12 to be fully absorbed. The diabetes drug *metformin* (Glucophage) also can reduce B-12 levels.

MEASURING DEFICIENCY

A common symptom of vitamin B-12 deficiency is neuropathy, a tingly and prickly sensation, sometimes felt in the hands and feet and occasionally in the arms and legs as well. People with B-12 deficiency also tend to have problems maintaining proper gait and balance. I recommend testing B-12 levels for a few groups of people, including those on PPIs for more than a few months...people having memory problems and/or often feeling confused—and this can include people of any age...those with neuropathy in the feet and/or legs...and those who have unexplained anemia.

As mentioned above, deficiencies of B-12 in older adults are nearly always a direct result of too little stomach acid, which is essential for absorption of B-12. This explains why powerful antacids trigger B-12 deficiency. Another problem is that sometimes, especially in older people, the stomach isn't making enough of a protein called intrinsic factor (IF) that is needed to break down B-12 effectively. There is no way to increase IF, and so the solution is to administer B-12 in large enough quantities to override the difficulty with absorption. Traditionally this has been done with injections of B-12, but more recently doctors have found that oral supplementation with high amounts of B-12 that dissolves under the tongue also is successful and certainly easier than regular injections. There is no reason to be concerned about "balancing" B vitamins as was once thought—B-12 is water soluble and the body can excrete what it doesn't need.

WHAT YOU CAN DO

Adults can easily get the recommended daily amount of 2.4 micrograms (mcg) of B-12 from dietary sources, which include all animal products. For example, just three ounces of steamed clams supplies 34.2 mcg and three ounces of salmon provides the necessary 2.4 mcg. However, this amount will not address the problems associated with aging and medications. Once again, the issue goes back to absorption—if you don't have enough stomach acid and/or IF to use the B-12 you ingest, it is almost irrelevant how much animal protein you eat. This is why the Institute of Medicine says that for people over age 50 and for vegetarians, the best way to ensure meeting your body's B-12 needs is to take a supplement or seek out foods fortified with it.

Reason: The body can more easily absorb the form of B-12 used for supplementation and fortification even in people who have low levels of stomach acid.

Caution: B-12 tests are sometimes insufficiently sensitive, especially for vegans. If your test indicates levels are fine in spite of symptoms, have your doctor order a different test that will evaluate whether your B-12 system is intact. There is no need to suffer from any kind of B-12 deficiency symptoms, let alone risk misdiagnosis of Alzheimer's, when the solution is so close at hand!

This Vascular Condition Causes Memory Loss… How to Stop It

Majid Fotuhi, MD, PhD, neurologist, medical director of the NeuroGrow Brain Fitness Center in McLean, Virginia, and affiliate staff at Johns Hopkins Medicine, Baltimore. He is also author of *The Memory Cure* and co-author of *The New York Times Crosswords to Keep Your Brain Young.*

Alzheimer's disease is the most widely recognized form of dementia. But there's another cause of memory loss that people should know about—but usually don't.

Vascular cognitive impairment (VCI), which is typically caused by multiple small strokes, has been estimated to affect 1% to 4% of adults over age 65. However, because there is no agreement on the exact definition of this condition, the actual number of affected individuals is not known. Most older adults with vascular risk factors—such as high blood pressure (hypertension) and diabetes—may have varying levels of VCI.

BLOOD VESSELS AND YOUR BRAIN

The brain requires a hefty amount of blood—about 20% of the heart's output—to function normally. Even a slight reduction in circulation—such as that caused by small strokes—can result in symptoms, including slowed thinking, that can mimic Alzheimer's disease.

While genetics can play a role in Alzheimer's disease, VCI is widely recognized as the most preventable form of dementia. Even if you've begun to suffer early signs of this form of cognitive impairment (see symptoms below), you may be able to avoid the devastating effects of full-blown dementia.

HIDDEN BLOCKAGES

Most people imagine stroke as a life-threatening event that causes dramatic symptoms. This is true of major strokes. It is not the case with mini-strokes, also known as transient ischemic attacks (TIAs).

When Johns Hopkins researchers looked for evidence of microscopic strokes—areas of brain damage that are too small to be visible on a magnetic resonance imaging (MRI) scan—they found that such strokes are extremely common. Millions of Americans with normal cognition, including healthy adults, have probably experienced one or more of these minor mini-strokes.

What happens: Small, transitory blood clots can momentarily prevent circulation to small areas of the brain. Or vascular hypertrophy, an abnormal growth of cells inside blood vessels, may impede normal circulation. In either case, certain parts of the brain receive insufficient blood and oxygen. The damaged areas can be much smaller than a grain of rice.

Symptoms—assuming that there are noticeable symptoms—tend to be minor. People who have experienced multiple mini-strokes that affect larger or more diverse areas of the brain are those most likely to develop dementia, but it might take years or even decades before the problem is severe enough to be diagnosed. *Symptoms to watch for…*

• **Specific symptoms of VCI depend on the part of the brain affected.** Patients who have suffered multiple mini-strokes may walk or think more slowly than they did before. Some have trouble following directions. Others may feel apathetic or confused.

• **Some mini-strokes,** however, affect only the part of the brain involved in decision-making and judgment. The changes might be so subtle that a patient isn't aware of them—at least, until subsequent mini-strokes affect larger or different areas of the brain.

GETTING THE RIGHT DIAGNOSIS

People who exhibit marked cognitive changes usually will be given an MRI or computed tomography (CT) scan. These tests sometimes reveal white, cloudy areas in the brain (infarcts) that have suffered damage from impaired circulation due to mini-strokes.

Often, however, the mini-strokes are too small to be detected. In these cases, patients may be incorrectly diagnosed with Alzheimer's disease. (The abnormal proteins that are characteristic of Alzheimer's cannot be detected by standard imaging tests.)

The distinction is important. There is no cure for Alzheimer's disease. In patients with VCI, there are a number of ways to stop the disease's progression and maintain long-term cognitive health.

BETTER VASCULAR HEALTH

Brain damage that's caused by mini-strokes can't be reversed. Medication—including cholinesterase inhibitors, such as *donepezil* (Aricept)—may modestly reduce some symptoms in patients with dementia but cannot cure it.

Preventive strategies, however, can be very effective in people with VCI alone. *Most important…*

•**Don't let high blood pressure shrink your brain.** Chronic hypertension is one of the main causes of dementia because the vascular trauma is constant. People with uncontrolled hypertension actually have smaller brains because of impaired circulation. Their risk of developing dementia is two to three times higher than that of people with normal blood pressure.

My advice: Blood pressure should be no higher than 120/80 mm Hg—and 115/75 mm Hg is better. Most people can achieve good blood pressure control with regular exercise and weight loss, and by limiting sodium and, when necessary, taking one or more blood pressure–lowering drugs, such as diuretics, beta-blockers or ACE inhibitors.

•**Avoid the other "D" word.** By itself, diabetes can double the risk for dementia. The actual risk tends to be higher because many people with diabetes are obese, which is also a dementia risk factor.

Important research: One study found that patients with multiple risk factors, including diabetes and obesity, were up to 16 times more likely to develop dementia than those without these risk factors.

My advice: By adopting strategies that prevent hypertension, including weight loss and regular exercise, you'll also help stabilize your blood sugar—important for preventing or controlling the health complications associated with diabetes.

•**Keep an eye on your waist.** Obesity increases the risk for hypertension and diabetes and has been associated with damage to the hippocampus (the brain's main memory center). Obese patients also have a much higher risk for obstructive sleep apnea, interruptions in breathing during sleep that can increase brain shrinkage (atrophy) by up to 18%.

My advice: Measure your waist. For optimal health, the size of your waist should be no more than half of your height. Someone who's 68 inches tall, for example, should have a waist measurement of 34 inches or less.

•**If you drink, keep it light.** People who drink in moderation (no more than two drinks daily for men or one for women) tend to have higher HDL, so-called "good," cholesterol… less risk for blood clots…and a lower risk for stroke and dementia.

My advice: If you already drink alcohol, be sure that you don't exceed the amounts described above. Drinking too much alcohol increases brain atrophy.

•**Get the right cholesterol-lowering drug.** People with high cholesterol are more likely to develop atherosclerosis (fatty buildup in the arteries) and suffer a mini-stroke or stroke than those with normal cholesterol levels.

My advice: Talk to your doctor about statins, such as *atorvastatin* (Lipitor) and *simvastatin* (Zocor). These drugs not only reduce cholesterol but also may fight blood-vessel inflammation. Other cholesterol-lowering drugs—such as resins, which bind in the intestines with bile acids that contain cholesterol and are then eliminated in the stool—don't provide this dual benefit.

Ask your doctor for a vitamin B-12 test. If your blood level is low, you may benefit from B-12 supplements or injections.

Alzheimer's Could Be Depression...or a Stroke

Zaldy S. Tan, MD, MPH, medical director, Alzheimer's and Dementia Care Program, and associate professor, David Geffen School of Medicine, University of California, Los Angeles. He is author of *Age-Proof Your Mind: Detect, Delay and Prevent Memory Loss—Before It's Too Late.*

Alzheimer's disease is a devastating condition for which there is no effective treatment.

What you may not know: Certain people who think they have Alzheimer's actually may have a condition that is treatable. Unless the misdiagnosis is identified, these people will not only be given ineffective and potentially dangerous treatment, but their real problem also will go untreated. *Conditions that can mimic Alzheimer's...*

DEPRESSION

Cognitive impairments due to depression are known as pseudodementia. Because of a depression-induced lack of attention, which makes it difficult to form and process effective memories, patients may forget appointments or have difficulty remembering names. They also may have trouble concentrating, learning new things and even recognizing faces. This type of dementia, unlike Alzheimer's, is potentially reversible.

Distinguishing signs: Sleep disturbances are more likely to occur with depression than with early-stage Alzheimer's disease. For example, depressed patients may have early morning awakenings or experience difficulty falling asleep at night (typically marked by tossing and turning in bed). They can also have unexplained tearfulness as well as a lack

of interest in things that they used to enjoy, a condition called *anhedonia.*

Treatment: If depression is the culprit, consider talk therapy or an antidepressant, such as *citalopram* (Celexa) or *sertraline* (Zoloft). An antidepressant can usually treat the forgetfulness associated with depression, but it may take several weeks to determine whether a particular drug/dose is going to work. You might also ask your doctor about Saint-John's-wort and other over-the-counter (OTC) natural remedies.

NPH

It's estimated that up to 200,000 older adults in the US have excessive accumulation of fluid on the brain, a condition known as normal pressure hydrocephalus (NPH). The fluid presses on the brain and can cause memory loss and other symptoms that may mimic Alzheimer's.

Distinguishing signs: Most patients with NPH have three main symptoms—an unsteady gait (in the early stages)...followed by urinary incontinence...and cognitive impairments (in later stages). With Alzheimer's, the order is reversed—memory loss and/or other cognitive problems occur first, followed in later stages of the disease by problems with bladder control and gait.

Treatment: NPH can potentially be corrected by inserting a shunt, a tube in the brain that drains excess fluid. However, the surgical procedure is not recommended until after the diagnosis is confirmed by an MRI of the brain and a trial removal of a small amount of fluid through a lumbar tap results in improved memory and/or gait. (For more information, see page 77 "This Brain Disorder Is Curable.")

STROKE

When a person has a series of mini-strokes (warning strokes), it can lead to a type of vascular dementia known as multi-infarct dementia, which can be mistaken for Alzheimer's.

Multi-infarct dementia occurs when damaged blood vessels in the brain slow (but don't completely stop) normal circulation. Reductions in blood and the oxygen it carries can damage brain cells and impair memory and other cognitive abilities—but usually without the motor deficits that accompany a stroke, such as weakness of a limb or slow and/or garbled speech.

Distinguishing signs: Multi-infarct dementia can cause rapid changes in mental functions, sometimes within a few weeks to a month. With Alzheimer's disease, these changes typically occur slowly but steadily over several years.

Treatment: Multi-infarct dementia usually can be diagnosed with a CT or MRI scan showing characteristic changes in the brain. Unfortunately, existing brain damage can't be reversed, although future damage may be avoided. The goal of treatment is to prevent additional vascular damage and cognitive declines by treating the underlying risk factors, such as high blood pressure.

Stengler's Medical Mystery: Surprising Cause of Memory Loss

Mark A. Stengler, NMD, a naturopathic medical doctor and leading authority on the practice of alternative and integrated medicine. Dr. Stengler is author of the *Health Revelations* newsletter, *The Natural Physician's Healing Therapies* and *Bottom Line's Prescription for Natural Cures.* He is also the founder and medical director of the Stengler Center for Integrative Medicine in Encinitas, California, and served as an associate clinical professor at the National College of Natural Medicine in Portland, Oregon. MarkStengler.com

Memory lapses—as in, what is her name?—are an uncomfortable but generally inevitable part of the aging process. Sometimes these lapses are amusing—but there's only anxiety and fear, no humor at all, when memory decline creeps into and interferes with everyday life. This is what had begun to happen to 69-year-old Brad, a financial consultant whose professional success had brought him the home and lifestyle that a high-level career affords. Rather suddenly, Brad began to have trouble remembering things he'd just been told. He sometimes got lost while driving in areas he'd

long known well. As a way to compensate he began to carry a pen and notepad at all times, constantly jotting down reminders about things people told him and tasks and errands he needed to do.

DIFFERENT DOCTORS, DIFFERENT ANSWERS

Always an active and forceful person, Brad wasn't the type to simply accept that dementia might be setting in. Because his cholesterol levels were moderately elevated and he worried about his heart, the physician he saw most regularly was a cardiologist. When he called her to discuss his increasingly frequent memory lapses, she referred him to a neurologist for an evaluation. This doctor examined Brad, ran standard tests and gave him the much-feared diagnosis—it appeared he was in early-stage dementia, perhaps from vascular problems or possibly as the first symptoms of Alzheimer's disease.

Facing this dire diagnosis prompted Brad to call Mark Stengler, NMD, in the hope that a physician trained and experienced in treating illness with natural substances might offer a way to strengthen his memory and perhaps even ward off dementia. Dr. Stengler first reviewed Brad's medical history, including when his memory problems started and how rapidly they had progressed. He quickly realized that this disturbing symptom first presented itself just a few months after Brad's cardiologist had put him on a statin drug (Lipitor) to lower his cholesterol. Knowing that statins have been anecdotally linked to a wide variety of side effects, including false dementia, Dr. Stengler decided to investigate if a more natural protocol to lower Brad's cholesterol could replace the drug. By stopping the Lipitor without endangering Brad's cardiovascular health, they would determine if his dementia was real or a side effect of the drug. His cardiologist was informed of the treatment plan.

NATURAL TREATMENT BEGINS

This wasn't going to be merely a matter of substituting a vitamin regimen for his prescription drug, however. The first step prescribed by Dr. Stengler was a diet to reduce Brad's LDL cholesterol (low-density lipoprotein, the potentially dangerous one). *It included…*

• **Regular consumption of soluble fiber,** including foods such as beans, barley, oats, peas, apples, oranges and pears. Soluble fiber reduces the absorption of cholesterol from the intestines into the bloodstream.

• **At least two servings a week (optimally four or more) of fish such as anchovies,** Atlantic herring, sardines, tilapia and ocean or canned salmon, specifically for their omega-3 fatty acids. This could also be accomplished with supplements.

• **A daily handful of nuts rich in monounsaturated fatty acids,** such as almonds and walnuts. A Spanish study found that a walnut-rich diet reduced total cholesterol by as much as 7.4% and LDL cholesterol by as much as 10%.

• **Ground flaxseeds**—up to a quarter-cup daily with 10 ounces of water or tossed into a salad or shake. This has been shown to reduce total and LDL cholesterol.

To manage his cholesterol, Dr. Stengler also had Brad double his number of weekly aerobic exercise sessions, from twice each week to at least four times. He prescribed plant sterols, shown to reduce LDL cholesterol by up to 14%, recommending Beta sitosterol, which works by inhibiting cholesterol absorption in the digestive tract by up to 50%, without disrupting the more beneficial HDL cholesterol. Dr. Stengler prescribed a 1.5 gram soft gel capsule to be taken with breakfast and dinner for a total of three grams daily. Brad would need to continue this regimen for life, since in taking his medical history Dr. Stengler had learned that his elevated cholesterol had genetic roots.

JUST REMEMBER THIS…MANY MEDS CAUSE FALSE DEMENTIA

Brad is now off Lipitor and into his new program and his memory has improved significantly. He has no need for memory-enhancing supplements, although he does take a multivitamin daily per Dr. Stengler's advice. Dr. Stengler also monitors Brad's cholesterol levels regularly. He says that they have remained in a normal range and Brad had no reason to return to statins.

Clearly Brad's memory problems were not symptoms of early dementia…but rather side effects of the statin drug. But statins are not the only drugs that may trigger side effects that mimic dementia. Other drugs that can cause these problems include tricyclic antidepressants and certain medications for Parkinson's disease—which is ironic in that PD itself can eventually cause dementia. Pain medications (narcotics such as OxyContin and Vicodin) can also cause memory problems, as can regular use of over-the-counter antihistamines including Benadryl, Chlor-Trimeton and Tavist.

These drugs have a common denominator: They all have anti-cholinergic properties, which means they suppress neurotransmitters that regulate certain aspects of mental functioning, especially those that relate to memory. This explains why anti-cholinergics can actually cause cognitive problems, and why the principal drugs to treat AD are in the pro-cholinergic category.

When concerned about memory lapses, many people today turn to a variety of supplements. A more effective strategy would be to schedule a visit to a naturopathic physician to review the medications they take regularly, both pharmaceutical and OTC, as these may be where the problem lies. In fact, a study published in the *British Medical Journal* reported on 372 elderly people without dementia who were taking anti-cholinergic medication. After following this group for eight years, the researchers found that 85% of this group had mild cognitive impairment, compared with 35% of the people in a second group who had never used the drugs. As Dr. Stengler says, this is an important reminder why people and their doctors should wonder whether symptoms of early dementia might relate to medication—and therefore be reversible. That's advice worth remembering.

How to Avoid "Statin Brain"

Statins can cause memory loss in some patients, despite a recent study that found they don't have cognitive side effects. The study was a generalized statistical study—not a personalized look at vulnerable patients. Some people who are susceptible do have "statin brain." Symptoms stop when the drug is stopped. These patients should talk to their doctors. Anyone considering starting a statin should ask about every-other-day rather than daily dosing.

Linda L. Restifo, MD, PhD, professor in the department of neurology at University of Arizona, Tucson.

This Brain Disorder Is Curable

Mark G. Luciano, MD, PhD, a neurosurgeon who is internationally known for his work in hydrocephalus. He is director, Cerebral Fluid Center and professor of neurosurgery, Johns Hopkins Medicine Baltimore.

The future can be bleak for patients with Alzheimer's disease or other forms of dementia because these conditions rarely can be reversed. Yet there's evidence that about 5% of patients diagnosed with dementia actually have an unrecognized—and treatable—condition.

It's believed that an estimated 700,000 people in the US have excessive fluid in the brain, a condition called normal pressure hydrocephalus (NPH). The fluid presses against the brain, causing poor balance, memory loss and other symptoms similar to dementia.

NPH occurs almost exclusively in adults 55 years old or older. It's called "normal pressure" because fluid accumulates so gradually that there isn't the sharp spike in pressure that occurs with acute hydrocephalus.

PROBLEM WITH BRAIN PLUMBING

Cavities within the brain called ventricles produce about a pint of cerebrospinal fluid a day. This fluid, which cushions the brain and spinal cord, is normally reabsorbed by tissues at about the same rate as it is produced.

In patients with NPH, the fluid is reabsorbed more slowly. This usually occurs because of scar tissue within brain membranes. The scarring, caused by factors such as inflammation, previous hemorrhages (strokes) or a traumatic head injury, impedes normal drainage. Excess fluid enlarges the ventricles.

Pressure from accumulated fluid presses against nerves and other brain tissues. It also can compromise blood vessels, decreasing blood flow to the brain.

Result: Dementia-like symptoms.

EASY TO MISS

Most patients with NPH exhibit three key symptoms…

- **Unsteady gait (they often walk with their feet far apart).**
- **Urinary incontinence.**
- **Cognitive impairments, including memory loss.**

Why it's missed: The same symptoms can be caused by many different conditions, including a stroke, Alzheimer's disease or other forms of dementia. Urinary incontinence could be due to a prostate problem. Balance problems often are due to spine diseases, diabetes or inner-ear problems.

A CT or MRI scan will show if a patient has enlarged ventricles, but this isn't always caused by NPH. It's normal, for example, for the ventricles to enlarge with age. It can be difficult to distinguish normal enlargement from ventricle changes due to fluid pressure.

IMPORTANT CLUES

Problems with gait and balance typically are the first symptom of NPH—memory loss usually comes later. This is the opposite of what happens with Alzheimer's, in which cognitive symptoms usually occur first.

If a neurologist suspects that a patient has NPH, an imaging test will reveal, to some degree, whether ventricular enlargement is caused by excess fluid.

Next step: The removal of excess fluid. If a patient has NPH, removing as little as 50 cubic centimeters (cc's), about 10 teaspoons, of fluid through a lumbar puncture (spinal tap) often will improve symptoms within a day.

Sometimes, a more involved procedure, lumbar catheter insertion, is necessary to diagnose NPH. A catheter is inserted into the area around the spinal cord. This permits continuous fluid removal (about a pint altogether) over 36 hours. The patient usually spends two nights in the hospital while fluid is removed from the brain. Then the catheter is removed, and he/she goes home for a few days. At a follow-up appointment, the neurologist re-tests the patient's balance, cognitive abilities, etc. The doctor also will ask friends or family members if they have noticed an improvement in the patient's symptoms.

If the patient improved significantly, then a diagnosis of NPH is virtually certain—particularly if the symptoms return when fluid levels in the brain gradually rise to pretreatment levels (within three to five days).

SURGICAL DRAINAGE

The only treatment for NPH is to insert a shunt, a silicone tube, in the brain that continuously drains excess fluid. Shunts are extremely durable and potentially can last for decades.

Best choice: A programmable shunt that allows the neurologist to fine-tune the settings and increase or decrease the rate at which fluid is removed from the brain. A doctor can make adjustments to the valve with an external device without additional surgery. The programmable shunt is more expensive but often is covered by insurance. Check with your provider.

The procedure to implant a shunt usually takes less than an hour. The device is inserted into the brain, and a drainage tube is implanted under the skin. This tube carries drained brain fluid into the abdominal cavity, where it's absorbed into the bloodstream. Both the shunt and tube are invisible to others, although patients might notice a small bump on the head where the valve is implanted and a bump where the tube passes over the collarbone.

About 80% of patients who undergo the procedure experience significant improvements in memory, gait, etc. The improvements tend to be most dramatic in those who are diagnosed and treated early, before fluid buildup permanently damages brain tissue.

Although any brain procedure carries risk, shunt insertion is relatively safe. About 25% to 50% of patients undergo additional procedures to remove blockages from the shunt or drainage tube over the next two years.

Unusual Memory Trouble

If you suddenly cannot remember where you are or how you got there, then your memory soon returns, what could be happening?

One possibility is that you had an attack of transient global amnesia (TGA). This is a temporary loss of memory that typically lasts for six to 12 hours. People who have TGA can perform physical tasks, such as driving, and can recognize familiar people, but they are unable to remember recent events. They often ask the same questions repeatedly even after those questions have been answered.

Neurologists don't know exactly what triggers TGA, but many believe it to be a type of migraine headache. It usually is a onetime event. Even though TGA is disturbing, it is a fairly benign condition. However, if this happens to you or someone you know, a neurological exam should be administered to rule out anything more serious, such as a stroke.

Louis R. Caplan, MD, professor of neurology, Harvard Medical School, Boston.

Stay Sharp as You Age— Surprising Causes of Memory Loss

Pamela W. Smith, MD, MPH, MS, founder of The Fellowship in Anti-Aging, Regenerative and Functional Medicine, Boca Raton, Florida...and codirector of the master's program in medical sciences with a concentration in metabolic and nutritional medicine, University of South Florida College of Medicine, Tampa. She is author of What You Must Know About Memory Loss & How You Can Stop It.

It is no secret that age and memory are intertwined. But age itself is not the sole reason that we forget things. Memory loss often can be traced to specific factors, including hormonal changes, inflammation and exposure to mercury and other toxins.

Common causes of memory loss—and what you can do to control them...

IMPAIRED CIRCULATION

If you have high cholesterol or other cardiovascular risk factors—you smoke, have high blood pressure, are sedentary, overweight, etc.—you probably have at least some atherosclerosis, fatty plaques in the arteries that reduce the flow of blood and oxygen to the brain.

What to do: In addition to the obvious—more exercise, weight loss, not smoking—I strongly advise patients to eat a Mediterranean-style diet. This features lots of fruits, vegetables and grains along with healthy amounts of olive oil and fish. A recent study found that people who closely followed this diet were 28% less likely to develop mild cognitive impairment and 48% less likely to get Alzheimer's disease.

Also helpful: Eating more soluble fiber (such as that found in oatmeal, beans, fruit and nuts) or taking a fiber supplement has been shown in both men and women to decrease hardening of the arteries and improve circulation.

EXPOSURE TO MERCURY

Americans are exposed to mercury all the time. It is present in soil, the water supply and some foods, including many fish. It also is used in many dental fillings. Over time, the mercury from fillings and other sources can cause inflammation and oxidative stress in the brain, both of which can damage the neurotransmitters that are essential for memory and other brain functions.

What to do: You can get tested for mercury and other heavy metals, but the tests will be positive only after long-term exposure. I advise patients to reduce their exposure long before it will show up on any test.

If you have dental fillings made of amalgam (an alloy of mercury and other metals), consider replacing them with fillings made from plastics or other materials. The work should be done by an environmental dentist who specializes in the safe removal of mercury.

Also important: Avoid eating shark, swordfish, king mackerel, marlin, orange roughy, ahi tuna and tilefish, which tend to accumulate mercury. Limit canned albacore tuna to three servings or less per month and canned light tuna to six servings or less per month.

Best: Cold-water salmon.

When a Hidden Infection Is the Culprit

The late Erno Daniel, MD, PhD, an internist and geriatrician in private practice at the Sansum Clinic in Santa Barbara, California. The author of *Stealth Germs in Your Body*, he lectured throughout the US on medical topics, including geriatrics and hidden infections.

All of us think that we know the telltale symptoms of an infection. Depending on the part of the body that's affected, there might be redness, warmth, swelling and tenderness at the infection site—or whole-body symptoms, such as a fever and/or chills.

Little-known fact: Many infections cause subtle, if any, symptoms and often are misdiagnosed. This is particularly true of low-level, smoldering infections—due to bacteria or viruses, for example—that are now thought to be a largely unrecognized cause of several diseases, including some forms of arthritis, dementia, hearing loss and digestive problems.

STEALTH GERMS

Our bodies contain more microorganisms (microbes) than human cells. Although many of these microbes are harmless, others are disease-causing (pathogenic). Our immune systems generally keep these harmful microbes in check, but mild infections still can be carried in the body—even when our immunity is strong—and persist for decades. These hidden infections can irritate and damage tissues throughout the body.

Example: Peptic ulcers were once thought to be caused by such factors as spicy foods or stress. It wasn't until the 1980s that researchers proved that the vast majority of these ulcers were caused by a bacterium, *Helicobacter pylori* (H. pylori), and could be treated with antibiotic therapy.

79

Conditions that can be caused by a hidden infection…

ARTHRITIS

People who develop joint pain after about age 50 usually assume that it is age-related arthritis. But pain and swelling in the joints also may be a sign of infection.

Suspect infection if: Joint pain (which may shift from joint to joint) develops after a flu-like illness. Swelling and fatigue as well as fever also may occur.

Possible cause: Lyme arthritis. This form of arthritis can affect people who have untreated, late-stage Lyme disease and typically occurs months after a bite from an infected tick. Without treatment, the pain can persist for years, sometimes with periods of remission.

What to do: The enzyme-linked immunosorbent assay (ELISA) test shows the presence or absence of antibodies to *Borrelia burgdorferi*, the bacterium that causes Lyme disease. The Western blot test is performed to confirm a diagnosis of Lyme disease.

Lyme arthritis is more likely to occur in areas of the US where the so-called deer tick is prevalent, including the Northeastern, North-Central and Pacific states.

Lyme disease is readily treated with oral antibiotics—usually *doxycycline* (Vibramycin) or *amoxicillin* (Amoxil)—typically taken for 14 to 21 days. For Lyme arthritis, your doctor may recommend a longer course of antibiotic treatment (typically 30 to 60 days). If the infection is more severe (or has persisted for months or longer), intravenous antibiotics may be needed.

DEMENTIA

Older adults who experience gradual mental decline are often assumed to have Alzheimer's disease. But some forms of more rapidly progressive dementia can be caused by exposure to harmful microorganisms.

Suspect infection if: Rapidly progressive memory loss, confusion or other cognitive disorders occur along with gastrointestinal (GI) symptoms, such as persistent diarrhea and/or unexplained weight loss.

Possible cause: *Tropheryma whippelii*, a bacterium that can cause a long-term infection, damages the intestine and spreads to other areas of the body (including the brain, where it can impair mental functions). The infection, known as Whipple's disease, can be treated.

Unfortunately, doctors don't tend to look for Whipple's disease, because it is rare and the same GI symptoms can be caused by medications—including cholinesterase inhibitors, such as *donepezil* (Aricept) and *rivastigmine* (Exelon)—that are used to treat Alzheimer's.

What to do: If you or a loved one has been diagnosed with dementia and has the symptoms described above, ask the doctor if Whipple's disease could be the cause. It's diagnosed with a small-intestine biopsy and can be treated with antibiotics—typically intravenous *ceftriaxone* (Rocephin) for two weeks, followed by long-term use of oral *trimethoprim-sulfamethoxazole* (Septra) to fully eradicate the bacterium from the brain.

HEARING LOSS

Most cases of gradual hearing loss are idiopathic—that is, there isn't a known cause. However, hearing loss that occurs suddenly might be due to a virus.

Suspect infection if: You wake up one morning and have virtually no hearing in one ear.

Possible cause: Certain herpes viruses can damage the nerves that control hearing, a condition known as sudden sensorineural hearing loss. (Often the virus has been dormant in the body for a long time and is activated for unknown reasons.)

What to do: The herpes viruses associated with hearing loss can be detected with blood tests and treated with antiviral drugs, such as *valacyclov*ir (Valtrex) or *acyclovir* (Zovirax), along with corticosteroids (such as prednisone). These drugs usually are taken for up to 10 days. Most patients will start to recover their hearing within a few days.

These herpes viruses also can cause vertigo, characterized by spinning dizziness. If you suddenly develop this symptom, ask your doctor if antiviral therapy would be appropriate.

Foggy and Forgetful? The Problem Could Lie in the Liver

Lisa M. Forman, MD, assistant professor of medicine in the division of gastroenterology and hepatology and the director of the Gastroenterology Fellowship Program at the University of Colorado School of Medicine in Aurora.

A woman started making so many mistakes at work that despite her decade of supercompetent service to the company, she was in danger of being fired. Noting her mother's growing confusion, concentration problems and uncharacteristic irritability, her daughter wondered if Alzheimer's was setting in. But then the mother's doctor diagnosed a completely different problem called hepatic encephalopathy (HE), a brain disorder that develops when the liver is unable to remove toxic substances from the blood. Toxins such as ammonia then build up and travel through the bloodstream to the brain, impairing cognitive function.

HE most often develops in people with cirrhosis (scarring of the liver) caused by hepatitis C, alcoholism or other conditions. (The woman above had contracted hepatitis many years before her concentration problems surfaced.) HE also can occur in the absence of cirrhosis in people who, for any of various reasons, develop acute liver failure. HE hospitalizes on average 200,000 individuals each year in the US. The condition can be acute or chronic.

Symptoms of HE can worsen gradually or suddenly. Mild HE symptoms include poor concentration, forgetfulness, mild confusion, mood problems, impaired math and handwriting skills, changes in sleep patterns and a musty, sweet odor to the breath. More severe symptoms include lethargy, apathy, disorientation, slurred speech, obvious personality changes, marked confusion and amnesia. In very severe cases, HE patients may experience brain swelling, then lapse into a coma and die.

Diagnosing the problem: The early symptoms of HE can be subtle, so it's easy for doctors to miss them. At a checkup, the patient might seem completely coherent—aware of the date and who the current president is, for instance. But then a family member will point out that the patient's driving reflexes are slow, almost as if she were driving while intoxicated, or that the patient is having trouble focusing, or that she sometimes stays awake at night and sleeps during the day. Another possible clue that can appear in the early or later stages is a phenomenon called asterixis, in which (for reasons that are not fully understood) the hands flap uncontrollably when the arms are extended.

While various tests can provide useful information, there is no laboratory or imaging test that can definitively diagnose HE. Thus, the diagnosis depends on excluding other possible causes for a patient's dementia-like symptoms, given that various conditions can mimic HE…and, in cases in which a liver problem had not been previously detected, identifying the underlying disorder.

Help for HE: In some cases of acute HE, the condition can be reversed by addressing the underlying cause of the liver dysfunction. For chronic HE, treatment centers on minimizing symptoms. *Treatment options may include…*

•**Avoidance of factors and/or prompt treatment of conditions that could increase the buildup of toxins in the bloodstream—**for instance, constipation, dehydration, electrolyte disturbances, kidney problems, infection or the use of medications that tax the liver.

•**Dietary changes that help reduce formation of ammonia and other toxins and/or speed the passage of food through the intestines.** For instance, patients may be instructed to limit animal protein and increase fiber consumption.

•**Medication.** Because the toxins responsible for HE arise from the gut, a laxative drug called lactulose may be used to speed the passage of food through the digestive tract and to help bind toxins so they can be eliminated in the stool. Antibiotics also may be prescribed to inhibit ammonia-producing bacteria in the gut.

Exciting development: The FDA recently approved the antibiotic *rifaximin* (Xifaxan) for treating HE. Rifaximin has been proven to decrease repeat HE episodes as well as hospitalizations and, unlike other antibiotics prescribed for HE, it has no serious negative side effects.

• **HE can lead to rapid deterioration**—so if the above measures are not enough to keep the condition under control, a liver transplant may be the best option. In that case, a patient should be referred to a transplant center to begin the evaluation process. For many transplant patients, receiving a new liver cures the HE.

Hidden Parathyroid Disease Can Weaken Bones, Cause Kidney Stones and Brain Fog

Shonni J. Silverberg, MD, professor of medicine, division of endocrinology, Columbia University College of Physicians and Surgeons, New York City. Her research has focused on investigation and management of disorders of bone and mineral metabolism, including the treatment of primary hyperparathyroidism.

You get a painful kidney stone and get treated, and your doctor tells you to drink more water to prevent another one.

You break a bone, and it turns out that you have osteoporosis, so your doctor talks to you about diet, exercise and prescriptions.

You're feeling nauseous, don't feel like eating and are experiencing constipation and diarrhea. Your doctor suggests various tests to see if you have a gastrointestinal condition.

You have trouble concentrating, find that your memory isn't as good as it used to be and, in general, feel like you're experiencing brain fog. Your doctor asks if you've been sleeping well lately.

But what if all these symptoms were caused by a little known disease...one that's entirely curable with surgery?

It's called primary hyperparathyroidism, a disease of the parathyroid glands, and it can cause havoc to the bones, kidneys and even the brains of sufferers.

A DISEASE WITH TERRIBLE SYMPTOMS... OR NO SYMPTOMS AT ALL

In a sense, you're lucky if you have symptoms. Some people have no symptoms at all even as the disease is causing serious harm. Fortunately, a common blood test for calcium levels that your regular doctor may routinely order can pick up the earliest signs. That's the first step to identifying the condition.

Unless you have symptoms, however, your doctor may not suggest surgery right away. Some physicians recommend watchful waiting for asymptomatic patients. But waiting while the disease may be damaging your body is controversial, even among experts.

Fortunately, the most current guidelines make it clear exactly who should get treated right away. *Here's what you need to know...*

A TINY GLAND CAN TURN YOUR WHOLE SYSTEM UPSIDE DOWN

About one in 1,000 Americans have primary hyperparathyroidism, three times as many women as men. It becomes increasingly more common over age 60. (Primary means it's not caused by another disease.)

A little background: Primary hyperparathyroidism is not a problem with the thyroid gland. Rather, it affects the tiny pea-sized parathyroid glands on or near the thyroid. There are four of them, but usually only one is overactive, signaling excessive release of parathyroid hormone. That hormone's purpose is to maintain the right level of calcium in the blood, and when it's overactive, it signals the body to pull too much calcium from the bones into the bloodstream. That can weaken bones and lead to osteoporosis and fractures...cause kidney stones...and create neurological issues that affect concentration and memory and lead to depression.

Until the 1970s, people with primary hyperparathyroidism would be diagnosed when they went to their doctors with serious complaints—bone pain, broken bones, abdominal pain and kidney stones. (Other symptoms of severe disease may include nausea, vomiting, loss of appetite, constipation and an increased need to urinate.) Since that time, the disease is generally caught earlier through calcium tests, which are now part of the routine blood test you get during an annual physical.

If you have any of the symptoms or conditions mentioned above and you haven't had a checkup recently, ask your doctor for a blood test. If the result shows a high calcium level in your blood, your parathyroid hormone level will be tested…and if it is high, you'll likely be diagnosed with parathyroid disease. It's usually caused by a noncancerous tumor on one of the glands.

Although medication is sometimes prescribed to manage the disease, there are no medications that can cure it or treat all of its effects. The only way to cure it is through surgical removal of the overactive gland or glands. Within the first year, your bones become stronger, kidney stones wane and you may find that the brain fog and mood issues get better, too.

But what if you get the diagnosis after a regular checkup but don't have any symptoms? Should you still get your diseased parathyroid gland removed?

THE SURGERY DECISION

Most people who show up at the endocrinologist with primary hyperparathyroid disease don't have any obvious symptoms, says Shonni J. Silverberg, MD, professor of medicine in endocrinology at Columbia University College of Physicians and Surgeons. When the calcium test was added to routine blood tests in the 1970s, patients began to be diagnosed when they were asymptomatic. The number of people diagnosed with the disease rose by a factor of four to five times.

Experts disagree about what to do if you don't have symptoms. Some recommend waiting because not everyone does develop clinical problems, and the disease progresses at different rates in different people…and more slowly in older adults. Other experts are concerned that those who don't receive surgery are needlessly putting themselves at risk for complications down the road.

Recently updated guidelines from an international group of experts can make that decision easier. Unless you are too frail for surgery, even if you have no clear symptoms you should have surgery if you are diagnosed with primary hyperparathyroidism and have any of these factors…

• **Very high blood calcium levels.** A normal blood calcium level for an adult ranges from 8.5 milligrams per deciliter (mg/dL) to 10.2 mg/dL, although there are slight variations based on different labs. If your calcium level is 1 mg/dL above the normal range, it's not just slightly but significantly elevated.

• **Silent kidney stones.** If you have kidney stones, you should have the surgery. When they're painful, you'll know you have them. But the new guidelines acknowledge that some people may have "silent" stones, meaning that they're there but not causing any symptoms. One study found that 15% of patients had kidney stones that were not causing symptoms. An ultrasound or other imaging test is recommended to detect any silent stones, and if any are found, you would be a candidate for parathyroid surgery.

• **Kidney trouble.** If your kidneys are not working well (impaired kidney function) for any reason, that's another reason to have surgery. This can be detected by a routine blood test as well.

• **Osteoporosis or fractures.** Patients with osteoporosis have low bone density and are at risk for fracture. Primary hyperparathyroidism can affect your bones, making them weaker. If you have low bone density, you should have surgery. Your physician can use a bone densitometry machine to noninvasively measure the density of your bones. The new guidelines now also recommend imaging of the spine to look for compression fractures, which can go undiagnosed but indicate that the bones are already fragile enough to have fractured…and support the need for surgery.

• **Early onset.** If you're under 50, you should have surgery because you are likely to develop symptoms in your lifetime.

Unlike many illnesses, primary hyperparathyroidism can be cured with surgery more than 95% of the time, so experts tend to recommend it. In most cases, you can go home the same day that you have the surgery, although it takes between one and three weeks to heal fully. Most of the time, you won't need any medication or further treatment (since you'll still have some working parathyroid glands) although you will have to have your blood calcium levels checked regularly and may need to take calcium/vitamin D supplements.

If you do opt for surgery, finding an experienced surgeon is key. The area is delicate and sometimes the glands are hard to find (or more than one is involved), so surgeons need to know how to respond in those circumstances. In general, a surgeon should do more than 50 parathyroid operations a year to be considered an expert. Don't be shy or embarrassed to ask how many of a certain type of operation a surgeon has done and if his/her complication rate is above the average, which is less than 1% for an experienced parathyroid surgeon.

Your Hormones May Be Out of Whack…

The late Alicia Stanton, MD, a physician who practiced antiaging and integrative medicine in the Hartford, Connecticut, area. She cowrote, with Vera Tweed, *Hormone Harmony: How to Balance Insulin, Cortisol, Thyroid, Estrogen, Progesterone and Testosterone to Live Your Best Life.*

When it comes to hormonal changes, women get the most attention. But hormones have a profound effect on the health of women and men.

In fact, these important chemical messengers, which constantly send instructions from one part of the body to another, may be at the root of mysterious and frequently undiagnosed health problems such as fatigue, insomnia, memory loss, depression and weight gain.

Hormones always act together, much like instruments in an orchestra. That is why a hormonal imbalance—too much or too little of one or more hormones—can trip up your health in many ways.

Six key hormones that may be out of whack…*

CORTISOL (ADRENAL GLANDS)

The hormone cortisol tells the body to respond to stress—both external stresses (such as traffic jams and financial troubles) and internal stresses (such as inflammation and infections).

The danger: Progesterone (a hormone that is produced by the adrenal glands as well as the ovaries and, in smaller amounts, by the testes) acts as a chemical building block for cortisol as well as estrogen and testosterone. If you are constantly under stress, you generate high levels of cortisol, depleting progesterone and, in turn, reducing the production of estrogen and testosterone. That is why effective stress management is essential to overall hormonal balance in women and men.

Common signs of imbalance: High cortisol levels can cause excess belly fat, high blood pressure, insomnia, irritability, low libido and weakened immunity. Low cortisol levels—from exhausted adrenal glands that can no longer manufacture enough of the hormone—can cause such problems as allergies, apathy and chronic fatigue.

My advice: Make stress management a priority. *Simple techniques…*

• **Breathe deeply.** Simply breathe in for a count of four, hold for a count of six and breathe out for a count of six. Do this five times whenever you're feeling stressed.

• **Create boundaries.** Feeling helpless and out of control is extremely stressful. Identify your major source of stress—such as a difficult relationship—and create boundaries to regain control. If a friend causes stress by al-

*If you experience any of the signs or symptoms of a hormone imbalance, ask your doctor about getting your hormone levels tested. *If you take a statin drug:* Cholesterol is a building block of testosterone—and cholesterol-lowering statin therapy also can lower levels of the hormone.

ways complaining, for example, tell her the topics you're willing to listen to—and those you're not.

• **Get enough sleep.** Sufficient sleep is crucial for balancing cortisol—and all other hormones. To improve sleep, keep your bedroom completely dark and a little cool…and don't watch TV at bedtime. End each day with a positive ritual, such as writing down things that you're grateful for or taking a warm bath.

INSULIN (PANCREAS)

Insulin regulates blood sugar (glucose), telling muscle cells to burn glucose for energy and fat cells to store it for future use.

Common signs of imbalance: Carbohydrate cravings, constipation, excess belly fat, poor memory, prediabetes and diabetes indicate high insulin levels, the most widespread insulin imbalance.

My advice: Balanced glucose levels lead to balanced insulin, and diet is the best way to balance glucose.

• **Eat six times a day.** Having healthful, smaller meals throughout the day balances glucose. Eat breakfast, a mid-morning snack, lunch, a mid-afternoon snack, dinner and a bedtime snack.

• **Include protein in snacks and at meals.** It helps keep glucose balanced.

Good protein sources: Nuts, cottage cheese, hummus and oily fish such as salmon and sardines.

• **Eat low-glycemic carbohydrates.** Slow-digesting carbohydrates that don't create spikes in glucose levels include nonstarchy vegetables, fruits, whole grains and beans.

THYROID HORMONE (THYROID GLAND)

This hormone regulates metabolism, including body temperature and heart rate.

Common signs of imbalance: Cold hands and feet, dry skin, fatigue, hair loss, slow heartbeat and/or weight gain could signal hypothyroidism, the most typical thyroid imbalance.

My advice: Reducing stress is key. Also helpful…**

**Check with your doctor before taking any of these supplements—some may react with certain drugs.

• **Avoid gluten.** Research now links gluten intolerance to thyroid problems.

To determine if you are sensitive to gluten: Give up gluten-containing foods for two weeks and gradually reintroduce them. If symptoms (such as abdominal pain, bloating and diarrhea) return, you are probably gluten-sensitive.

• **Take zinc.** A daily dose of zinc (30 mg) helps restore normal thyroid levels. (Also take 2 mg of copper—zinc supplements can deplete copper.)

• **Take selenium.** A daily dose of selenium (100 mcg), a potent antioxidant, helps to improve thyroid function.

• **Test for iodine.** If you have symptoms of thyroid imbalance, ask your doctor to test your iodine level. This mineral is crucial for production of thyroid hormone. If levels are low, eat more iodine-rich foods, such as sushi that contains seaweed.

ESTROGEN AND PROGESTERONE (OVARIES, ADRENAL GLANDS, TESTES)

These hormones work together to regulate functions in the brain, heart and every other organ.

Common signs of imbalance: For most premenopausal women, estrogen is too high and progesterone is too low. Symptoms include bloating, breast tenderness, heavy menstrual bleeding and moodiness. High estrogen also increases risk for breast cancer. For perimenopausal and menopausal women, estrogen is usually low, and symptoms can include hot flashes, urinary incontinence and vaginal pain and dryness.

In men, low libido, increased belly fat and breast size, depression and erectile dysfunction may occur with imbalances of these hormones.

My advice: Controlling stress and following the eating habits described earlier in the insulin section are two of the best ways to balance estrogen and progesterone.

TESTOSTERONE (TESTES, OVARIES)

Testosterone affects sex drive and muscle mass in men and women.

What's often overlooked: In men, low testosterone levels are linked to higher rates of heart disease, type 2 diabetes, Alzheimer's disease, osteoporosis, prostate problems—and death from any cause.

Signs of imbalance: Fatigue, low libido, decrease in strength, erectile dysfunction, irritability, anxiety, depression, poor concentration, memory loss and weight gain.

My advice: To boost testosterone, don't smoke or drink alcohol excessively (for men, no more than two drinks a day). *Also helpful...*

• **Lose weight.** For men who are overweight, weight loss is one of the most effective ways to boost testosterone. Emphasize filling, low-calorie foods, such as vegetables, fruits, whole grains and beans.

• **Resistance training.** Lifting weights three times a week stimulates the production of testosterone.

• **Interval training.** This type of exercise also helps boost testosterone levels.

What to do: Exercise to maximum capacity for one minute...slow down until normal breathing is restored (usually about one minute)...then repeat that two-part cycle for 20 minutes.

For women: Low testosterone can lead to weight gain and loss of sex drive. The self-care methods described above for men also work for most women. This includes no excessive drinking (for women, no more than one drink a day).

If you take a statin drug: Cholesterol is a building block of testosterone—and cholesterol-lowering statin therapy also can lower levels of the hormone.

If you're taking a statin and have signs of testosterone imbalance, ask your doctor to test your total testosterone. If levels are 400 ng/dL or below in men, testosterone-replacement therapy should be considered. In women, a total testosterone level of 15 ng/dL or below is considered low.

Your Drugs May Give You Dementia

Sam Gandy, MD, PhD, professor of neurology and psychiatry at the Mount Sinai School of Medicine in New York City.

A diagnosis of dementia could be your worst nightmare, but what may be even more troublesome is the possibility of being told you have dementia, when in fact one simple step could reverse it quite simply. "Pseudodementia" is far more common than you'd guess...and the cause can often be found in your medicine cabinet.

Sam Gandy, MD, PhD, professor of neurology and psychiatry at the Mount Sinai School of Medicine in New York City, sees many elderly patients who seem to be suffering from Alzheimer's disease (AD) or other forms of dementia...but may not be. He said he believes as many as 10% of those 65 and older believed to have dementia may actually be experiencing side effects from medication.

Sleeping pills are a common culprit. A good night's sleep often becomes increasingly elusive for aging men and women, leading doctors, sympathetic to their plight, to prescribe drugs such as *zolpidem* (Ambien). These drugs trigger mental and physical lethargy—that's why they work—but in some people that state of mind and body carries over to the next day and impairs function, says Dr. Gandy. It's not just prescriptions, either—over-the-counter sleep-aids, which seem as innocent as popping a vitamin, can also cause this problem. OTC sleep-aids (including brands like Unisom SleepTabs, Tylenol PM and Nytol QuickCaps caplets) contain antihistamines, virtually all of which can cause dementia-like symptoms.

Yet another common type of drug prescribed to elderly patients to promote sleep and/or calm nerves are tranquilizers in the benzodiazepine class. This includes *lorazepam* (Ativan), *clonazepam* (Klonopin), *alprazolam* (Xanax), *diazepam* (Valium) and many more. Occasional use is okay, Dr. Gandy said, but when people take such medications often, they can build up in the system, leading to dementia-type symptoms. Dr. Gandy said if you are going to take a "benzo," look for one with a short half-life such as Ativan or Xanax rather than, say, Valium, which lingers much longer in the body, thus making accumulation more likely.

BEYOND SLEEPING PILLS—WHAT ELSE?

Still other drugs used to treat frequent medical problems in the elderly can slow cognition. These include some beta blocker drugs, prescribed for a wide variety of problems such as high blood pressure, irregular heart rhythm, migraine, angina and glaucoma. Also, anticholinergic drugs are a problem—these are prescribed to treat Parkinson's disease, chronic obstructive pulmonary disease (COPD), some gastrointestinal problems, urine retention and more. Although some studies seem to have shown that statin drugs (the world's top-selling pharmaceuticals, prescribed to lower cholesterol levels) help prevent dementia, there is considerable anecdotal evidence of people developing dementia symptoms after taking them—with symptoms then vanishing when they stop the drug. Drugs are often life-savers, but not all that much is known about what happens in the body when they are used over long periods, and most especially in combination with other medications. This is one of the most important reasons why it is smart to take as few medications as possible.

Yet another frequent cause of pseudodementia is not a drug, but rather depression—a condition that is particularly complicated in the elderly, Dr. Gandy pointed out, because they tend to isolate themselves and often their depression symptoms closely resemble early-stage dementia. In fact, he said he has had experiences of trying to set up a clinical trial for Alzheimer's disease, only to discover that candidates referred by their physicians actually suffered clinical depression, not AD at all. Treating these patients with antidepressants also improved their cognition, Dr. Gandy said.

WHAT YOU CAN DO

The resounding message is that no one should be quick to accept a diagnosis of dementia as the cause of memory loss and/or confusion, especially in an elderly individual.

Call your doctor if you develop memory problems soon after starting a new drug. Have your doctor scrutinize all medications to see if one or the combination might be causing the symptoms. Be sure your pharmacist has a complete list of all medications taken, especially if they aren't all filled at the same pharmacy. If it turns out that one or several of the drugs you take could be the cause, Dr. Gandy advised working out a plan with your doctor to withdraw from the drug or drugs for a month or so to see if symptoms change. Finally, be very careful about any sleep aids, whether OTC or prescription.

Best Drug Self-Defense

Armon B. Neel, Jr., PharmD, a certified geriatric pharmacist, adjunct instructor in clinical pharmacy at Mercer University College of Pharmacy and Health Sciences in Atlanta and founder of the Georgia-based MedicationXpert, LLC, a private practice focused on pharmaceutical care for outpatients and institutional geriatric patients. Dr. Neel is also coauthor of *Are Your Prescriptions Killing You? How to Prevent Dangerous Interactions, Avoid Deadly Side Effects, and Be Healthier with Fewer Drugs.* MedicationXpert.com

If you're over age 60—especially if you take more than one medication or suffer drug side effects—it's a good idea to ask your physician to work with a consulting pharmacist who is skilled in medication management. A consulting pharmacist has been trained in drug therapy management and will work with your physician to develop a drug management plan that will avoid harmful drugs. These services are relatively new and may not be covered by insurance, so be sure to check with your provider.

To find a consulting pharmacist in your area, go to the website of the American Society of Consultant Pharmacists, ASCP.com, and click on "Find a Senior Care Pharmacist."

Also helpful: Make sure that a drug you've been prescribed does not appear on the "Beers Criteria for Potentially Inappropriate Medication Use in Older Adults." Originally developed by the late Mark Beers, editor of *The Merck*

Manual of Medical Information, the list has been recently updated by The American Geriatrics Society. To download the list for free, go to GeriatricsCareOnline.org (search Beers Criteria).

Over-the-Counter Drug-Induced Memory Loss

Answer from Malaz Boustani, MD, MPH, associate director, Indiana University Center for Aging Research, Indianapolis.

A reader asks: I usually don't take any medication, but I started using an antihistamine for my allergies. I seem to be forgetting things lately. Could there be a connection?

Yes. Drug-induced memory loss may occur after just 60 days of antihistamine use. These anticholinergic drugs are in a class of medication that also includes many blood thinners, antidepressants and medications used for overactive bladder, heart disease and chronic obstructive pulmonary disease.

In a recent study of 3,690 adults, those who took a daily dose of a strong anticholinergic drug, such as *diphenhydramine* (Benadryl),

for 60 days had mild cognitive impairment, including memory loss.

If you regularly take an anticholinergic: Talk to your doctor about switching to a different drug. *Cetirizine* (Zyrtec) has far fewer anticholinergic side effects and can be used for allergies.

How Often Is Alzheimer's Misdiagnosed?

As many as two in 10 cases of Alzheimer's may be misdiagnosed, according to recent research.

Reason: There is no medical test that can definitively diagnose Alzheimer's. Instead, diagnosis is based on symptoms. Men seem to develop Alzheimer's at an earlier age than women, who typically develop it in their 70s or later…and men's symptoms may be behavioral or involve motor problems, while women's are more likely to involve memory issues.

Melissa Murray, PhD, is assistant professor of neuroscience at Mayo Clinic, Jacksonville, Florida, and leader of a study of the brains of more than 1,600 people, presented at a recent Alzheimer's Association International Conference.

CHAPTER 4

Treatments and Care for Alzheimer's and Dementia

We're Closing in on a Cure for Alzheimer's Disease

Whenever the subject of Alzheimer's disease comes up, the discussion always includes a line that there is no cure. Those affected are told to get their finances, wills, living arrangements and do-not-resuscitate (DNR) instructions in order for when others will be making decisions for them after they literally have lost their minds. But if you've been following health-related news stories, maybe you've noticed reports on potential crossover drugs—drugs already on pharmacy shelves—that may be repurposed or pave the way to halt Alzheimer's disease. Among these is a currently available drug for Lou Gehrig's disease.

Although it is unlikely that doctors will begin prescribing these drugs to treat dementia in the very near future, the possibility of being able to participate in clinical trials of these drugs for Alzheimer's—either for you or for a loved one—is now very real.

FINDING NEW TRICKS FOR OLD DRUGS

The truth is that we are in a high-stakes race for a cure. More than 5.4 million Americans have Alzheimer's disease, and that number is going to substantially increase because the population as a whole is aging and living longer. The Alzheimer's drugs we now have treat the symptoms poorly, and none slow down the disease. We need a treatment that prevents and stops it.

Enter *riluzole* (Rilutek), which is used to slow Lou Gehrig's disease (also known as amyotrophic lateral sclerosis, or ALS), a condition whereby excess of a neurotransmitter called glutamate destroys brain cells responsible for

Kristina Endres, PhD, head of biochemical laboratory, Clinic of Psychiatry and Psychotherapy/University Medical Centre, Johannes Gutenberg Mainz, Germany. Her study on *acitretin* was published in *Neurology*.

Ana C. Pereira MD, clinical investigator, Laboratory of Neuroendocrinology, The Rockefeller University, New York. Her study on *riluzole* was published in *PNAS* (*Proceedings of the National Academy of Sciences*).

muscle function. A neurotransmitter is a chemical that carries messages across synapses through dendrites, branches protruding from brain cells that connect to communicate with other brain cells. Glutamate excess also has been implicated in damaging and destroying brain cells related to cognition.

Because riluzole inhibits glutamate overload, researchers affiliated with the Icahn School of Medicine at Mount Sinai Medical Center and at The Rockefeller University in New York City examined what it could do in rats that had natural age-related memory loss.

Along with their normal diets, either plain water or water treated with riluzole was fed to elderly, cognitively impaired rats for 17 weeks. During this time, memory and other cognitive functioning of these rats and a group of young rats were periodically tested by putting the rats through various maze exercises. They were then euthanized and their spines examined so that correlations between cognitive performance and structural brain changes could be made.

The results: The untreated elderly rats had terrible memory performance during the maze exercises—in fact, their performance swiftly and dramatically declined during the 10-minute tests. In contrast, the performance of the treated elderly rats nearly matched that of young rats. They noticed and retained memory of changes to the maze set-up from one exercise to the next and also had a much greater ability to recognize objects and remember where they could be expected to be found in the maze. And their performance significantly increased instead of decreased across a 10-minute maze exercise. Further, the dendrites in the spines of rats drinking riluzole-laced water were more clustered than those of untreated rats, significantly increasing synaptic strength…the communication between neurons.

HOW YOU CAN GET ON BOARD

The riluzole researchers are now conducting a clinical trial in patients with mild Alzheimer's disease. If you or a loved one want to get on board, you may be able to. First, be aware that, like other powerful drugs, riluzole can cause side effects, which include but are not limited to stomach upset, dizziness, drowsiness,

fatigue and numbness/tingling around the mouth. Then, if being part of an experiment to improve treatment for Alzheimer's disease is still calling to you, talk to your doctor about getting in on the clinical trial being conducted through The Rockefeller University in New York City. Its coordinators are actively recruiting people with mild Alzheimer's who are 60 to 85 years old. More information on the trial can be obtained by contacting the Rockefeller recruitment office at 800-RUCARES (800-782-2737) or RUCARES@rockefeller.edu.

The New Alzheimer's "Prescription"

Dean Sherzai, MD, a neurologist and director of the Alzheimer's Disease Prevention Program at Cedars-Sinai Medical Center in Los Angeles. For more on brain health, follow him on Facebook at Team Sherzai.

Every now and then, researchers announce yet another "breakthrough" drug to halt mental declines or clear away the sticky brain plaque (beta-amyloid) that's the hallmark of Alzheimer's disease.

Unfortunately, the enthusiasm tends to fade as limitations of these drugs become apparent. The handful of medications that help ease the cognitive symptoms of Alzheimer's (such as memory loss and confusion) do not stop the disease's progression.

What most people don't realize: Even though medication plays a role in treating Alzheimer's symptoms, certain lifestyle changes actually can slow the progression of Alzheimer's disease by 30% or more—something that is impossible with even the newest drugs.

Dean Sherzai, MD, one of the country's leading authorities on Alzheimer's disease, explained…

THE NEURO APPROACH

When I treat a person at risk for dementia or newly diagnosed with this disease or mild cognitive impairment (a condition that often precedes Alzheimer's), I recommend a set of lifestyle changes I call NEURO. This stands for Nutrition…Exercise…Unwind…Restful sleep… and Optimize mental/social activities.

People who practice each of these steps—and who also address health conditions, especially high blood pressure and diabetes, that increase the risk for and symptoms of Alzheimer's—can significantly slow the disease from progressing. Regardless of whether the person is also taking an Alzheimer's medication, these lifestyle steps are crucial.

What you need to know about the five-step NEURO approach…

STEP 1: Nutrition. With few exceptions (see below), I don't often recommend individual vitamins, antioxidants or other supplements—the totality of your diet is more important because healthy foods contain a complex mix of nutrients that work together to give maximum benefit.

Best choice: A Mediterranean-style diet. This diet includes lots of fruits, vegetables, whole grains, beans, fatty fish and monounsaturated fats (such as olive oil). Research has shown that a version of this diet that emphasizes certain brain-healthy foods (such as berries and leafy-green vegetables) is especially effective.

Important findings: In a study that was published in *Archives of Neurology*, researchers tracked nearly 1,400 people—482 of whom had already been diagnosed with mild cognitive impairment—for an average of more than four years. They found that those with this condition who were most careful about following a Mediterranean diet were 48% less likely to develop full-fledged Alzheimer's disease than those who were more lax in their eating habits. And those who were still healthy at the start of the study were 28% less likely to develop symptoms in the first place.

Will supplements help when you are already eating well? Maybe—but the evidence isn't conclusive. *Supplements to consider…*

• **Vitamin B-12.** I've found that Alzheimer's patients with B-12 blood levels even at the lower end of the normal range (typically around 180 ng/L) sometimes have fewer cognitive symptoms when they take B-12 supplements.

• **Omega-3s.** Increasing blood levels of omega-3 fatty acids might help as well.

• **Vitamin D.** If vitamin D levels are low, a supplement may improve symptoms and help slow Alzheimer's progression.

STEP 2: Exercise. Exercise can slow progression by about 30% or more. Exercise works on multiple levels—it stimulates growth factors that maintain neurons (brain cells)…and increases circulation of blood in the brain, which promotes healthy cognitive function.

My advice: Get 30 minutes of exercise five or more times weekly.

What works well for some people: Riding a recumbent bike while watching TV.

STEP 3: Unwind. People who experience a lot of stress are up to two-and-a-half times more likely to develop Alzheimer's disease than those who have less or who deal with it more effectively.

Why? No one's sure, although it seems likely that the stress-related surge in cortisol and other hormones is harmful to the brain.

Exercise and volunteering are great stress reducers. Some people manage stress by keeping busy with hobbies…practicing yoga…and/or enlisting help from friends/relatives to deal with daily responsibilities. Do what works best for you—and make stress reduction a priority.

STEP 4: Restful sleep. Many Alzheimer's patients don't sleep well. Experts once assumed that poor sleep was merely an Alzheimer's symptom. But recent research suggests that a lack of restful sleep may play a role in the development and progression of the disease.

Important finding: A study in *JAMA Neurology* that looked at 70 older adults found that those who got less than five hours of sleep a night had higher brain levels of beta-amyloid than those who slept more than seven hours. Researchers speculate that poor sleep impairs the body's ability to clear beta-amyloid or other toxic molecules from the brain.

Also: Sleep apnea, a very common (and underdiagnosed) condition in which breathing intermittently stops and starts during sleep, reduces brain oxygen and is strongly linked to Alzheimer's.

If you frequently snore or snort during sleep, or you're tired in the morning despite having what you thought was a good night's sleep, your doctor might suggest a sleep study that measures brain waves and blood oxygen levels to detect apnea and other sleep disorders.

STEP 5: Optimize mental/social activities. People who stay mentally busy with hobbies, for example, and do other stimulating activities (such as playing challenging video games that require memory, problem-solving, hand-eye coordination, etc.) have smaller declines in memory and other cognitive functions...less Alzheimer's-related brain damage...and slower disease progression. They have a deeper "cognitive reserve," the neural connections (and brain size) that can forestall future impairments.

Once people start doing these new activities, it's both motivating and rewarding because the positive changes—including improved cognitive functioning—can occur within a matter of weeks.

MEDICATION CHOICES FOR ALZHEIMER'S

The drugs that are FDA-approved for treating Alzheimer's disease affect brain chemicals and can improve memory, alertness and concentration. *The two classes of these medications...*

•**Cholinesterase inhibitors** (Aricept, Exelon and Razadyne). These drugs block an enzyme that breaks down acetylcholine, a neurotransmitter that's vital for memory, language, learning and other cognitive functions. There are no serious side effects, but some patients may experience nausea, vomiting, diarrhea or other problems. If this occurs, an Exelon patch can be used.

•**N-Methyl-D-Aspartate (NMDA) receptor blocker** (Namenda). This drug affects glutamate, another brain chemical. It's approved for treating moderate-to-severe Alzheimer's, but it can also help patients with milder forms of the disease. In some patients, Namenda, which may cause side effects such as dizziness and/or headache, works best when combined with Aricept or another cholinesterase inhibitor.

Alzheimer's Symptoms Reversed!

Dale Bredesen, MD, the Augustus Rose Professor of Neurology and director of the Mary S. Easton Center for Alzheimer's Disease Research, the Alzheimer's Disease Program and Neurodegenerative Disease Research in the David Geffen School of Medicine, UCLA. He is founding president of the Buck Institute for Research on Aging in Novato, California.

C an Alzheimer's symptoms be reversed? A breakthrough treatment suggests that they can. In a study recently published in the journal *Aging*, Dale Bredesen, MD, director of the Alzheimer's Disease Program at UCLA's David Geffen School of Medicine, presented an all-natural, multicomponent treatment program that reversed memory loss in four people with Alzheimer's and in five people with either subjective cognitive impairment or mild cognitive impairment (the stages of memory loss that typically precede Alzheimer's). *Here he describes the breakthrough...*

RECENT THINKING

The current, widely accepted theory of Alzheimer's says that the protein beta-amyloid forms plaques outside neurons in the brain... somehow triggering the production of abnormal tau tangles inside neurons...thereby interfering with synapses, the information-laden connections between neurons that create memory and other mental activity.

Recent development: Normal mental function depends on a balance between synaptoblastic (synapse-making) and synaptoclastic (synapse-destroying) activity. If there is more synaptoclastic activity, memory loss may ensue. If there is chronic synaptoclastic activity, our research suggests that Alzheimer's occurs.

My colleagues and I have identified 36 unique synapse-affecting factors (including beta-amyloid). Addressing only one or two of these factors—with a drug, for example—will not reverse Alzheimer's. But addressing many factors—10, 20 or more—can effectively reverse the symptoms.

Here are several key factors in what we call the MEND (Metabolic Enhancement for Neuro Degeneration) program—factors anyone can use to prevent, slow, stop or potentially even reverse memory loss…

RESTORING MEMORY

Synapse-making and synapse-destroying factors function in a "loop" that develops momentum, like a snowball rolling downhill. In the synapse-destroying momentum of Alzheimer's, you gradually lose memories, ultimately even basic ones such as the faces of loved ones. But because the synapse-making factors in the MEND program are so effective, they can reverse the momentum of Alzheimer's. The more of them that you incorporate into your daily life, the more momentum there is to protect and restore memory.

• **Optimize diet.** Eliminate simple carbohydrates such as anything made from white flour and/or refined sugar. Don't eat processed foods with either "trans fats" or "partially hydrogenated vegetable oil" on the label. If you're sensitive to gluten, minimize your consumption of gluten-containing foods, such as wheat and rye (there are simple tests to determine whether you are indeed gluten-sensitive). Emphasize fruits and vegetables. Eat nonfarmed fish for neuron-protecting omega-3 fatty acids.

Why it works: This dietary approach reduces inflammation and high levels of insulin (the hormone that regulates blood sugar), both of which are synapse-destroying.

Important: Dietary changes have more impact than any other factor in preventing or reversing memory loss.

Helpful: Four books that have diets consistent with MEND are *Eat to Live* by Joel Fuhrman, MD…*The Blood Sugar Solution* by Mark Hyman, MD…*The Spectrum* by Dean Ornish, MD…and *Grain Brain* by David Perlmutter, MD.

• **Have a nightly "fast."** Don't eat three hours before bedtime. Ideally, 12 hours should pass between the last time you eat at night and when you eat breakfast.

Example: Dinner ending at 8:00 pm and breakfast starting at 8:00 am.

Why it works: This eating pattern enhances autophagy (the body's ability to "clean up" dysfunctional cells, such as beta-amyloid) and ketosis (the generation of ketones, molecules that can help protect neurons). It also reduces insulin.

• **Reduce stress.** Pick a relaxing, enjoyable activity—walking in the woods, yoga, meditation, playing the piano, etc.—and do it once a day or every other day for at least 20 to 30 minutes.

Why it works: Stress destroys neurons in the hippocampus, the part of the brain that helps create short- and long-term memory. Stress also boosts cortisol, a synapse-damaging hormone. And stress increases corticotropin-releasing factor (CRF), a hormone linked to Alzheimer's.

• **Optimize sleep.** Sleep seven to eight hours every night.

Why it works: Anatomical changes during sleep flush the brain of toxic, synapse-damaging compounds. If you have trouble sleeping, we have found that 0.5 mg of melatonin at bedtime is the best dose for restorative sleep.

• **Exercise regularly.** I recommend 30 to 60 minutes per day, four to six days per week. Combining aerobic exercise (such as brisk walking) with weight-training is ideal.

Why it works: Among its many benefits, exercise produces brain-derived neurotrophic factor (BDNF), a powerfully synaptoblastic compound.

• **Stimulate your brain.** Brain-training exercises and games stimulate and improve your ability to remember, pay attention, process information quickly and creatively navigate daily life.

Why it works: Just as using muscle builds muscle, using synapses builds synapses. (Scientists call this ability of the brain to change and grow plasticity.)

Helpful: Brain HQ (BrainHQ.com) and Lumosity (Lumosity.com) are good, science-based online programs for stimulating your brain.

• **Take folate, vitamin B-6 and vitamin B-12.** These three nutrients can reduce blood levels of the amino acid homocysteine, which is linked to an increase in tau, increased age-related shrinkage of the hippocampus and double the risk for Alzheimer's disease.

However: To work, these supplements must undergo a biochemical process called methylation—and many older people don't "methylate" well, rendering the supplements nearly useless. To avoid the problem, take a form of the supplements that already is methylated (or activated)—folate as L-methylfolate, B-6 as pyridoxal-5-phosphate and B-12 as methylcobalamin.

• **Take other targeted supplements.** Along with the three B vitamins, there are many other supplements that target synaptoblastic and synaptoclastic factors. Check with your doctor about the right dosages. The supplements include vitamin D-3 (low levels double the risk for Alzheimer's)…vitamin K-2…vitamin E (as mixed tocopherols and tocotrienols)…the minerals selenium, magnesium and zinc (zinc, for example, lowers copper, which is linked to Alzheimer's)…DHA and EPA (anti-inflammatory omega-3 fatty acids)…coenzyme Q10, N-acetyl-cysteine, alpha-lipoic acid (they nourish mitochondria, energy-generating structures within cells)…and probiotics (they improve the microbiome, helping to strengthen the lining of the gut, reducing body-wide inflammation).

Also, certain herbs can be helpful. These include curcumin (1 gram per day), ashwagandha (500 mg once or twice per day) and bacopa monnieri (200 mg to 300 mg per day). These have multiple effects, such as reducing inflammation and amyloid-beta peptide and enhancing neurotransmission.

Brain-Power Boost for Dementia Patients

Bob Woods, MSc, a professor of clinical psychology of the elderly and codirector of the Dementia Services Development Centre Wales at Bangor University in Bangor, Wales, and lead author of a study on dementia published in *Cochrane Database of Systemic Reviews.*

M astering a new language, learning to play a musical instrument and other such complex mental tasks may help keep our brains sharp as we age—and may even provide some protection against dementia. But what about less challenging activities, such as putting together puzzles, tending to plants or chatting about the past? Such pursuits are pleasurable, sure…but can they protect brain power for those who need help most—people who already have dementia?

Researchers from the UK decided to find out by pooling the results of 15 randomized controlled trials involving a total of 718 patients with mild-to-moderate dementia. Patients in the various studies' cognitive stimulation groups participated in a wide range of activities that aimed to stimulate thinking and memory generally. Examples included discussing past and present events, playing word games, doing jigsaw puzzles, listening to music, baking and indoor gardening. Typically these were done as group activities involving trained staff plus a handful of dementia patients, though in some cases family caregivers provided the cognitive stimulation to their relatives on a one-to-one basis. Activities averaged 45 minutes, three times per week…and continued for anywhere from one month to two years.

Findings: Patients who participated in the cognitive stimulation activities reported improved quality of life and well-being…were found to communicate and interact with others better than they had previously…and their scores on tests of memory and thinking improved, too. The beneficial effects were seen not only at the end of treatment, but also during the study follow-up periods, which ranged from one to three months.

Brain gain: If a loved one has mild-to-moderate dementia, make a point of initiating stimulating discussions and involving the person in interesting group activities.

Protect yourself, too: Even for people who don't have dementia, lack of cognitive stimulation appears to hasten mental decline over the years—so pull out the jigsaw puzzles and Scrabble board and invite a few friends over for some brain-building fun.

For Mild Cognitive Impairment, Dementia Drugs Don't Help…and May Hurt

Sharon E. Straus, MD, physician, St. Michael's Hospital, Toronto, and professor, department of medicine, and director, geriatric medicine, University of Toronto, Canada. Her study was published in *CMAJ*.

It's very scary to feel like your memory is slipping and you can't think as clearly as you once did…and to wonder whether you've started down the path toward dementia. This condition is called mild cognitive impairment (MCI). And unfortunately, within two years of an MCI diagnosis, an estimated 11% to 33% of patients do progress to full-blown dementia.

So it's no wonder that a growing number of people with MCI are asking for prescription drugs in an attempt to keep their minds sharp. These drugs, called cognitive enhancers, support the production and performance of memory-related neurotransmitters, and they sometimes help patients who already have dementia. And doctors in some countries, including the US and Canada, are giving these drugs to patients who don't have dementia.

The hope is that the medications might help MCI patients in the short term by enhancing memory…and in the long term by reducing dementia risk.

Is the strategy working? Or are the drugs doing more harm than good for patients with MCI? *A recent study has the answer…*

EXAMINING THE EVIDENCE

Researchers from Canada examined existing studies that involved a total of more than 4,500 patients with MCI who were given either a placebo or one of the cognitive-enhancing drugs. They identified eight high-quality studies that were conducted between 1999 and 2007 in various parts of the world.

The goal was to gauge the safety and effectiveness of four medications—*donepezil* (Aricept), *rivastigmine* (Exelon), *galantamine* (Razadyne) and *memantine* (Namenda). These drugs are widely prescribed for dementia patients to improve mental functioning—memo-ry, attention, mood, reasoning, language and ability to perform activities of daily living. The drugs work by increasing the amount of naturally occurring neurotransmitters in the brain or by decreasing abnormal brain activity.

Disheartening results: Not a single one of the medications brought about significant improvement in short-term cognitive performance for MCI patients…nor did any of the drugs help in the long term to help stave off the progression to full-blown dementia. What the drugs did do was cause unpleasant side effects, including diarrhea, nausea, vomiting and headaches. Worse, the researchers found a link between the medications and an elevated risk for cardiac problems—specifically, the drug galantamine was associated with a higher incidence of bradycardia (slow heart rate), which can be dangerous.

Bottom line: It's understandable that people with MCI would be desperate to try just about anything that might reduce their risk of progressing to full-blown dementia…but this study shows that taking what are essentially Alzheimer's drugs is not the answer, because they don't help with MCI and can cause harm.

What does help: Anyone who wants to reduce dementia risk is best off living a healthy lifestyle—eating properly, exercising, and staying mentally and socially active. A plethora of studies show that these measures really can help keep us fit in both body and mind.

Combination Treatment for Alzheimer's

Marwan Sabbagh, MD, director of Alzheimer's and Memory Disorders Division and professor, department of neurology, Barrow Neurological Institute, Phoenix. Dr. Sabbagh is author or coauthor of more than 70 scientific articles on Alzheimer's and author of *The Alzheimer's Answer*.
Alzheimer's Research & Therapy.

Medications can slow the development of Alzheimer's symptoms. Research now shows that combining certain drugs maximizes their effectiveness. The FDA has approved two types of drugs to treat Alzheimer's—cholinesterase inhibitors, such as *donepezil* (Aricept), which work by slowing the breakdown of acetylcholine, a neurotransmitter that helps brain cells communicate... and *memantine* (Namenda), which calms excitotoxicity, a type of cellular hyperactivity that harms neurons.

In a 30-month study of nearly 400 people with Alzheimer's, researchers at Harvard Medical School found that taking both drugs together is more effective in reducing Alzheimer's symptoms than taking either a cholinesterase inhibitor alone or a placebo. According to more recent research, published in *Alzheimer's Research & Therapy*, the combination appears to be most effective for moderate-to-severe forms of Alzheimer's.

In December 2014, the Food and Drug Administration approved a combination pill for moderate-to-severe Alzheimer's disease. The medication, called Namzaric, combines Namenda (memantine) and Aricept (donepezil). This combo my help to improve the symptoms of Alzheimer's, but there is no evidence that Namzaric prevents or slows the underlying progression of the disease in patients who have been diagnosed.

WHAT DOESN'T WORK

The following do not seem to be effective against Alzheimer's...

•**NSAIDs.** Some studies have linked regular intake of a nonsteroidal anti-inflammatory drug (NSAID)—such as aspirin, *ibuprofen* (Advil), *naproxen* (Aleve) and *celecoxib* (Celebrex)—with lower rates of Alzheimer's. But in the Alzheimer's Disease Anti-Inflammatory Prevention Trial (ADAPT)—a study conducted by more than 125 researchers, involving more than 2,000 people age 70 and older—celecoxib didn't reduce the risk for developing Alzheimer's. Naproxen had a minor effect that was outweighed by the fact that it increased the rate of heart attacks and strokes.

•**Ginkgo biloba.** A team of dozens of researchers led by scientists at University of Pittsburgh studied more than 3,000 people age 75 and older, dividing them into two groups.

One group took a daily dose of 240 milligrams (mg) of ginkgo biloba extract, which is widely touted for invigorating the brain and improving memory. A second group took a placebo. Those taking ginkgo did not have a lower rate of developing Alzheimer's.

•**B vitamins.** Elevated blood levels of the amino acid homocysteine have been linked to Alzheimer's. Because B vitamins can lower homocysteine, scientists wondered if B vitamins could slow the development of Alzheimer's.

Researchers in the department of neurosciences at University of California, San Diego, studied 340 people with mild-to-moderate Alzheimer's disease for about four years and found that B vitamins reduced homocysteine levels but didn't slow the progression of Alzheimer's disease.

•**Antipsychotics.** Alzheimer's patients often develop behavioral disturbances, such as wandering, agitation, aggression, paranoia, delusions, anxiety and hallucinations. A standard treatment is an antipsychotic drug, such as *risperidone* (Risperdal), *ziprasidone* (Geodon), *olanzapine* (Zyprexa), *quetiapine* (Seroquel) or *aripiprazole* (Abilify).

Danger: For three years, researchers in England studied 165 Alzheimer's patients who had taken antipsychotics—continuing the drug in half the patients and switching the other half to placebos. After three years, 59% of those on the placebo were alive, compared with 30% on the medication. In other words, those who continued the drug had twice the risk of dying.

Recent approach: Researchers at Indiana University Center for Aging Research reviewed nine studies on the use of a cholinesterase inhibitor to manage behavioral symptoms and found it to be a "safe and effective alternative" to antipsychotics.

Magnet Therapy for Alzheimer's and Parkinson's Patients

Irving Reti, MBBS, associate professor, psychiatry and behavioral sciences, and director, Brain Stimulation Program, Johns Hopkins University, Baltimore.

Would the world be excited to hear about a treatment that helps people with Alzheimer's disease, Parkinson's disease and depression…and one that doesn't involve either surgery or medication? The answer is yes. This therapy, called transcranial magnetic stimulation (TMS), now has research backing its usefulness.

Several years ago, the FDA approved the therapy for patients with severe, intractable depression. Its name describes it quite well. Specially designed machinery delivers a series of magnetic pulses aimed at a particular region in the brain. (For patients with depression, that's the prefrontal cortex—the part of the brain responsible for mood regulation.) More than half of the patients with previously treatment-resistant depression experienced a 50% improvement after six weeks of TMS, and 33% experienced full remission of symptoms.

TMS FOR NEUROLOGICAL DISEASES

Italian research published in *Britain's Journal of Neurology, Neurosurgery, and Psychiatry* reports that TMS helped boost memory in patients with Alzheimer's. Other research has found that TMS improved motor symptoms in people with Parkinson's disease. Irving Reti, MBBS (that's the Australian equivalent of an MD), associate professor of psychiatry and behavioral sciences and director of the brain-stimulation program at Johns Hopkins Hospital, said that he, too, is encouraged by this research.

Dr. Reti stressed, however, that using TMS to treat patients with Alzheimer's, Parkinson's and other neurological disorders is still in the investigative stage. Right now, there's just one kind of FDA-approved machine made by one manufacturer (NeuroStar, NeuroStar.com), with technology specifically designed to treat patients with depression. It may be that effective TMS treatment for other neurological issues would require adjusting the technology or even designing some specialized equipment—there are many as yet unanswered questions.

JUMP-STARTING THE BRAIN

TMS treatment takes about 40 minutes per session, five days a week for about six weeks —some patients get additional follow-up treatments afterward on an as-needed basis. Having a treatment is sort of like having an MRI while seated in a recliner. A magnetic coil positioned over your head delivers a series of rapid-fire magnetic pulses. It's loud, so patients wear earplugs. TMS affects the nerves in the scalp, so some patients experience discomfort there, including feelings of twitching or tingling—but these symptoms typically fade after the first week. Some patients experience a headache after treatment—for relief, they can take over-the-counter pain relievers such as ibuprofen.

Dr. Reti explained that the magnetic signals create improvement by exciting underperforming neurons in the appropriate region of the brain, somewhat like giving them a jump-start. These signals don't penetrate all that deeply, just a centimeter or two, but Dr. Reti said that they are nonetheless very effective. Interestingly, however, he said that "functional imaging studies of the brain with people who have had the treatment clearly show effects in deeper regions, so there are secondary effects as well."

There are some safety considerations. TMS carries a remote risk for seizures, and it should be used with great caution for people with pacemakers, metal implants and implanted or wearable cardioverter defibrillators.

At present, a six-week course of TMS treatment costs around $12,000, and insurers are covering it for depression only on a case-by-case basis. Dr. Reti said that research will be required to establish whether it is a viable therapy for other neurological illnesses, and clinical trails are now under way.

If you'd like to learn more about the treatments, or if you suffer from treatment-resistant depression and are interested in exploring TMS, you can find clinics offering the FDA-approved treatment by visiting the manufacturer's website at NeuroStar.com.

Resveratrol for Alzheimer's Treatment: Time to Celebrate?

Study titled "A randomized, double-blind, placebo-controlled trial of resveratrol for Alzheimer disease" by researchers at Georgetown University, Washington, DC, University of California, San Diego, Wake Forest University, Winston-Salem, North Carolina, Yale University, New Haven, Connecticut, and Roper St. Francis Healthcare, Charleston, North Carolina, published in *Neurology*.

You'd have to drink 1,000 bottles of red wine to get the amount of the antiaging compound resveratrol that's used in a recent Alzheimer's study. Scratch that idea. But it may be worth uncorking a bottle to celebrate the positive findings of the longest and largest human resveratrol study to date.

Researchers gave 119 people with mild-to-moderate Alzheimer's super-concentrated synthetic resveratrol supplements for a year. It was safe. It got into their brains. It arrested "biomarkers" that indicate the disease is progressing. And there was a modest improvement in the ability to do daily tasks. Next stop on this clinical train—a larger study specifically designed to study effectiveness.

The researchers say it's too early to recommend supplements yet for Alzheimer's patients. Certainly anyone being treated for the disease should discuss any supplement with his/her doctor first.

Don't Let Dementia and Age-Related Diseases Catch You Off-Guard

Jullie Gray, MSW, LICSW, CMC, co-owner of Aging Wisdom, a life-care management firm in Seattle, president National Academy of Certified Care Managers, and past president, National Association of Professional Geriatric Care Managers.

Few situations could be more tragic for older adults than being treated as if they have Alzheimer's disease when they real-ly have a treatable health issue, such as a drug side effect or depression. Equally troubling is not knowing what is happening or where to turn if Alzheimer's or a movement disorder, such as Parkinson's disease, is setting in. This is especially true for older people who live alone and away from family. It happens every day to thousands of mature adults. They end up malnourished and living in squalor, forgotten in suboptimal nursing facilities—or on the street.

Help is available—help that can ensure you get the right diagnosis and treatment. And, just like estate planning, it can assist you in making arrangements in advance for health and physical needs if you have the beginnings of an incurable and progressive age-related disease.

WHEN DAILY LIVING BECOMES A CHALLENGE

The doorway to help is through a process called a geriatric assessment. Besides physical and psychological health, a geriatric assessment evaluates whether activities of daily living are becoming challenging. Activities include ordinary tasks such as eating, bathing and dressing as well as taking medications, keeping appointments, paying bills and getting around.

The first step is to make an appointment with your primary care physician for a geriatric assessment. The doctor will give you a physical exam and interview you to assess activities of daily living. If an age-related health issue is found, the doctor may act as the point person for a team of specialists who will take care of your health needs and help you plan for the future, whether that be making arrangements for physical therapy, optimizing your home to help you live there safely, getting transportation or a visiting nurse service or home-delivered meals, or arranging for nursing home care. Or the doctor may refer you to a geriatric specialist to assess your health and act as the point person for multispecialty care.

KNOW WHEN TO GO

A recent health alert by the division of geriatrics and palliative medicine at University at Buffalo, The State University of New York, gave guidance about when to arrange for a geriatric assessment of a parent, spouse or sibling by observing how that person manages the activities of daily living. It's easy to see when someone close to you is becoming frail and physically or mentally challenged—but what about when you have to make that decision about yourself? *A geriatric assessment may be wise if you answer yes to even one of these questions…*

• **Are you more forgetful, distracted and irritable than usual, and are you worried that your memory is failing?**

• **Do you feel not as steady on your feet, resulting in having a fall?**

• **Is taking care of your house, paying your bills and taking care of your health becoming more challenging?**

• **Do you have more than one chronic health problem?**

• **Are you worried about changes in your health and feel confused about what to do or who to turn to for help?**

PREPARING FOR AGING

Whether or not you decide to have a geriatric assessment, there are ways to ease age-related challenges that you can do on your own, such as optimizing your living space with better lighting, grab rails, easy-to-reach cabinets and drawers, elevated toilets and open showers.

DICE Promises to Improve Life for Dementia Patients and Caregivers

Helen C. Kales, MD, professor of psychiatry, director, section of geriatric psychiatry and Program for Positive Aging, University of Michigan, Ann Arbor. Her study appeared in the *Journal of the American Geriatrics Society*.

Although we casually think of Alzheimer's as memory loss, any caregiver will tell you that it's far more than that—depression, anxiety, agitation, delusions, hallucina-

tions and apathy are all symptoms, and they all can take a great toll on the caregiver. How to cope with this often martyring challenge?

A strategy that goes by the acronym DICE and is forged by a partnership between patient, caregiver and health-care provider has gotten a lot of buzz in the health-care community. The Centers for Medicare and Medicaid Services will include DICE in their training and resource modules for health-care providers. If you are the caregiver of someone with dementia, DICE really can improve life for you and the person you care for.

FOUR STEPS TO WORK IT OUT

DICE is a four-step process in which the patient, caregiver and a health-care provider—it could be a geriatrician, geriatric psychiatrist, nurse practitioner or physician assistant, social worker or similar professional trained in dementia care—work as a team to identify the real causes of a patient's "bad behavior" in any given situation and come up with solutions.

The four steps are…

• **D…escribe.** Encouraged by the health-care provider, the caregiver describes a specific event that exemplifies the patient's behavior problems to the health-care provider in a way that gets the caregiver to relive the episode with all its details and feelings. One way of doing this is to describe the event as if it were a movie scene. This conversation may take place in person or over the phone, and the patient may also be present. The caregiver may be encouraged to record episodes of problem behavior in a journal so that one or another episode can be easily remembered and discussed when meeting with the health-care provider. Unless dementia in the person being cared for is so severe that he or she can't communicate anymore, the health-care provider also gets that person's version of the story. The provider then helps the caregiver think about what led up to the event being discussed and its aftermath to get insight about the context and patterns underlying it.

• **I…nvestigate.** The health-care provider then investigates the cause of the problem. Issues to be probed include whether another medical or psychiatric condition is at play, whether the patient's behavior is related to side effects of medications, whether he or she is in pain or not getting enough sleep or is frightened, depressed, bored, etc. or whether the dementia is simply getting worse. Much of this can be learned from a physical and psychiatric exam. Followup laboratory work may also help shed light on underlying causes (such as a urinary tract infection). The caregiver's expectations and any social or cultural issues, such as economic status, education level, ethnic traditions and religious beliefs, of the caregiver and patient might also be examined.

• **C...reate.** Together, the caregiver and health-care provider—with participation from the patient, if possible—create a plan for positive change. The plan begins with the health-care provider addressing problems discovered during the investigation. For example, a medication might be discontinued if it is thought to be causing a behavioral side effect...pain management might be started if pain is the issue...more intensive psychiatric care might begin and any other newly discovered health need of the patient will be attended to.

The caregiver will be directed toward education resources and support groups, and the caregiver and health-care provider will work together to improve communication with the patient, simplify caregiver tasks, create structured routines and establish meaningful activities for the patient (such as revival of a hobby or participation in an adult day-care program) to help minimize his or her boredom, frustration, fear or other difficult emotions.

• **E...valuate.** The health-care provider then evaluates the plan as time goes by. Is the caregiver using it? Is it working? If so, great! If not, a reassessment takes place to tweak and optimize the plan.

A SIMPLE EXAMPLE IN PRACTICE

This example illustrates a problem situation that DICE is meant to address.

Imagine that you're the caregiver of a relative—maybe your mom—with Alzheimer's disease. You're preparing to bathe her and think you are being gentle as you lower her into a tub, but she physically and verbally lashes out at you, exclaiming that she's in pain. Well,

you've been through this before with her and think that she's intentionally giving you a hard time. How could she possibly be in pain? You were handling her with kid gloves!

These misunderstood problem behaviors also referred to as noncognitive neuropsychiatric symptoms, are often so stressful for caregivers that families sometimes put loved ones in nursing homes much sooner than they really want to.

With the DICE approach, you would relate the event in detail during an appointment with a specialist trained in dementia care. The specialist would get you thinking about what might be causing this repeated problem and would also get your mother's take on the situation. The specialist would arrange for Mom's physical and psychiatric evaluation and, in examining her living space, might question you about whether the tub has grab bars, nonslip mats or other fixtures that would make bathing less stressful for her.

Suppose that, during the physical examination, it's discovered that your mother has arthritis but isn't on medication for it. The specialist explains that Mom means it when she says she's in pain. Pain medication is prescribed, and your mother is referred for physical therapy. Meanwhile, you get to work outfitting the bathroom and other parts of the home to make them more user friendly for your mother. The specialist also provides you with educational counseling, reading material and referrals to support resources to help you better understand what your mother is going through...and to help you feel less alone.

PLAYING WITH THE DICE APPROACH

The DICE approach is only recently being rolled out in a formal way. Its real value and feasibility won't be fully known until its use becomes more widespread and clinical trials are completed to scientifically prove its value, ease of use and cost effectiveness. If you would like to try the DICE approach, start by asking your loved one's health-care providers whether they are familiar with it—they may be able to refer you to a specialist or a practice that provides a similar service. Also contact a geriatric psychiatrist, whose training makes it more likely that he or she will apply an approach similar to DICE when working with dementia patients and their caregivers. You might even find that some or all of this is covered by insurance, depending on your loved one's coverage.

Music and Cooking Help Behavioral Problems in Alzheimer's Patients…

Pauline Narme, MD, Neuropsychology of Aging, Paris Descartes University, Boulogne-Billancourt, in collaboration with the University of Lille and the University Medical Center of Reims, all in France.

Dealing with a loved one who is agitated and aggressive is never easy—but it's especially tough when that person has Alzheimer's disease and can no longer understand what is "appropriate" behavior and what isn't. Such behavioral issues are very common in Alzheimer's patients…and medication helps little while potentially causing side effects.

This places a tremendous burden on family caregivers. In fact, behavioral problems are a primary reason why people with Alzheimer's end up in nursing homes. And even if you're just visiting your loved one in a nursing home rather than delivering around-the-clock care yourself, it's still upsetting to witness and try to deal with that person's distress.

So what can be done about these difficult behavioral issues? According to a recent study, activities involving music and cooking can help patients and their caregivers. *Here's why…*

ENGAGING THROUGH SONG AND FOOD

Forty-eight nursing home residents with moderate-to-severe Alzheimer's disease were randomly assigned to one of two group-activity programs—music or cooking. The goal was to see whether either or both programs would help reduce behavioral problems in patients and ease caregiver stress.

Before beginning the programs, each resident's caregiver (the nursing home staff member assigned to that resident) completed a questionnaire. The point was to gauge the frequency and severity of the patient's problem behaviors—including aggression, agitation, delusions, disinhibition (loss of inhibitions that would normally govern behavior) and sleep abnormalities (frequent awakenings, sleeping during the day instead of at night, etc.)…and to measure how much emotional or psychological distress the patient's behavior caused for the caregiver. The higher the scores, the worse the problems. The questionnaire was repeated halfway through the programs and four weeks after the programs ended. The caregivers did not know which program the residents were enrolled in. (Though this study looked at professional caregivers, it's reasonable to suppose that family caregivers—who typically would have less caregiving training and a deeper emotional attachment—would experience even greater stress when trying to manage a loved one's behavioral problems.)

Two one-hour sessions were held each week for four weeks. In the music group, CDs were played featuring classical music and popular songs from the 1950s through 1980s. Participants were encouraged to listen, sing along and/or keep the beat on a small drum. In the cooking group, all participants cooperated in preparing various foods—for instance, by measuring, mixing, etc.—depending on their capabilities. Participants were invited to express their feelings and to recall memories that were evoked by the music or the food preparation.

The results were encouraging. Both programs helped reduce the severity of behavioral disorders and caregiver distress, with the music program being especially effective. *Specifically, in terms of…*

●**Severity of patients' behavioral problems.** In the music group, patients' average score improved by 74% during the program… and four weeks after the program ended, there was still a 37% improvement. In the cooking group, the patients' average behavioral score improved by 57%…and four weeks after the program ended, there was still a 32% improvement.

• **Caregiver distress levels.** Among caregivers of patients in the music group, the average distress score improved by 78% during the program…and four weeks after the program ended, there was still a 44% improvement. In the cooking group, caregivers' average distress score improved by 65% during the program…and four weeks after the program ended, there was still a 34% improvement.

MUSIC TO THEIR EARS

According to the Alzheimer's Foundation of America, music has the power to improve patients' mood and cognitive function and to stimulate positive interaction because the part of the brain that responds to auditory cues requires little cognitive functioning. That's why, even in advanced dementia, the ability to engage in music by singing along may remain intact.

Although this study showed greater benefits from music than from cooking, the benefits from the cooking were significant…and it's possible that a patient who had a lifelong interest in cooking would respond more positively to a cooking activity than to a music activity.

Advice for caregivers: The supervisors who led the programs in this study were not professional music therapists or chefs—and in fact, one of the researchers' goals was to look for nonmedical care strategies that could easily be adapted for use at home by family caregivers. So why not try re-creating the programs' positive effects yourself when you're with the Alzheimer's patient you care for?

For instance, play some CDs when you're together, choosing a style of music that is familiar and soothing, and encouraging your loved one to sing, clap or drum along to the tune. Or spend time together in the kitchen, preparing a simple recipe (such as pancakes) and inviting your loved one to handle safe and easy tasks, such as measuring, mixing and pouring. You might include other family members, too, to more closely duplicate the social aspect of the study's group activities. You may end up doing everyone involved a world of good.

How Healing Hands Provide Sleep for Dementia Patients

Michael Reed Gach, PhD, founder of Acupressure.com. He is based in Kihei, Hawaii, and is author of numerous books and self-healing CDs on the topic of acupressure and health, including the fully guided CD *Sleep Better.*

If you live with someone who has Alzheimer's disease or another type of dementia, he or she may be keeping you up at night—even keeping you up all night—with restlessness just as a newborn baby would. But the feeling of dealing with an Alzheimer's patient overnight is worlds apart from that of dealing with a beautiful new baby's nighttime fussing. In fact, it can be maddening, exhausting and frustrating for caregivers.

Difficulty falling or staying asleep as well as "sundowning" (becoming agitated in the late afternoon or early evening) are common among people with dementia. Although medication can help calm agitation in a person with dementia, it won't necessarily improve his or her sleep quality. In fact, medication for sleep can make patients drowsy at the wrong times and unsteady on their feet, causing falls. It also can increase confusion and reduce a patient's self-care abilities. But there is a safe, effective nondrug technique that can relieve dementia-related sleep problems—acupressure. And if you are a caregiver, you can easily learn it and do it at home.

Acupressure is based on the same principles as acupuncture—but no needles are used. Acupressure simply involves using the fingers and hands to press certain parts of a person's body. The pressure is applied to meridian points, a highway of human energy flow, explained Michael Reed Gach, PhD, acupressure educator and founder of Acupressure.com, an online hub for self-healing. Acupressure can release stress and tension, increase circulation and reduce pain—all of which leads, as you might imagine, to better sleep.

PROVEN TO IMPROVE SLEEP

Acupressure was recently shown, in a scientific study from Turin, Italy, to relieve sleep problems in nursing home residents who had insomnia and either Alzheimer's disease or mild cognitive impairment (a mild form of dementia that may or may not worsen to full-blown dementia). The study included 129 people between the ages of 69 and 96 who received acupressure on a pressure point called HT7 every day for eight weeks. (To find HT7, follow a line on the palm side of the hand from the space between the little finger and ring finger to the crease where the hand and wrist meet.) Residents were much better able to fall asleep and stay asleep and also got more overall hours of sleep when they had acupressure treatment. Plus, the need to use sedative drugs for sleep among these residents decreased.

ACUPRESSURE TECHNIQUES FOR YOU

Although having some formal training in acupressure is ideal, anyone can learn the basics of this hands-on therapy to help another person—including a person with dementia. *Here is some guidance from Dr. Gach to improve sleep…*

When the person with dementia is in bed and ready for sleep, sit beside him or her and…

• **Locate the two main acupressure points for relief of agitation, anxiety and sleep problems.** These are HT7 (the spot on the wrist in line with the space between the little finger and ring finger) and a spot on the forearm, called P6, that's in line with the middle finger but about two inches (three fingers' width) below the wrist.

• **Apply firm, steady pressure to each point, one after the other** (which point is first doesn't matter), using a finger, thumb or, if you have arthritis that makes this uncomfortable, a knuckle. For P6, Dr. Gach suggests clasping the person's forearm so that you press your thumb on the P6 point while pressing your fingertips into the corresponding spot on the other side of the arm.

How much pressure to apply? It should be the kind that "hurts good," similar to the kind of smarting relief you feel from a nice massage of sore muscles. Although it mildly hurts, it also feels good. So when doing acupressure on a person with dementia, you will have to carefully observe and patiently ask the person about his or her comfort level and not go be-

yond it. (Explaining that this "massage" will help with sleep can be a good strategy, too.)

• **Hold the pressure for two to three minutes on each spot,** and, if possible, encourage the patient to breathe slowly and deeply. "But even if the patient doesn't understand what acupressure is or why you are doing it, it will still have the desired effect," said Dr. Gach. "The body will respond even if the brain doesn't fully comprehend the purpose of it."

Also, although you might think anxiety and aggression are symptoms that might get in the way of giving acupressure to a person with dementia, studies have shown that acupressure and similar hands-on healing techniques, such as massage therapy, are well-tolerated and symptom-relieving solutions for people with dementia. In addition to improving sleep, acupressure relieves anxiety and agitation and decreases aggression and combativeness.

EMPOWER YOURSELF

Of course, you can use these acupressure techniques on anyone, including yourself, to help the body naturally fall asleep and sleep well. But these techniques are particularly empowering for caregivers of people with dementia, who may feel helpless in the face of a disease that can only get worse, said Dr. Gach. "Even if you can't stop the disease or reverse it, you can at least be empowered to help with the symptoms."

"Golden Oldies" Trigger Memories for Dementia Patients

Concetta M. Tomaino, DA, MT-BC LCAT, executive director/cofounder, Institute for Music and Neurologic Function, senior vice president, music therapy services, CenterLight Health System, Bronx, New York. She is past president of the American Association for Music Therapy.

You've surely had this experience—you're driving somewhere and a song from 20 or 30 years ago comes on the radio…and you remember every word. Not only that, it brings to mind a host of great memories, too.

Music therapists at CenterLight Health System in the Bronx are using old-time tunes in this way to help people with dementia sharpen their memories. Here, Concetta M. Tomaino, DA, director of the Institute for Music and Neurologic Function (IMNF) tells more, including how families of dementia patients might be able to use this technique on their own.

MUSICAL MEMORIES

Music can serve as a gateway into the brain that actually stimulates its function. In one study at the University of California at Irvine, researchers found that listening to Mozart helped Alzheimer's patients improve their scores on memory tests. And, in a study conducted by Dr. Tomaino and her colleagues and published in *Music and Medicine*, 45 patients with mid- to late-stage dementia who participated in a music-based reminiscence program three times a week for 10 months boosted their scores on cognitive function tests by 50%. After several sessions, one patient even recognized his wife for the first time in many months.

Music can reach people who are unreachable by other means. Often an Alzheimer's patient who cannot recall a close family member's name is able to summon the words of a favorite old song and recapture seemingly lost memories. Sometimes therapists stop singing and patients fill in the words...and some are even able to learn new songs. At Beth Abraham, music therapists most commonly use music from patients' teen years and early 20s, finding that listening to these familiar tunes can help them to...

• **Improve memory and cognitive skills.**

• **Increase attention, motivation, focus and awareness of self and others.**

• **Reduce agitation.**

• **Perform daily activities such as eating, toileting and bathing.**

USE AN IPOD AND TRY IT YOURSELF

Aging patients don't need formal music therapy to reap benefits from listening to music from the past. The Institute for Music and Neurologic Function's international Music and Memory program (MusicAndMemory.org)

provides custom-tailored playlists for people who have memory impairment. (People must provide their own MP3 player or iPod.) Favorites from the 1940s, for example, that you might want on your list include "Unforgettable," "Some Enchanted Evening" and "Que Sera, Sera."

You can play old-time music as often as your loved one seems to enjoy it—but whatever type of music you choose and however you play it, try to listen together. Even fleetingly, you can recapture a sense of closeness by singing together, holding hands, dancing or just quietly listening to the music and enjoying the memories it unlocks.

Finally…There's a Way to Connect with a Loved One Who Has Dementia

Gerontologist Tom Brenner, MA, cofounder, with his wife, Karen Brenner, MA, of Brenner Pathways, a consulting and educational company in Chicago that specializes in the Montessori Method for Positive Dementia Care. He and his wife are also coauthors of *You Say Goodbye and We Say Hello: The Montessori Method for Positive Dementia Care.*

Henry had been diagnosed with early-onset Alzheimer's and was quiet and withdrawn. When he was younger, he had collected vintage cars, so his caregiver gave him some old hubcaps and polish. After 30 minutes of polishing, Henry began talking with a great deal of emotion about his time as a soldier. Perhaps the process of polishing the hubcaps reminded him of polishing his boots, and an important memory was triggered. This activity enabled Henry and his caregiver to connect, even if only for a short time.

One of the most heartbreaking and frustrating aspects of caring for a loved one with dementia is the loss of meaningful interaction.

But there's good news on this front: The Montessori Method for Positive Dementia Care, a nondrug approach (often used in combination with medication), is now being used by some caregivers in home-care settings and nursing homes with dramatic results.

Through basic Montessori principles (see below), this method offers ways to be in the moment with a dementia patient and possibly have a deep connection. Patients become more secure, confident and calm. And caregivers are less likely to get frustrated and burn out.

Recent research: In a study involving nine residential facilities in Melbourne, Australia, dementia patients were two times more actively engaged when participating in Montessori-based activities than when they were not doing these activities.

Background: Developed more than 100 years ago as a method of teaching "unreachable" children with learning disabilities, the Montessori approach encourages the use of all five senses to stimulate different areas of the brain and the use of "muscle memory"* to develop small-muscle coordination and promote confidence. The Montessori method also advocates an environment that meets the specific physical and emotional needs of those using it.

Montessori classrooms for children are uncluttered but homey and filled with natural light and materials to promote use of the senses. Students are free to move about and engage in activities that appeal most to them. This sets the stage for focused and calm activity. Research has shown that Montessori pupils learn to excel at problem solving, adapting to change and social skills—all areas that are difficult for adults with dementia.

Key Montessori tenets and how they can help dementia patients...

•**Emphasis on environment.** The surroundings of the dementia patient should be familiar and comforting and designed to foster as much independence as possible. For example, the layout of a facility, or your home if a loved one is living with you, should be uncomplicated so there is less potential for confusion.

•**Muscle memory stimulation.** While the mind of a dementia patient might be faltering, the muscles often "remember" how to do an activity that was done repetitively and enjoyably in the past. The key is to discover a patient's unique strengths, passions and interests—not only tapping muscle memory but strong emotions as well. Focusing on a physical task and having success helps dementia patients feel more secure and confident and less angry and agitated.

A caregiver might take a former golfer to the driving range to jump-start his/her muscle memory. Or a long-retired handyman might be given a toolbox with a tape measure, paintbrushes and a level so that he can tinker.

These activities also build muscle coordination and can simply make life more pleasant and enriching for a dementia patient.

•**Sharing stories.** This is one of the most effective tools for helping dementia sufferers stay connected. Moments when patients share their stories, even if the time is fleeting, can enable the patient and caregiver to feel a deep connection, boosting the patient's sense of security.

To encourage a patient to share a story: A caregiver might give him a meaningful object to hold—something important from the patient's life or an object from nature. This simple act can help spark a memory and get the patient talking.

•**Art therapy.** Painting, singing and playing an instrument can provide patients new avenues of self-expression and strengthen their spirits. These activities also can give patients the opportunity to engage their senses.

Good activity: Flower arranging. Patients are encouraged to feel and smell the flowers, cut stems and pour water. This exercise calls on small motor skills, essential for independence and range of motion. Key areas of the brain are also exercised when deciding how to arrange the flowers.

•**The Knobbed Cylinder.** This classic Montessori tool—a long wooden block with 10 different-sized holes in which the user places matching cylinders—builds focus and small-muscle coordination. Dementia patients might be asked to fill only two holes—the point is

---

*Sometimes called procedural memory, this involves physical movements fixed into memory through repetition (think of riding a bike or playing a musical instrument).

for the patient to feel success and build confidence through this activity.

•**Finish a phrase.** Old sayings may never leave our minds. With this technique, the caregiver holds up the first half of a statement on a piece of paper ("The whole nine…") and asks the patient to finish the saying ("…yards"). It's astonishing to see dementia sufferers suddenly become very vocal and involved.

Benefits for the caregivers: The Montessori method gives the caregiver more tools to care for a dementia patient. It encourages the caregiver to use his imagination and allows him to act more like a guide than a director. Plus, patients are less agitated and aggressive, so they are easier to be with. All this helps minimize caregiver burnout and frustration.

How to Talk to Those with Dementia so They Can Hear You

Kristine N. Williams, RN, PhD, former associate professor, University of Kansas School of Nursing, Kansas City, Kansas.

Have you noticed how loudly some people talk when attempting to communicate with a person who doesn't speak English? They seem to think turning up the volume will bridge the language gap. Similarly it is common for many, including trained professional caregivers, to use "elderspeak" with people who are old and infirm. It sounds a lot like baby talk, with simplified grammar and vocabulary and liberal use of terms of endearment, such as honey, sweetie and dearie. Though it may be done with the best intentions, a recent study finds that when elderly patients are spoken to in this way, they often become angry, less responsive and harder to care for.

The study, led by researcher Kristine N. Williams, RN, PhD, while she was an associate professor at the University of Kansas School of Nursing, videotaped interactions between

caregivers (nursing assistants, nurses, therapists and social workers) and 20 nursing home residents with moderate dementia. Using a measure called the "Resistiveness to Care Scale" to quantify the intensity of care-disrupting behaviors (acts of withdrawal or aggression, such as grabbing onto a person or pulling one's own limbs tightly into the body, hitting, crying and kicking), researchers reviewed the tapes. When they witnessed such episodes, they rewound the tapes to see what kind of communications occurred in the preceding seven seconds. Often (55% of the time), it turned out that the caregivers had been using "elderspeak," compared with the 26% of the time these behaviors arose when caregivers used normal adult communication. It seemed that the elders objected to being talked to in this childlike way. The researchers hypothesized that this form of communication sends a negative message of incompetence, which ends up irritating rather than soothing listeners.

RESPECT YOUR ELDERS

The National Institute on Aging and Dr. Williams offer these tips for communicating with those who have Alzheimer's disease or dementia…

•**Before speaking,** gain the person's full attention. Use his/her name.

•**While interacting,** turn off distractions such as the TV or radio.

•**Speak in a tone that is calm and gentle, without infantilizing.** Dr. Williams also points out that nonverbal cues such as establishing eye contact convey your focus and willingness to communicate.

•**Use simple words and short, clear sentences**—but not baby talk.

•**If someone is having trouble finding the right words,** it's fine to help him/her out by gently making suggestions.

•**Be patient,** providing ample time to think and respond. It is important to give people with dementia time to compose and communicate their thoughts, says Dr. Williams. When you are patient, it shows you believe that what they have to say is important and that you are paying attention to them.

•**Do not talk about a person with AD or dementia in front of him/her as if he/she was not present.**

It's not so hard, actually. It's pretty much all about treating every human with dignity, no matter what their cognitive ability.

When a Patch Is Better Than a Pill—Topical Meds Often Are Safer for Alzheimer's

Jack E. Fincham, PhD, RPh, a registered pharmacist and professor in the division of pharmacy practice and administration at the University of Missouri, Kansas City, where he is also an adjunct professor in the Bloch School of Management.

If you take medication, chances are it's a pill. But topical versions of many widely used drugs (in the form of patches or a topical gel or cream) are often more effective—and safer—than pills.

What's new: Topical medications now are available to treat a wide range of conditions, including high blood pressure, chest pain (angina), depression, Alzheimer's disease and hormonal deficiencies.

Why use a patch? Let's say you have arthritis and often take a nonsteroidal anti-inflammatory drug (NSAID), such as *ibuprofen* (Motrin) or *diclofenac* (Voltaren), to control pain. If you experience gastric bleeding—a side effect of NSAIDs and a common reason for hospitalization—the topical version of the drug may be a much better choice for you.

Medicated patches also are a good choice for patients with swallowing difficulties… those who forget to take their pills…or those who can benefit from steady dosing.

WHY THE SKIN?

The skin is one of the best organs for administering drugs into the bloodstream, where the drug's active ingredients are then distributed throughout the body. With oral medications, the active ingredient is metabolized (broken down) in the digestive tract, liver and kidneys, which often leads to side effects. While topicals also pass through the liver and kidneys, they don't go through the digestive tract. *Advantages of topical medications…*

•**Lower doses.** When you take an oral medication, some of the active ingredient may be destroyed by acids in the digestive tract or reduced when broken down in the liver and kidneys. In fact, with some oral drugs, only about 10% of the active ingredient reaches its intended target—the bloodstream, then a specific organ or system. As a result, you must take a high dose to offset losses. Higher doses mean more complications and side effects.

•**Fewer side effects.** Topical medications are not risk-free. But side effects are typically limited to minor skin irritation. Oral medication side effects are a major cause of hospitalization and sometimes even death.

Example: Topical medications can be helpful for patients who need narcotic painkillers. Oral narcotics often cause constipation and stomach upset. Patches are much less likely to cause these types of side effects.

•**Steadier dosing.** When you take an oral drug, you achieve a high initial blood concentration of the active ingredient. Then, the levels slowly decline until you take the next dose. With a patch, drug levels are more evenly sustained throughout the day—or even for days at a time.

Time-released oral medications can mimic this effect, but they're unpredictable. Many factors—the acid in your stomach, what you've eaten, etc.—can affect how quickly the medication is released. There's less variability with patches.

•**More convenient.** It's estimated that 55% of older adults don't take their medications the way they're supposed to—because of forgetfulness or limited mobility, for example. Some patches can be applied once a week. It's easier to remember once-a-week dosing than multiple daily pills.

Downside: The main drawback of topicals is the cost. They are more expensive than pills because they're more complicated to manufacture.

PATCHES NOW AVAILABLE

Medicated patches you should know about...*

•*Clonidine* **(Catapres-TTS) patch for high blood pressure.** Because it is applied just once a week, it is much easier to use—and easier to remember—than daily oral drugs.

•*Deponit* **for angina.** Patients who have angina due to coronary artery disease can take a nitroglycerin tablet for quick relief. Deponit, the same medication used in patch form, delivers a steady dose of the medication and can prevent these attacks from happening. It is applied for 12 to 14 hours at a time, with 10 to 12 hours off.

•**Exelon patch for mild-to-moderate Alzheimer's disease.** This patch, applied once every 24 hours, provides the same benefits as the equivalent oral drug *rivastigmine* (Exelon), with less nausea and/or vomiting.

Check first with your doctor if you have heart or lung disease, bladder problems or seizures—the Exelon patch may worsen these conditions. Caregivers often prefer the patch because they can see that they have given the medication.

•*Oxybutynin* **(Oxytrol) for overactive bladder.** Applied twice weekly, this medicated patch helps patients achieve better control by inhibiting involuntary contractions of the bladder. It is less likely than the oral medication to cause other side effects such as constipation or dry mouth.

•**Testosterone patch,** applied once every 24 hours—generally between 8 pm and midnight to match a man's daily hormonal cycles. Men who suffer from fatigue, low libido or other symptoms of testosterone deficiency can use a patch (Androderm or Testoderm) that delivers a steady supply of the hormone—with less risk for liver damage than oral drugs.

*Talk to your doctor if you take any medications (patches could interact with them). Some patches, such as Catapres-TTS, contain aluminum and have been reported to cause skin burns during MRI. Remove patches before MRIs.

Better Mealtimes for Dementia Patients

Family-style meals with caregivers and others can help prevent dehydration and weight loss in dementia patients, a recent study of more than 2,200 people with the disease has found. Patients ate and drank more and were less likely to become agitated when they weren't alone.

Other ways to manage mealtime: Spend more time at the table, play soothing music and talk with the person who has dementia.

Lee Hooper, PhD, senior lecturer in research synthesis & nutrition, University of East Anglia, Norwich, UK.

The Healing Power of Animals

Bill Benda, MD, an emergency medicine physician at Big Sur Health Center and Mee Memorial Hospital in King City, California.

We've all seen those highly trained, four-legged helpers assist a blind person in navigating a street crossing.

What's new: Scientists now are discovering that dogs and other types of animals can actually help promote the healing process in people with a wide range of medical conditions... even Alzheimer's. Sound far-fetched?

So-called animal-assisted therapy (AAT) is also increasingly incorporating an even broader range of animals. For example, horseback riding is being used by people with health problems such as multiple sclerosis and Parkinson's disease. Even rabbits, llamas, birds and other types of animals are being used to promote physical, emotional and social well-being.

WHY IT HELPS

Support for the therapeutic effects of animals continues to grow...

Landmark findings: Among 92 patients hospitalized for a heart condition or heart attack, only 6% of pet (mostly dog) owners died within one year of discharge, versus 28% of people who did not own pets. In a study of 48 New York City stockbrokers, those who owned a dog or a cat had half the increase in blood pressure associated with stressful situations as those without pets.

More recently, research focusing specifically on AAT suggests that interacting with animals may have salutary effects because it increases levels of the hormone oxytocin, which is believed to have powerful effects on the body's ability to heal and grow new cells.

HOW IT WORKS

With AAT, the animals are not there to simply play with the patients. Instead, the animal, whose temperament has been evaluated by a national animal therapy organization, helps a patient achieve specific treatment goals.

For example, a physical therapist may use a dog (owned by a volunteer who has participated in training or, in some cases, the facility where the therapy takes place) to help a stroke patient regain the ability to stand and walk. The stroke patient may walk the dog for short distances (the dog owner may use a double-handle leash to accompany the dog and patient).

AAT can help reduce agitation and depression in Alzheimer's patients, and it can curb a cancer patient's perception of pain and fatigue.

Patients who have AAT receive individualized treatment plans with the animal…sessions are scheduled at set intervals…and the health-care provider makes notes on the progress that is made by the patient during each session. In some cases, AAT may be covered as part of a physical therapy program.

GETTING STARTED

If you would like to try AAT, speak to your doctor. If he/she gives you the go-ahead, contact Pet Partners (formerly Delta Society), 425-679-5500, PetPartners.org. This nonprofit organization, which registers therapy animals and their owners, can help you locate a facility that offers AAT.

People who are not able to leave their homes may also receive AAT. A family member or health-care provider should contact Pet Partners for a referral to a trained animal

owner who provides AAT on a volunteer basis. In these instances, therapy visits should be arranged and overseen by a home health-care provider.

Important: If you have reduced immunity—for example, due to an autoimmune disease or if you are on chemotherapy, high-dose steroids or other immune-suppressive medications—AAT may not be appropriate for you.

Animals that participate in AAT are required to be clean and well groomed and must undergo a thorough veterinary checkup. However, patients with reduced immunity often are advised to limit unnecessary contact with animals—and humans—to help them avoid exposure to infectious agents.

With Dementia, a Little Humor Goes a Long Way

The late Peter Spitzer, MB BS, Churchill Fellow, a physician in private practice, and medical director and cofounder of the Humour Foundation, Australia.

The sad truth is that dementia patients don't just lose their mental acuity—many also lose control of their behavior. As many as 70% to 80% experience agitation, symptoms of which include irritability, pacing, rummaging, yelling, cursing, hitting, biting and kicking. These symptoms are often treated with antipsychotic medications, but such drugs have terrible side effects, including sudden death in dementia patients. And while the drugs may indeed quell symptoms of agitation, they don't seem to make patients feel any happier—and, after all, shouldn't that also be a goal?

The good news is that a recent Australian study presented at the National Dementia Research Forum in Sydney, Australia, has shown that humor therapy can reduce symptoms of agitation in patients with mild-to-severe dementia and do it with no side effects. And it seemed to make them happier.

A STUDY THAT MAKES YOU SMILE

Mainstream humor—like the kind that dementia patients see on TV sitcoms and talk shows—doesn't really connect with them, according to Peter Spitzer, MD, medical director and cofounder of the Humour Foundation. So health-care workers had to "find the key that would open the door to the patients' humor." During each session, the workers would wear red clown noses and attempt to engage patients by using mime, music, massage, touch, stories and magic tricks. In many cases, they would ask a simple question like, "Which way is the bathroom?"…and then, after the patient gave the correct answer, the worker would play the fool and purposefully walk in the wrong direction. This might elicit a laugh—but there was another positive effect, too. For patients who have already lost so much independence, this type of humorous play can give them a brief but uplifting sense of personal power and control, said Dr. Spitzer.

The study didn't just make patients smile—its results made the researchers smile. Immediately after 12 weeks of humor therapy—and even six months after treatment ended—frequency of overall patient agitation as measured by standard psychological surveys was down by 20%, on average, compared with measurements taken at the beginning of the study. Since the patient population included some people who were already being treated for agitation with antipsychotic meds, the results are promising—especially because they seem to last, which is remarkable. "These findings suggest that humor therapy may be as effective as antipsychotic drugs in reducing agitation—while providing more happiness and no dangerous side effects," said Dr. Spitzer. Controlled studies that compare antipsychotic medications to humor therapy need to be done in the future.

MAKE A PATIENT LAUGH

Right now, one of the few organizations in the US providing humor therapy for seniors in nursing homes is Big Apple Circus's Vaudeville Caravan in Chicago and Montrose, New York. Dr. Spitzer suspects that as more "psychosocial" research is done with dementia pa-

tients, more resources will become available. Dr. Spitzer added that humor therapy could be effective in a residential setting, too. So if you're caring for a dementia patient at home who has agitation, Dr. Spitzer said to try goofy humor to play and ease symptoms—even if you don't have formal training—so you can bring a smile to your loved one's face.

Could Dementia Villages Come to the US?

Dayne DuVall, LMT, CAEd, CRTS, certified Alzheimer educator and former chief operating officer, National Certification Board for Alzheimer Care, Chicago.

Amazing things happen when people with dementia have the freedom to do things they enjoy, in familiar environments, surrounded by people who watch out for them and help them feel accepted.

In the Netherlands, a dementia village has become an international model of what can happen when people with dementia are given extraordinary freedom in a safe, structured environment. Meanwhile, in England and now in the US, many communities are exploring ways to become dementia-friendly so that people at earlier stages of memory-robbing conditions can remain actively involved in social and cultural activities.

Contrast that to what typically happens: We care for loved ones at home for as long as possible, and then the alternative is often an assisted-living facility or a nursing home. But when loved ones get there, they are often isolated, lonely, scared and oversedated—all of which accelerates their cognitive and physical decline. Assisted-living facilities are now what nursing homes used to be, and nursing homes are really hospitals.

A NEW MODEL: A VILLAGE BUILT FOR PEOPLE WITH DEMENTIA

Imagine an environment where someone with dementia can leave his house and take a walk whenever he wants, shop, take in a movie and eat with neighbors in a family-style dining room. The town looks like the kind of place he may have once lived in.

That's the experience in Hogewey in the Netherlands, a residential facility outside Amsterdam where elderly people with dementia live in a seemingly normal community, complete with parks, a grocery store, a restaurant, a theatre, post office, barbershop and other amenities. The residents are generally people with "moderate-stage" dementia.

Although they are restricted to the facility's grounds, the 152 residents are free to roam around the community, which has on-site geriatric nurses and caregivers dressed in street clothes who provide around-the-clock care. The residents live in groups of six to eight to a home, with one or two caretakers on site. Residents also manage their own homes, including cooking, cleaning and laundry—with some help. For safety's sake, cameras monitor the residents 24/7, and there's only one door in and out of "town," so there's little risk that residents will wander off the premises.

To some, it's a little disquieting to have a community where residents are essentially deceived into believing that they are living in a normal community—a real-life version of *The Truman Show*, as it were. But the benefits are that residents can maintain social engagement and much more independence. "There has to be some oversight—somebody has to be monitoring what's going on," says Dayne DuVall, LMT, CAEd, CRTS, a certified Alzheimer educator. "To me, the simulation connotes safety."

The benefits are many. Research shows that putting people with dementia into environments that mimic their familiar, formative experiences helps them cope better. So Hogeway mimics traditional towns from 50 or so years ago. There are even living clusters for different lifestyles such as urban, homemaker, trade/craft, upper class…and Indonesian.

According to CNN's chief medical correspondent Sanjay Gupta, MD, whose reporting helped create international interest in the Hogewey model, the residents take fewer medications and eat better than others of the same age and condition—and live longer, too. "On a mental level, they also seem to have more joy," he reported. "It's a difficult thing to measure, but that is the most important thing here at Hogewey."

WHAT WE CAN LEARN FROM HOGEWEY

The Hogewey model has inspired international interest. There are dementia villages being planned in Switzerland, England and Canada—and in Florida, where the Miami Jewish Health Systems is actively planning a Hogeway-like expansion of their dementia care facilities.

There are obstacles to widespread adoption of the model here, however. The primary one is cost. It's very expensive. In the Netherlands, Hogewey is heavily subsidized by the government, which covered almost all of the nearly $25 million dollars it cost to build and subsidizes operating expenses, too. Even then, the families of residents need to pay as much as $3,600 a month. In the US, a dementia village on that scale may be affordable only for the rich.

But sometimes, great ideas create change in surprising ways. The example of a more humane way to treat people with dementia, one that gives them more freedom and dignity than was thought possible, is inspiring. And it's just one example…many communities in the US are striving to find better ways to provide care. There may be elements of the Hogewey model—environments that mimic an earlier time, professionally staffed movie theaters that look like the real thing—that assisted-living facilities may adopt.

CHAPTER 5

Help for Cancer and Other Brain Dangers

How a Top Brain Doc Protects His Own Brain from Cancer

A large study that examined data over a 20-year period found that the incidence of brain tumors had increased by 200% in older adults. In children age 14 years and younger, primary brain tumors are now the most common cause of cancer. But is brain cancer really on the rise—or simply more likely to be detected? *A noted expert discusses the research and what he does to protect his own brain...*

IS THE INCREASE REAL?

CT scans are an important tool for diagnosing brain tumors. Before they were introduced in the 1970s, many patients with tumors might have been misdiagnosed as having strokes or other neurological diseases. The increased use of CT scans—along with MRIs and brain biopsies—may have caused an apparent increase in brain tumors.

Using research that took into account better imaging technology, scientists at the National Brain Tumor Registry concluded that the incidence of new tumors has remained stable. The National Cancer Institute Brain Tumor Study found a slight decrease in the incidence of brain tumors between 1990 and 2002.

However, the data is murky. There does appear to be an increase in brain tumors in some populations, but it still is unclear if this is due to better diagnostic tests or other factors (such as extended cell-phone use...see next page).

We know that secondary brain tumors (those that originate in other parts of the body) are about five times more common than primary tumors (ones that originate in the brain and tend to stay in the brain)—in part, because

Keith Black, MD, chairman of the department of neurosurgery and director of Maxine Dunitz Neurosurgical Institute at Cedars-Sinai Medical Center, Los Angeles. He is author, with Arnold Mann, of *Brain Surgeon: A Doctor's Inspiring Encounters with Mortality and Miracles.*

many people with cancer now are living long enough for the cancer to spread to the brain.

About 30% of those who die from breast cancer are later found to have evidence of brain cancer. With lung cancer, about 60% will be found at autopsy to have had the cancer spread to the brain.

REDUCE THE RISK

Primary brain cancers are relatively rare, accounting for about 2% of all cancers. The American Brain Tumor Association estimates that 26,000 malignant cases will be diagnosed in 2017. Sadly, only about one-third of patients with brain or other nervous system cancers survive more than five years.

Brain tumors are difficult to treat. Surgery isn't always possible or effective, because these tumors tend to grow rapidly and invade large areas of brain tissue. Unlike other blood vessels in the body, those in the brain are selective in what they allow to pass. This so-called blood-brain barrier makes it difficult to deliver chemotherapeutic drugs to brain tumors.

The causes of brain cancer are largely unknown, but there are some clear risk factors…

•**Dental X-rays.** Most dentists routinely use X-rays during checkups.

The danger: Radiation scatters and can potentially irradiate—and damage—brain cells. Even low-dose X-rays may increase the risk for gliomas (a type of brain tumor) and meningiomas (tumors that develop in the membranes that cover the brain and spinal cord).

I tell my dentist, flat-out, that I don't want X-rays. An occasional X-ray probably isn't harmful, but no one should get them routinely.

•**Air pollution.** At Cedars-Sinai, we're doing a study now to look at the association between air pollution and brain cancers. We see molecular changes in the brains of rats after three months of exposure to air pollution that are similar to the changes we see just prior to the development of brain cancer.

•**Electromagnetic radiation from cell phones, cellular antennas and the like.** A Swedish study found that the risk for brain cancer is 250% higher in those who used a cell phone for up to an hour a day for 10 years.

This is controversial. Other, shorter-term studies have found no risk from cell-phone use. But we know that it typically takes 20 to 30 years before toxic exposures lead to cancer. Cell phones haven't been around long enough to know what the long-term consequences might be. (See page 115 for more studies on cell phones and brain cancer.)

My advice: Use a wireless earpiece when talking on a cell phone. If you don't use an earpiece, hold the phone as far away from your head as possible. The amount of radiation that reaches the brain drops significantly with distance.

Caution: Children have thinner skulls than adults. It's easier for electromagnetic radiation from cell phones to penetrate a child's skull and reach the brain. It's possible that even low levels of electromagnetic radiation can produce cancer-causing changes in brain cells. Children and young adults should always use an earpiece.

•**Hot dogs and other processed meats usually contain nitrites,** substances that have been linked with brain tumors. I like a hot dog as much as anyone, but moderation is important. Also, whenever possible, buy nitrite-free hot dogs, bacon and other processed meats.

•**Heating plastic in the microwave.** There isn't direct evidence that using plastic containers in the microwave can increase brain tumors, but we know that the vinyl chloride in some plastics is a risk factor. Personally, I don't use plastic containers or cover foods with plastic wrap in the microwave.

Pregnant women should be especially careful. We've found in animal studies that adult females exposed to vinyl chloride or other carcinogens might not develop brain tumors themselves, but their offspring face a much higher risk.

Advice About Dental X-Rays

Keith Black, MD, chairman of the department of neurosurgery at Cedars-Sinai Medical Center in Los Angeles.

D oes your dentist take X-rays every time you get a checkup? If so, there's a recent study that you should know about.

Researchers from Yale and Brigham and Women's Hospital found that people (mean age 57) who received "bitewing" exams (using X-ray film held in place by a tab between the teeth) yearly or more frequently over their lifetimes were 50% more likely than a control group to develop a meningioma, a noncancerous brain tumor that can cause headaches, vision problems and loss of speech, during a five-year period. People who had been given "panorex" exams (X-rays that show all of the teeth on one film) one or more times a year had triple the risk.

It is true that modern dental X-rays use less radiation than in the past, but any exposure is risky.

"I go to the dentist two or three times a year, but haven't had an X-ray in probably 10 years," says Keith Black, MD, chairman of the department of neurosurgery at Cedars-Sinai Medical Center in Los Angeles. *Dr. Black's advice…*

• **Refuse "routine" X-rays.** If your dentist has examined your teeth and deemed them healthy, don't allow him/her to take an X-ray "just to be safe." Risk for a brain tumor increases with every X-ray.

• **Limit the exposure.** If you have a cavity or other problems, ask your dentist to X-ray only that area.

• **Less is more.** The American Dental Association recommends that adults get their teeth X-rayed every two to three years (children— one X-ray every one to two years). Unless your dentist needs to evaluate a specific problem or plan a procedure, you don't need an X-ray.

---

4 Supplements That Can Impair Your Brain

Cynthia Kuhn, PhD, professor of pharmacology, cancer biology, psychiatry and behavioral sciences at Duke University School of Medicine in Durham, North Carolina. Dr. Kuhn is also coauthor of *Buzzed: The Straight Facts About the Most Used and Abused Drugs from Alcohol to Ecstasy.*

I t is hardly news that supplements—just like drugs—can often cause physical side effects and reactions with prescribed medicines.

Recent development: Researchers are now learning more and more about unwanted mental changes that can occur when taking popular supplements (such as herbs and hormones).

These supplements can be a hidden cause of depression, anxiety, mania and other mental changes because patients—and their doctors—often don't realize how these products can affect the brain.

Supplements that may cause unwanted mental changes…

MELATONIN

Melatonin is among the most popular supplements for treating insomnia, jet lag and other sleep disorders. Melatonin is a natural hormone that's released by the pineal gland at night and readily enters the brain. Unlike many sleep aids, it doesn't render you unconscious or put you to sleep—it causes subtle brain changes that make you "ready" for sleep.

Studies have shown that people who take melatonin in the late afternoon or early evening tend to fall asleep more quickly when they go to bed. The amount of melatonin used in scientific studies ranges from 0.1 mg to 0.5 mg. However, the products in health-food stores typically contain much higher doses—usually 1 mg to 5 mg. Supplemental melatonin also may become less effective over time, which encourages people to increase the doses even more.

Effects on the brain: In people with depression, melatonin may improve sleep, but it may worsen their depression symptoms, according to the National Institutes of Health.

What to do: Melatonin can help when used short term for such problems as jet lag. It is not particularly effective as a long-term solution for other causes of insomnia.

ST. JOHN'S WORT

St. John's wort is probably the most studied herb for treating depression. Researchers who analyzed data from 29 international studies recently concluded that St. John's wort was as effective as prescription antidepressants for treating minor to moderate depression.

St. John's wort appears to be safe, particularly when it's used under the supervision of a physician. However, it can cause unwanted mental changes.

Effects on the brain: St. John's wort may increase brain levels of "feel good" neurotransmitters, including serotonin and dopamine. But unwanted mental changes that may occur in anyone taking St. John's wort include anxiety, irritability and vivid dreams. It may also lead to mania (a condition characterized by periods of overactivity, excessive excitement and lack of inhibitions)—especially in individuals who are also using antipsychotic drugs.

Caution: This supplement should never be combined with a prescription selective serotonin reuptake inhibitor (SSRI) antidepressant, such as *sertraline* (Zoloft) or *paroxetine* (Paxil). Taking St. John's wort with an SSRI can cause serotonin syndrome, excessive brain levels of serotonin that can increase body temperature, heart rate and blood pressure—conditions that are all potentially fatal. It also can interact with certain drugs such as oral contraceptives and immunosuppressant medications.

What to do: If you have depression, do not self-medicate with St. John's wort. Always talk to your doctor first if you are interested in trying this supplement.

TESTOSTERONE

Older men whose testosterone levels are declining (as is normal with aging) are often tempted to get a prescription for supplemental "T," which is advertised (but not proven) to improve their ability to get erections. Some women also use testosterone patches or gels (in much lower doses than men) to increase sexual desire and arousal.

Effects on the brain: If your testosterone is low, taking supplemental doses may cause a pleasant—but slight—increase in energy. However, with very high doses, such as those taken by bodybuilders, side effects may include aggression and mood swings. Men and women may experience withdrawal symptoms—such as depression and loss of appetite—when they stop taking it.

Testosterone replacement for men is FDA approved only for those with a clinical deficiency—defined as blood levels under 300 nanograms per deciliter (ng/dL).

What to do: Testosterone has been shown to increase sexual desire in women—it is not FDA approved for women but may be prescribed "off-label." The evidence supporting testosterone's ability to improve sexual function and well-being in normally aging men is weaker—unless they have been proven on more than one occasion to have low testosterone and related symptoms. Both men and women should take testosterone only under the supervision of a doctor.

WEIGHT-LOSS SUPPLEMENTS

Two ingredients that are commonly used in weight-loss supplements, beta-phenylethylamine (PEA) and P-synephrine, are said to increase energy and metabolism and burn extra calories.

Effects on the brain: Both PEA and P-synephrine (a compound found in supplements made from bitter orange) can make you feel jittery and anxious, particularly when they are combined with stimulants such as caffeine.

Many weight-loss and "energy" products are complicated cocktails of active ingredients that haven't been adequately studied—nor have they been approved by the FDA. They're risky because they've been linked to dangerous increases in blood pressure.

Important: There is little evidence that any of these products is particularly effective as a weight-loss aid.

What to do: Don't rely on weight-loss supplements. To lose weight, you need to decrease your food intake and increase your exercise levels—no supplement can accomplish that!

Can Your Cell Phone Cause Cancer?

Devra Davis, PhD, MPH, president of Environmental Health Trust, a nonprofit scientific and policy think tank focusing on cell-phone radiation. She is author of *Disconnect: The Truth About Cell Phone Radiation.* EHTrust.org

You may have heard that cell phones have been linked to cancer but wondered if that could really be true. A recent study offers strong evidence that this is the case—cell phones and other wireless devices emit a type of microwave radiation termed radiofrequency radiation (RFR) that can cause brain cancer and other cancers.

Here are the findings and what to do to minimize this risk to your health…

THE NEWEST EVIDENCE

The government's National Toxicology Program (NTP) conducts scientific studies on toxins to see how they might affect the health of Americans. More than 90 studies show that the radiation emitted by cell phones and other wireless devices can damage DNA, the first step on the road to cancer.

In May 2016, the NTP published preliminary results from a two-year animal study on the health effects of cell-phone radiation—this was the largest study on animals and cell-phone radiation ever published.

One out of every 12 of the animals studied were affected by the radiation. Some of those that were exposed to daily, frequent doses of cell-phone radiation from birth developed glioma, a rare, aggressive type of brain cancer already linked to cell-phone use in people. (Glial cells surround and support neurons.) Other animals had precancerous changes in glial cells. And some developed rare tumors of the nerves around and within the heart called schwannomas. In contrast, a control group of animals not exposed to wireless radiation had no gliomas, no precancerous changes in glial cells and no schwannomas.

There are two crucial takeaways from this recent study…

1. For decades, many scientists and governments have embraced the following scientific dogma—the only unsafe radiation is "thermal" radiation that heats tissue, such as an X-ray. "Nonthermal" RFR doesn't heat tissue and therefore is safe. The latest study—during which animals exposed to RFR were monitored to ensure that there was no heating of tissue—contradicts this dogma.

2. Epidemiological studies that analyze health data from hundreds of thousands of people have linked gliomas and schwannomas to long-term cell-phone use—and this latest study found the same type of cancers in animals exposed to wireless radiation, strengthening the link.

EVEN MORE DANGERS

Gliomas and schwannomas aren't the only dangers. *Research links wireless-device use to a range of other cancers, diseases and conditions…*

• **Meningioma.** A recent study published in *Oncology Reports* showed that heavy users of mobile and cordless phones had up to twice the risk for meningioma, cancer in the protective coverings that surround the brain.

• **Salivary gland (parotid) tumors.** Salivary glands are below the ear and in the jaw—exactly where many people hold cell phones during conversation. A study published in *American Journal of Epidemiology* showed a 58% higher risk for these (usually) noncancerous tumors among cell-phone users.

• **Acoustic neuroma.** Studies show that heavy or longtime users of cell phones have nearly triple the risk of developing acoustic neuromas (also called vestibular schwannomas), noncancerous tumors on the nerve that connects the inner ear to the brain. Symptoms can include gradual hearing loss and tinnitus in the affected ear, along with balance problems, headaches and facial numbness and tingling.

• **Breast cancer.** A study published in *Case Reports in Medicine* describes four young American women, ages 21 to 39, who had tucked their smartphones into their bras for up to 10 hours a day for several years. Each of them developed breast tumors directly under the antennas of their phones. None of the women had the cancer-causing BRAC1 or BRAC2 gene, a family history of cancer or any other known risk factors.

• **Male infertility and potency.** Several studies link close contact with wireless devices—wearing a cell phone on the hip or using a laptop computer on the lap—with fewer sperm, sluggish sperm, abnormally shaped sperm, sperm with damaged DNA and erectile dysfunction.

• **Sleeping problems.** Research shows that people who use cell phones and other wireless devices in the hours before bedtime have more trouble falling asleep and staying asleep. Both wireless radiation and the "blue light" from screens suppress melatonin, a sleep-inducing hormone.

HOW TO PROTECT YOURSELF

Every step you take to reduce radiation is protective because exposure to radiation is cumulative—the higher the exposure, the higher your risk for cancer and other health problems.

The devices you should be concerned about include cell phones, cordless phone handsets and bases, Wi-Fi routers, wireless computers, laptops, iPads and other tablets, smartwatches, wireless fitness bands, iPods that connect to the Internet, wireless speakers, cordless baby monitors, wireless game consoles and any other type of wireless device or equipment such as thermostats, security networks, sound systems and smart meters.

•**Keep it at a distance.** To decrease your exposure to wireless radiation, keep wireless devices as far away from you as possible. *Just a few inches can make a big difference…*

•Never put the phone next to your head. Instead, use the speakerphone function or a wired headset or an earpiece.

•Never place a turned-on device in a pocket or jacket or tucked into clothing. Keep it in a carrier bag, such as a briefcase or purse. Never rest a wireless device on your body. This includes laptops and tablets—keep them off your lap.

•Never fall asleep with your cell phone or wireless tablet in the bed or under your pillow. Many people fall asleep streaming radiation into their bodies.

•**Prefer texting to calling.** And avoid using your cell phone when the signal is weak—radiation is higher.

•**Turn it off.** Putting your cell phone in "airplane" mode stops radiation. Also, look for the function key on your wireless device that turns off the Wi-Fi. Turn it off when the device isn't in use. There's also a function key to turn off Bluetooth transmissions. If you must use a Wi-Fi router at home, locate it as far away from your body as possible. And turn it off at night.

To stop a gaming console from emitting radiation, you need to turn it off and unplug it.

•**Don't use your cell phone in metal surroundings such as a bus, train, airplane or elevator.** Using the phone creates radiation "hot spots" that increase exposure.

Exception: It is OK to use a cell phone in a car if your phone is hooked into the car's Bluetooth system—this reduces radiation to the user.

•**Trade in the cordless phone.** Cordless phones and wireless routers that use a technology called DECT emit as much radiation as cell phones whether you are using them or not. At home, install telephones that get their signal by being plugged into a jack. Forward your cell phone to your landline whenever you're home.

Radiation from Your Washing Machine? Hair Dryer? How to Stay Safe

David O. Carpenter, MD, director of the Institute for Health & Environment and a professor of environmental health and toxicology at the University at Albany, New York.

You've probably heard about the scientific studies linking cell phones to a variety of tumors, including brain cancer. The World Health Organization has now classified cell phones as a "possible carcinogen."*

What's being largely overlooked: Electromagnetic radiation—from electrical appliances, such as hair dryers, microwave ovens and washing machines…as well as that from wireless signals for computers—also may contribute to cancer risk independent of cell-phone use.

What you need to know…

*A team of 31 scientists from 14 countries analyzed peer-reviewed studies before classifying radiofrequency electromagnetic fields from wireless cell phones as "possibly carcinogenic to humans" based on an increased risk for glioma, a type of brain cancer.

INVISIBLE POLLUTION

Every electrical appliance in your home emits electric and magnetic fields (EMFs) of energy. An appliance that is plugged in has an electric field even when it is turned off. The appliance produces a magnetic field when it is turned on and the electrical current is flowing. However, the EMFs from appliances are considered extremely low frequency (ELF), meaning that the radiation flows at very low levels.

Still, some studies show that regular exposure to even low levels of ELF electromagnetic radiation, such as 3 milligauss (mG), may increase the risk for leukemia in children—and possibly, to a lesser degree, in adults. Preliminary research has also linked this form of energy to Alzheimer's disease and Lou Gehrig's disease, but this association is still being debated.

Some experts maintain that the electromagnetic radiation from cell phones and electrical appliances is too weak to cause the types of cell damage that can lead to cancer. But evidence is emerging that even weak forms of energy may interfere with normal cell functions, perhaps contributing to the development of cancer and other diseases.

SAFER POWER

Appliances that use the most electrical current, such as handheld hair dryers, emit the highest levels of ELF radiation. But even small appliances, such as coffeemakers, produce some. (See next page for other examples.)

Important: ELF fields are strongest at the point where the electrical wires enter the device. The fields diminish to almost nothing within a foot or two.

To test electromagnetic radiation around your appliances: Use a gauss meter—available online for about $100 to $500.

Important: ELF fields are directional—if you hold the meter to the right of a washing machine, for example, the reading might be zero, but it may be much higher a foot to the left. For accurate readings, test in different locations around the electrical appliance within a radius of a few feet.

Electrical wiring in the walls also can be an issue.

What I've found: In my son's bedroom, most of the wiring that carries electricity to lights and electrical outlets is in one of the walls. When we tested with a gauss meter, the EMFs were highest near his bed, so we moved his bed to the other side of the room.

In general, electrical wiring in walls generates high ELF only when the current is flowing or there is a ground current created by faulty wiring. However, the ELF exposure from wiring adds to the total exposure from appliances.

To reduce exposure…

• **Don't linger near appliances when they're running.** Even though the ELF levels are typically highest at the back of an appliance where the electrical cord plugs in, the magnetic field directly in front of a typical washing machine can reach 20 mG. You'll be exposed to only normal background levels by moving a foot or two away.

Important: Even the best microwave ovens leak some of the radiation they use to heat the food, so stand at least four feet away from the front of the oven when it's running. Microwave ovens also produce high levels of ELF electromagnetic radiation from the electricity used to power the oven, so there's a double risk.

• **Towel-dry your hair.** Hair dryers are among the most dangerous sources of magnetic fields because they use a lot of power and the motor/heater is held close to the head. Although using a low-fan and/or low-heat setting helps some, it's better to avoid hair dryers altogether.

If towel-drying is not convenient, consider using a low-EMF hair dryer such as the Chi Ceramic Low EMF Ionic Hair Dryer available for about $100 online…or a low-EMF wall-mounted hair dryer for about $100 from the EMF Safety Superstore, Lessemf.com.

• **Use the electric blanket before you get into bed.** Electric blankets don't draw a lot of electrical current, but they expose your entire body to ELF radiation for the entire night if you leave them on. If you want a warm bed, turn on the blanket half an hour before bedtime, then turn it off when you get into bed.

• **Get a new bedside clock.** Old-style alarm clocks—analog clocks with lighted dials—produce surprisingly high levels of electromagnetic radiation.

My advice: Get a digital bedside clock, which emits almost no ELF.

• **Throw out your cordless phones.** Cordless phones emit electromagnetic radiation whether or not they are being used. That's why I recommend replacing cordless phones with corded phones.

SAFER COMPUTER USE

Most computers give off electromagnetic radiation. If you use a desktop model, position it toward the back of your desk. Most monitors, which produce lower levels of electromagnetic radiation than computers, have conductive screens to block the ELF exposure. But it's still wise to position your monitor as far away from you as possible.

What I've found: I once measured the fields near my secretary's desk. The reading was about 10 mG, which is extremely high. I realized that the high-powered electrical wiring used by the computer was behind the wall closest to her. We had to move her desk 10 feet to get out of range.

Also, virtually every modern computer (including laptops) is designed to receive wireless signals. If you have a wireless router, which connects to a cable and wirelessly "routes" this connection to one or more computers in your home, your exposure to electromagnetic radiation is constant.

To be safer…

• **Hardwire the computer to the modem.** Use cables to connect computers to your modem rather than using a wireless signal, so you can forgo the router. If more than one person uses a computer at home, however, this approach may not be practical.

• **Turn off the router when it's not in use.** If you do use a router, turn it on only when you need the signal for using the Internet, streaming video to the TV, etc.

• **Disable Wi-Fi settings on your computer if you don't use a router.** Otherwise, the computer—or any device that operates wirelessly, such as some printers—will constantly emit electromagnetic radiation as it tries to find the nearest wireless source. Shut down your computer when it's not in use to reduce ELF radiation in your home.

RADIATION FROM APPLIANCES IN YOUR HOME

The following table lists the median electromagnetic fields for household appliances as measured from varying distances in milligauss (mG)*…

Source	Distance from Source			
	6 inches	1 foot	2 feet	4 feet
Electric shaver	100	20	--	--
Hair dryer	300	1	--	--
Microwave oven	200	40	10	2
Electric range	30	8	2	--
Television	n/a	7	2	--
Air conditioner	n/a	3	1	--
Washing machine	20	7	1	--
Vacuum cleaner	300	60	10	1
PC with color monitor	14	5	2	--

*The dash (--) means that the magnetic field at this distance was indistinguishable from background measurements taken before the appliance was turned on. *Source*: Environmental Protection Agency.

Don't Stand in Front of the Microwave…and Other Radiation Dangers in Your Home

Magda Havas, PhD, associate professor of environmental and resource studies at Trent University in Peterborough, Ontario, Canada. She is coauthor, with Camilla Rees, of *Public Health SOS: The Shadow Side of the Wireless Revolution*.

Virtually everything with a cord or battery emits electromagnetic radiation—but some devices emit much more than others. The official exposure limit for electromagnetic radiation, set by the Federal

Communications Commission, is based on old research that considered tissue heating to be the danger threshold.

Recent research: Radiation levels up to 1,000 times lower than the FCC's guidelines have been shown to affect our health.

Magda Havas, PhD, one of the leading experts in this field, explains what to do...

MICROWAVE OVENS

Medical technicians leave the room when X-rays are taken. People should be just as cautious with microwave ovens.

Reason: Just about every microwave oven that I have tested, including the newest models, leaks radiation. In my home, I could detect electromagnetic radiation from the microwave 20 feet away.

Self-test: Put your cell phone inside the oven, and close the door (do not turn on the microwave). Call the cell-phone number. If you hear the phone ring, the cell-phone signal was able to pass through the walls of the oven—meaning that microwaves are able to pass out.

Self-defense: Leave the kitchen when the microwave is on.

DIRTY ELECTRICITY

Household electricity normally is delivered at 60 cycles per second. Along with this stable current, however, come higher frequencies— spikes in power that cause surges of radiation from appliances and even unused electrical outlets.

This so-called "dirty electricity" has been linked to fatigue, headaches, difficulty concentrating and even cardiac symptoms in people who are sensitive (known as electrohypersensitivity).

Self-defense: Surge protectors, commonly used to protect computers and other electronic equipment, will "clean" household current to some extent.

Better: Stetzerizer Filters. These devices filter electrical "noise." You just plug them into wall outlets. They're designed to clean up entire circuits in the house. The average North American home needs about 20 filters. When you plug the filters in, you can use a micro-surge meter to measure the levels of dirty electricity and try to get the levels below 40 GS units. The filters and meters are available at some hardware stores and online at Stetzer Electric.com and Lessemf.com.

Cost: About \$35 for a filter, \$125 for a meter.

PLASMA TELEVISIONS

Plasma TVs generate high levels of dirty electricity. Using one filter won't solve the problem—people with plasma TVs might have to use three or more filters to clean up the power, compared with just one filter for an LCD TV.

Self-defense: LCDs produce nearly as good a picture and produce less dirty electricity than plasma TVs.

Don't Ignore That Headache or Stumble

Marie Savard, MD, former medical contributor for ABC News. A board-certified internist, she is author of several books, including *How to Save Your Own Life*.

Amy P. Abernethy, MD, director, Duke Cancer Care Research Program, Durham, North Carolina.

A painful headache may occur because you are prone to tension headaches or migraines, which are more common in women. *But watch out for...*

• **Brain tumor**—if you recently started having headaches, especially in the mornings, or have experienced a change in headache patterns.

Action: Call your doctor immediately. An MRI or CT scan can rule out a brain tumor.

• **Meningitis**—if the headache is accompanied by a fever and stiff neck. This deadly infection causes inflammation of the membranes around the brain and spinal cord.

Action: Go to the ER immediately. You need a lumbar puncture (spinal tap) to check for white blood cells and bacteria in the cerebrospinal fluid.

• **Bleeding in the brain**—particularly if head pain is sudden and extremely severe. Possible causes include a cerebral aneurysm (a bulging, weakened area in a brain artery)...subarachnoid hemorrhage (bleeding beneath the tissues covering the brain)…or hemorrhagic stroke.

Action: Call 911. You need magnetic resonance angiography (MRA), which produces detailed images of blood vessels…and a lumbar puncture to check for red blood cells in the cerebrospinal fluid.

Watch out also for tumbles or falls: If you suddenly become "clumsy," it may signal a neurological problem, such as nerve damage from diabetes or multiple sclerosis, or it could be a sign of a brain tumor.

It may be cancer if: Your clumsiness is accompanied by confusion, difficulty concentrating and an inability to move your arms and/or legs. Although paralysis is an obvious sign that something is wrong, it is rarely the first sign of a brain tumor. Check with your doctor immediately if your body's basic functions change in any way.

Cholesterol and Brain Cancer

Researchers have discovered that lethal brain malignancies known as glioblastomas require cholesterol to grow. Removing cholesterol with medications could promote the death of cancer cells.

American Association for Cancer Research.

What If It's a Brain Tumor?

Alessandro Olivi, MD, a professor of neurosurgery and oncology and director of neurological oncology at Johns Hopkins University School of Medicine and chairman of neurosurgery at Johns Hopkins Bayview Medical Center, both in Baltimore.

No one wants to hear a doctor say, "It's a brain tumor." But what most of us don't realize is that for the majority of people who hear these words, the diagnosis is not a death sentence.

Meningioma is the most common kind of brain tumor—and the majority of these, 85%, are benign. This does not mean that these tumors are not harmful or do not cause serious problems. But understanding of these tumors has advanced, and research is ongoing to determine why these tumors occur and in whom—and this has produced new detection and treatment options.

New findings you should know about…

WHAT ARE MENINGIOMAS?

Meningiomas are tumors that do not grow within the brain tissue itself, but on the meninges, the membrane that covers the brain and lines the spinal cord. Commonly, meningiomas develop between the upper surface of the brain and the skull.

Meningiomas also can occur on the skull base—including forming in the bones at the bottom of the skull and the bony ridge in the back of the eyes.

Symptoms can occur as the meningioma grows large enough to exert pressure on the brain or if it irritates the surrounding areas. Depending on its location and which brain areas and nerves are disrupted, symptoms may include blurred vision, impaired hearing or sense of smell, loss of balance or facial pain or numbness. Symptoms such as headaches, seizures, muscle weakness and/or memory loss may also occur.

WHO IS AFFECTED?

Meningiomas are two to three times as common in women as in men and are found more frequently in blacks than in any other ethnic group. The higher rate among women has led scientists to wonder whether hormones might play a role—and whether hormone treatment may increase risk.

So far, the data from large population studies in both the US and Finland have found no connection between oral contraceptives and meningiomas and no more than a weak association between postmenopausal hormone-replacement therapy (HRT) and the occurrence of brain tumors.

A large 2011 study that looked at lifestyle factors suggested that the risk for meningioma after menopause rose for women who were overweight but dropped slightly for active women.

THE CAUSE IS UNKNOWN

Researchers are still working on what causes meningiomas. One area of interest is radiation. Several studies have shown that very large amounts of radiation appear to increase the risk for these tumors. Most susceptible are children and young adults who had high doses of radiation to treat a previous cancer. A connection between cell-phone use and meningioma has not yet been determined.

Now researchers at Brigham and Women's Hospital and Yale University are using genetic analysis to help understand why some individuals develop meningiomas after radiation exposure while other people do not.

A study that was published in the journal *Cancer* in 2012 suggested that there may be a connection between bitewing dental X-rays and meningioma, but the evidence is not definitive. For now, the best advice is simply to have dental X-rays no more often than is necessary.

DIAGNOSIS OF MENINGIOMAS

Sometimes, meningiomas are diagnosed by accident, even before they cause symptoms— for example, in the course of examination for an unrelated problem such as head trauma.

For other patients, meningiomas are not diagnosed until they have been growing for years and reached a substantial size. Slow-growing tumors are almost always benign and rarely become cancerous.

When symptoms (such as those mentioned earlier) make physicians suspect a meningioma, they turn to computed tomography (CT) and magnetic resonance imaging (MRI), with contrast dye to better see the tumor, for diagnosis.

Recent progress: The development of powerful magnets has made MRI scans far more precise than they were in the past—and they are able to detect brain tumors that might have been missed a few years ago.

TREATMENT STRATEGIES

Once found, not all meningiomas need to be treated. Physicians may opt for the "watchful waiting" approach for small, benign tumors that do not create symptoms.

Researchers are studying these benign tumors. At Johns Hopkins, they are looking at the genetic differences between benign meningiomas that stay benign and those that become malignant. This will help doctors determine which tumors need treatment and when it is safe to wait and watch a tumor.

Surgery may become necessary if symptoms develop or if periodic brain scans show that the tumor is starting to grow rapidly. The usual surgical treatment is removal of the entire tumor.

Major advances: With image-guided surgery, the surgeon uses CT or MRI as a kind of 3-D internal GPS to tell him/her just where the tumor ends and to navigate around blood vessels and neural structures.

This type of advance makes it possible to remove tumors that would previously have been considered too risky to remove, and to remove them more completely, making recurrence less likely. The use of intraoperative CT and MRI in the operating room enables surgeons to verify that the entire tumor has been removed.

Sometimes the location of the tumor makes surgery impossible. For instance, a meningioma in the middle of the skull base is likely to be surrounded by crucial nerves and blood vessels that make surgery too risky.

In cases like these, radiation therapy (also called radiotherapy) is used. Radiation therapy has also advanced. Today, stereotactic radiosurgery uses imaging and computerized programming to precisely target high-intensity radiation to the tumor while limiting damage to nearby brain tissue. Gamma Knife, CyberKnife and similar methods deliver this type of concentrated radiation. Stereotactic radiosurgery usually keeps tumors from growing but only occasionally shrinks them.

One possible side effect is brain swelling, which can cause symptoms such as headaches or neurological problems such as seizures or loss of balance.

Chemotherapy plays a small role in meningioma—it is reserved for aggressively malignant or recurrent tumors that cannot be treated effectively with surgery or radiotherapy alone.

Research is ongoing to develop new drugs. At Johns Hopkins, scientists have identified a molecular pathway within meningioma cells that spurs their growth—and this could lead to the development of drugs to block their growth.

Researchers at Harvard Medical School, Memorial Sloan-Kettering Cancer Center and elsewhere also are testing medications approved for pancreatic and gastrointestinal cancers with hopes of identifying more effective chemotherapy for those meningiomas that do become aggressive or recurrent.

Starve Cancer to Death with the Ketogenic Diet

Thomas N. Seyfried, PhD, a professor of biology at Boston College and author of *Cancer as a Metabolic Disease: On the Origin, Management, and Prevention of Cancer.* His numerous scientific articles have appeared in *Nature Medicine, Science, The Lancet Oncology, Proceedings of the National Academy of Sciences, Journal of Oncology, Cancer Letters, Journal of Neurochemistry* and many other medical and scientific journals.

A 65-year-old woman with brain cancer had surgery to remove the tumor, but the operation couldn't remove it all. The woman started following the ketogenic diet—a diet very high in fat, moderate in protein and very low in carbohydrate. She also had chemotherapy and radiation. After six weeks on the diet, a brain scan showed that the tumor had disappeared. A brain scan five months later showed it was still gone. However, the patient stopped the diet—and a scan three months later showed that the tumor had returned.

Yes, a special diet called the ketogenic diet can fight cancer. It is being used to manage brain cancer and advanced (metastatic) cancer, which is when the disease has spread beyond the original tumor to other parts of the body (such as breast cancer that spreads to the liver and bones). It may be effective in fighting most, if not all, cancers, but it must be done under the supervision of an experienced oncological nutritionist.

Here, what you need to know about this little-known therapy for cancer...

HOW IT WORKS

The ketogenic diet is very high in fat—the ratio is four grams of fat to one gram of protein/carbohydrate. It has long been used to control epilepsy and is offered as an epilepsy treatment at hundreds of hospitals and clinics around the world, including The Johns Hopkins Epilepsy Center, Mayo Clinic and Mattel Children's Hospital at UCLA.

It eases epilepsy by stabilizing neurons (brain cells). It does so by reducing glucose (blood sugar), the main fuel used by neurons, and increasing ketones (beta-hydroxybutyric acid and acetoacetic acid), a by-product of fat metabolism used by neurons when glucose levels are low. Reducing glucose and increasing ketones play key roles in fighting cancer as well.

The typical American diet is about 50% to 60% carbohydrate (fruits, vegetables, breads, cereals, milk and milk products, and added sugars in sweetened foods and beverages). The body turns carbohydrate into glucose, which is used for energy.

Cancer cells gorge on glucose. Eating a ketogenic diet deprives them of this primary fuel, starving the cells, which stop growing or die. Also, ketones are a fuel usable by normal cells but not by cancer cells, so this, too, helps stop cancer growth. *In addition, the diet...*

• **Puts you into a metabolic state similar to that of fasting**—and fasting has repeatedly been shown to arrest cancer.

• **Lowers levels of insulin** (the glucose-regulating hormone) and insulin-like growth factor—both of which drive tumor growth.

CASE HISTORIES

The first case report about the ketogenic diet for cancer appeared in *Journal of the American College of Nutrition* in 1995. The ketogenic diet was used by two children with advanced, inoperable brain cancer who had undergone extensive, life-threatening radiation and chemotherapy. They both responded remarkably well to the diet.

A case report that I coauthored, published in *Nutrition & Metabolism* in 2010, told the story (see beginning of this article) of the 65-year-old woman with glioblastoma multiforme—the most common and most aggressive type of brain tumor, with a median survival of only about 12 months after diagnosis. Standard treatment—surgery to remove as much of the tumor as possible, plus radiation and/or chemotherapy—extends average survival time only a few months beyond that of people who aren't treated.

My viewpoint: In animal research, the ketogenic diet is the only therapeutic approach that deprives tumors of their primary fuel…stops tumor cells from invading other areas…stops the process of angiogenesis (blood supply to tumors)…and reduces inflammation, which drives cancer. The diet also could reduce the need for anticonvulsant and anti-inflammatory medications in brain cancer patients.

Considering how ineffective the current standard of care is for brain cancer (and for metastatic cancer), the ketogenic diet could be an attractive option for many cancer patients.

WORKING WITH AN EXPERT

The ketogenic diet for cancer is not a diet you should undertake on your own after reading a book or other self-help materials. It requires the assistance of an oncological nutritionist or other health professional who is familiar with the use of the regimen in cancer patients. Ask your oncologist for a referral.

Important aspects of the ketogenic diet include…

• **Measuring glucose and ketone levels.** For the management of cancer, blood glucose levels should fall between 55 mg/dL and 65 mg/dL, and ketone levels between 3 mmol and 5 mmol. In order to monitor those levels—and adjust your diet accordingly—you need to use methods similar to those used by patients with diabetes. These methods include glucose testing several times a day with a finger stick and glucose strip…daily urine testing for ketones…and (more accurate) home blood testing for ketones, perhaps done weekly.

• **Starting with a water-only fast.** If you are in relatively good health (aside from the cancer, of course), it is best to start the ketogenic diet with a water-only fast for 48 to 72 hours, which will quickly put you in ketosis—the production of a therapeutic level of ketones. This fast should be guided by a health professional.

If you are fragile or in poor health, you can skip the water fast and initiate ketosis with the ketogenic diet, reducing carbohydrates to less than 12 grams a day. This should produce ketosis within two or three weeks.

• **Macronutrient ratios and recipes.** Working with a nutritionist, you will find the fat/protein/carbohydrate ratio that works best for you to lower glucose and increase ketones… and the recipes and meal plan that consistently deliver those ratios. A food diary, a food scale and the use of a "KetoCalculator" (available on websites such as KetoDietCalculator. org) are necessary tools to implement the ketogenic diet.

Helpful: The oncological nutritionist Miriam Kalamian, EdM, MS, CNS, managed her own son's brain tumor with the ketogenic diet, and she counsels cancer patients around the world in the implementation of the diet. You can find more information on her website, DietaryTherapies.com.

CAN THE DIET PREVENT CANCER?

Cancer survivors and people with a family history of cancer may wonder if they should go on the ketogenic diet as a preventive measure. It is not necessary for people to follow the diet if they do not have cancer. A six-to-seven-day water-only fast done once or twice a year—under a doctor's supervision—can be effective in reducing the risk for recurrent cancer in survivors and in those individuals with a family history of cancer. Fasting reduces glucose and elevates ketones.

CLINICAL TRIALS

Currently, there are several clinical trials being conducted using the ketogenic diet for cancer.

You can find out more about these trials at ClinicalTrials.gov. Enter "Ketogenic Diet" into the search engine at the site for a complete listing of cancer trials and trials testing the ketogenic diet for other conditions, including epilepsy, amyotrophic lateral sclerosis (ALS), autism, mild cognitive impairment, Parkinson's disease and obesity.

Better Brain Cancer Test

According to a recent study, a newly developed test called GlioSeq correctly identified all known genetic alterations in 54 adult and pediatric brain tumor samples, allowing physicians to tailor drug treatment for best response and possibly improved survival. The test may be covered by insurance.

Marina N. Nikiforova, MD, director, molecular & genomic pathology laboratory, University of Pittsburgh Medical Center.

When to Try "Keyhole" Surgery

David F. Jimenez, MD, FACS, chairman and professor in the department of neurosurgery at The University of Texas Health Science Center at San Antonio. He is the editor and a coauthor of *Intracranial Endoscopic Neurosurgery*, a textbook published by the American Association of Neurological Surgeons.

No one likes the thought of undergoing brain or spine surgery. Traditionally, a neurosurgeon would create a four- to six-inch incision and peel back the scalp before drilling through the skull to expose the brain...or make a similar-sized incision in your back, where muscles are then moved to expose the spine.

Recent development: Endoscopic, or minimally invasive, surgery, which has long been offered for such common procedures as gallbladder removal and knee surgery, is now widely available at major US medical centers for neurosurgical operations that involve the brain, spine and peripheral nerves.

Whether it's the removal of a brain tumor or the repair of herniated disks, spinal stenosis or carpal tunnel syndrome, neurosurgeons can now use sophisticated instruments to operate through an incision that's smaller than a dime or even through a natural opening such as a nostril.

This approach allows for a faster recovery and less pain and swelling than the traditional "open" procedures. Older patients frequently respond better to surgery that has minimal blood loss and requires less time under general anesthesia.

Why this matters: Even though endoscopic (sometimes known as "keyhole") neurosurgery is now available, not all surgeons have the training and experience to perform it. This means that you may not be offered endoscopic neurosurgery when it would be a better option than a traditional procedure—or a surgeon may attempt the endoscopic operation without adequate training and/or experience. *What you need to know...*

A NEW GENERATION OF NEUROSURGERY

What makes most types of surgery so challenging has less to do with repairing a problem—whether it's replacing a joint or removing an appendix—than simply getting access to the specific body part.

With endoscopic neurosurgery of the brain, the surgeon makes one or two incisions ranging from one-third to three-quarters of an inch and drills into the skull. A tube (endoscope) is passed through the narrow opening. Everything that's needed to complete the procedure, such as a lighted camera and cutting and scraping tools, is guided into place through the endoscope. Surgeons enter through the nostrils or above the eyebrow to operate on pituitary adenomas and tumors in the front of the brain.

The benefits of endoscopic surgery are largely due to the smaller incision, which is obviously less painful than a large one and has less risk for infection. Since there is less blood loss, there is less need for blood transfusion—another benefit.

Because endoscopic procedures can usually be done faster than traditional surgeries, patients also spend less time under general anesthesia, which reduces postoperative complications, such as cognitive dysfunction and nausea, and improves recovery.

In my practice, at least 30% of brain surgeries (including treatment for hydrocephalus—buildup of fluid in the brain that is drained via a shunt...and removal of skull-base tumors) are minimally invasive. Deep areas of the brain cannot be accessed with endoscopic neurosurgery. Most of our spine surgeries and virtually all carpal tunnel procedures are done this way.

Examples of when endoscopic neurosurgery can be used...

•**Herniated disk.** Computerized image guidance creates a three-dimensional image of the spine so surgeons can achieve a superb view of the operating field with an endoscopic incision that's barely more than a half-inch long. They use microinstruments to remove the damaged part of the disk.

•**Spinal stenosis.** This narrowing inside the spinal canal (usually due to arthritis) often causes leg pain or other symptoms. It's relatively easy to "open up" the spinal space with endoscopic surgery. Patients often make a full recovery within a month—and may be symptom-free almost immediately—while traditional surgery usually requires a recovery period of at least three months.

IS IT FOR EVERYONE?

In general, endoscopic surgery is a good option for most patients, especially those who are too old, ill or frail to have traditional surgeries.

One patient's story: My oldest patient was a 96-year-old woman whose spinal stenosis was so bad she could barely walk. She might not have done well with a lengthy open procedure, but I knew that I could complete the operation in about 90 minutes—half the usual time. Her pain was gone almost instantly—and a month later, she was bowling and dancing with her boyfriend.

The complication rate (infections and/or bleeding) for endoscopic surgery is at least as good as—and sometimes better than—that of traditional procedures. The numbers will only get better as surgeons gain experience and new approaches and technologies are developed.

FIND THE RIGHT SURGEON

Before agreeing to any type of neurosurgery, ask the surgeon whether the procedure will be open or minimally invasive. While some operations, such as certain brain tumors, still require a traditional approach, most do not.

Chances are that you'll recover much more quickly—and experience less postoperative pain—if you go with endoscopy. If your surgeon doesn't do endoscopic surgery, get a second opinion. You can find a surgeon at the American Association of Neurological Surgeons, AANS.org.

Experience and training are crucial for surgeons who perform endoscopic surgeries. Compared with traditional operations, endoscopic surgeries require the surgeon to overcome such issues as poor depth perception (from the endoscopic camera) and limited range of motion to manipulate surgical instruments. Make sure your surgeon has several years of experience in performing the procedure you'll be getting and has received endoscopic neurosurgical training.

Dr. Mark Hyman's "UltraMind" Strategy for Brain and Mental Health

Mark Hyman, MD, author of *The UltraMind Solution: Fix Your Broken Brain by Healing Your Body First, UltraMetabolism* and *The UltraSimple Diet*. Dr. Hyman is founder and medical director of The UltraWellness Center in Lenox, Massachusetts. DrHyman.com

---

Mental illness is on the rise, and conventional medicine cannot cure it. That's the message from Mark Hyman, MD, who offers an alternative answer in his recent book, *The UltraMind Solution: Fix Your Broken Brain by Healing Your Body First.* He notes that an epidemic of "broken brains" affects millions of people worldwide, taking many forms—anxiety, depression, dementia, addictions, attention deficit hyperactivity disorder (ADHD), autism, etc. The common model for addressing these disorders is drug therapy…but drugs alone fail to address the underlying causes of mental disease.

THE SHORTCOMINGS OF DRUG THERAPY

The real cure for brain disorders lies outside the brain, Dr. Hyman explains. If you suffer from depression, for example, you are not suffering from a "Prozac deficiency" in spite of the fact that doctors may prescribe it or other antidepressants. Mainstream medicine's approach is to make a diagnosis based on symptoms, then suppress those symptoms with a medication rather than identifying the cause and fixing that. For example, many cases of depression are actually rooted in nutritional deficiencies or imbalances, including vitamin D, B-12, an omega-3 fatty acid deficiency, or a problem with digestive function or some other biological deficit. And, just about all these can be corrected without antidepressants. In fact, Dr. Hyman points out that most people who take antidepressants find that they offer only partial relief, lose effectiveness over time or simply don't work. These drugs also cause side effects such as weight gain and loss of sex drive, and more than half of people who take them quit within months.

In reality, everything that affects the body affects the brain, since it is one of the most vital organs of the body, and everything that affects the brain affects the rest of the body. Simply taking an antidepressant for depression—or Ritalin for ADHD, or an anti-anxiety medication and so forth—fails to take this basic body-mind connection into account. In Dr. Hyman's opinion, a new paradigm for mental illness must take a wider view of a person, not merely focus on the brain, since there are myriad causes of mental illness. This view should replace the shortsighted approach to treatment where a doctor marks down a diagnostic code on a patient's chart and prescribes the corresponding pill.

DR. HYMAN'S ULTRAMIND SOLUTION

According to Dr. Hyman, there are seven key influences affecting your brain, your memory, attention, mood and behavior—nutrition, hormones, inflammation, digestion, detoxification, energy metabolism and the mind-body connection. When one or more of these are thrown off-kilter, imbalances develop, which can manifest in mental and/or emotional illness. Identifying and addressing imbalances thusly enables the body's natural healing mechanisms to take over, bringing about dramatic improvements in mood, memory, attention, concentration, cognition and other brain functions.

Dr. Hyman recommends a three-pronged strategy for brain wellness: His book has quizzes to help identify which of your seven underlying systems isn't working…suggestions on how to fix the underlying problem causing the imbalance…and ways to nourish all these aspects so they can function optimally as an integrated system. We took a brief look at how each of the seven key systems affects mental health, and what you can do to help keep them in balance.

• **Are you eating right?** Inadequate nutrition is at the root of many illnesses, both mental and physical. If your diet is loaded with fatty fast foods, processed foods and refined carbohydrates (e.g., white bread and pasta) you're not only missing the nutrients your brain requires to function properly, but also creating other chemical imbalances. To restore balance, eat a diet based on a variety of whole, unprocessed foods.

• **Is there a hormonal issue?** Improper diet is among the factors that can lead to a hormone imbalance—specifically, eating sugar and refined carbohydrates causes the body to pump out an overload of the hormone insulin into the bloodstream. Too much insulin can cause mood swings and behavior disturbances such as depression, anxiety, panic attacks and insomnia. Other hormonal imbalances are caused by swings in sex hormones, which can be a natural result of aging, or an improperly functioning thyroid gland, etc. See your physician to identify and treat hormonal issues.

• **Do you need to cool down inflammation?** If the body is inflamed, the brain is too. Brain inflammation is implicated in nearly every brain disease, from Alzheimer's to autism to depression to schizophrenia. Sources of inflammation include refined carbohydrates, food allergens, stress and anxiety—but on the bright side, Dr. Hyman reminds us that these are all fixable problems. In addition to eating healthier whole foods, getting plenty of omega-3 fatty acids, and taking steps to control stress, you can also add anti-inflammatory herbs such as turmeric, ginger and rosemary to your diet.

• **Is there a digestive problem?** One of the most powerful ways you can fix your brain is to fix your gut, says Dr. Hyman. For example, if your digestive enzymes malfunction, undigested gluten from wheat or casein from milk can harm brain function. Strategies to resolve digestive problems might include eliminating food allergens, considering digestive enzymes and taking probiotics to bring digestive colonies of microbes back into proper balance.

• **Do you need to detox?** Toxic chemicals in the environment such as mercury and lead underlie many neurological diseases. Limit exposure to these toxins to the greatest degree possible. For example, do not eat (or rarely eat) large fish such as swordfish or tuna that is likely to contain higher levels of mercury. If you live in an older house, be sure the water and paint are not contaminated with lead.

• **How's your energy metabolism?** Mitochondria are the miniature energy factories in your body's cells, including those in the brain. The single most important thing you can do to support your mitochondria and boost your energy is to exercise. For energy problems specifically related to stress, toxicity or aging, Dr. Hyman prescribes supplements such as Acetyl-L-Carnitine, Alpha-lipoic acid, Coenzyme Q10, magnesium, riboflavin and niacin.

• **Are you stressed out?** Closely examine your life, Dr. Hyman urges. Stress robs you of energy, so take action to more effectively manage it. For instance, make a promise to yourself that this week you will eliminate one thing that causes anxiety and add one that helps you heal and thrive.

Drugs can provide a temporary fix for brain problems, says Dr. Hyman, but these are not the long-term solution. As usual, it takes more work than popping a pill, but in the long run a healthy mind and body are worth it.

Medical Disorders That Cause Mental Problems

Barbara Schildkrout, MD, psychiatrist and assistant clinical professor of psychiatry, Harvard Medical School and the Beth Israel Deaconess Medical Center, both in Boston. She is author of *Unmasking Psychological Symptoms: How Therapists Can Learn to Recognize the Psychological Presentation of Medical Disorders*. BarbaraSchildkrout.com

If you develop anxiety or depression, your first thought might be to call a therapist.

What you should do instead: See your doctor. Many physical problems masquerade as mental health issues. For example, patients with a treatable thyroid disorder often experience intense anxiety. Some seizure disorders may cause intense emotional experiences. And manic behavior could be a medication side effect.

Frightening statistic: Up to 40% of patients in some nursing homes and mental health facilities have mental symptoms that are caused—or made worse—by underlying medical disorders.

According to Barbara Schildkrout, MD, a psychiatrist and leading expert on this subject, mental/physical issues are often intertwined. For example, a former football player suffering from midlife depression may have suffered multiple concussions in the past. Such head trauma may trigger depression...even years later.

Problem: Many primary care physicians don't spend enough time with patients to know their psychological histories, and mental health professionals may wrongly assume that a doctor has thoroughly considered a physical cause of mental symptoms. *Before you conclude that you have a mental health problem, ask yourself…*

• **Did it start quickly?** If you're fine one day and suffering from depression or another mental health symptom the next, you should suspect that there might be a physical cause.

• **Does your mood match your life?** It's understandable that someone who is recently divorced or having financial problems might be depressed. But if everything in your life is fine and you still feel lousy, you might have a physical disorder.

• **Are you experiencing any other symptoms, even if they seem unrelated?** Timing is important. A patient who is hallucinating might be psychotic. But hallucinations could also be symptoms of a seizure disorder or the sleep disorder narcolepsy.

CONFUSING CONDITIONS

More than 100 medical conditions cause symptoms (indicators of a disease or disorder that are detected by the patient) and signs (indicators detected by a physician) that may be misinterpreted to be the evidence of a mental illness. *Examples…*

• **Drug side effects versus mood disorder.** You would expect to experience mood changes when taking a sedating medication, such as codeine. But depression is a common side effect of many medications, including some of those used to treat asthma, elevated cholesterol and high blood pressure. Birth control pills also can cause depression.

Other drugs may trigger mania, a symptom of certain psychiatric conditions, such as bipolar disorder. Mania is marked by racing thoughts, euphoria and lack of sleep. Corticosteroids (such as *hydrocortisone* and *prednisone*) may cause mania. Some antidepressants, including selective serotonin reuptake inhibitors, such as *fluoxetine* (Prozac), and monoamine oxidase inhibitors, such as *phenelzine* (Nardil), may trigger an episode of mania.

What to look for: The *timing* of mood changes. If you've recently started a new medication and you're suddenly feeling depressed, talk to your doctor.

What to do: Make a list of all the medications that you take, and ask your doctor if they could be responsible for your mood changes. He/she may advise you to switch medications and/or take a lower dose.

• **Hyperthyroidism versus anxiety.** Patients who produce too much thyroid hormone (*hyperthyroidism*) may experience intense anxiety. Some spend months or even years in therapy before they discover that they have a physical problem. The diagnosis is easy to miss because, unlike many other psychological symptoms caused by physical ailments, the symptoms come on *gradually*, sometimes over a period of years.

What to look for: Feelings of anxiety that don't correspond with what's happening in your life. Patients who suffer from psychological anxiety will usually be worried or concerned about something in particular. One exception is patients with *generalized anxiety disorder*, who have excessive worry about everyday matters.

The anxiety caused by thyroid disorders will *feel* physical. Your heart might be pounding…you might sweat a lot…or have shaky hands. Patients *interpret* these sensations as anxiety even though they may just be physical symptoms.

What to do: If you experience these symptoms or you've been told that you have anxiety, make sure that your doctor has considered the possibility of thyroid disease. It's diagnosed with a blood test. Hyperthyroidism is treated with medication and sometimes surgery.

• **Seizures versus intense emotional episodes.** Emotional outbursts are a common symptom of mental illness, including psychotic disorders. But intense emotional experiences—feelings such as fear, a sense of impending doom, rage or déjà vu experiences—can sometimes be caused by seizures. In addition, seizures can disrupt sleep, which, in turn, may lead to irritability and more likely emotional outbursts.

What to look for: Intense emotional reactions when there's no clear reason. Patients with mental illness can usually describe what makes them angry, anxious, etc. With seizures, emotional outbursts "come out of the blue." Depending on the type of seizure, the episodes are usually brief, often only a minute or two. The short duration often indicates a physical rather than a psychological problem.

What to do: Ask your doctor/therapist if you should have an electroencephalogram, a test that measures electrical activity in the brain. A negative test doesn't mean that you don't have seizures—it just means that your brain activity was normal at the time of testing. If symptoms continue, a repeat test might be needed. If a seizure disorder is diagnosed, symptoms usually improve with medication.

Important: Certain types of seizures cause only subtle changes in consciousness—for example, a moment of unresponsiveness that may be misinterpreted as, say, a problem with attention. Some seizure disorders are also associated with various types of hallucinations, including auditory, visual and olfactory.

• **Normal pressure hydrocephalus (NPH) versus depression.** NPH is an enlargement of the fluid-filled ventricles of the brain that often causes symptoms such as apathy and depression along with cognitive and memory impairments. Some people who are diagnosed with Alzheimer's disease actually have NPH.

What to look for: NPH symptoms include apathy, depression and mental slowing, along with the development of an unsteady gait and urinary incontinence. With Alzheimer's, any trouble with walking or incontinence occurs only at very advanced stages of the disease.

What to do: If you or a loved one has any of these symptoms, there's a chance that the mental health problems have a physical origin. From a simple CT scan, a neurologist can tell whether a person might have NPH. The diagnosis must then be confirmed by further tests including a lumbar puncture in which a small amount of fluid is drained. Doctors then observe whether the patient's gait improves. If so, the diagnosis has been confirmed, and the condition is treated with the surgical insertion of a shunt to drain fluid from the brain.

Autoimmune Encephalitis: the Brain Disease That Makes People Seem Crazy

Souhel Najjar, MD, chair, neurology, Lenox Hill Hospital, New York City, and chair and professor of neurology, Hofstra Northwell School of Medicine, Hempstead, New York.

Ricki had it all—a great job, great little Manhattan apartment, great life. Only in her early 20s, she already had accomplished much in the fashion world.

But over the course of barely more than a month, all that blew up as Ricki developed increasingly weird and worrisome behaviors.

First, there were memory problems. She couldn't recall simple things, such as where she normally kept her car keys or the names of her coworkers. The following week, her speech slowed, her body felt numb and her movements became awkward. Soon after, Ricki began hallucinating and a psychiatrist put her on medication.

A week later, she had a seizure and was hospitalized. A huge battery of tests, including a spinal tap and brain MRIs, revealed nothing except a little inflammation…doctors were stumped.

Then Ricki began having violent spells, leaping at nurses and orderlies. Said to be psychotic, she was transferred to a psychiatric hospital. And there she might have stayed for the rest of her life—if not for a stroke of luck.

Ricki's father, a retired physician, did not believe that the daughter who had always been so sweet, smart and sane could have become, in a matter of weeks, seriously and irrevocably mentally ill. So he diligently researched her symptoms and discussed her condition with his doctor friends. Fortunately, one of the father's colleagues suggested consulting Souhel Najjar, MD, a neurologist at Lenox Hill Hospital in New York City.

Dr. Najjar gave the young woman a thorough examination, including a special blood test that revealed antibodies targeting certain receptors in the brain—and within days, he had made the diagnosis. Ricki was suffering from a rare autoimmune disorder called anti-NMDA receptor encephalitis.

DEADLY "DEMONIC" DISEASE

Encephalitis, or inflammation of the brain, usually is the result of a viral infection, but it also can be caused by bacteria, fungi or parasites—or, as doctors now realize, by an autoimmune disorder.

In the case of anti-NMDA receptor encephalitis, severe brain inflammation occurs when the immune system attacks special proteins on the surface of nerve cells in the brain called NMDA receptors. These receptors control various cognitive functions, mood, behavior and personality traits—so when they are compromised, the brain malfunctions.

The resulting symptoms include mood and personality changes, violent outbursts, paranoia, psychosis, memory loss, speech problems, numbness, seizures, involuntary movements, increased heart rate, irregular heart rhythm, slowed breathing and/or decreased levels of consciousness. Patients sometimes sink into an unresponsive catatonic state that may last for weeks. Some experts even suspect that anti-NMDA receptor encephalitis is the true cause underlying many cases of "demonic possession" described in the Bible!

This disease is largely unknown, having first been reported in medical literature only about a decade ago. It typically strikes in early adulthood, but it has been diagnosed in children as young as one and in seniors as old as 85. It can strike both genders, though more than 75% of those affected are female.

Dr. Najjar explained more about this disturbing and devastating disease. He said that, though considered rare, anti-NMDA receptor encephalitis may be more common than is currently recognized, with many patients being misdiagnosed with severe psychiatric disorders. "These patients act aggressive, belligerent, violent, psychotic and paranoid. Yet now that we know what the real problem is, we have to wonder how many people have been locked up in psychiatric units for years after they were misdiagnosed," Dr. Najjar said.

Sadly, some patients with anti-NMDA receptor encephalitis die from medical and neurological complications related to irregular heart rhythm, very low blood pressure, slowed breathing, prolonged convulsions and/or persistent coma.

BRAIN-SAVING TREATMENT

The earlier that anti-NMDA receptor encephalitis is diagnosed and treated, the better the outcome tends to be. Treatment includes immunotherapy—a heavy-duty dose of steroids and other drugs aimed at suppressing the body's attack on itself. Typically, Dr. Najjar said, the treatment is effective, and most severe symptoms improve within three to four weeks after treatment begins. However, patients often need physical, occupational and/or cognitive therapies to regain their ability to walk, talk and function normally, and full recovery may take up to two years.

What causes this disease? That's not entirely clear. As with other autoimmune disorders, such as lupus or rheumatoid arthritis, a genetic predisposition may contribute to an individual's risk, Dr. Najjar said.

A certain type of ovarian tumor called a teratoma appears to play a key role, particularly in females of childbearing age. Bizarrely, teratomas often contain skin, hair, tooth and/or brainlike cells. A recent study from the University of Pennsylvania found that up to 55% of female patients under 18 years of age who had anti-NMDA receptor encephalitis also had teratomas in their ovaries. The body's immune system may be provoked into producing antibodies that attack the abnormal brainlike cells in the tumor, Dr. Najjar explained. Since the antibodies don't distinguish between the brainlike cells in the tumor and cells in the brain itself, the patient's brain becomes a battlefield. If a teratoma is found in a patient's ovary, the ovary needs to be surgically removed.

What's puzzling is that anti-NMDA receptor encephalitis also can develop in patients who do not have teratomas. Such cases may be the result of some kind of virus that damages the blood/brain barrier, allowing antibodies to enter the brain, Dr. Najjar said. These patients are at greater risk for recurrence, even many years after the initial episode. For instance, the University of Pennsylvania researchers reported that, of the 20% of anti-NMDA receptor encephalitis patients who experienced a relapse, most had not had teratomas.

Lucky lady: Ricki is recovering nicely, thanks to timely intervention. But here's what all of us should remember from her story...

If a loved one suddenly starts exhibiting psychiatric symptoms that are way out of character, Dr. Najjar said, it is vital to consult a neurologist and ask whether anti-NMDA receptor encephalitis could be the culprit.

Warfarin Danger

Warfarin risk is greater than previously believed among patients with dementia and certain other conditions, reports John Dodson, MD.

Recent finding: One in 50 US veterans over age 75 who took the anticoagulant warfarin for atrial fibrillation (irregular heartbeat) developed severe bleeding inside the skull. Newer anticoagulants are available, but they have risks of their own.

John Dodson, MD, assistant professor, department of medicine, and director of the Geriatric Cardiology Program at NYU Langone Medical Center, New York City.

Lyme Disease Alert

Richard S. Ostfeld, PhD, a senior scientist and disease ecologist at Cary Institute of Ecosystem Studies in Millbrook, New York. He is author of *Lyme Disease: The Ecology of a Complex System.*

In some parts of the country, tick season appears to be starting earlier and ending later. It's not merely that summers are getting warmer. Winters, on average, are less cold than they used to be. Warmer winters are known to allow tick populations to expand northward and to higher elevations.

Self-defense...

• **Check for ticks.** Check yourself, your children and your pets after spending time outdoors. To reduce risk on hikes, stay on trails. If you plan to leave the path, wear light-colored clothing to make ticks easier to spot. Wear long sleeves, and tuck long pants into your socks.

Also, use insect repellent containing DEET on exposed skin.

• **Know the symptoms.** Tick-related illnesses often are accompanied by flulike symptoms such as fever, fatigue, aches and pains, memory and concentration problems. Lyme and other tick diseases also can cause distinctive rashes. See your doctor if you develop any of these symptoms, particularly if you develop flulike symptoms when it's not flu season.

Most victims of tick-borne illnesses can be cured with antibiotics, particularly when the infection is detected and treated early.

Herbal Help for Chronic Lyme Disease

Richard Horowitz, MD, board-certified internist and medical director of the Hudson Valley Healing Arts Center, an integrative medical center based in Hyde Park, New York.

If acute Lyme disease goes untreated or if antibiotic treatment is unsuccessful, patients can develop an array of persistent symptoms in the following weeks and months. The CDC's symptom list includes palsy (loss of muscle tone) on one or both sides of the face...severe headaches and neck stiffness due to meningitis (inflammation of membranes covering the brain and spinal cord)...heart palpitations...dizziness due to changes in heartbeat...severe joint pain and swelling...shooting pains, numbness or tingling of the hands and feet...irritability...and problems with concentration and memory.

Though some patients have symptoms that last for years, chronic Lyme disease is a controversial issue. In fact, *The Journal of Pediatrics* recently reported that half of physicians surveyed question the existence of chronic Lyme disease—even though there are numerous scientific articles proving the existence of persistent infection despite both short-term and longer-term antibiotic use.

HERBS IN ACTION

Numerous clinical studies have demonstrated the effectiveness of including certain herbs in the treatment of chronic Lyme disease. Why do herbs help achieve what antibiotics alone cannot? Because chronic Lyme disease can involve not only the main spirochetal infection, but also multiple bacterial, viral and/or parasitic coinfections transmitted by the same tick bite. Herbs typically prescribed for chronic Lyme are able to combat these various infections because they have antispirochetal, antibacterial, antiviral, antiparasitic and/or antimalarial properties. They also help reduce inflammation...protect the heart...support the liver...aid kidney function...provide antioxidants....and/or boost the immune system.

Herbs to ask your doctor about: Herbal extracts usually are taken in capsule or tablet form. *Among the herbs most commonly prescribed for chronic Lyme are....*

- **Andrographis paniculata**
- **Astralagus**
- **Banderol**
- **Polygonum cuspidatum**
- **Samento**
- **Sarsaparilla**

Lyme patients should take herbs only under the guidance of a health-care practitioner who knows their benefits, side effects and interactions...who can determine which of the various herbal protocols that have been developed for Lyme would be most appropriate for an individual patient...and who can prescribe the right dosages.

Referrals: Visit LymeDiseaseAssociation. org and click on "Doctors Referral."

Note: Certain herbs should not be used by patients who have particular medical conditions (such as gallbladder disease), who take certain medications (such as *cyclosporine*, cortisone drugs or blood thinners), who are or plan to get pregnant, or who are breast-feeding.

Some herbs initially can cause gastrointestinal side effects, such as constipation or nausea, so patients may start with a small dosage and increase gradually over several weeks... maintain the top dose for several months or so...then reduce the dosage incrementally as their chronic Lyme disease symptoms subside at last.

Brain Killer Lurking in the Water...

Jonathan S. Yoder, MSW, MPH, team leader for the Domestic Water, Sanitation, and Hygiene Epidemiology Team in the National Center for Emerging Zoonotic and Infectious Diseases at the Centers for Disease Control and Prevention, Atlanta. CDC.gov

The single-cell organism *Naegleria fowleri* is found in freshwater lakes, rivers, streams and hot springs. It is not found in the ocean or other bodies of saltwater. It rarely causes infection—but when it does, the infection is deadly.

This amoeba thrives in warm, untreated water and can survive in temperatures up to 115°F. It has been identified most often in southern states in the US.

But a few recent cases have occurred in northern regions (such as Indiana, Kansas and Minnesota)—areas that were typically too cold for the amoeba to survive. Scientists aren't sure if the warming of the planet has extended the amoeba's range, but it is one possibility. From 2006 to 2015, 37 cases were reported in the US, according to the Centers for Disease Control and Prevention. This is a slight increase over the previous 10-year span.

What happens: The amoeba enters the body through the nose, usually when people are swimming or diving in contaminated water. It then travels to the brain, where it literally consumes brain tissue.

Symptoms start one to seven days after exposure. The disease progresses rapidly, and there are no effective treatments. The fatality rate is more than 99%.

The organism can cause infection only when it enters the nasal cavities. There is no risk from drinking a glass of water or from typical showering.

Self-defense…

• **When swimming in warm fresh-water lakes, rivers, ponds or streams, wear nose plugs or keep your head above water.** Hold your nose shut, or use nose plugs when jumping or diving into the water.

• **If you use a Neti pot or a bulb syringe to flush congestion from your nose, always use boiled, properly filtered or sterilized water.** Officials recently found Naegleria in a municipal water system in Louisiana, where it caused two deaths—in both cases, the patients had performed nasal flushing.

Is It a Concussion?

Diane Roberts Stoler, EdD, a neuropsychologist and board-certified health and sport psychologist with a private practice in North Andover, Massachusetts. A brain injury patient herself, she is coauthor, with Barbara Albers Hill, of *Coping with Concussion and Mild Traumatic Brain Injury.* DrDiane.com

With all the recent talk about football players suffering concussions that have caused permanent brain damage, you might think that these brain injuries occur only on sports fields.

But that's far from the truth. Anyone can suffer a concussion. More than 40% of concussions are caused by falls…and 14.3% by car accidents.

So how can you tell when a concussion might lead to permanent damage…or will simply heal on its own? *Here's what you need to know to make that call…*

WHY THE BRAIN IS VULNERABLE

Most people imagine that the brain is firmly anchored inside the skull. Actually, it floats on cushions of fluid and air, with plenty of room to move. This means that if you bang your head hard enough, or if your head is "whipped" during a car accident, the brain can slam against the skull. The violent movement stretches and shears nerve fibers.

What most people don't realize: Even if your head feels fine, there might be areas of microscopic damage that impair normal brain functions and may cause headaches, dizziness, fatigue and other symptoms for weeks or longer.

Fortunately, a single concussion is unlikely to cause long-term problems, and symptoms usually begin to improve within hours. Most people recover completely within a month to six weeks.

The risk: Once you've had a concussion, you're more likely to get another one if you suffer an additional brain injury—and the brain is more susceptible to long-term damage if you do.

For example, recent studies have linked repeated concussions to Parkinson's-like symptoms, such as hand tremors and gait problems, and other cognitive problems, such as memory loss. People who have suffered repeated concussions may also experience concussion symptoms (sometimes years after the last brain injury) if they receive anesthesia or medication that affects the central nervous system, such as pain medications and steroids. Repeated concussions, such as those suffered by some football players and boxers, can even lead to progressive, life-threatening dementia.

IS IT A CONCUSSION OR NOT?

You may assume that you don't have a concussion if you didn't "black out." In fact, a concussion may not cause a noticeable loss of consciousness. You're more apt to be dazed… unaware of where you are…or briefly confused.

Because injuries to the brain can feel minor even when they're life-threatening, I would advise anyone who's been in a car accident that caused significant head movement, taken a hard fall or been hit hard on the head to go to a hospital emergency department.

Doctors can usually diagnose a concussion in a few minutes. You'll be given a quick, in-office neurological exam to assess the degree—and location—of brain damage.

Examples: You might be asked to recite numbers backward and forward...and/or recall what the doctor just said. You will also be given tests to check your balance, reflexes, vision and hearing.

If you have acute symptoms—for example, severe headaches and/or repeated vomiting—you may be hospitalized for further tests, such as an MRI or a CT scan, which also check for conditions that are even more serious, such as hemorrhagic (bleeding) stroke or subdural hematoma (in which blood collects on the surface of the brain).

If these tests are inconclusive and your symptoms suggest a concussion, you can ask your doctor for a specialized test called diffusion tensor imaging. It's a type of MRI that can identify extremely small areas of nerve damage, blood clots or bleeding in the brain.

However, unless you are planning a personal injury or workers' comp claim, you probably don't need to prove your diagnosis with these imaging tests. If you have symptoms of a concussion, your doctor will probably advise you just to wait it out. Symptoms usually subside within six weeks.

LET YOUR BRAIN HEAL

If you suffer a concussion, getting enough rest—including mental rest—is crucial. Until you've recovered, use your television, computer and smartphone only when absolutely necessary and for no more than two hours a day for the first few weeks after a concussion.

Also important...

• **Focus on your sleep.** Many people who have had concussions complain that they sleep fitfully or sleep too little or too much.

To promote sleep: Go to bed and get up at the same time every day...avoid bright lights in your bedroom...and create a soothing atmosphere.

Helpful: Try Bach Flower Rescue Remedy, which promotes the calm and relaxation that's needed to heal the brain.

• **Soothe the inflammation.** Because the brain is inflamed after a concussion, avoid foods that promote inflammation, such as sugar and other refined carbs. Instead, eat plenty of anti-inflammatory foods, such as omega-3–rich salmon and sardines.

Also: Give up all alcohol while a concussion is healing because it can increase the severity of your symptoms.

WHEN SYMPTOMS PERSIST

Concussion symptoms may linger for three months or longer, especially if you've had multiple concussions. If you have post-concussion syndrome (PCS)—continued symptoms may include sleep problems, difficulty concentrating, memory problems, sensitivity to lights or sounds, or unexplained emotional ups and downs—see a neurologist with training in traumatic brain injury. For a referral, consult the American Academy of Neurology, Patients. AAN.com/FindaNeurologist, and click on "Traumatic Brain Injury" under "Subspecialty."

Blood Test for Brain Trauma

Army Colonel Dallas Hack, MD, MPH, director, Combat Casualty Care Research Program, US Army Medical Research and Materiel Command, Fort Detrick, Frederick, Maryland.

Army doctors have made a tremendous breakthrough developing a simple blood test that can detect mild brain injury and concussion. This has been a dream of our armed forces doctors—especially in recent years, as they work with such a high percentage of soldiers injured in bomb blasts during combat operations. If a concussion is misdiagnosed—even a mild one—and then a second concussion occurs soon after the first, permanent brain damage is more likely to result. And this breakthrough test is going to help anyone who might one day receive a mild concussion—not just soldiers on a battlefield, but teen athletes, car accident victims or any of us.

A little background: Certainly a first concussion can cause brain damage, but doctors tend to worry about a second concussion as most likely to do significant harm. Until now, brain injury could be accurately detected only with X-rays, CT scans and/or MRI scans…and even then, only moderate to severe brain trauma was revealed. Mild brain injuries could easily be missed. Doctors have had to depend on a patient's medical history and neurologic exams—from simple in-office visits to EEGs, MRIs and brain scans, to attempt a diagnosis.

But now the Army has identified unique proteins that spill into the blood when brain cells are damaged. Earlier on, scientists had assumed proteins did not cross the blood-brain barrier, but through laboratory tests on rats, Army researchers found proteins normally present only in the brain that were clearly measurable in the body afterward. Next, they found the same thing held true in humans.

A NEW FIELD OF STUDY

Army Colonel Dallas Hack, MD, MPH, Combat Casualty Care Research Program director, US Army Medical Research and Materiel Command, said that the study of proteins in the body—called "proteinomics"—has advanced greatly in the past decade. The search for a brain trauma protein was inspired by the momentous 1970s' discovery of a protein released into the blood by damaged cardiac tissue, which changed the way doctors identify heart disease. After years of rigorous trials, that test was approved by the Food and Drug Administration in the 1980s, became available to the whole medical field—and is now run routinely to diagnose cardiac injury.

To win FDA approval for the new brain trauma blood test, the Army will have to conduct three successive phases of testing on humans. Phase I was concluded in early 2010, and Phase II in late 2010. Phase III will include about 1,200 subjects at civilian trauma centers around the country.

Dr. Hack said that the new blood test for the brain trauma protein is "very accurate, very sensitive and very specific." Tests for other biomarker proteins have been discovered that may be able to screen for subacute and chronic brain injury and will enable military doctors to make early diagnoses and monitor brain injury over time. Dr. Hack eventually wants to

see test results sent directly from the lab to the battlefield.

THIS WILL CHANGE THE WHOLE FIELD

It isn't hard to imagine the tremendous effect this test may have on civilian health, too. In fact, we don't have to just imagine—Dr. Hack's team is already working with the National Football League to define requirements for concussion screenings in its players. School athletes will also benefit tremendously from such a clear-cut diagnosis. All too often symptoms such as dizziness, headache and disorientation are downplayed by athletes who risk serious injury when they continue playing.

The test will be equally useful for people who have been in vehicle accidents…children who bang their heads on playgrounds…elders who fall…and even people who simply have persistent, unexplained headaches, which can be a symptom of a mild blow to the head—one that actually is a concussion—that someone might not even remember sustaining.

And finally, there will be safety measures that can be taken, whether it's giving someone on the bomb squad a desk job, taking a soldier out of combat—or an athlete off the field.

So there you go: A piece of good news for all of us that is, in fact, a game changer.

Concussion/Dementia Link

Even a mild concussion after age 65 can boost risk for dementia. The older brain appears to be particularly vulnerable to traumatic brain injury.

To reduce the risk for dementia once you've recovered from a concussion: Exercise, be mentally active and maintain an active social life.

Raquel Gardner, MD, clinical research fellow, San Francisco Veterans Affairs Medical Center, and leader of a study published in *JAMA Neurology*.

Little-Known Dangers of Head Injury

Alex B. Valadka, MD, professor and chair of the department of neurosurgery at the University of Texas, Houston, Health Science Center. He directs the neurotrauma services at Memorial Hermann Hospital, also in Houston, and has authored more than 100 papers on brain injury.

E ach year, more than one-third of Americans over age 65 fall. Although hip fracture is a well-known consequence, few people are aware of the seriousness of a blow to the head.

Especially in older adults, a head injury—whether it occurs during a fall, a car accident or a sports activity—can trigger potentially deadly bleeding inside the skull. That's because the brain shrinks as we age, increasing tension on the bridging veins, which run from the brain's surface to its outer lining (dura). As a result, the bridging veins become more vulnerable to rupture. The situation is often worsened by the use of blood thinners, which are commonly prescribed to help prevent heart attack and stroke. An estimated 50,000 Americans die each year as a result of head injuries.

Caution: It can be difficult to determine the seriousness of a head injury from outward signs alone. For example, bleeding inside the skull may not cause symptoms until days, or even weeks, after the head injury occurred.

Red flags: Increasing sleepiness…a severe headache that keeps getting worse…confusion…difficulty walking…impaired memory…slurred speech…blurred vision…and/or vomiting.

Important: People who have suffered a minor head injury don't necessarily have to see a doctor—but they should get to an emergency room immediately if any of the above symptoms occur…even if it's days after the injury.

Main types of head injuries…

SKULL FRACTURES

A skull fracture is a break in the skeleton of the head (skull) and typically is caused by a fall or a car accident. A skull fracture is among the most dramatic-looking head injuries because it may be accompanied by copious external bleeding.

In most cases, however, a skull fracture isn't very serious as long as there isn't an accompanying brain injury and/or bleeding. In fact, a skull fracture may protect the brain. When the skull fractures during an accident, it absorbs part of the blow, and less of the trauma reaches the brain itself.

Physical signs of a skull fracture include bruises around the eyes (raccoon's eyes) or behind the ears, or the leaking of clear cerebrospinal fluid from the nose or ears.

Treatment: Many skull fractures heal on their own. Hospitalization may be required for overnight observation. Patients also may be given imaging tests, such as a computed tomography (CT) scan, to check for bleeding inside the skull.

CONCUSSION

A concussion is a head injury that does not cause visible physical damage and is often characterized by headache, confusion and/or amnesia. The brain damage that occurs—which is thought to involve disruptions in blood flow or nerve impulses, or temporary damage to axons (nerve fibers)—may not show up on CT scans or other imaging tests. Doctors rely on a medical history and the concussion symptoms listed above to make a diagnosis.

Most concussions are caused by a fall, car accident or athletic injury. Patients usually recover completely within a few hours—or, at most, a few days.

Treatment: Anyone with concussion symptoms following a blow to the head should get to an emergency room, especially if there is any loss of consciousness, confusion or memory loss.

The patient probably will be given a CT scan to check for bleeding in the skull or brain. If the test is normal—and most are—the patient will be advised to avoid strenuous physical activity, such as heavy lifting or climbing stairs, for a few days to aid healing of the brain. *Acetaminophen* (Tylenol) is prescribed for pain.

CONTUSIONS/LACERATIONS

Contusions (bruises) and lacerations (tears) of brain tissue are potentially more serious than a concussion. Both contusions and lacerations may be caused by a sudden blow to the head, which often occurs during a fall, physical assault or when the head moves very rapidly, causing the brain to hit the inside of the skull, such as often occurs in a car accident.

Symptoms may include severe headaches, dizziness, vomiting, irritability, agitation and/or confusion.

Minor contusions/lacerations usually clear up on their own within a few days.

Warning: Patients who experience severe, persistent headache, decreased alertness or consciousness, weakness in a limb, or one pupil larger than the other may have sustained a serious brain injury and should get immediate attention.

Treatment: Emergency surgery will probably be required if the CT or magnetic resonance imaging (MRI) scan shows significant bleeding/bruising, and the patient is also exhibiting the neurological symptoms described above. The surgeon will make an incision in the skull over the area of the injury. He/she will remove damaged brain tissue, along with any blood/fluids that may be present, to reduce brain swelling and pressure inside the skull.

INTRACRANIAL HEMATOMAS

An intracranial hematoma occurs when blood accumulates inside the brain, or in the area between the brain and the skull, due to an injury.

With a hematoma, the brain may be injured by the pressure caused by a blood accumulation (clot). This pressure can cause neurological problems, such as seizures, visual problems and/or weakness in a limb. Additional symptoms of an intracranial hematoma, including headache, loss of consciousness and one dilated pupil, are similar to those caused by other head injuries.

Treatment: Small hematomas, which can be detected by MRI or CT scans, often clear up on their own without subsequent treatment. Patients with larger hematomas, however, may require emergency surgery to stop bleeding and remove blood that could increase pressure on the brain.

How to Help Your Brain Heal

Laurie Steelsmith, ND, naturopathic doctor and acupuncturist in private practice, Honolulu.

News stories about concussions have brought this brain injury to the top of our minds—their number has doubled between 2005 and 2012 among young athletes (according to a recent study published in *American Journal of Sports and Medicine*), and researchers are looking closely at a pattern of deadly brain disease in former NFL players, trying to discern whether a history of concussions plays a role in its development.

But don't make the mistake of thinking this is a problem only for those playing sports. The truth is that a concussion can be the result of banging your head on a piece of furniture, being in a minor car accident or even tripping over your dog in a dark hallway and bumping your head against the wall. About one million concussions occur in the US each year, according to reports of hospital admissions, and there are likely many more people who have them and don't seek help—in short, we're all at risk.

There has been some fascinating research based on work done with soldiers who had suffered brain injuries. It concluded that one of the most important things to do for someone who has suffered a concussion (or a far more serious traumatic brain injury) is to feed him or her as soon as possible. It seems that making sure patients get at least 50% of their usual calorie intake within 24 hours—including a higher-than-usual amount of protein, which should be continued for two weeks—is vital to healing. A healthy diet makes sense. But what other natural treatments might help heal a hurting brain?

WHAT YOU NEED TO KNOW

First, it's important to review what we should know about concussion, which is like a bruise that results from your brain colliding with your skull. Anyone who has had a blow to the head should consider himself at risk, most especially if there was even a momentary loss of consciousness.

Other signs of concussion: Headache, nausea, difficulty concentrating and/or short-term memory loss. One or more of these symptoms should trigger a call to your doctor, who will determine if further testing is required.

Laurie Steelsmith, ND, a naturopathic doctor and acupuncturist based in Honolulu, believes that naturopathic medicine can offer natural ways to help the tissues heal after a concussion. *Here are the natural remedies Dr. Steelsmith revealed…*

• **Load up on antioxidants.** Eat a healthy diet with abundant protein (as mentioned above) and also eat lots of blueberries during the two weeks following the injury.

The reason: Blueberries contain potent flavonoid antioxidants that help to strengthen blood vessel walls, including in the brain. Supplement the fruit's antioxidants by taking up to 3,000 mg a day of vitamin C, which also helps reduce the oxidative stress in the brain associated with head trauma. According to Dr. Steelsmith, buffered powder (vitamin C combined with small amounts of calcium, magnesium and potassium) is most easily absorbed—she suggested mixing the powder with juice.

• **Drink fluids.** Make sure the body is well-hydrated, as that allows the brain to heal more quickly.

How much to drink: Dr. Steelsmith said to drink one ounce of fluid (nonalcoholic and preferably noncaffeinated—water is best) per day per two pounds of body weight, so a person who weighs 100 pounds should drink 50 ounces over the course of the day for the critical two weeks.

• **Take arnica (Arnica montana).** You are probably familiar with arnica cream, made from a plant that has served medicinal purposes for more than 500 years and used for sore muscles, sprains and bruises. But arnica also comes in the form of homeopathic pellets, which help to expedite healing of bruised

brain tissue, Dr. Steelsmith said. Place three homeopathic arnica 30c pellets (available at health stores and online) under your tongue within 15 minutes of the trauma or as soon as you can get them. Continue this dosage every hour for the rest of the day, reducing frequency on the second, third and fourth days to three doses—one in the morning, one at lunch and one in the evening, says Dr. Steelsmith.

• **Double dose of fish oil—fast.** While the general recommendation for most people is to take one to two grams daily of high-potency fish oil, Dr. Steelsmith said that it is a good idea for people who have suffered head injuries to take up to four grams as quickly as possible after the injury and to continue taking four grams once daily for up to seven days afterward. This advice is based on a recent animal study from West Virginia University School of Medicine reported in the *Journal of Neurosurgery*, which demonstrated that taking high-potency fish oil that contained large amounts of the omega-3 fatty acids EPA and DHA (such as Nordic Naturals Omega-3D, which contains 825 mg EPA and 550 mg DHA per one-teaspoon serving), can assist in healing concussion. This will help decrease brain inflammation and with it the fogginess, memory loss and headaches that are often a part of concussion.

Note: If there is evidence of bleeding in your brain (see below), do not take fish oil.

DANGER ZONE

It is important to realize that the danger zone following a concussion can last up to 48 hours, with the first 24 hours being the most critical. The danger is that bleeding will occur in the brain (especially likely if a person is taking an anticoagulant medication such as *warfarin*) or that a blood clot can form. The following symptoms should be seen as a medical emergency, warranting a call to 9-1-1 and a visit to the emergency department of the nearest hospital:

• **A headache that gets continually worse**
• **Vomiting**
• **Slurred speech**
• **One pupil larger than the other** or other visual disturbances

- **Change in sleeping pattern**—such as sleeping more than normal
  - **Seizure**
  - **Confusion and restlessness**
  - **Amnesia**

Luckily, severe problems are quite rare. Most concussions are much less threatening, and most people can heal safely and completely at home.

Can a Concussion Cause PTSD?

Study titled "Association of Symptoms Following Mild Traumatic Brain Injury With Posttraumatic Stress Disorder vs. Postconcussion Syndrome," published in *JAMA Psychiatry.*

After a concussion, even a mild one, many people feel completely out of sorts. They're discombobulated, jittery, depressed, irritable, unable to sleep well—for weeks, months or even years. Doctors call this experience post-concussion syndrome… but they should be calling it something else. That's because it could actually be post-traumatic stress syndrome—yes, the same thing that war vets and crime victims get. *Knowing this can help you and your doctor take important steps to treat these symptoms and get back on track after a concussion…*

THE PTSD LINK

Symptoms of post-concussion syndrome can include headache, dizziness, fatigue, light sensitivity, irritability, anxiety, sleeplessness, loss of memory and lack of concentration. All of these are also symptoms of PTSD. Now a team of French physicians has evidence that post-concussion syndrome may really be a form of PTSD.

The researchers followed 1,361 patients who had had traumatic injuries due to assaults, car crashes, falls or some other cause for three months from the time the injuries occurred. A total of 534 patients had concussions and 827 patients had other (nonhead) injuries. Three

months after the injury, 21% of the concussed patients and 16% of patients who did not have a head injury had symptoms that qualified for a diagnosis of post-concussion syndrome.

The team then created graphs that plotted out the symptoms of post-concussion syndrome and PTSD in their patients, both concussed and those without head injuries. The graphs became potent visuals to confirm that a diagnosis of "post-concussion syndrome" was not specific to having a concussion. The graphs also showed that symptoms of post-concussion syndrome fit into those of a certain form of PTSD called hyperarousal-type PTSD. They ultimately concluded that "post-concussion syndrome" is a redundant diagnosis and is really a form of PTSD.

BEING PREPARED

Most people don't know that they should seek medical help for psychological symptoms after a concussion. Standard treatment for post-concussion syndrome is actually similar to that of PTSD. Patients may be prescribed a limited course of an antidepressant, such as *amitriptyline*, to ease symptoms, including irritability, dizziness, depression and headache. They also may be referred to a mental health specialist for psychological counseling. This may be all a person needs, or a regimen specifically used for PTSD may be better.

Although different types of psychotherapy are used to treat PTSD, cognitive behavioral therapy is considered the most effective. It focuses on identifying and changing faulty thinking (such as misinterpretation of traumatic events) and replacing negative, self-sabotaging thoughts, feelings and behaviors with positive, empowering ones.

Amitriptyline may be prescribed for relief of chronic headache and other symptoms, or a type of antidepressant called a selective serotonin reuptake inhibitor may be given to patients to help them feel less worried and depressed. Selective serotonin reuptake inhibitors include drugs such as *paroxetine* (Paxil) and *sertraline* (Zoloft). Of course, no patient offered antidepressant therapy should feel that no other options exist. Naturopathic physicians have a toolbox of natural approaches to anxiety and depression, as well. And therapy doesn't go on indefinitely. Most people complete cognitive behavioral therapy in three to six months. As for SSRI therapy, treatment to reverse symptoms typically lasts up to three months after which a person may continue taking a lower dose of the medication for up to a year, if needed.

If you or anyone you know suffers a concussion, don't feel confused or alone if symptoms described above emerge and linger. You might well have post-traumatic stress disorder. You can best help yourself get through it by seeking mental health care.

Don't Suffer with OCD

James Greenblatt, MD, an integrative psychiatrist board-certified in child and adult psychiatry. He is chief medical officer, Walden Behavioral Care, Waltham, Massachusetts, and an assistant clinical professor of psychiatry at Tufts University School of Medicine in Boston. JamesGreenblattMD.com

You wash your hands so often that they're red and raw. Perhaps you repeatedly rearrange the food in your kitchen cabinets so that all items are facing a certain way.

Or you may check over and over again to make sure that your front door is locked. Perhaps you hoard newspapers and other everyday objects until your house is filled with junk—or count to yourself whenever you drive through a stoplight.

If you or someone you know experiences these or similar symptoms, it could be a red flag for obsessive-compulsive disorder (OCD).

Inside the mind of an OCD sufferer: People with this disorder have disturbing, unwanted thoughts, such as the belief that they are contaminated by germs or are about to be in a horrible car crash. These obsessive thoughts cause intense anxiety that the sufferer attempts to ease with compulsive behaviors (or rituals) such as repeated hand-washing or counting in unusual patterns.

Suffering in silence: For people who have never experienced OCD, the symptoms seem entirely irrational. The irony is, even those who

have the disorder know that their thoughts and behaviors are irrational but, for unknown reasons, they just can't stop them. As a result, people with OCD are usually ashamed of their symptoms and often go to great lengths to hide them from their friends, family or doctor. Unfortunately, more than half of Americans with this disorder never receive treatment.

Even when a person with OCD sees a doctor for it, the condition is very difficult to treat. The conventional approach—usually, an antidepressant and psychological counseling called cognitive behavioral therapy—reduces the severity of symptoms by about 50%, according to research, but achieves complete recovery in only 20% of cases.

New approach: A technique called integrative psychiatry—using conventional treatments and natural therapies such as nutritional supplements—is likely to produce far better results than conventional treatment alone. *Best approaches…*

SEROTONIN BOOSTERS

• **Serotonin is a neurotransmitter** (brain chemical) that plays a key role in regulating mood, appetite and sleep. Low levels of serotonin are believed to be a contributing cause of OCD. Many factors can reduce serotonin. For example, it's thought that serotonin levels can be lowered by a diet high in processed foods, sugar and fat…stress…and chronic inflammation.

• **Selective serotonin reuptake inhibitor (SSRI) antidepressants** help OCD by blocking the absorption of serotonin in the brain, which keeps levels in the body higher. Medication is quite helpful for some OCD patients, while others find that it increases their obsessive thinking.

The integrative approach: Several nutritional supplements boost serotonin and thereby help reduce or eliminate OCD symptoms.

Work with your doctor to determine which of the following supplements (one or more may be recommended) would be the most useful for you. To find an integrative doctor near you, go to IMMH.org.

Helpful supplements...*

• **Vitamin B-12.** A deficiency of this serotonin-boosting B vitamin is common in people with OCD. If you have this disorder, your doctor should test your blood levels of vitamin B-12.

My advice: Most conventional doctors consider blood levels of 200 pg/mL to 1,100 pg/mL to be "normal," but I treat any patient with a level below 500 pg/mL with weekly B-12 injections until his/her blood level reaches 900 pg/mL. B-12 is also available in sublingual and liquid forms. Some patients have a dramatic decrease in OCD symptoms with this treatment alone.

• **Folate.** This B vitamin is also crucial for serotonin production and can boost the effectiveness of antidepressants. However, some OCD patients can't absorb folate properly due to a genetic abnormality.

My advice: For patients with OCD, I typically recommend having an MTHFR test (methylenetetrahydrofolate reductase mutations) to check for the enzymes that are necessary to process folate. If the test is positive, you may need to take 7.5 mg to 15 mg daily of a medication called L-methylfolate (Deplin) that supplies a high dose of the nutrient.

• **Omega-3s.** The brain is nearly 60% fat. To work optimally, it needs healthful fats such as the omega-3 fatty acids EPA and DHA found in fish oil. Omega-3s can be obtained by eating fatty fish two or three times a week, but I have found that OCD patients often have an aversion to fish.

My advice: Try a daily supplement containing 3 g of omega-3 fatty acids with an EPA to DHA ratio of 2:1.

• **5-HTP (5-hydroxytryptophan)** is a compound that boosts serotonin levels.

My advice: I typically recommend a daily dose of 100 mg to 300 mg of 5-HTP for OCD sufferers.

Important: Serotonin syndrome is a potentially dangerous condition (with agitation, rapid heart rate, blood pressure fluctuations and hot flashes) that can develop when patients take 5-HTP in addition to some painkillers and cough medicines. 5-HTP should not be used with an antidepressant unless the patient is under the guidance of a medical professional.

• **Inositol.** In some OCD patients, supplementing with inositol (a vitamin-like compound that plays a role in serotonin receptors on cells) improves symptoms of the condition dramatically.

My advice: I typically have OCD patients start with 1 g to 3 g a day and increase slowly to 10 g to 12 g daily. The dose should be divided so it's taken two to three times a day. (Taking too much inositol too quickly can cause digestive trouble.)

SLOW DOWN THE INFLAMMATION

Inflammation anywhere in the body disrupts serotonin metabolism—and people with OCD are often in a state of chronic, low-grade inflammation.

To reduce chronic inflammation...

• **Get enough vitamin D.** Ask your doctor to test you for vitamin D deficiency (which I define as a blood level below 30 ng/mL). If you're deficient, take 2,000 international units (IU) to 4,000 IU of vitamin D daily to reach the level recommended by your doctor.

• **Take magnesium.** This mineral is also thought to reduce inflammation. In addition, it's required to balance levels of the stress hormone cortisol. If you have OCD, ask your doctor if you should take a magnesium citrate or magnesium glycinate supplement.

Important: Don't take magnesium supplements if you have kidney disease, since you may not be able to excrete excess magnesium.

• **Get better sleep.** Treat insomnia with the basics—for example, go to bed at the same time every night and get up at the same time every morning, giving yourself at least seven hours in bed.

• **Reduce stress.** Stress not only causes inflammation but also worsens the symptoms of OCD. Reduce stress with mindfulness-based stress-reduction techniques, such as meditation, yoga, playing a musical instrument and/or exercise.

*Check with your doctor before trying these or any other nutritional supplements. Some may interact with prescription medications or affect medical conditions.

WHAT IS OCD?

Obsessive-compulsive disorder (OCD) is a psychiatric illness that affects more than two million Americans.

The condition is characterized by repetitive, upsetting thoughts (obsessions) and an overwhelming urge to perform behaviors or rituals (compulsions) to help alleviate related anxiety. The cause is unknown, but genetics may play a role.

PROBIOTICS FOR OCD

The toxic gut bacteria Clostridia can generate HPHPA, a compound that disrupts normal brain function. High levels of HPHPA are a feature of many psychiatric diseases, including OCD. If OCD symptoms increase after use of an antifungal or antibiotic (both of which may allow HPHPA growth), ask your doctor about testing for HPHPA.

Your doctor can order a urine test for HPHPA from a lab that specializes in digestive disorders, such as the Great Plains Laboratory, GreatPlainsLaboratory.com, or Genova Diagnostics, GDX.net. If HPHPA is detected, consider trying high-dose probiotics that supply 50 billion to 300 billion CFUs (colony-forming units) daily. Consult your doctor for any additional treatment you may need.

Schema Therapy: Effective Treatment for Borderline Personality Disorder

Joan Farrell, PhD, director of the Schema Therapy Institute Midwest–Indianapolis Center, and coauthor, with Ida Shaw, of Group Schema Therapy for Borderline Personality Disorder.

Borderline personality disorder (BPD), a mental illness marked by difficulty managing emotions, extreme fears of abandonment and self-destructive behaviors has continued to be notoriously difficult to treat—until recently. BPD patients can get the help they need, thanks to a novel form of psychotherapy called schema therapy. (Unhealthy or early maladaptive "schemas" are self-defeating, core themes or patterns that we keep repeating throughout our lives.)

The research is encouraging. In one study, for instance, one group of BPD patients received the typical treatment consisting of weekly individual psychotherapy sessions—but after eight months, 84% of these patients still met the diagnostic criteria for the disorder. However, a second group received the typical treatment plus weekly sessions of schema therapy—and after eight months, only 6% still had BPD.

Who develops BPD? Though not as well-known as bipolar disorder or schizophrenia, BPD is actually more common, affecting from 2% to 6% of US adults. People who develop BDP tend to have sensitive, reactive temperaments. Often their core emotional needs were not met during childhood. Perhaps they had an unstable home environment…did not form a secure attachment with a caregiver…and/or were physically, sexually or emotionally abused. Genetics also may play a role, as the disorder appears to run in families.

Although more US women than men are treated for BPD, this could be due to a gender bias in diagnosis. For instance, men with certain BPD symptoms, such as intense anger and aggressiveness, often are diagnosed instead with antisocial personality disorder (a long-term pattern of manipulating and exploiting others). In many cases, for both women and men, BPD goes unrecognized.

Signs of the disorder: BPD symptoms often first appear in adolescence. The diagnosis generally is made if a person exhibits five or more of the typical symptoms. *For instance, he or she may…*

• **Make frantic efforts to avoid real or imagined abandonment.**

• **Have tumultuous, intense relationships** in which he or she alternates between idealizing and disliking the other person.

• **Have an unstable self-image** (signs include difficulty choosing friends or sticking to a career path).

• **Act impulsively and self-destructively** (overspending, binge eating, excessive drinking, risky sex).

- **Experience intense mood swings and excessive emotional reactions.**
- **Have chronic feelings of emptiness.**
- **Feel intense rage or have difficulty controlling anger.**
- **Experience brief episodes of being out of touch with reality.**
- **Engage in self-injury** (such as cutting) or make repeated suicide attempts.

The treatment that can help: Schema therapy combines cognitive behavioral and emotion-focused techniques. It centers on helping patients change longstanding, negative self-images and self-defeating behaviors, incorporating methods such as role-playing, letter writing, assertiveness training, anger management, guided imagery, relaxation, gradual exposure to anxiety-producing situations and challenges to negative thoughts and beliefs.

A unique key element of schema therapy is limited reparenting in which, within the bounds of a professional relationship, the patient establishes a secure attachment to the therapist. "Many patients with BPD missed some critical emotional learning as children. They were not adequately validated and encouraged to express their emotions and needs. In schema therapy, the therapist meets some of those core childhood needs—for example, by setting limits, expressing compassion and providing nurturance," Joan Farrell, PhD, director of the Schema Therapy Institute Midwest-Indianapolis center, said. The goal is for patients to become emotionally healthy and autonomous enough that eventually they no longer need the therapist to meet these core needs—because they learn to do so themselves.

Do you think that you or someone you love might benefit from schema therapy for BPD? Dr. Farrell recommended working with a therapist certified by the International Society of Schema Therapy.

Referrals: SchemaTherapySociety.org.

Schema therapy usually is done in one-on-one sessions. However, research from Dr. Farrell and colleagues demonstrates a high level of effectiveness from a group-therapy version, and a large international trial is under way

to further test this model. A combination of group and individual schema therapy may prove to be the optimal way, Dr. Farrell said, to go beyond the symptom control of other behavioral approaches to improve the quality of BPD patients' lives—and even lead to remission of the disorder.

What a Fainting Spell Could Really Mean...

Lewis A. Lipsitz, MD, a professor of medicine at Harvard Medical School, vice president for academic medicine and director of the Institute for Aging Research at Hebrew SeniorLife in Boston. He is the chief of the gerontology division at Beth Israel Deaconess Medical Center, also in Boston.

Even though some people faint for seemingly harmless reasons, such as the sight of blood, there are several potential causes. This temporary loss of consciousness that lasts no more than a few minutes can occur any time the brain isn't getting enough oxygen-rich blood.

What you need to know about the most common causes of syncope (pronounced "SIN ko-pe"), the medical term for fainting...

- **Heart conditions.** Arrhythmias, in which the heart beats too fast (tachycardia), too slow (bradycardia) or in an irregular pattern, cause fainting in up to 12% of older adults who suffer from syncope. With an arrhythmia, ineffective pumping of blood can result in an insufficient amount of blood going to the brain.

Typical treatment: Medication to help control the underlying heart condition.

- **Medications.** Certain drugs, such as medications for high blood pressure, heart failure, depression and Parkinson's disease, can cause fainting, especially when you first start taking them and/or if the dosage is too high. Men who take excessive doses of medication for an enlarged prostate, such as *tamsulosin* (Flomax), also may faint.

Typical treatment: Your doctor may lower the dosage or prescribe a different medication.

Never stop taking a prescription drug without speaking to your physician.

●**Orthostatic (postural) hypotension (low blood pressure).** Standing up after sitting or lying down shifts your center of gravity and causes blood to pool in the legs—often reducing blood flow to the brain. Normally, blood vessels constrict in response to this postural change, ensuring that your brain continues to get enough blood. But in people with orthostatic hypotension, this mechanism is defective.

Typical treatment: Drinking enough water (which increases blood volume and prevents dehydration)…avoiding alcohol (which is dehydrating)…and wearing support hose (to prevent blood from pooling in the legs). Some people may be prescribed *fludrocortisone* (Florinef) to increase blood volume (including that to the brain) and *midodrine* (ProAmitine) to constrict blood vessels.

●**Postprandial hypotension.** After a meal (postprandial), blood pools in the intestines, thus reducing blood flow to the brain. In healthy people, the body responds by increasing heart rate and constricting blood vessels to maintain normal blood pressure. This mechanism fails in people with postprandial hypotension.

Typical treatment: Eat smaller, more frequent meals with fewer carbohydrates.

●**Vasovagal syncope.** This type of fainting, which can be triggered by emotional distress, exertion (such as straining on the toilet), heat or the sight of blood, leads to an exaggerated bodily process. The heart rate slows and blood vessels in the legs widen, allowing blood to pool in the legs. This lowers blood pressure, reduces blood flow to the brain and can result in fainting.

In some people, vasovagal syncope results from overly sensitive reflexes involved in swallowing, urinating or defecating. Vasovagal syncope also can occur in people who have a condition known as carotid sinus hypersensitivity, which causes fainting when excess pressure is placed on the carotid (neck) artery—for example, when a shirt collar is too tight.

Typical treatment: Avoiding situations that trigger vasovagal syncope. In people with swallowing syncope, eating smaller, more frequent meals can help. Men should sit on the toilet while urinating if they have this form of syncope. Adding more fiber to your diet helps prevent constipation.

●**Illnesses.** In people with anemia (deficiency of red blood cells), fainting may occur if they bleed excessively (due to an injury, for example), because blood loss can trigger a sharp drop in blood pressure. Hypoglycemia (low blood sugar), which can occur in people with or without diabetes, also can lead to fainting.

Typical treatment: People who have anemia should see their doctors regularly for treatment and monitoring of the condition. People with diabetes should control their blood sugar levels.

IDENTIFYING THE CAUSE

Syncope is sometimes misdiagnosed as a stroke, brain tumor or seizure—all of which can cause loss of consciousness. But strokes, tumors and seizures are more apt to also cause slurred speech and/or vision loss. According to a recent study, doctors often rush to perform costly heart tests, such as cardiac enzyme tests, which measure possible heart damage, while overlooking much less expensive postural blood pressure testing.

Simple test: When assuming a standing position after lying down, you may have orthostatic hypotension if systolic (top number) blood pressure drops by more than 20 mm/Hg or if systolic pressure drops below 100 mm/Hg.

Another important tool: The tilt table test. For this test, you lie down and are strapped to a table, which is then tilted to raise the upper body to simulate what happens when you go from a lying to a standing position. Your body's response to the change in position may indicate whether you have orthostatic hypotension.

The tilt table test may be used in addition to postural blood pressure testing (mentioned above).

If your doctor suspects that your fainting is due to a heart problem, you may receive an electrocardiogram (which measures electrical activity of the heart) and an echocardiogram (a type of ultrasound test that helps detect abnormalities in heart rate or rhythm).

IF YOU OR SOMEONE ELSE FAINTS

If you're feeling faint: Lie or sit down immediately. If you're sitting, put your head between your knees to help restore blood flow to your brain.

If someone else faints...

•**Get the person into a supine position** (lying down with the face up). Raise the legs so they're higher than the head to bring blood back to the heart and head.

•**Check breathing.** If breathing has stopped, call 911 and perform cardiopulmonary resuscitation (CPR)—about 100 uninterrupted chest compressions per minute.

The Secret to Curing Dizziness

Jack J. Wazen, MD, a neurotologist (an ear, nose and throat doctor) who specializes in microsurgical procedures, removal of tumors, and hearing devices at the Silverstein Institute. He is coauthor of *Dizzy: What You Need to Know About Managing and Treating Balance Disorders*.

If you go to a doctor complaining of dizziness, chances are one in five that your condition will be misdiagnosed. Even though dizziness is one of the most common medical problems—affecting up to 15 million Americans each year—it is also one of the most complex.

Problem: Many people downplay the significance of dizziness and end up suffering unnecessarily for months or even years. But when dizziness is chronic (occurring for more than three weeks), it could indicate a serious health problem, such as heart failure, a brain tumor, diabetes or a thyroid disorder.

If dizziness develops suddenly, it could be due to an inner-ear disorder or even signal an emergency such as a transient ischemic attack (TIA)—also known as a "ministroke"—or a full-blown, life-threatening stroke. (Dizziness

that is due to a stroke typically is accompanied by other neurological symptoms, such as double vision, slurred speech or weakness or numbness in the face or limbs.)

Solution: Fairly simple, noninvasive therapies are now available for most forms of chronic dizziness, including some that were previously thought to be incurable or correctable only through surgery.

What you need to know...

WHAT'S CAUSING YOUR DIZZINESS?

Dizziness is a general term used to describe vertigo (a spinning sensation), light-headedness and/or imbalance. This wide variety of symptoms is due, in part, to the fact that dizziness can have many possible causes.

What your symptoms may mean...

•**Vertigo can be caused by inner-ear disorders such as Ménière's disease,** in which fluid buildup (due to an unknown cause) affects the inner-ear function and often is accompanied by tinnitus (ringing in the ears) and/or hearing loss in one or both ears...a viral or bacterial infection...allergies...or head trauma. Vertigo also can be caused by migraine...a TIA or stroke...a brain tumor...or certain medications. If one of the underlying conditions mentioned above is causing the vertigo, it will generally go away when the condition is treated. If dizziness is caused by medication, such as aspirin or antihistamines, it usually stops when the drug is discontinued. However, the damage may be permanent if the dizziness is caused by medications, such as the cancer drug *cisplatin* (Platinol), that have a toxic effect on the inner ear.

Improved therapy: The antibiotic *gentamicin* (Garamycin) can effectively treat Ménière's disease, not through its antibacterial effects, but rather by destroying the nerves causing the vertigo while leaving other nerve cells intact. The drug is administered to the inner ear over several days while the patient's hearing and balance are carefully monitored. In about half of cases, tinnitus symptoms are improved.

Gentamicin therapy for Ménière's disease has revolutionized treatment for this condition, which formerly required surgery that involved removal of the inner-ear system or the balance nerve.

Caution: Gentamicin therapy has about a 20% risk for some hearing loss.

Another common cause of vertigo is an inner-ear disorder known as benign paroxysmal positional vertigo (BPPV).

What happens: Calcium carbonate crystals break loose from the part of the inner ear that senses gravity and move into the area that senses movement, sending the brain a distorted signal when a person changes the position of his/her head—such as while looking up, bending over, lying down or turning over in bed.

This harmless condition usually can be alleviated by avoiding the head movements that trigger BPPV or by receiving a treatment known as the Epley maneuver, in which a doctor gently moves the patient's head into specific positions that can dislodge the calcium crystals and move them back to where they belong.

The Epley maneuver has an 85% success rate. Before this technique was adopted, the only cure for BPPV was open-ear surgery. Now such operations are rare.

• **Light-headedness (without vertigo) can be caused by a circulatory problem,** such as high or low blood pressure…hardening of the carotid arteries leading to the brain…cardiac arrhythmia (heart rhythm disturbance) or heart failure…a metabolic problem such as hormonal imbalances (including those due to menopause) or low blood sugar (glucose)…diabetes…or a thyroid disorder such as hypothyroidism (underactive thyroid). Treating the underlying condition usually eliminates the feeling of light-headedness.

Exciting recent discovery: A newly identified cause of dizziness, called a superior canal fistula, results from a hole in the superior semicircular canal (a balance receptor in the inner ear). The condition causes a vague feeling of light-headedness, imbalance and muffled hearing—especially after coughing or blowing one's nose. Previously it was written off as being untreatable, but this disorder can now be identified via a magnetic resonance imaging (MRI) or computed tomography (CT) scan and cured by placing a tiny patch made of bone dust and soft tissue over the hole—an operation that often can be performed without an overnight stay in a hospital.

• **Imbalance may be severe enough to make a person stumble or even fall.** It can be caused by an inner-ear disorder, such as vestibular neuritis (inflammation due to an infection in the inner ear)…a TIA or stroke…diabetic neuropathy (in which sensation is lost in the legs and feet)…acoustic neuroma (a tumor that can affect the balance nerve)…multiple sclerosis…or Parkinson's disease.

When the condition that is causing imbalance is treated, the dizziness usually goes away. In other cases, imbalance can be due to age-related degeneration of the nervous system.

Best therapy: Vestibular rehabilitation therapy to treat imbalance or non-vertigo dizziness. This technique involves working with a specially trained physical therapist to enhance neurological connections between the inner ear, the visual system and the legs. For example, the patient might practice walking down a hallway while looking right and left at pictures on the walls.

Prior to the development of this technique, the only therapy for these disorders were drugs prescribed for dizziness, such as *meclizine* (Antivert), which often cause unpleasant side effects, including drowsiness and dry mouth.

WHO SHOULD EVALUATE YOU?

Many primary care doctors can start the diagnostic process by taking your medical history and referring you to the right specialist.

Don't forget to tell your doctor about: All the medications you take. Also be sure to mention any allergies you have and note exactly when symptoms occur.

Depending on your symptoms, your physician may refer you to…

• **A cardiologist** if circulatory problems are suspected.

• **A neurologist** if the dizziness seems linked to a neurological problem, such as multiple sclerosis or Parkinson's disease.

• **An otolaryngologist** (ear, nose and throat, or ENT, specialist) if the inner ear is involved.

Best option: If your dizziness persists for 10 days or more, I recommend seeing a neurotologist (an ENT doctor specializing in inner-ear disorders) for a complete exam, including audiological and balance testing. An MRI or CT scan also may be performed.

Because neurotologists are trained to understand all forms of balance disorders, these specialists are well-equipped to identify the underlying cause and treat you or refer you to a cardiologist or neurologist. To find a neurotologist near you, contact the American Academy of Otolaryngology—Head and Neck Surgery (703-836-4444, EntNet.org).

What Is Face Blindness?

Galia Avidan, PhD, senior lecturer in psychology, Ben-Gurion University of the Negev, Be'er Sheva, Israel.

Prosopagnosia, also known as face blindness, is a disorder characterized by the brain's inability to perceive and remember faces. Individuals with this condition typically cannot recognize faces, often including familiar ones such as close friends and family members—and in extreme cases one's own face in the mirror.

Face blindness is often an inherited condition but can also result from a stroke or traumatic brain injury. It is not caused by learning disabilities, vision problems or memory loss. Once thought to be rare, face blindness is estimated to occur to some degree in one out of 50 people in the US.

There's currently no cure for the disorder, but people with this condition often learn to compensate by using other cues to recognize people, such as voice, body shape or other characteristics. For an online face blindness self-test, go to the site FaceBlind.org/facetests.

When Stuttering Strikes in Adulthood

Jane Fraser, president of The Stuttering Foundation of America, based in Memphis. She is editor of *Counseling Stutterers and Stuttering Therapy: Transfer and Maintenance* and coauthor, with Stanley Ainsworth, PhD, of *If Your Child Stutters: A Guide for Parents* (all from The Stuttering Foundation of America).

Most people think of stuttering as a speech problem. But when it occurs in an adult who has no history of stuttering, there are a variety of possible causes.

Here's what stuttering can mean if you or a loved one experiences it in adulthood…*

FINDING THE ROOT CAUSE

Every word that you speak is preceded by thousands of neuromuscular events. Anything that interrupts this complex—and lightning-fast—progression of steps can interrupt the normal flow of speech.

When researchers looked at adults who began stuttering, stroke was found to be the main cause. Adult-onset stuttering can also be caused by head injuries, brain tumors or neurodegenerative diseases such as Parkinson's disease and multiple sclerosis (MS). The stuttering in these cases develops as the disease progresses.

A number of drugs also can affect the brain's ability to coordinate the different components involved in speech. There have been reports of new-onset stuttering in adults taking a stimulant, such as *methylphenidate* (Ritalin), as well as selective serotonin reuptake inhibitor (SSRI) antidepressants, such as *sertraline* (Zoloft). Once the drug is discontinued, the stuttering typically stops.

If you experience a sudden change in speech: Always discuss it with your doctor so that he/she can investigate the cause.

WHAT IT SOUNDS LIKE

Adult-onset stuttering may sometimes be similar to the developmental stuttering that occurs during childhood—but there are some differences. *When an adult stutters, it may…*

*For more information on stuttering, call The Stuttering Foundation's toll-free hotline at 800-992-9392 or check the website at StutteringHelp.org.

• **Affect any part of a word.** Children with a stutter usually trip over the first letter: "I want to g-g-go." With adults, stuttering can occur on the second, third or fourth syllables: "I like that rest-t-aurant."

• **Be marked by interjections.** Some adults who stutter begin using interjections in their speech. For example, a sentence might be peppered with extraneous (nonword) sounds, such as "ahhh." An interjection can also be a long silence or hesitation between words or within a word.

• **Include rapid bursts of speech.** With neurological disorders, speech may be affected in this way. These bursts of speech might be unintelligible...or include the repetition of certain words or phrases.

FRUSTRATING BUT TEMPORARY

If the underlying problem improves, the stuttering will naturally get better—but it can take a long time. Someone who's had a mild stroke will probably regain normal speech within a few months. It can take much longer for those with more serious types of brain injuries. It might never go away in patients with MS, Parkinson's or other progressive neurodegenerative disorders.

WHAT YOU CAN DO

If you have a stutter that's caused by a neurological problem, including stroke, MS or Parkinson's disease, your doctor will probably refer you to a speech-language pathologist who specializes in stuttering. Sessions usually last about an hour and may be covered by insurance.

In addition to guiding a patient through strategies such as those described below, a therapist may help him identify disruptions in speech patterns and instruct him in the use of more appropriate patterns. If the patient has anxiety about his speech, therapy may include counseling to help change harmful perceptions about stuttering.

What helps most...

• **Speak slowly.** This is among the most effective ways to deal with a stutter. Super-slow speech will make you less likely to stumble over initial sounds. It can also help you reduce the frequent (and often unconscious) use of "filler" sounds, such as "um" or "ahh."

• **Ask others to slow down.** Many neurological diseases slow the rate at which you process information. It's easy to become overwhelmed when you're faced with a barrage of rapid speech from others—and you'll also tend to reciprocate with your own rapid-fire speech. Encourage people to speak more slowly. Take your time when you're listening as well as speaking.

Also, minimize background noise whenever possible to avoid getting overwhelmed by sounds—for example, keep the volume of the TV and radio in your home on low.

• **Maintain eye contact when speaking.** This will help both the person who stutters and the listener tune in to the conversation.

• **Use short sentences.** It will help your speech keep pace with your thoughts. Avoid complex sentences, such as "I really like the food at the new Chinese restaurant, and it's only three miles away, so let's go." Keep it short—"I like the new Chinese restaurant. It's close. Let's go."

• **Ease into words.** Word initiation can be a challenge for adults who stutter. My last name, "Fraser," will often come out "F-F-Fraser." You can get past this with a technique called easy onset. Speaking slowly, you say the first letter gently, then ease into the rest of the word—keep your lips slightly parted, as though you're puffing out a breath of air. The words will sound "softer," but they'll be easier to get out.

• **Loosen up.** If your posture feels tense, loosen up. And consciously relax the muscles in your face and throat. Breathe normally—and softly—while you speak.

• **Speak more.** It's natural to want to interact less with people when you're embarrassed about your speech. But the fact is, you need to speak more to overcome a stutter.

When you meet someone new, tell him that speech is a challenge. Say something like, "I have MS and a bit of a stutter. I need to speak slowly. OK?" You'll probably get an encouraging smile. Acknowledging your disability up front will make you feel less self-conscious.

Eye Symptoms That Mean Brain Danger

Neil Shulman, MD, associate professor in the department of internal medicine at Emory University School of Medicine, Atlanta, and Jack Birge, MD, medical director for performance improvement at Tanner Medical Center in Carrollton, Georgia. They are authors, with Joon Ahn, MD, of *Your Body's Red Light Warning Signals*. RedLightWarningSignals.com

Many serious health problems are first diagnosed from changes in the eyes. *Never ignore these eye symptoms…*

•**Sudden eyelid droop.**

What it may mean: If you notice that one of your eyelids has abruptly drooped lower than the other (possibly accompanied by double vision), it could indicate an aneurysm—a ballooning-out of a blood vessel in the brain. This is particularly likely when a patient's pupils are unequal in size. An aneurysm can press against nerves that control both eyelid position and pupil size.

Aneurysms aren't always dangerous, but those that rupture can cause brain damage or death. It's estimated that up to 5% of Americans have a brain aneurysm.

Causes: Most brain aneurysms are due to a natural weakness in an artery wall. Less often, they're caused by head trauma.

What to do: Get to an emergency room immediately.

Treatment: Aneurysms that are large and/or are causing symptoms are typically clipped—a neurosurgeon uses a metal clip to prevent blood from flowing through the aneurysm. Small aneurysms often are best left alone.

•**A haze, blur or darkness in the field of vision.**

What it may mean: A clot in a blood vessel may be blocking circulation to the retina, optic nerve or brain. Patients with this type of clot may be suffering from a stroke or be at high risk for a subsequent stroke—possibly within hours or days. (Other conditions that can cause these symptoms include inflamma-tion in the blood vessels, a retinal detachment or inflammation of the optic nerve.)

Causes of stroke: The same risk factors for cardiovascular disease, such as diabetes, high blood pressure and smoking, also increase the risk for stroke. The optic nerve and retina are very sensitive to changes in blood flow. Even a partial blockage can cause visual changes—and these changes may occur long before an actual stroke.

Important: Small clots that cause visual changes often dissolve on their own. Symptoms disappear—but the stroke risk still is there. Also, if you're having a stroke, you may not be aware of any symptom—an onlooker may be the one to alert you to a shift in behavior.

What to do: Get to an emergency room, even if the symptom is fleeting.

Treatment: Patients with clots (or a history of getting them) usually are treated with clot-dissolving (or clot-preventing) therapies. These include aspirin, *heparin*, *warfarin* or tissue plasminogen activator (TPA).

A procedure called carotid endarterectomy may be recommended for patients with large amounts of plaque in the carotid arteries. Fatty buildups in these arteries, which run from the neck to the brain, increase the risk for subsequent strokes. A test called the carotid doppler can be used to detect and measure the plaque.

EYE SYMPTOMS THAT ARE ALWAYS AN EMERGENCY

•**Sudden drooping of one or both eyelids.**

•**Pupils that are suddenly of unequal size.**

•**Severe pain within the eyeball.**

•**Rapid vision changes,** such as blurred vision or swarms of floaters or flashing lights.

What You Must Know About Unruptured Brain Aneurysm Removal

Seppo Juvela, MD, PhD, neurosurgeon, department of neurosurgery, University of Helsinki, Finland. His study was published in *Stroke*.

What if you had some reason for needing a brain scan? Maybe you got shook up in a car accident or maybe you have ringing and pressure in one of your ears that affects your hearing. So you get the scan, and the doctor comes back with good and bad news...

It turns out that you don't have a brain injury or an acoustic neuroma (a tumor in the ear that affects hearing) or whatever you had the brain scan for, but you do have an unruptured intracranial aneurysm (UIA)—a bulging blood vessel smack in the middle of your brain! An estimated six million people in the United States have a UIA, and one of those UIAs bursts every 18 minutes. If you have a UIA and it bursts, causing a hemorrhagic stroke, there's a 40% chance you won't survive more than 30 days. So surgery to remove it before it bursts sounds pretty attractive. Yet, when small UIAs (one-quarter inch or smaller) are found on brain scans, docs usually leave them alone, believing that their risk of bursting is small. In fact, the unruptured aneurysm lodged in your brain might not ever burst—but not necessarily because of its size. A Finnish study found that certain telltale characteristics determine whether or not a UIA should be removed. And this is a key point that American doctors have not been in the know about. For them, size is what matters most, even though small aneurysms have been known to burst, too.

TOP REASON TO HAVE THAT UIA REMOVED

So which people with UIAs are really most at risk for a hemorrhagic stroke? Being a cigarette smoker topped the list. Compared with ex-smokers and nonsmokers, smokers had three times the risk. Since most of us don't know if we are walking around with UIAs, the findings of this study make smoking even

more of a game of Russian roulette. If warnings about lung cancer, heart disease and premature aging aren't incentive enough to quit, the risk of brain damage or death from hemorrhagic stroke should be.

It also turns out that women, smokers or not, are more vulnerable than men when it comes to a bursting UIA. Age at diagnosis is also a big factor—men and women who were younger than 50 when the UIA was diagnosed were more than three times as likely to suffer a hemorrhagic stroke as people who were older than 50. If nothing else, these findings are clear—if you are a smoker or younger than 50 and told you have a UIA, you ought to have it removed no matter what the size, according to the researchers. If you are a nonsmoker and older than 40, especially if you are a man, you probably can safely take that watch-and-wait approach, they said.

GETTING RID OF UIAs

Microsurgical clipping and endovascular coiling are two common ways that UIAs are surgically taken care of. In microsurgical clipping, a hole is drilled through the skull to get to the aneurysm. Then a small metal clip is permanently placed at the base of the aneurysm to stop blood flow into it. Endovascular coiling, on the other hand, doesn't involve open brain surgery. Instead, a microcatheter is snaked through an artery in the groin to the site of the aneurysm in the brain. An x-ray technology called fluoroscopy is used to guide the microcatheter into place and make it release one or more tiny platinum coils attached to it into the aneurysm. The coils cause the blood in the aneurysm to clot, cutting off blood flow into the bulge.

The most serious complication of these procedures is rupture of the aneurysm. Incidence is not that common, occurring 2% to 3% of the time. And, naturally, recovery for microvascular clipping is longer than it is for endovascular coiling because microvascular clipping involves open brain surgery.

After clipping, most patients spend a night in the intensive care unit and then a few days in a private hospital room. Although patients will be able to be up and about after they leave the hospital, they do have to take it easy for the next four to six weeks to fully recover.

After endovascular coiling, patients also spend a night in the intensive care unit but get to go home the next day. Within a few days, they are fully back to all of their normal activities. One drawback to endovascular coiling, though, is that the UIA can come back. So patients having this procedure are required to visit their doctors for imaging tests on occasion to make sure all is well.

In any case, no matter what your health status, sex or age, there's no guarantee that a brain aneurysm won't burst, and it's ultimately up to you to decide whether to have surgery. The Finnish researchers came to their conclusions after they examined 118 people given a diagnosis of UIA before 1979 and followed them until they had hemorrhagic strokes or died of old age or other causes. The Finns were in a unique position to study what happens to people when UIAs, large or small, are just left alone. Up until 1979, instead of remov-ing at least large UIAs, Finnish doctors just left them alone.

Their study found that women, especially women who smoke and have large UIAs (more than one-quarter of an inch in size) are most at risk for a hemorrhagic stroke. In fact, the risk of hemorrhagic stroke in women with large UIAs was 73%. If the woman also smoked, her risk increased to 100%. Meanwhile, men who smoked and had an aneurysm of this size had half the risk of their female counterparts...50%. Risk was virtually nil for men who didn't smoke regardless of the size of their aneurysms...and nonsmoking women had a 31% risk.

Importantly for those people who learn that they have a UIA, this information can help them and their doctors make crucial decisions about whether to go through a risky procedure to remove it. If you do not have any of the risky characteristics, your safest option may be to do nothing at all—be sure to have a thorough discussion about this with your doctor.

CHAPTER 6

Help for Neurological Disorders: Parkinson's, MS, Epilepsy and More

Best Nondrug Approaches for Parkinson's

The telltale tremors, muscle stiffness and other movement problems that plague people with Parkinson's disease make even the mundane activities of daily living—such as brushing teeth, cooking and dressing—more difficult.

What's new: Even though medication—such as *levodopa* (L-dopa) and newer drugs including *pramipexole* and *selegiline*—have long been the main treatment to control Parkinson's symptoms, researchers are discovering more and more nondrug therapies that can help.

Among the best nondrug approaches (each can be used with Parkinson's medication)…

EXERCISE

For people with Parkinson's, exercise is like a drug. It raises neurotrophic factors, proteins that promote the growth and health of neurons. Research consistently shows that exercise can improve motor symptoms (such as walking speed and stability) and quality of life.

For the best results: Exercise 30 to 60 minutes every single day. Aim to work hard enough to break a sweat, but back off if you get too fatigued—especially the following day (this indicates the body is not recovering properly). Parkinson's symptoms can worsen with over-exercise. *Smart exercise habits…*

For better gait speed: Choose a lower-intensity exercise, such as walking on a treadmill (but hold on to the balance bars), rather than high-intensity exercise (such as running), which has a higher risk for falls and other injuries.

A recent study showed that a walking group of Parkinson's patients performed better than a group of patients who ran.

Michael S. Okun, MD, professor and chair of the department of neurology and codirector of the Center for Movement Disorders and Neurorestoration at the University of Florida College of Medicine in Gainesville. He is also the medical director at the Nation[...]son Foundation and has written more th[...] journal articles. Dr. Okun is autho[...] *Therapies for Parkinson's D[...]*

Important safety tip: Parkinson's patients should exercise with a partner and take precautions to prevent falls—for example, minimizing distractions, such as ringing cell phones.

• **For aerobic exercise**—Use a recumbent bicycle or rowing machine and other exercises that don't rely on balance.

• **For strength and flexibility**—Do stretching and progressive resistance training.

Excellent resource: For a wide variety of exercises, including aerobic workouts, standing and sitting stretches, strengthening moves, balance exercises and fall-prevention tips, the National Parkinson Foundation's *Fitness Counts* book is available as a free download at Parkinson.org/pd-library/books/fitness-counts.

• **For balance**—Researchers are now discovering that yoga postures, tai chi (with its slow, controlled movements) and certain types of dancing (such as the tango, which involves rhythmic forward-and-backward steps) are excellent ways to improve balance.

COFFEE AND TEA

Could drinking coffee or tea help with Parkinson's? According to research, it can—when consumed in the correct amounts.

Here's why: Caffeine blocks certain receptors in the brain that regulate the neurotransmitter dopamine, which becomes depleted and leads to the impaired motor coordination that characterizes Parkinson's. In carefully controlled studies, Parkinson's patients who ingested low doses of caffeine—about 100 mg twice daily—had improved motor symptoms, such as tremors and stiffness, compared with people who had no caffeine or higher doses of caffeine.

My advice Have 100 mg of caffeine (about the amour ___ ne six-ounce cup of home-brewed c ___ vo cups of black or green tea) twi ___ e in the morning and once i ___ n.

N ___ coffee has about 10 ___ cup.

___ supple-
___ help
___ ost

the effects of levodopa, but large studies have failed to prove that these supplements provide such benefits.

However, because Parkinson's is a complex disease that can cause about 20 different motor and nonmotor symptoms that evolve over time, the existing research may not apply to everyone. *Some people with Parkinson's may benefit from…*

• **Coenzyme Q10 (CoQ10).** This supplement promotes the health of the body's mitochondria ("energy generators" in the cells), which are believed to play a role in Parkinson's. In a large study, people with Parkinson's who took 1,200 mg per day showed some improvement in symptoms over a 16-month study period. However, follow-up studies found no beneficial effects.

• **Riboflavin and alpha-lipoic acid** are among the other supplements that are continuing to be studied.

Important: If you wish to try these or other supplements, be sure to consult your doctor to ensure that there are no possible interactions with your other medications.

MARIJUANA

A few small studies have concluded that marijuana can improve some neurological symptoms, but larger studies are needed to show benefits for Parkinson's patients, especially for symptoms such as depression and anxiety.

However: Marijuana is challenging for several reasons—first, it is illegal in most states. If you do live in a state that allows medical marijuana use, it has possible side effects—for example, it can impair balance and driving…it is difficult to know the exact dosage, even if it's purchased from a dispensary…and with marijuana edibles (such as cookies and candies), the effects may take longer to appear, and you may accidentally ingest too much.

If you want to try marijuana: Work closely with your doctor to help you avoid such pitfalls.

SEEING THE RIGHT DOCTOR

For anyone with Parkinson's, it's crucial to see a neurologist and, if possible, one who has advanced training in Parkinson's disease and movement disorders.

Important recent finding: A large study showed that patients treated by a neurologist had a lower risk for hip fracture and were less likely to be placed in a nursing facility. They were also 22% less likely to die during the four-year study.

Neurologists are best equipped to treat the ever-changing symptoms of Parkinson's. For optimal care, see the neurologist every four to six months. The National Parkinson Foundation's Helpline, 800-4PD-INFO (473-4636) can assist you in finding expert care.

Early Signs of Parkinson's Disease

Long before people exhibit the tremors, slowness and stiffness of Parkinson's, they often have other problems. Some of the potential risk factors for Parkinson's are loss of smell (about 80% of Parkinson's patients lose most of their sense of smell before they have problems with their motor skills)...chronic constipation...sleeping problems, in which patients act out violent dreams and may injure themselves or their bed partners...and feelings of fear and anxiety that develop for the first time in life.

Tanya Simuni, MD, professor of neurology, Northwestern University Feinberg School of Medicine, Chicago.

Easy Way to Ward Off Parkinson's

Xiang Gao, MD, PhD, assistant professor of medicine, Harvard Medical School, and associate epidemiologist, Brigham and Women's Hospital, both in Boston. He is leader of a study that was published in *Neurology*.

If you're at high risk for Parkinson's disease, then you probably want to do everything in your power to reduce your chance of getting this debilitating condition.

And now there is something you can do, according to some very exciting research out of Harvard.

This recent study suggests that eating a certain type of food may help stave off Parkinson's and the shaking, balance and movement problems that go along with it.

What's the fabulous food, you ask?

You'll be pleased to know that it's delicious!

EATEN ANY GOOD FLAVONOIDS LATELY?

The study took place at the Harvard University School of Public Health in Boston. A class of nutrients called flavonoids had been shown by previous research to protect certain neurons in the brain from damage and death. Since Parkinson's is a disease that affects the nervous system (including the brain and the spinal cord), the researchers decided to see whether eating high amounts of flavonoids and/or eating certain flavonoid-rich foods might reduce the risk for Parkinson's. They started by asking subjects to fill out food questionnaires.

They found that men who ate the most flavonoid-rich foods (five or more servings per week) had a 40% lower risk for developing Parkinson's within 20 to 22 years, compared with those who ate the least (less than one serving of flavonoid-rich foods per week). That's a huge reduction in risk.

However, women who ate the most total flavonoids were not at any lower risk, compared with women who ate the least.

But wait a minute, women—there is something valuable for you in this study. Researchers also analyzed the data more closely to see what they could tell about the effect of consuming specific flavonoid-rich foods. These included all kinds of teas, apples, strawberries, blueberries, red wine, oranges and orange juice. What they found was that, for female participants, eating two or more servings per week of strawberries and/or blueberries, in particular, was associated with a 22% lower risk of getting Parkinson's, compared with women who ate the least strawberries and/or blueberries (less than one serving per month).

For men, each of the flavonoid-rich foods mentioned above (not just strawberries and blueberries) seemed to reduce Parkinson's risk.

POWERFUL PROTECTORS

Lead researcher Xiang Gao, MD, PhD, explained why there were different results for each gender. It could be due to the different ways that men's and women's bodies work—such as hormones or metabolism—or it could be due to chance, Dr. Gao said.

Regardless, strawberries and blueberries worked for both genders, with at least two servings per week being associated with less Parkinson's for both genders. Dr. Gao didn't study whether other types of berries (such as blackberries and raspberries) would have a similar effect, but he noted that all berries contain similarly high levels of flavonoids, so there's a chance that they would.

A BERRY GOOD DIET

Future research will need to look at whether eating strawberries, blueberries and other flavonoid-rich foods helps those who already have Parkinson's. In the meantime, this study is one more good reason to eat more strawberries and blueberries.

Parkinson's Prevention

Xiang Gao, MD, PhD, research scientist, Harvard School of Public Health, Boston.

If an immediate family member had Parkinson's (such as a parent)...Is there anything you can do to help protect yourself from developing it?

Previous studies have shown that healthy dietary patterns (fruits, vegetables, whole grains, nuts and moderate amounts of alcohol), coffee consumption and exercise could be helpful. Furthermore, a recent study of 136,197 men and women shows that those who took *ibuprofen* regularly (twice weekly) for six years had a 40% lower risk for Parkinson's disease than those who took no ibuprofen.

Ibuprofen is believed to activate a pathway that inhibits brain inflammation, which may lead to Parkinson's disease.

If you are at increased risk for Parkinson's disease (due to family history or ongoing pesticide exposure, another Parkinson's risk factor), ask your doctor about taking ibuprofen as a potential preventative.

Caution: It's important to weigh your Parkinson's risk against heart disease risk. Taking a nonsteroidal anti-inflammatory drug (NSAID) other than aspirin, such as ibuprofen, may increase heart attack risk. All NSAIDs increase risk for bleeding.

Surprising Symptoms of Parkinson's Disease

Tien K. Khoo, PhD, senior lecturer, Griffith University School of Medicine, Australia. He completed this research while a research fellow at Newcastle University in England. His study was published in *Neurology*.

When people think about Parkinson's disease, what comes to mind are the characteristic movement problems—shakiness, rigidity, slowness. Yet even very early in the disease, Parkinson's brings other symptoms that have nothing to do with impaired movement.

Though these symptoms can lower quality of life, many Parkinson's patients don't mention them to their doctors, perhaps mistaking them for normal signs of aging...and doctors fail to ask about them. This is a shame, since many of these nonmotor symptoms are treatable. *A recent study highlights what patients should know about these other Parkinson's symptoms...*

• **The study.** Participants included 159 adults with early-stage Parkinson's plus 99 healthy adults. In both groups, the average age was in the late 60s. All participants answered a questionnaire that screened for 30 different nonmotor symptoms, including gastrointestinal and urinary problems...sexual dysfunc-

tion…emotional and cognitive troubles…sleep difficulties and more.

• **Findings.** On average, people with early Parkinson's disease had 8.4 of these nonmotor symptoms, while the healthy participants had only 2.8 of the symptoms. The most common symptoms in the Parkinson's group were drooling…urinary urgency…impaired sense of smell…anxiety…and constipation.

You might be thinking that some of these symptoms are common complaints that come with age. And that's true—but the symptoms were much more common among the Parkinson's patients than among the other people in the study. For example, among Parkinson's patients, 56% had problems with drooling, 46% experienced urinary urgency and 42% had constipation…but among the healthy participants, only 6% drooled, 19% had urinary urgency and 7% had constipation.

Even if you have not been diagnosed with Parkinson's, it is important to be aware of this research because the nonmotor symptoms of the disease sometimes are the first to appear. Bringing these symptoms to a doctor's attention may lead to a speedier and more accurate diagnosis.

What you can do: To take the Parkinson's Disease Nonmotor Symptoms Questionnaire, go to PDNMG.com and click on PD NMS Questionnaire (under Downloadable Tools to the right). Fill it out, then show it to your doctor. Many of these nonmotor symptoms of Parkinson's disease can be treated—but first, you and your doctor must recognize them for what they are.

Vitamins for Parkinson's

Vitamin D may protect against Parkinson's disease. Helsinki-based researchers found that people with the highest blood levels of vitamin D had a 67% lower risk for Parkinson's disease than those with the lowest levels of the vitamin. The vitamin's antioxidant activity and its role in regulating calcium to improve nerve conduction in the brain could provide the benefit. Have your vitamin D level checked annually, and supplement accordingly.

P. Knekt, et al., "Serum Vitamin D and the Risk of Parkinson's Disease," *Archives of Neurology* (2010).

You Need Vitamin B-6

A lack of vitamin B-6 is associated with Parkinson's disease risk.

Recent study: Japanese researchers have found that reduced levels of vitamin B-6 may raise risk for Parkinson's disease by about 50%. A deficiency of vitamin B-6 may increase levels of homocysteine, an amino acid that is potentially toxic to brain cells.

Good food sources of vitamin B-6 include eggs, walnuts, bananas and whole grains. Have your doctor test your homocysteine level. If it is elevated, supplement with vitamins B-6 and B-12 and folate.

K. Murakami, et al., "Dietary Intake of Folate, Vitamin B6, Vitamin B12 and Riboflavin and Risk of Parkinson's Disease: A Case-Control Study in Japan," *British Journal of Nutrition* (2010).

Dark Hair Advantage

The darker your hair, the lower your risk for Parkinson's disease. Blondes have a 60% higher risk for Parkinson's than people with black hair…and redheads have twice the risk.

Way to reduce risk: Drink caffeinated coffee. A recent study found that drinking one to four cups of coffee a day lowered Parkinson's risk by 45%.

Xiang Gao, MD, research scientist, department of nutrition, Harvard School of Public Health, Boston, and lead author of a study of more than 132,000 people, published in *Annals of Neurology*.

Look to Your Feet for Possible Signs of Neurological Disorders

If you pull your feet away because you're oversensitive to your podiatrist's* touch (such as when he/she cuts your toenails), this may be a sign of hyperreflexia. This condition can be an early indicator of Parkinson's disease or multiple sclerosis.

*To find a podiatrist, go to the website of the American Podiatric Medical Association, APMA.org.

Johanna S. Youner, DPM, a board-certified podiatrist in private practice, Park Avenue Laser Treatment, and director of the podiatric clinic at New York University Downtown Hospital, both in New York City. She serves as a spokesperson for the American Podiatric Medical Association.

ED May Mean Parkinson's

Erectile dysfunction may be an early sign of Parkinson's disease. Men with erectile dysfunction (ED) are 3.8 times more likely to develop Parkinson's disease than men without ED. In its early stages, Parkinson's alters brain circuits that control involuntary functions, including sexual arousal. This can occur years before the first Parkinson's symptoms appear.

Self-defense: Men experiencing ED should discuss the problem with their doctors. Also, consider drinking two cups of caffeinated coffee daily. Men who do so are less likely to develop Parkinson's.

Xiang Gao, MD, research scientist, department of nutrition, Harvard University, Boston, and leader of a 16-year study of 32,616 men, published in *American Journal of Epidemiology*.

Berries Lower Parkinson's Disease Risk

A recent study found that men who ate the most berries—along with tea, apples, or-anges and other major sources of healthful flavonoids—were about 40% less likely to develop Parkinson's than men who ate the least amount. Women and men appear to have a lower risk for the disease mainly due to anthocyanins, a type of flavonoid found in berries.

Xiang Gao, MD, PhD, a research scientist at Harvard School of Public Health and assistant professor of medicine at Harvard Medical School, both in Boston, and leader of a study presented at the American Academy of Neurology's 63rd Annual Meeting.

Handwriting Gives an Early Warning Sign of Parkinson's Disease

Study titled "Handwriting as an objective tool for Parkinson's disease diagnosis," published in *Journal of Neurology*.

Doctors usually diagnose Parkinson's disease after patients complain of the telltale symptoms—tremors, rigidity, slowed movements, impaired balance. These signs typically don't appear until this degenerative neurological disease is at a relatively late stage. In its early stages, however, Parkinson's often goes unnoticed…which is a problem, because early diagnosis maximizes the treatment options.

Breakthrough: There's a simple clue that can help detect Parkinson's in the early stages, long before obvious symptoms appear, a recent study reveals. *All that's required is putting pen to paper…*

SMALL WRITING, BIG CLUES

The study included 20 patients who had been diagnosed with early-stage Parkinson's disease and did not yet have obvious signs of motor impairment…plus 20 healthy people (the control group) who were matched for age, gender, education level and hand dominance. All of the participants were asked to write their names and copy an address. You may think that this is a very simple task, but actually it's quite complex—because it involves manual dexterity as well as cognitive, sensory and perceptual-motor abilities.

For this study, the participants wrote on regular lined paper attached to an electronic tablet that could measure the amount of pressure applied. The writing utensil was a wireless, electronic pen with a pressure-sensitive tip. A computer assessed the pressure applied by the pen, the placement and angle of the pen's tip, and the length of time it took to prepare and place the strokes of the pen. The length, height and width of the letters each person wrote also were measured.

Findings: Compared with the healthy control group, the patients with early-stage Parkinson's...

• **Spent more time with their pens in the air between strokes** (as if strategically planning their next move, the researchers said).

• **Applied less pressure when writing.**

• **Required more time to complete the handwriting task.**

• **Wrote smaller letters.**

Simplest clue revealed: Next, the researchers determined that it was possible to identify, with 97.5% accuracy, which writing samples were produced by people with early-stage Parkinson's based solely on the size of the letters! Researchers who were unaware of which writing samples came from which participant correctly identified 19 out of the 20 Parkinson's patients as having the disease...and correctly identified all 20 of the healthy controls as not having the disease.

People with Parkinson's frequently notice changes in their thinking ability before they notice any loss of motor skills. That's why a handwriting test that also engages cognitive skills—as opposed to one that focuses strictly on motor skills, such as drawing spirals (an assessment test doctors often use)—could well help doctors diagnose the disease in its early stages.

This was a fairly small study, so the results will need to be replicated in larger studies before the handwriting test could become a standard diagnostic tool. But in the meantime, why not test yourself? Write your name and copy several addresses, then compare what you've written to a sample of your handwriting from years ago. If your letters have become notice-

ably smaller, bring this fact to your doctor's attention, show him/her this article and ask whether you might benefit from being evaluated for Parkinson's.

Constipation Concern

Constipation may signal Parkinson's disease. In a study of 392 adults, those with Parkinson's disease were about twice as likely to report a history of constipation as those without the disease.

Theory: Parkinson's may begin to affect the autonomic nervous system—which controls digestion, bowel movements and other body functions—years or even decades before motor symptoms of the illness (such as tremors and rigid muscles) appear.

Self-defense: If you have a history of constipation and are suffering Parkinson's-like symptoms, see your doctor.

Walter A. Rocca, MD, MPH, professor of epidemiology and neurology, College of Medicine, Mayo Clinic, Rochester, Minnesota.

Depression May Increase Parkinson's Risk

The more severe the depression, the higher the risk for the disease. Parkinson's disease is three times more common among people with depression than people without it. Among those with depression, people who were hospitalized or whose depression was recurrent were at higher risk.

Possible reason: Depression may damage the brain in such a way that Parkinson's becomes more likely...and drugs used to treat depression may raise a person's risk.

Study of 140,688 people with depression and 421,943 people without depression over seven years by researchers at Umeå University, Umeå, Sweden, published in *Neurology*.

Parkinson's-Metals Link

Parkinson's may be caused by certain metals, we hear from Allison Wright Willis, MD.

Recent finding: Long-term residents of areas with industries that emit high levels of manganese have a 78% increased risk for Parkinson's. People in areas with factories that emit copper are at 11% higher risk. Parkinson's is a progressive disorder of the nervous system that affects movement. The way that these metals cause or accelerate Parkinson's is not understood.

Self-defense: Don't settle in an urban area with metal-emitting industries, especially if you have a genetic susceptibility to the disease.

Allison Wright Willis, MD, assistant professor of neurology at Washington University School of Medicine in St. Louis and leader of an analysis of data on 35,000 Medicare patients, published in *American Journal of Epidemiology*.

A Painkiller That Protects Against Parkinson's Disease

Xiang Gao, MD, PhD, assistant professor of medicine at Harvard Medical School, research scientist at Harvard School of Public Health and an associate epidemiologist at Brigham and Women's Hospital, all in Boston.

Researchers have discovered that people who regularly take the popular painkiller *ibuprofen* (such as Advil and other brands) seem to be at lower risk for Parkinson's.

WHICH PAINKILLERS WORK?

Xiang Gao, MD, PhD, assistant professor of medicine at Harvard, has been examining the association between painkillers and Parkinson's disease for nearly a decade. In fact, the Harvard researchers identified a link between lower Parkinson's risk and nonsteroidal anti-inflammatory drug (NSAID) painkillers as early as 2003. Then in 2005, they found that ibuprofen appeared to be the only NSAID that protected against Parkinson's. This more recent study has confirmed that finding and added some more detail.

The study: After examining the medical records of 136,197 participants (none of whom had Parkinson's at the start) in the Nurses' Health Study and the Health Professionals Follow-up Study over a six-year period, Dr. Gao found that 291 participants developed the disease…and participants who used ibuprofen at least twice a week had a one-third lower risk for Parkinson's than those who did not take it as often. Dr. Gao then did a secondary meta-analysis of six other studies concerning Parkinson's and ibuprofen and learned that their results were almost identical to his, showing a risk reduction for ibuprofen users of about 30%. His study also confirmed that the decreased risk was not found among people using any other painkillers, including aspirin or *acetaminophen* (Tylenol).

WHAT ELSE WORKS?

Dr. Gao theorizes that ibuprofen reduces the risk for Parkinson's disease by activating a signaling pathway called the peroxisome proliferator-activated receptor (PPAR-gamma) that in turn inhibits nerve cell death, oxidative stress and inflammatory damage in the brain. While it seems safe to say that ibuprofen has some specific protective property, Dr. Gao emphasized that we don't yet know what it is. And, he added, it's important to note that ibuprofen can cause troubling side effects, including gastrointestinal distress and bleeding. In high doses, it has been known to worsen kidney and cardiovascular problems as well. People who have a family history of Parkinson's disease should discuss with their doctors whether and how much ibuprofen to take.

In general, Dr. Gao says, he prefers to see people bolster their health with a heathful diet and exercise. In fact, in another recent study, he discovered that the antioxidants in berries were as effective as ibuprofen in lowering Parkinson's risk—people who ate at least two cups of berries per week had a one-fourth lower risk than those who didn't eat berries. And their only side effect was to make people want more!

New Hope for Parkinson's Patients

A cholesterol-lowering drug has been shown to affect the protein clumping that occurs in Parkinson's patients. A multicenter clinical trial to test the effects of *simvastatin* (Zocor) in Parkinson's patients is now under way.

Plymouth University, United Kingdom.

Essential Tremors...When It's Not Parkinson's

Elan D. Louis, MD, professor of neurology and epidemiology and chief, division of movement disorders, Yale school of Public Health, New Haven, Connecticut.

M any diseases can cause tremors, involuntary shaking/muscle movements that can make it hard to drink a glass of water, hold a knife or fork, or write a note. The most common is essential tremor, a difficult-to-treat disorder that causes uncontrollable shaking of the hands, head and/or other parts of the body.

An estimated seven million Americans have the disorder, as did the late Katharine Hepburn. According to the National Institutes of Health, essential tremor may affect as many as 14% of people over the age of 65.

Essential tremor can be so mild that it is merely an inconvenience, or it can progress to the point that patients struggle with any activity that requires hand control, such as buttoning a shirt.

Little was known about essential tremor until recently. Elan D. Louis, MD, a pioneering neurologist and epidemiologist, describes what we know now about the disorder...

RECENT FINDINGS

We have learned from recent brain studies that patients with essential tremor have about a 40% reduction in Purkinje cells. These are brain cells that produce an inhibitory neurotransmitter known as gamma-aminobutyr-

ic acid (GABA). Lower-than-normal levels of GABA could cause, or contribute to, a loss of muscle control.

Healthy Purkinje cells are packed with protein structures (neurofilaments) that are linearly shaped and neatly arranged. In patients with essential tremor, these structures more often look messy and chaotic. The disruption in these structures could inhibit the transport of essential substances within the nerve cells.

About half of all cases of essential tremor are thought to be due to a genetic mutation. Exposure to lead may be a factor. Also, a substance called *harman* could contribute to the disorder. Harman is naturally produced in the body—it also is present in many foods, especially meat. We have found, in some studies, that patients with essential tremor sometimes have levels of harman that are 50% to 100% higher than in people without the disease.

Levels of harman rise when meat is cooked at high temperatures or for long periods of time. However, the research is too preliminary at this stage to advise people to change their cooking and/or eating habits to avoid essential tremor.

IS IT PARKINSON'S?

Essential tremor usually is easily distinguished from Parkinson's disease. In patients with Parkinson's, the hands mainly shake when they are at rest. With essential tremor, the shaking occurs when the hands are in use. With Parkinson's disease, shaking often occurs in the legs as well, whereas in essential tremor, the head and voice often shake.

Until recently, doctors mainly looked for action tremors (shaking while the hands were being used) to diagnose essential tremor. We have learned in the last few years that these patients tend to have other issues as well, including abnormal eye movements, problems with coordination and possibly cognitive changes (such as memory loss).

Though essential tremor is different from Parkinson's disease, the underlying causes may be linked in some fashion. We have found that Parkinson's disease occurs about four times more often in those with essential tremor than in those without it.

Postmortem (after-death) studies show that patients with Parkinson's disease as well as some patients with essential tremor have abnormal clumps of proteins (Lewy bodies) in the brain. However, the clumps occur in different areas depending on the disease.

TOP TREATMENTS

There is nothing we know that individuals can do to prevent essential tremor. Nor can it be cured. Treatments can help but, due to side effects, are recommended only when the tremor is severe enough to interfere with daily life or cause embarrassment.

•*Propranolol* (Inderal) or other beta-blocker drugs. Commonly used to treat cardiovascular diseases such as hypertension, these drugs interfere with adrenaline and can reduce the severity of tremors by 10% to 50%. Only about half of patients who take a beta-blocker will achieve a significant reduction in essential tremor symptoms. These drugs cause side effects in many patients, including inability to exercise (due to a slower heart rate), a worsening of asthma and sometimes depression/fatigue.

•*Primidone* (Mysoline), an anti-seizure drug, is about as effective as a beta-blocker. It is used as frequently as beta-blockers. Again, it is effective only in about half of cases. The main side effects are nausea and drowsiness—the drowsiness, though, often diminishes over time.

Deep-brain stimulation can reduce tremors in most patients by 70% to 90%. Slender electrodes are surgically implanted in the brain and powered by a battery-run unit, implanted under the collarbone, that a patient can control. This is the best treatment that we now have for essential tremor, but patients often are reluctant to undergo brain surgery. There is a risk for stroke (if the surgeon accidentally nicks a blood vessel) during the procedure, but this is extremely rare. The operation is performed with "waking" anesthesia.

Any patient who can't control essential tremor with medications (assuming that the symptoms are significant) should talk to his/her doctor about this procedure.

Drug-Free Therapy for Relieving Tremors

Scott Theirl, DC, a functional neurologist in private practice at Functional Restoration in Glendale, Wisconsin, a diplomate of the American Chiropractic Neurology Board and a fellow of the American College of Functional Neurology. He uses noninvasive therapies to treat patients with movement disorders, chronic pain, brain injuries, balance difficulties, learning problems, autism and other neurologic conditions. YourBestBrain.com

The razor slips, cutting your leg...the spoon misses your mouth, spilling the soup...the pen wavers, leaving your note illegible For people with essential tremor (ET)—a chronic neurological disorder in which the hands, head and/or other parts of the body tremble uncontrollably—such frustrating experiences occur daily. Some people, unable to handle job duties or tired of other people's curious glances, retreat into social isolation.

If ET hasn't affected you (or someone you love), the day may come. ET can develop at any time but becomes more common with age, affecting up to 14% of people over 65, according to the National Institutes of Health. ET's cause is unknown, though genetics may play a role. Symptoms result from abnormal impulses in areas of the brain that initiate and coordinate muscle movement. Unfortunately, when it comes to conventional treatment with drugs or surgery, there is much room for improvement—yet many ET patients are never told about safer alternative therapies.

Problems with conventional treatments: The antiseizure drugs and blood pressure-lowering beta-blockers prescribed for ET work for only about half of patients and can cause serious side effects, such as slow heartbeat, dizziness, fainting and blurred vision (which may explain a recent study reporting that nearly one-third of ET patients stop taking their medication). For severe ET, the conventional treatment is deep-brain stimulation, in which electrodes are surgically implanted in the brain to deliver electrical impulses to areas that control movement. This procedure carries risks for brain hemorrhage, stroke and infection.

Safer options: A functional neurologist, usually a chiropractor or medical doctor with advanced training in neurology, can treat ET without drugs or surgery. So why don't patients know this? According to functional neurologist Scott Theirl, DC, a diplomate of the American Chiropractic Neurology Board, many conventional doctors are unfamiliar with these options because they haven't had the specialized training. Also, the treatments do not lend themselves to large clinical trials, Dr. Theirl said, "given that they are specific to each patient and change with each visit to reflect the patient's current condition." Nevertheless, he added, many ET patients report significant improvement with the following three therapies, especially when the techniques are used together. *Here's what ET patients should know about...*

• **Neurotransmitter optimization.** Neurotransmitters are chemicals that allow nerve cells to communicate with each other. Some are excitatory, stimulating the brain...others are inhibitory, calming the brain. Dr. Theirl explained that ET symptoms can be exacerbated when stress—physical, cognitive or emotional—causes neurotransmitters to elevate initially and then decline over time, creating imbalances of excitatory and inhibitory neurotransmitters and impairing the function of neurotransmitter receptors.

Using the results of urine tests that measure levels of various neurotransmitters, a functional neurologist devises an individualized program of supplementation with specific amino acids (precursors from which neurotransmitters are synthesized), such as 5-hydroxytryptophan (5-HTP), tyrosine, theanine and taurine. "These supplements help rebalance neurotransmitter levels naturally, replenishing the patient's metabolic 'fuel tank' and letting the nervous system function at a higher level," Dr. Theirl explained.

• **Brain-based therapy.** First the doctor conducts neurologic and orthopedic tests to assess which particular areas of a patient's brain and body are contributing to ET. "The act of moving a muscle is complicated. Generally, the prefrontal association cortex first decides what to move...the premotor cortex decides how to move...the primary motor cortex initiates movement...the cerebellum coordinates the smoothness of movement...and the primary somatic sensory cortex senses how the movement happened. When one area malfunctions, there is a 'miswiring' of the brain. Brain-based rehabilitation aims to retrain the brain and body back to the original wiring," Dr. Theirl said.

Specialized exercises help by stimulating specific areas of the brain.

Examples: Moving a hand or foot to the beat of a metronome exercises brain regions that improve muscle speed and decrease tremors...listening to slow-tempo music in one ear improves signals to muscles on that side of the body...eye-movement exercises target areas that reduce muscle spasms and improve neck muscle coordination.

But brain-based rehabilitation is not a one-size-fits-all therapy, Dr. Theirl emphasized. Each patient's routine must be based on the types and amount of stimulation needed—otherwise the exercises could fatigue the brain, worsening ET symptoms rather than improving them.

• **Hands-on therapy.** Manual techniques—for instance, chiropractic manipulation, physical therapy or therapeutic massage, depending on an individual patient's response—can improve muscle tone and promote relaxation of tight muscles affected by ET. Consequently, there is better feedback to the brain from the muscles and joints.

Bonus: Manual therapies also ease the muscle pain and tenderness that accompany ET.

To find a functional neurologist: Visit the website of the American Chiropractic Neurology Board at acnb.org and click on "doctor locator."

Natural Ways to Quiet Tremors

Monique Giroux, MD, a neurologist and medical director and cofounder of the Movement & Neuroperformance Center of Colorado in Englewood, Centerfor Movement.org. Dr. Giroux was formerly a clinical fellow in integrative medicine at The University of Arizona and movement disorders at Emory University. She is author of *Optimal Health with Parkinson's Disease.*

N atural therapies can help calm tremors by easing the stress and altering the brain chemicals and emotional responses that exacerbate the condition.

Important: Before trying natural remedies, be sure to avoid caffeine, smoking and/or excess alcohol—all of which can worsen tremors. Also, make regular exercise (especially strength training) a priority—tremors are more common when muscles become fatigued. *Natural treatments to tame any type of tremor...**

AROMATHERAPY

Breathing in the aroma of certain flowers and herbs can reduce tremors by enhancing brain levels of gamma-aminobutyric acid (GABA), a widely circulated neurotransmitter with proven stress-fighting effects. Raising GABA levels helps calm the overexcited neurons that can worsen tremors. *What to try for tremors...*

•**Lavender.** This fragrant blue-violet flower has been shown in a number of small studies to produce calming, soothing and sedative effects when its scent is inhaled. Lavender essential oil is widely available and can be inhaled in the bath (add five to eight drops to bath water for a long soak) or by dabbing a drop on your neck or temples.

SUPPLEMENTS

Certain supplements can ease tremors by enhancing muscle relaxation and/or reducing the body's overall stress levels or load of inflammatory chemicals, which can play a role in tremors caused by neurodegenerative diseases. *Check with your doctor to make sure these*

supplements don't interact with any medication you may be taking and won't affect any chronic condition you may have...**

•**Magnesium.** This mineral helps to regulate nerve impulses and muscle contraction. Magnesium-rich foods include sesame seeds, beans, nuts, avocados and leafy greens. To ensure that you're getting enough magnesium, consider taking a supplement.

Typical dose to ease tremors: 200 mg to 400 mg daily.

•**Fish oil.** The omega-3 fatty acids in fish oil offer proven anti-inflammatory effects—systemic inflammation is implicated in neurodegenerative diseases such as MS and Parkinson's disease. Fish oil is abundant in fatty fish such as salmon, albacore tuna, mackerel and herring. Aim for two servings per week. If you don't like fish, consider trying a supplement.

Typical dose to ease tremors: 1,000 mg to 1,500 mg daily.

•**Valerian, skullcap and passionflower.** These calming herbs have been successfully used as part of a regimen to ease tremors. The supplements can be found in combination products, including capsules, teas and tinctures. Follow instructions on the label.

BEAT TREMORS WITH YOUR MIND

If you suffer from tremors, it's common to think—Oh no...my arm (or other body part) is shaking again...this is so embarrassing! I hate this! While such thoughts are perfectly natural when tremors emerge, they are potentially destructive when trying to calm your condition.

What helps: Mindfulness can reset this negative thought pattern so that you stop viewing tremors as a problem, which only leads to distress that often worsens the condition.

Mindfulness is more than just relaxation. Often done in conjunction with deep-breathing exercises, mindfulness helps you simply observe your thoughts, feelings and sensations and let them pass without judging them, labeling them or trying to control them. By re-

---

*Consult your doctor before trying these therapies to determine the cause of your tremors and for advice on the approaches best suited to your situation.

**Because supplements aren't regulated by the FDA for purity, I advise looking for products that bear the "USP-verified" stamp on the label—this means they have met rigorous testing standards to ensure quality by the scientific nonprofit US Pharmacopeial Convention.

ducing the distress you feel about the tremors, you are no longer fueling the condition.

You can learn mindfulness from CDs or books.

My recommendations: Consult your local hospital to see if it offers mindfulness-based stress-reduction classes. Also consider trying other mind-body therapies that may help, such as hypnosis, biofeedback and breath work.

Better Treatment for Early Parkinson's Disease

In a recent study, 251 Parkinson's patients (average age 52) with early motor symptoms, such as tremors, were given either standard medical treatment (the drug *levodopa*) or neurostimulation (a therapy involving an implanted device that blocks brain signals that cause motor problems).

Result: Quality of life in the neurostimulation group improved by 26% over two years, compared with a 1% worsening of quality of life in the medical treatment group.

Conclusion: Neurostimulation is an established treatment for advanced Parkinson's but may be effective for early cases as well.

Gunther Deuschl, MD, professor of neurology, University of Kiel, Germany.

Cholesterol-Lowering Drugs May Help Reduce Risk for Parkinson's

People who stopped taking fat-soluble statins were almost 58% more likely to suffer from Parkinson's disease than people who kept taking them.

Theory: Fat-soluble statins, such as *simvastatin* (Zocor) or *atorvastatin* (Lipitor), reduce inflammation and alter dopamine pathways in the brain that are linked to Parkinson's. Water-soluble statins, such as *rosuvastatin* (Crestor) and *pravastatin* (Pravachol), do not provide the same benefit. People taking water-soluble statins develop Parkinson's at about twice the rate as people taking fat-soluble statins.

Self-defense: If you are taking a statin and have a family history of Parkinson's, ask your doctor if you should be taking a fat-soluble statin.

Study of 43,810 statin users from 2001 to 2008 by researchers at National Taiwan University Hospital, Taipei, published in *Neurology.*

Coffee Combats Parkinson's Disease

Ronald B. Postuma, MD, researcher in neurosciences, McGill University Health Centre, and associate professor, department of neurology, McGill University, both in Montreal.

Caffeine—everyone's favorite stimulant—has been shown in past studies to help prevent Parkinson's disease.

Now recent research shows that it may do even more than we previously thought.

It may also help people who already have Parkinson's.

If you or a loved one is coping with this progressive motor disorder, which can cause slow movement, muscle stiffness, shaking and balance problems, grab a coffee mug.

CAFFEINE JOLT EASES SYMPTOMS

Does it matter where the caffeine comes from (coffee…tea…chocolate)? And how much is needed to see relief? Recent research answers these questions…

In the study, scientists split Parkinson's patients into two groups. One group received a placebo pill, while the other took a 100-milligram (mg) caffeine pill twice a day for three weeks and then a 200-mg caffeine pill twice a day for another three weeks. (To give you an idea of how much caffeine that is, one eight-ounce cup of coffee contains roughly 100 mg of caffeine.) Many participants had already

165

been consuming caffeine before the study—up to a maximum of 200 mg (two eight-ounce cups of coffee) per day. They were allowed to maintain their prior habits throughout the study as long as they didn't change their intake amounts.

Results: Debilitating symptoms such as stiffness and slow movement were reduced by 10% to 15% among those taking the caffeine pills, whereas the placebo group saw no significant symptom relief.

More good news: Many of those taking the caffeine noticed improvements within the first few days of the study. Both doses worked about equally well, and neither dose increased patients' bothersome tremors, as you might have expected.

What's at play here? Caffeine likely blocks a brain receptor called adenosine-2A, which may contribute to some Parkinson's symptoms, said lead researcher Ron Postuma, MD.

A SUPPLEMENT NOT A REPLACEMENT

Despite this promising finding, however, caffeine's effects aren't so strong that it can replace Parkinson's drugs, Dr. Postuma cautioned. But, if you have Parkinson's, caffeine could be a helpful supplement to whatever medication you're on, he said.

Dr. Postuma said that caffeine in any form—including pills, coffee, tea or chocolate—is likely to work the same way. (And flavors, sweeteners or creams mixed with the caffeinated beverages won't reduce its effect.)

So how much caffeine should you consume per day if you have Parkinson's? Dr. Postuma said that the research is too preliminary for him to give a specific recommendation, but study subjects benefited by consuming up to a total of 400 mg (four eight-ounce cups) per day from both pills and any coffee that they already drank. (If you already drink four or more eight-ounce cups of coffee a day, it's unknown whether consuming extra caffeine will help.)

Most Parkinson's patients should have no problem consuming up to 400 mg of caffeine, said Dr. Postuma. If you're worried that it might stop you from sleeping, be sure to have your last "dose" no later than early afternoon. If you have heart rhythm problems, uncon-

trolled high blood pressure or ulcers, talk to your doctor before consuming any caffeine.

Dr. Postuma would like to eventually study the long-term effects of caffeine on Parkinson's—which are still unknown—and determine whether consuming caffeine might help Parkinson's patients take less medication. A 200-mg caffeine pill costs about seven cents, he noted, while new Parkinson's drugs typically cost between $3,000 and $5,000 per year. "Caffeine is incredibly low-cost and could save patients lots of money," he said. "It's also extremely well-tolerated, so it has great potential."

Black Tea and Parkinson's

When researchers analyzed health data for 63,257 adults, they found that those who drank at least 23 cups of black tea monthly (caffeinated or decaffeinated) had a 71% lower risk for Parkinson's disease over a 12-year period than those who drank less black tea. Intake of green tea had no effect on Parkinson's risk.

Theory: Black tea contains complex antioxidants that may help protect against Parkinson's disease.

Louis C. Tan, MD, senior consultant, department of neurology, National Neuroscience Institute, Singapore.

Is This Parkinson's Disease Cure on Your Spice Rack?

Kalipada Pahan, PhD, professor of neurological sciences, Floyd A. Davis Professor of Neurology, Rush University Medical Center, Chicago. His study appeared in the *Journal of Neuroimmune Pharmacology*.

The Bible makes several references to it. The ancient Egyptians used it to preserve their mummies. The ancient Greeks and Romans used it to help them digest their feasts of lamb and wine. We know it's great for diabetes and glycemic control.

And now we find out that this substance fights Parkinson's disease. What is it? Cinnamon.

Besides being a commonly used spice, cinnamon has a long history as a medicine. Medieval physicians used it to treat arthritis, coughing, hoarseness and sore throats. In fact, it was once so valuable, wars were fought over it.

Cinnamon can prevent symptoms of Parkinson's disease that include tremors, slow, jerky movement, stiffness and loss of balance. Or at least my research has shown that cinnamon has this effect in mice acting as experimental models of Parkinson's disease.

Mouse studies often translate to humans when further research is done—so, given how devastating Parkinson's disease can be…and how familiar and safe cinnamon is…these cinnamon studies merit our attention right now. If these results are repeatable in Parkinson's disease patients, it would represent a remarkable advance in the treatment of this neurodegenerative disease.

The first thing to know is that we are not talking about just any kind of cinnamon, but a specific, authentic kind.

Two types of cinnamon are sold in the United States—Chinese cinnamon (sometimes sold as Saigon cinnamon) and Ceylon cinnamon. Chinese cinnamon, or cassia, is the more common, less expensive type of cinnamon and is what you generally find in supermarkets. You know it—the usual cinnamon powder or that hard, aromatic curl of wood that you plunk into hot apple cider or cocoa. But this is not really "true" cinnamon and does not have its health benefits. Ceylon cinnamon is true cinnamon, and its sticks are softer and flakier than those of Chinese cinnamon. The powder is also lighter and sweeter smelling. There is virtually no way of knowing whether the powdered cinnamon you buy is true cinnamon or cassia or a mix unless it is specifically marked. Ceylon cinnamon is the spice of choice in medicinal research. So even just for general health, keep that in mind the next time you head out to the grocery store to replenish your spice rack—you may need to go

to a higher-end market or even order online to get Ceylon cinnamon.

HOW DOES IT WORK?

As you may know, cinnamon is loaded with antioxidants. It may be therapeutic in Parkinson's disease because its antioxidant effects counteract nitric oxide, a free radical that attacks proteins essential to supporting adequate levels of dopamine. Dopamine is the chemical in our brains that not only makes us feel happy and motivated but also controls many of our muscle and limb movements.

It's known that the amount of proteins like DJ-1 and Parkin decrease in the brains of patients with Parkinson's disease. We have found that these proteins also decrease in the brains of mice with Parkinson's disease because of nitric oxide production. After the mice ate ground cinnamon, their livers turned the cinnamon into an element, or metabolite, that cinnamon breaks down into during digestion, called sodium benzoate. Once the sodium benzoate got to the brain, it decreased the production of nitric oxide, which stopped the loss of Parkin and DJ-1, protected brain cells and allowed the mice to move around more normally, with steadier legs and less need for rest and downtime. It's possible that cinnamon could also prevent or lessen the symptoms of other diseases, such as types of palsy and Lewy body dementia, which are also caused by dopamine dysfunction.

HOW TO USE CINNAMON

These findings are potentially great news for people with Parkinson's disease and those who worry that they carry the potential for it in their genes. As it stands, Parkinson's disease patients must rely on drugs, such as *levodopa*, to replace dopamine, but these drugs neither cure nor change the course of the disease. They only provide temporary relief. Over time, symptoms become increasingly harder to control, and the drugs often have a wide range of serious side effects.

Cinnamon, however, and its metabolite sodium benzoate, could potentially be among the safest approaches to stop the progression of Parkinson's disease once it's diagnosed.

Sodium benzoate is a common food preservative found in salad dressings, juices, condiments and cosmetics. The National Institutes of Health's National Center for Complementary and Integrative Health has concluded that sodium benzoate and true cinnamon are safe and that true cinnamon is safe even in large amounts—but this is not true for cassia (Chinese cinnamon) because it contains coumarin, which, besides being a blood thinner, can damage the liver.

Unless you're allergic to cinnamon, take one teaspoon a day. But don't attempt to just swallow a teaspoon of dry cinnamon powder "straight-up"! It will make you gag and could cause you to cough and inhale the powder into your lungs, which is dangerous. Instead, mix cinnamon into food or drink.

You can bet there's much more research coming on cinnamon and Parkinson's—meanwhile, generous helpings of this richly antioxidant spice could be well worth trying.

CoQ10 for Parkinson's

Vitamin-like coenzyme Q10 (CoQ10) aids energy production in cells. In a study of 80 Parkinson's patients, those who took 1,200 mg of CoQ10 daily for 16 months showed significantly less decline in motor function than other patients. A larger study is now testing an even higher dose.

Patients: Ask your doctor about CoQ10.

Katie Kompoliti, MD, neurologist, Rush University Medical Center, Chicago, and researcher in an ongoing multicenter clinical trial of 600 Parkinson's patients.

Better Balance for Parkinson's Patients

Dancing the tango improved balance and functional mobility in 40 Parkinson's patients who took twice-weekly classes for 12 weeks. Dancers also reported better cognitive function and less fatigue.

Why: The rhythmic forward-and-backward steps of the tango stimulate cognitive functioning and promote better balance.

Silvia Rios, Romenets, MD, research associate, McGill University, Montreal, Canada.

Parkinson's Drug Warning

Withdrawal symptoms from Parkinson's drugs can be similar to those of cocaine addicts. Dopamine agonists (DAs) are given in combination with the drug L-DOPA, the primary treatment for Parkinson's. But DAs have side effects, including uncontrolled, compulsive behaviors such as overeating, hypersexuality, compulsive shopping and gambling.

Recent study: Reducing the dose of DAs can cause dopamine agonist withdrawal syndrome—whose symptoms include anxiety, panic attacks, depression, sweating, nausea, pain and fatigue. Patients should let their physicians know if they experience impulse-control problems—stopping the DAs immediately may prevent withdrawal symptoms.

Melissa J. Nirenberg, MD, PhD, former associate director, Parkinson's Disease & Movement Disorders Institute, New York-Presbyterian Hospital/Weill Cornell Medical Center, New York City, and leader of a study published in *Archives of Neurology.*

Ulcers and Parkinson's

Adults with the ulcer-causing Helicobacter pylori bacterium are more likely to develop Parkinson's disease.

Possible reason: A neurotoxin linked to Parkinson's is almost identical to a substance produced by H. pylori.

Louisiana State University Health Sciences Center.

Parkinson's Patients Have Difficulty Recognizing Other People's Feelings

Parkinson's by itself tends to make emotion recognition more difficult, and this can be exacerbated by deep brain stimulation—a treatment for Parkinson's patients who no longer respond to medication. It may further affect patients' ability to recognize emotions in other people's faces and voices. In particular, they have more trouble recognizing negative emotions, such as fear and sadness.

For caregivers: Strengthen other forms of communication when dealing with Parkinson's patients as a way to limit the negative effects of the disease and its treatment.

Example: Articulate feelings using words ("I am feeling sad right now"), rather than relying on facial expressions or tone of voice to get your point across.

Heather Gray, PhD, research associate, Cambridge Health Alliance, Harvard Medical School, Boston, and coauthor of an analysis of 34 studies involving 1,295 patients, published in *Neuropsychology*.

A Better Way to Treat Advanced Parkinson's Disease

John T. Slevin, MD, professor of neurology and molecular and biomedical pharmacology, department of neurology, University of Kentucky Medical Center, Lexington. His study appeared in the *Journal of Parkinson's Disease*.

The drug Sinemet relieves Parkinson's disease symptoms such as tremor, difficulty swallowing and an awkwardly shuffling gait, but it becomes less effective over time.

Breakthrough: There's a new way of getting Sinemet's active ingredient, *levodopa*, to last longer and more consistently to control Parkinson's symptoms. It has been available in Canada, Australia and throughout Europe for a few years and, finally, it is now available here in America.

IMPROVING A DRUG'S STAYING POWER

Parkinson's disease happens when certain brain cells degenerate and produce less dopamine, a chemical necessary to control muscle movement. Levodopa is meant to replace that lost dopamine, but it wears off within minutes. The pill Sinemet contains levodopa plus a drug called *carbidopa* that helps the levodopa last longer and get to where it needs to go—the brain. It is initially very effective in controlling Parkinson's symptoms, but within four to six years of starting treatment, it's effectiveness wears off for roughly 40% of patients. By nine years, 90% of patients are showing troublesome symptoms again. And besides the Parkinson's symptoms, the body begins to react poorly to the unevenness of levodopa levels…erratic muscle movements (a condition called dyskinesia) begin to occur either when the level of levodopa peaks in the body after taking a dose or when it wears off between doses.

A better—albeit invasive—way to receive levodopa that minimizes these problems was finally approved by the FDA in January 2015 after being available for several years in many other countries around the world. The treatment is a process called carbidopa-levodopa enteral suspension (CLES), marketed as Duopa. It involves surgery to insert a tube through the abdomen into the small intestine. The tube is connected to an external portable pump that a person can carry in his or her pants pocket or some other wearable pouch while the pump delivers a constant flow of the carbidopa-levodopa during waking hours.

THE BENEFITS AND RISKS

Although studies have shown that the CLES system works well to control Parkinson's symptoms in people with advanced disease, how safe and tolerable is it over the long term? A team of researchers from three top medical institutions—University of Kentucky Medical Center, Cleveland Clinic and Northwestern University Feinberg School of Medicine—along with researchers associated with

169

the drug's manufacturer, AbbVie Inc., closely examined symptoms and patient quality of life before and after beginning CLES. Side effects of CLES were also examined.

In the first part of the study, which lasted three months, patients on Sinemet were compared with patients receiving CLES. In the second part of the study, the patients who had been on Sinemet were switched to CLES, and all the patients—those who had been on CLES and those new to it—were followed for a year.

The results: Patients put on the CLES system during the first part of the study averaged 12 symptom-free hours a day, compared with an average of 10 hours for patients on Sinemet. Once patients on Sinemet were switched to the CLES system, they also improved to meet the sustained 12-hour window of symptom control. Symptoms were less severe, and dyskinesia—the main debilitating side effect of Sinemet—was much less common once the patients were switched to CLES.

Most side effects were related to surgery rather than CLES use. In fact, serious side effects, such as intestinal perforation during surgery, were common, occurring in 23% of patients. In addition, infection at the surgical site occurred in 18% but cleared up with antibiotic therapy.

Besides surgical side effects, the most common side effects for those new to CLES were abdominal pain, which affected 42% of the patients. Nausea was also common, as was skin redness at the site of the tube insertion, which cleared up in some patients over time.

Since CLES is relatively new, doctors don't yet know exactly how long, in terms of years, the therapy will provide symptom control for patients with Parkinson's disease. The lead author of the study, John T. Slevin, MD, from the University of Kentucky Medical Center, said that it is expected that, as the disease progresses and more brain cells that produce dopamine are lost, the benefits of CLES will eventually ebb. CLES simply helps extend symptom control and quality of life longer when other treatments lose their effectiveness.

If you or a loved one has an interest in CLES to control worsening Parkinson's disease, consult an experienced neurologist who specializes in movement disorders who will work with a gastroenterologist skilled in gastrointestinal surgery. You can find Parkinson's Disease Centers of Excellence through the National Parkinson Foundation, Parkinson.org.

Brain Pacemaker for Parkinson's

In a recent finding, Parkinson's patients who received low-frequency (60 Hz) deep-brain stimulation (DBS), in which an implanted "brain pacemaker" sends electrical impulses to the brain, had significant improvements in swallowing difficulty and in their walking gait—problems that were not resolved with standard treatment, including high-frequency (130 Hz) DBS or medication, such as *carbidopa* and *levodopa*. The patients in the study received daily low-frequency treatments for six weeks.

Tao Xie, MD, PhD, associate professor of neurology, The University of Chicago.

Music Can Aid Parkinson's Patients

Music, in combination with physical therapy, improves upper-body mobility and makes it easier for people with Parkinson's to walk. A rhythmic beat works as a timekeeper for the motor system, helping to coordinate muscles so that they move in time and work efficiently together. Music also can help patients who have had strokes or suffered traumatic brain injury.

Kimberly Sena Moore, board-certified music therapist and neurologic music therapist and director of Neurosong Music Therapy Services, Warrensburg, Missouri. MusicTherapyMaven.com

Gentle Treatment for Parkinson's

Fuzhong Li, PhD, senior research scientist, Oregon Research Institute, Eugene.

Imagine feeling so unstable that you are afraid of falling from the minute you get out of bed in the morning. That's what life can be like for many patients who are suffering from Parkinson's disease.

And while medications can help with the tremors and stiffness caused by Parkinson's, there is no pill to help with feeling unstable and unbalanced.

But recent research shows that there is a natural treatment that might help—tai chi. Past studies have shown that tai chi, an ancient Chinese exercise known for its slow and graceful movements (think yoga meets martial arts), can improve balance and stability in people with Parkinson's. But no studies comparing tai chi with other types of physical activity had been done before. So researchers set out to see how tai chi fared against resistance training (using weighted vests and ankle weights) and stretching—and to find out, in particular, which might help Parkinson's patients improve their balance.

Guess which wins…

YOGA MEETS MARTIAL ARTS

Fuzhong Li, PhD, a senior research scientist at Oregon Research Institute in Eugene, Oregon, explained the new research.

The researchers recruited 195 men and women with Parkinson's between the ages of 40 and 85. They all had either mild or moderate Parkinson's, but not severe, because those with severe Parkinson's are unable to stand unassisted so they wouldn't have been able to do the exercises. The participants were randomly assigned to one of three different exercise programs—tai chi, resistance training or stretching. All groups participated in a twice-weekly, 60-minute class for six months.

The tai chi program emphasized slow, continuous movements with multiple body parts moving at the same time, such as hand movements, trunk rotation and weight shifting from foot to foot. The resistance-training program focused on strengthening muscles of the hips, knees and ankles. The stretching program included light walking…arm, leg and neck circles…and deep abdominal breathing.

At the end of the six-month study, the researchers measured balance by looking at maximum excursion (which measured how far the person could lean over while standing without stumbling or falling)…directional control (which measured the amount of "intentional" movement toward a target compared with "uncontrolled" movement) while walking…and length of walking stride. *Here's what they discovered…*

• **Tai chi participants increased their maximum excursion by 13%,** while the resistance-training group improved by only 6% and the stretching group saw no improvement.

• **The tai chi group increased their directional control by 11%,** but neither the resistance-training group nor the stretching group saw any improvement.

• **Those in the tai chi group had 67% fewer falls** than those in the stretching group and marginally fewer falls than those in the resistance-training group.

• **Length of stride improved for the tai chi participants by 10 centimeters (cm),** compared with 4 cm for the resistance-training group and no improvement for the stretching group.

In other words, doing tai chi really helped these people with their balance and mobility! The research was published recently in *The New England Journal of Medicine*.

NATURAL HEALING

It's powerful…simple…and safe. If you have Parkinson's and you're interested in trying tai chi, mention it to your doctor (who will almost certainly say "by all means"), and then simply enroll in a class near you. Many gyms, YMCAs and community centers offer tai chi. Or you can rent or buy a tai chi DVD. Tai chi doesn't require special equipment or fancy gym clothes, and it can be done indoors or outside. If you are unable to devote 60 full minutes to it twice a week, just remember, said Dr. Li, that any amount is better than no amount.

Exercise for Parkinson's

Low-intensity exercise improves Parkinson's patients' ability to walk.

Recent finding: Gait and mobility improved more among Parkinson's patients who walked on a treadmill at a comfortable speed for 50 minutes three times a week than among patients who walked at a higher speed for 30 minutes three times per week.

Lisa Shulman, MD, professor of neurology, University of Maryland School of Medicine, codirector of Maryland Parkinson's Disease and Movement Disorders Clinic, University of Maryland Medical Center, both in Baltimore.

Cycling Improves Parkinson's

Michael D. Phillips, MD, section head of imaging sciences and vice chairman of research and academic affairs, Imaging Institute, Cleveland Clinic. His study was presented at the annual meeting of the Radiological Society of North America.

What do actor Michael J. Fox, evangelist Billy Graham, former US Attorney General Janet Reno and the late Muhammad Ali have in common?

Answer: Parkinson's disease, a chronic degenerative disorder of the central nervous system that kills off or impairs the brain cells responsible for the body's ability to move.

You've probably recognized Parkinson's patients by their shaking hands and awkward gait. Sadly, as the disease progresses, patients also develop behavioral and cognitive problems, including dementia.

It's not just older folks who are affected. Though the disease usually strikes after age 50, it can begin sooner—Michael J. Fox was just 30 when he was diagnosed.

There is no cure for Parkinson's…and though a new type of brain surgery technique is promising, it is invasive and not without risk.

Enough with the bad news. Here's some good news—a commonplace activity that is actually fun and safe can improve brain function and mobility in Parkinson's patients. The secret is to go fast.

PEDAL TO THE METAL

The revelation comes from a recent study that focused on the effects of using stationary exercise bikes. For eight weeks the participants, all of whom were in the middle stages of Parkinson's, rode stationary bikes three times weekly for 40 minutes per session. One group pedaled at their preferred pedaling rate while making sure they were still in their target heart rate zone. The other group rode stationary cycles with motors and control systems to monitor pedaling rate—and with the assistance of the motors, they pedaled approximately 30% faster than their preferred rate. In effect, this assistance from a motor "forced" riders to move their legs faster than their disease would normally allow.

At the start of the study, after the eight-week exercise sessions and again four weeks later, all participants underwent brain-imaging tests called functional connectivity MRIs. These scans assessed changes in blood oxygen levels in different parts of their brains, which allowed researchers to look at the connections among the various brain regions involved in Parkinson's.

What the researchers found: After eight weeks of cycling, patients whose motorized cycles had helped them pedal faster showed greater strengthening of connections in brain areas tied to motor function than patients who had pedaled only as fast as they could without assistance…and these positive effects were still evident four weeks after the exercise sessions ended. The results weren't tied to increased aerobic fitness, the researchers reported. What mattered most was how fast the participants had moved their legs—because this seemed to train the brain to allow better movement.

Interestingly, the types of brain changes brought about by the faster pedaling were similar to those that result from deep brain stimulation, an effective but invasive (not to mention expensive) therapy for Parkinson's in which a device is surgically implanted in the brain to deliver electrical stimulation to brain areas that control movement and block the abnormal nerve signals that cause tremors. In comparison, fast pedaling offers a very attractive, risk-free, low-cost alternative.

What about improvement in actual symptoms? This study and an earlier non-MRI study by the same researchers found that patients in the "forced" exercise group did indeed show improvements in motor function—including in the upper body, even though the lower body was doing the work. (*Fun fact:* The inspiration for the study arose when one of the researchers partnered with a female Parkinson's patient on a long-distance tandem bike ride. The researcher could pedal faster than the patient, which forced her to pedal faster as well—and afterward they noticed improvement in her motor skills!)

More research is needed to determine how long the effects might last and whether other exercise activities, such as rowing, would have similar benefits. The Cleveland Clinic is partnering with an exercise company to develop a motor-driven cycle to replicate the effects of the research.

In the meantime, Parkinson's patients who want to try this therapy themselves should first get the go-ahead from their doctors. Then patients are encouraged to exercise on a stationary cycle at as fast a rate as they can, turning down the resistance and ramping up their pedaling speed.

Alternative: They can get a tandem bicycle, go out on a beautiful day and ask a fit friend to set a brisk pace while cycling with them.

Simple Stretches That Really Do Relieve Pain

Ben Benjamin, PhD, a sports medicine and muscular therapy practitioner since 1963. The founder of The Benjamin Institute in Cambridge, Massachusetts, BenBenjamin.com, he conducts seminars and workshops on Active Isolated Stretching across the US and is author of several books, including *Listen to Your Pain: The Active Person's Guide to Understanding, Identifying, and Treating Pain and Injury*.

If you suffer from pain or stiffness due to an injury, arthritis or even a neurological disorder, such as Parkinson's disease or mul-

tiple sclerosis, a type of bodywork known as Active Isolated Stretching (AIS) may give you more relief than you ever thought possible.

What makes AIS different: While most other stretching techniques recommend doing each stretch for 30 seconds or longer, AIS uses brief, two-second stretches that are done eight to 10 times each.

What's the advantage of quick, repeated stretches? This approach gives the muscle a full stretch without triggering its stretch reflex—an automatic defense mechanism that causes the muscle to contract and ultimately undo many of the stretch's benefits. The result is that muscles stretch more efficiently and avoid the buildup of waste products that lead to muscle soreness.

Developed by American kinesiologist Aaron Mattes about 35 years ago, AIS also stretches each muscle group at a variety of different angles, thus stretching all muscle fibers equally.

A MINI REGIMEN

To get a sense of AIS, try the stretches in this article. While doing each one, slowly count to yourself "one-one thousand, two-one thousand"—never any longer than two seconds. Always exhale while performing the stretch and inhale as you return to the starting position.

The first repetition of each stretch should be gentle...the second should go up to the point where you begin to feel resistance. Subsequent repetitions should push just beyond this point (with the help of your hands, a rope or other aid, if necessary) to go a few degrees further each time, thus providing a maximum stretch. If you feel discomfort during a stretch, stop the stretch at that point. If a stretch feels painful from the start, then skip it.

Daily AIS exercises that help relieve common types of pain...*

SHOULDER STRETCHES

Purpose: To help prevent muscle strain and joint sprain by increasing flexibility.

1. With your right elbow bent, position your right arm at a 90° angle in front of your body. Place your right palm on the back

*Check with your doctor before performing these movements.

of your right shoulder. Exhale and extend your flexed arm upward as far as possible. Gently assist the stretch with your left hand. Repeat eight to 10 times on each side.

2. With your right elbow bent and your right arm positioned at a 90° angle in front of your body, place your right palm on the back of your right shoulder. Drop a two- to three-foot rope over your right shoulder and grasp the bottom of it with your left hand. Gently pull the rope to move your right arm upward behind your neck at a 45° angle for a maximum stretch. Return to the starting position after each repetition. Repeat eight to 10 times on each side.

NECK STRETCHES

Purpose: To help prevent neck injuries, relieve stiffness and improve range of motion.

1. Tuck your chin as close to your neck as possible. Put both your hands on the back of your head and, while keeping your back straight, gently bend your neck forward, bringing your chin as close to your chest as you can. Return to starting position. Repeat 10 times.

2. Gently bend your head to the right side, moving your right ear as close as possible to the top of your right shoulder. Exhale and place your right hand on the left side of your head to gently extend the stretch. Keep your left shoulder down. Focus your eyes on a point directly in front of your body to keep your head in an aligned position. Repeat 10 times on both sides.

GETTING STARTED

For people who are new to AIS, I advise working with an AIS practitioner for hands-on instruction. If the movements are done incorrectly, you will get no benefits and could even hurt yourself. To find a practitioner near you, go to StretchingUSA.com and click on the "Find a Therapist" link. Sessions are not typically covered by insurance and usually range from $50 to $150 per session. The website also offers books, including *Specific Stretching for Everyone*, and DVDs if you prefer to learn a complete AIS regimen on your own.

Got Parkinson's? MS? Ballroom Dancing Can Help—Really

Alexander Ng, PhD, associate professor, Program in Exercise Science, Marquette University, Milwaukee. His study, "Dancing with MS: Benefits of Ballroom or Recreational Social Dance for Persons with MS," was presented at the Consortium of Multiple Sclerosis Centers 2015 Annual Meeting.

When you have a chronic condition, you may not feel like dancing the night away. But dancing with a partner actually may be the best thing you can do for body and mind. Studies show that partnered dancing offers tremendous benefits to people with Parkinson's disease, Alzheimer's and other forms of dementia, and those recovering from a stroke.

Here's a new condition to add to the list—multiple sclerosis (MS). The progressive chronic central nervous system disease, which can alternate between flare-ups and periods of remission, can cause fatigue, muscle weakness and balance problems. It often affects the ability to walk unaided.

Whether it's the waltz, fox-trot or salsa, partnered dancing is a perfect activity for people with MS. "If you're with a partner, you might be able to do movements that you wouldn't ordinarily be able to do if you have issues with balance or impaired movement," says study author Alexander Ng, PhD, a professor of exercise science—and a recreational ballroom dancer himself. The partner offers physical support and can be somewhat of a coach, encouraging the patient to push him or herself.

To test the theory, Dr. Ng included 12 people with MS who were able to walk at least 25 feet on their own and stand for at least five minutes without assistance. Some had no noticeable movement problems at all, while others needed the help of a cane or walker to get around. Six participated in hour-long dance classes…twice a week…for six out of eight weeks (to give participants flexibility around summer vacations). The other six people, the control group, didn't dance but received the same routine medical care as the dancers. Dances included the waltz, fox-trot, rumba and swing. (In the next study they will also be including salsa, tango and merengue.) Before and after the dance program, both groups underwent a battery of tests such as walking unaided for 25 feet, getting up from a chair and walking three yards and then sitting down quickly (a measure of mobility), and tests for walking balance, which predicts the risk of falling.

The results: Dancers had higher scores on those tests for balance, mobility and endurance. They also had improvements in self-reported fatigue and depression (which tend to afflict people with MS) as well as cognitive benefits related to the ability to stay focused, while the control group did not.

It's a small, preliminary study, although another small study has found similar benefits when people with MS learn salsa dancing. As it turns out, there is a good body of research backing up partnered dancing for chronic conditions.

HOW SOCIAL DANCING WORKS AS THERAPY

At a minimum, dancing is aerobic exercise, which has been demonstrated to improve both physical and cognitive function in people with neurological disorders. Dance is also a complex activity that uses a combination of physical and mental tasks. Physically, dance requires balance, flexibility, speed and coordination—all skills that diminish in people with MS. And it calls on brain power—you have to remember and repeat steps, work with a partner and coordinate your movements together. Plus, it's social, which engages yet another part of the brain, and, last but not least, it's joyful. "When you're focused on dancing," says Dr. Ng, "troubles that may otherwise occupy your brain are shunted aside, so that you finish mentally refreshed."

Indeed, neuroimaging studies have shown that frequent dancing increases activity throughout the brain. When you're in the groove, it seems, your whole brain just lights up.

The strongest evidence for the benefits of partner dancing is in Parkinson's disease, another neurological condition in which move-ment is affected. Partner dancing actually echoes many of the key elements recommended in physical therapy for Parkinson's, such as responding to cues, learning new ways to move and engaging in balance exercises.

Studies show that partnered dancing helps people with Parkinson's develop a better gait while walking, have less rigidity in their movements, improve their ability to use their arms and hands and, in general, helps with functional mobility. One non-profit organization, Dance for Parkinson's (DanceforParkinsons. org) offers resources in more than 120 communities in 16 countries.

Perhaps its strongest appeal is that it's fun, creative and social. Says Dr. Ng, "People don't tend to view dance as exercise or physical therapy...so they're more likely to want to do it." Nor do you need to find special classes for people with MS or other chronic conditions. While it's a good idea to get lessons in ballroom dancing if you're unfamiliar with the steps, it's not a requirement. Says Dr. Ng, "Partnered dance for people with MS isn't rehabilitation per se but a fun option for physical activity."

Living Well with Multiple Sclerosis

Patricia K. Coyle, MD, professor and vice chair of the department of neurology at Stony Brook University Medical Center, and director of the Stony Brook Multiple Sclerosis Comprehensive Care Center.

The term multiple sclerosis (MS) conjures up frightening images of life in a wheelchair—but thanks to recent advances, an MS diagnosis no longer means that disability is inevitable. This is especially good news for women, given that MS is two to three times more common in women than men.

It is now possible to detect MS earlier...begin effective treatment just about as soon as symptoms appear...and slow the disease's progression. Yet despite this encouraging news, MS often goes undiagnosed for months or years—narrowing the window of opportunity that early treatment provides.

What women must know to protect themselves...

MS EXPLAINED

With MS, the immune system's white blood cells mistakenly attack the myelin (nerve fibers' protective coating) and nerve fibers themselves in the brain, spinal cord and optic nerves. This impairs the nerves' ability to transmit messages.

Women's greater vulnerability to MS may be related to hormones. MS typically strikes young adults, but it can appear as late as in one's 70s. People of northern European descent are more genetically predisposed to MS. Parents, siblings and children of MS patients have a 2% to 5% chance of developing it, too. Genes alone don't bring on the disease, however. Something in the environment—such as exposure to the Epstein-Barr virus (which causes mononucleosis) or vitamin-D deficiency at a young age—seems to help trigger MS.

DIAGNOSIS DIFFICULTIES

MS diagnosis often is delayed because the first symptoms can be vague. Patients tend to attribute them to a minor problem, such as a pinched nerve...doctors may mistake MS for spinal disk disease, vitamin B-12 deficiency or anxiety.

Any of the symptoms below merit a call to the doctor. If MS is suspected, a neurologist or MS center can run tests.

Referrals to a specialist: National Multiple Sclerosis Society, 800-344-4867, NationalMs Society.org...The Consortium of MS Centers, 201-487-1050, Mscare.org.

Initial symptoms...

- **Clumsiness, loss of balance**
- **Double vision, blurred vision**
- **Eye pain, facial pain**
- **Numb face, limbs or torso**
- **Shocklike sensations upon bending the neck**
- **Stiffness, muscle spasms**
- **Weakness, extreme fatigue**

Later symptoms...

- **Bladder or bowel incontinence**
- **Difficulty becoming sexually aroused or climaxing**

- **Paralysis, typically in the legs**
- **Poor concentration and memory**
- **Speech or swallowing problems**

Diagnosis is based on a patient's medical history, a neurological exam and magnetic resonance imaging (MRI) to check for damaged tissue in the brain and spinal cord. *There are four types of MS...*

- **Relapsing-remitting MS,** which affects about 85% of patients, is characterized by sudden flare-ups (relapses) of symptoms followed by periods of improvement, during which patients are stable.

- **Primary progressive MS accounts for about 10% of MS cases.** Symptoms worsen progressively from onset with no improvement.

- **Progressive-relapsing MS,** which affects about 5% of patients, involves steady worsening of symptoms from onset, plus later flare-ups.

- **Secondary progressive MS refers to relapsing-remitting MS that transitions to slow worsening.** Patients get increasingly disabled instead of stabilizing between flare-ups.

MS is rarely fatal. Except when vital brain stem functions (such as breathing and heart rate) are affected or the disease has led to severe disability, most patients have a near-normal life expectancy.

MS TREATMENT TODAY

New disease-modifying therapy (DMT) drugs are key to treatment. Starting a DMT soon after MS develops can lower the risk for long-term disability...cut the number of relapses...and lessen symptom severity during flare-ups. DMTs cannot reverse existing damage but can forestall future damage and significantly reduce the likelihood that relapsing MS will transition to progressive MS. For patients who have had MS for years, DMTs also are helpful so long as relapses are still occurring.

Each MS medication has its own pros and cons, so doctors work with each individual patient to determine the optimal treatment. *Options...*

- ***Glatiramer*** **(Copaxone) and *interferon betas* (Avonex, Betaseron, Rebif)** are DMTs that reduce nervous system inflammation and protect nerve cells. They are given by self-injection once or more weekly.

• *Natalizumab* (Tysabri), a monthly DMT given by intravenous infusion (IV drip) at an infusion center, targets errant white blood cells.

• *Mitoxantrone* (Novantrone), an intravenous chemotherapy drug, suppresses the immune system.

• **Prescription steroids are used during flare-ups to calm symptoms.**

Natural therapies also ease MS symptoms. *Examples...*

• **Dietary changes.** MS patients may benefit from eating less saturated fat and more vitamin B-12 (found in dairy foods, eggs, meat, poultry and shellfish)...vitamin D (found in dairy foods and fish)...omega-3 fatty acids (found in fatty fish, cod liver oil and flaxseed oil)...and omega-6 fatty acids (found in safflower seed oil and sunflower oil). If blood tests show a deficiency, supplements may be recommended.

• **Exercise.** Aerobics help reduce fatigue, stress and incontinence...stretching eases stiffness.

Recommended: Yoga, tai chi, aquatics.

• **Acupuncture.** For many patients, this eases pain, numbness, spasms and incontinence.

• **Massage.** This may reduce pain, stiffness and spasticity.

On the horizon: Though still a long way off, novel therapies—such as oral DMTs and a DNA vaccine to treat MS—hold some promise that, in the future, MS may become a thing of the past.

New Thinking on MS

Rob Motl, PhD, associate professor in the department of kinesiology and community health, College of Applied Health Sciences at the University of Illinois at Urbana-Champaign. He chairs the advisory committee on patient management care and rehabilitation for the National Multiple Sclerosis Society and has published more than 180 research studies on MS.

Until recently, if you were diagnosed with multiple sclerosis (MS), treatment options were extremely limited. Doctors prescribed powerful drugs to reduce the number of new harmful brain lesions that characterize MS...to help control relapses...and to perhaps even slow progression of the disease.

Unfortunately, these medications, available only by injection, were often inconvenient to use and not always effective. Newer medications (such as Gilenya, Aubagio and Tecfidera) are now available in pill form. But is that enough?

New thinking: Even though medication is still believed to be important for most people with MS and should begin soon after diagnosis (when it is likely to be most effective), researchers are now identifying nondrug therapies that can also help.

BEYOND THE RX

With MS, the immune system mistakenly attacks the myelin sheaths that insulate the nerves, resulting in weakness, tingling, spasticity (marked by stiff or rigid muscles), balance problems and dizziness.

The nondrug therapies below have been shown to help people with MS have the best possible outcomes. Try as many as possible.

• **Walking.** Inactivity is dangerous for a person with MS—it can lead to muscle weakness, shallow breathing and other problems that can be exacerbated by the illness.

In studies of people with MS, walking (a great exercise because it can be adapted to various fitness levels) has been shown to reduce symptoms of fatigue, depression and pain...and improve sleep quality. Walking also may improve cognitive functioning, which can decline with MS, and improve balance, reducing one's risk of falling.

My advice: Walk for at least 15 to 30 minutes three to five times per week. Use a cane or walker if MS symptoms include leg weakness or numbness, spasticity and/or balance problems.

• **Strength training.** Research shows that muscle-strengthening exercises increase bone health and improve bladder and bowel control—all of which can be compromised with MS.

My advice: Twice a week, use weights that target the major muscle groups (such as quads, hamstrings, calves, biceps, triceps, shoulders and core). Do 15 of these exercises for each muscle group per session, and slowly add more repetitions and/or heavier weights.

Important: Speak with your physician before starting an exercise regimen. If you have problems with balance, consider working out with a physical therapist, friend or personal trainer for extra support.

• **Cooling strategies.** Increased activity and warmer temperatures can raise the core body temperature in people with MS. Even a slight increase may temporarily worsen their symptoms. With regular exercise, however, the body becomes more efficient in regulating its temperature, and heat sensitivity decreases.

My advice: While your body is becoming conditioned to respond efficiently to heat during your exercise program, take steps to prevent overheating. For example, exercise in an air-conditioned environment…use fans…wear loose-fitting clothing…and stay well hydrated. Cooling products such as vests, headbands, shirts and hats can help keep your core temperature stable.

Good cooling products include: Vests from GlacierTek (GlacierTek.com) or Coolture (Coolture.net), which range in price from $100 to $400. The cost may be covered by insurance. Cooling vests and neck, ankle and wrist wraps are also available from the Multiple Sclerosis Association of America (MyMSAA.org)—free to those who meet income limits.

• **Salsa dancing.** In a pilot study, people with MS who did salsa dancing for 40 minutes twice a week for four weeks improved their balance and gait and increased their activity levels. The front-to-back and side-to-side movements used in salsa dancing are believed to be especially helpful for those with MS.

My advice: If salsa dancing sounds appealing, ask your doctor whether he/she thinks lessons and regular practice sessions would be appropriate for you. Ballroom dancing and the video game *Dance Dance Revolution* have also been shown to help MS patients.

• **Acupuncture.** Acupuncture has been found to help with MS symptoms such as bladder problems, sleep disorders and tingling.

My advice: If you want to try acupuncture, look for a licensed acupuncturist. To find one near you, consult the National Certification Commission for Acupuncture and Oriental Medicine, NCCAOM.org.

• **Massage.** In a recent study, MS patients who received a 45-minute massage twice a week for five weeks improved their physical and social functioning and suffered less depression. By relaxing the muscles and increasing blood flow, massage may also alleviate spasticity, cramping and pain.

My advice: Consider trying Swedish massage, which uses long strokes and a light touch. Avoid using a table warmer or hot packs during the session, since people with MS tend to get overheated.

Caution: Some people with MS take corticosteroids, which may increase their risk for osteoporosis. If you have osteoporosis, massage may not be advisable unless your physician recommends it.

Mercury and MS

Mercury may cause autoimmune diseases. Mercury found in swordfish, king mackerel, tilefish and other seafood can impair the immune system, especially among women of childbearing age. The higher the level of exposure to mercury, the more proteins, called "autoantibodies," which can be an indicator of autoimmune disease. Autoimmune disease causes the immune system to attack healthy cells, which then leads to such diseases as lupus, rheumatoid arthritis and multiple sclerosis.

Study of government data from the National Health and Nutrition Examination Survey of women ages 16 to 49 by researchers at University of Michigan, Ann Arbor, published in *Environmental Health Perspectives*.

Dr. Terry Wahls's Brain-Boosting Diet Helped Her Conquer Multiple Sclerosis

Terry L. Wahls, MD, an internist and clinical professor of medicine at the University of Iowa Carver College of Medicine in Iowa City and president of the Wahls Foundation, TheWahlsFoundation.com, which supports research and provides education to the public about managing multiple sclerosis and other chronic diseases. She is author of *Minding My Mitochondria: How I Overcame Secondary Progressive Multiple Sclerosis and Got Out of My Wheelchair.*

A t age 44, I was diagnosed with multiple sclerosis (MS). Three years later, when I became dependent on a wheelchair, my MS was classified as "secondary progressive," meaning that the disease was steadily progressing with no periods of improvement. I kept getting weaker, even though I was receiving widely used treatments for MS including chemotherapy and immune-suppressing medications.

Now: Thanks to the regimen I designed, I haven't needed a wheelchair or even a cane for more than three years. I ride to work on my bicycle, my energy is good and I've stopped taking medication to treat my MS. What happened?

Here's what I credit for my dramatic turnaround—and a description of how it might help you, as well. Because MS is a neurological disease, this program is designed to also help people who are concerned about dementia or Parkinson's disease, have depression or have suffered a traumatic brain injury or stroke.

FINDING A SOLUTION

With the help of my medical training, I began poring over the medical literature and designed my own treatment protocol in 2007 based on my theories of what allowed MS to develop and progress.

In people with MS, immune cells damage the myelin sheath, protein and fatty substances that surround nerve cells in the brain and spinal cord. This results in slower nerve signals, which lead to muscle weakness, a lack of balance and muscle coordination, bladder or bowel spasms, blurred vision and other symptoms.

Medications can reduce symptoms, but they don't accelerate nerve signals. As a result, MS patients battle physical and neurological disability—experienced either episodically or in a steady, unrelenting course. The disease often continues to worsen despite therapy. Within 10 years of initial diagnosis, half of MS patients are unable to work because of disabling levels of fatigue, and one-third need a cane, scooter or wheelchair.

After thoroughly reviewing the research, I decided to put myself on a diet that increases the efficiency of mitochondria, units within cells that supply the energy that's needed for nerve activity. Although the effect of diet on MS was unproven, I firmly believed that this was my best hope for fighting MS.

My eating plan was designed to improve the balance of neurotransmitters and supply the mitochondria with the building blocks needed for healthy nerve activity.

MY BRAIN-HEALTH DIET

People who follow this diet typically notice improvements in neurological symptoms within weeks.*

Because natural foods contain a variety of nutrients that can work synergistically, I recommend taking supplements only when you are unable to get the following nutrients in your diet. Be sure to discuss the supplements (and dosages) with your doctor if you take blood-thinning medication—some supplements may have a blood-thinning effect.

In addition to taking such general steps as avoiding sugary and/or processed foods that are low in key nutrients, make sure you get enough...

•**Sulfur vegetables.** Cabbage, kale, collard greens and asparagus are excellent sources of sulfur, which is used by the body to produce gamma-aminobutyric acid (GABA). This "inhibitory" neurotransmitter counteracts the early brain-cell death that can occur if the neurotransmitter glutamate reaches excessive levels.

*Consult your doctor before trying the diet and/or supplements described here—especially if you take any medication or have kidney or liver disease.

My advice: Consume three cups of greens each day, including one to three cups of sulfur-rich vegetables daily.

Also: To get other important nutrients, consume one to three cups of brightly colored vegetables or berries each day.

• **Coenzyme Q-10.** Exposure to environmental toxins, such as detergents, pesticide residues and mercury, has been linked to MS and other neurological conditions, such as dementia and Parkinson's disease. Coenzyme Q-10 is a fat-soluble compound that helps minimize the effects of these toxins while increasing the amount of energy produced by mitochondria.

Organ meats, such as calf liver and chicken liver, are among the best sources of coenzyme Q-10. I particularly recommend organ meats for older adults because coenzyme Q-10 production declines with age. It's also suppressed by cholesterol-lowering statin drugs.

My advice: Eat organ meats at least once a week. If you don't like organ meats, sardines, herring and rainbow trout are also high in coenzyme Q-10. Coenzyme Q-10 is available in supplement form, too.

• **Omega-3 fatty acids.** The omega-3 fatty acids in cold-water fish, such as salmon and sardines, are used by the body to produce the myelin that insulates brain and spinal cord cells. Myelin is also used to repair damage caused by MS. Omega-3s are concentrated in the brain and are necessary to help prevent depression and cognitive disorders.

My advice: To avoid concern about mercury and other toxins in cold-water fish, such as salmon, get your omega-3s from fish oil supplements that are purified.

Recommended dose: 1 g to 3 g daily.

• **Kelp and algae.** These detoxify the body by binding to heavy metals in the intestine and removing them in the stool.

My advice: Take supplements—one to two 500-mg to 600-mg capsules of kelp and one to four 500-mg capsules of algae daily. Or, as an alternative, add about a tablespoon of powdered algae—different types include Klamath blue green algae, spirulina and chlorella—to morning smoothies.

• **Green tea.** It's high in quercetin, an antioxidant that reduces inflammation. Green tea also changes the molecular structure of fat-soluble toxins and allows them to dissolve in water. This accelerates their excretion from the body.

My advice: Drink several cups of green tea daily.

Best choice: Finely milled Matcha green tea. It has more antioxidants than the typical tea brewed with dried leaves.

Note: Most types of green tea contain caffeine—on average, about 25 mg per cup.

The Vitamin That MS Patients Need

Ellen Mowry, MD, associate professor of neurology, Johns Hopkins University School of Medicine, Baltimore. Andrew L. Rubman, ND, founder and medical director, Southbury Clinic for Traditional Medicines, Southbury, Connecticut. SouthburyClinic.com

People with multiple sclerosis (MS) want to do everything possible to prevent the autoimmune disease's uncomfortable and disabling consequences, including weakness, numbness, blurred vision and bladder problems.

What's wonderful is that recent research has found that consuming more of a certain nutrient found in foods and supplements might slow the progression of the disease.

The study's lead author, Ellen Mowry, MD, explained more about this vitamin and how much of it exactly might help my readers who are living with MS…

"D-CIPHERING" THE RESEARCH

The nutrient in question is vitamin D.

Dr. Mowry and her colleagues analyzed people with MS during a five-year period. They gauged their blood levels of vitamin D from all sources—sunlight, foods and/or supplements. (Patients weren't told to consume specific amounts of vitamin D.) Researchers used MRI scans on the patients to look for two particular types of lesions in the brain—new

T2 lesions and gadolinium-enhancing lesions. These lesions indicate that MS is advancing—the development of lesions in MS patients is associated with long-term disability.

Dr. Mowry and her team found an intriguing association—the higher the level of vitamin D in the blood, the lower the number of both types of lesions. Each increase of 10 nanograms per milliliter of vitamin D in the blood was linked to a 15% lower risk for new T2 lesions and a 32% lower risk for gadolinium-enhancing lesions.

Researchers also tracked the progression of disability in patients and found that the higher the levels of vitamin D, the less disability a person would subsequently have.

This doesn't mean that consuming more vitamin D will definitely prevent MS from progressing (this study did not show cause and effect—only an association with blood levels), but there's a chance that it could.

THE BEST DOSE OF D

How much vitamin D should MS patients take? Dr. Mowry and Andrew Rubman, ND, founder and medical director of the Southbury Clinic for Traditional Medicines in Connecticut, answered this question…

Both said that beyond getting vitamin D through foods and sunlight, people with MS often need to take an additional 2000 IU to 4000 IU of the vitamin each day in supplement form. (Keep in mind that not all experts agree yet on what is optimal. Plus, vitamin D may interact negatively with certain drugs and exacerbate certain health conditions. So check with your doctor before taking any vitamin D.)

Both also advised having your blood levels of vitamin D measured by your doctor before starting supplementation. This way, if you have MS, you can see whether your measurement falls between the 40 and 60 nanograms per milliliter that Dr. Mowry counsels her MS patients to shoot for. You can then adjust your vitamin D dosage to reach that range.

Drug for Early-Stage MS

The drug BG-12, which is taken orally, reduced relapse rates in early-stage multiple sclerosis (MS) by nearly 50%...compared with a reduction of about 30% in patients treated with the current first-line treatment of choice, interferon and *glatiramer acetate*, which must be given by injection. BG-12's side effects—such as skin flushing and gastrointestinal upset—typically are mild.

Robert Fox, MD, staff neurologist at the Cleveland Clinic Mellen Center for Multiple Sclerosis and lead author of a study of BG-12, published in *The New England Journal of Medicine*.

How Stents May Help MS

Robert Fox, MD, staff neurologist, Mellen Center for Multiple Sclerosis at Cleveland Clinic, Cleveland.

Multiple sclerosis (MS) has been incurable and intractable for so long that there was a collective gasp from the medical community in 2009 when an Italian vascular surgeon, Paolo Zamboni, MD, published a study in the *Journal of Vascular Surgery* describing a new surgery that, he said, relieved two major MS symptoms—fatigue and brain fog—and also might help ameliorate other symptoms as well, including improving energy level.

If you have or know someone who has MS, you might have picked up on this apparent breakthrough back then—but curiously there has been little said about it in the mainstream health media since the announcement. Even many people who follow health news closely wouldn't be able to say whether Dr. Zamboni's procedure has really turned out to be a godsend for MS patients. This disease of the central nervous system is so widespread and so insidious, it's definitely time we found out—so let's see where things stand right now.

A CONTROVERSIAL MATTER

Some doctors believe that stenosis (narrowing) of the principle veins that carry blood from the brain, a condition that is also known as chronic cerebrospinal venous insufficiency (CCSVI), slows drainage of the blood from the brain and spinal cord, and even causes the blood to reflux back into both. And some think that, left uncorrected, the reflux may lead to oxygen deprivation and iron deposits in the brain tissue and theorize it may contribute to—or even cause—MS. The controversial new surgery Dr. Zamboni brought to light is called transluminal angioplasty and helps to correct the stenosis by opening those principle veins and widening them with stents.

However, many doctors are not convinced that reflux blood is a problem—if it exists at all. Nor for that matter are they sure how many MS patients actually have CCSVI or even how specific the condition is to the disease. Furthermore, doctors worry that the surgery for CCSVI carries considerable risk. Not surprisingly, this has caused a huge controversy in the MS world.

Dr. Zamboni's study investigated 109 MS patients and 177 people without MS and found that all participants with MS had CCSVI while not one of the others did. Other studies have not replicated these findings, however. For example, in a large follow-up study at the University of Buffalo, just over half of MS patients were found to have CCSVI and, even more surprising, nearly 25% of the healthy "controls" also had CCSVI but with no symptoms.

Dr. Zamboni also reported that the surgery, which he performed on 65 MS patients, was quite successful, in particular for patients with relapsing-remitting (RR) MS, the most common form of the disease in which occasional relapses or flare-ups are interspersed with longer periods of disease remission. At a reassessment 18 months after surgery, RR MS patients had "significant improvement" in physical and mental quality-of-life measures compared with their condition before surgery.

However, there is little information to date about results of similar surgeries performed for CCSVI, and several alarming problems have emerged. One concerns use of angioplasty stents for the surgery. Neurologist Robert Fox, MD, staff neurologist at the Mellen Center for Multiple Sclerosis at Cleveland Clinic, explained that angioplasty stents are designed for placement in arteries, which get progressively smaller the further they are from the heart, whereas veins grow larger as they get closer to the heart. This increases the likelihood that a stent placed in a vein will travel, a circumstance that can be quite dangerous—and indeed, one MS patient in the US ended up having emergency surgery to remove a stent from her heart.

In spite of these problems and the questions surrounding CCSVI, in general, a number of doctors in the US and abroad continue to perform the surgery on MS patients. Clearly, though, we need much more information to guide people in the MS community. A Canadian CCVSI clinical trial of the angioplasty procedure in people with MS is nearing completion.

DR. FOX'S ADVICE

Acknowledging the difficulty of doing so, Dr. Fox urges people with MS to hang on while researchers work to close the information gap between what patients want to be true and what we know is true. *We discussed some of the specific questions people have regarding this controversial therapy...*

What causes the vein blockages in MS patients?

We don't know—the ongoing studies are taking a step back to establish the true role blockages do or do not play in MS, along with what may or may not be different about them in MS patients and people without the disease. We want to find out if CCSVI is a possible cause of MS or is a result of it. MS, as well as other neurological conditions, cause the brain to atrophy, becoming what we call a "sick brain," and that alone may create vascular changes. If a sick brain is behind CCSVI, the condition, when it exists, may not be a factor in causing MS, but rather a result.

Still, if MS patients' doctors find blockages, why not just have them fixed?

Not only are we not certain whether CCSVI has anything to do with MS, we also believe that the body is typically able to manage damaged veins by putting other veins to work. This means there may be no reason to open a vein and no benefit to be gained from it.

Shouldn't MS patients at least be tested for CCSVI?

We are not recommending this yet—we do not yet know what imaging techniques are most effective for making a careful diagnosis. And if a test does show CCSVI, we don't yet have the information we need to know what to do about it.

The Internet is filled with offers for "medical-tourism" vacations overseas, some of which say this surgery is guaranteed as successful with no risk. While such claims are clearly exaggerated, could any of this be helpful?

CCSVI surgery has generated a great deal of buzz in social media and on medical-tourism websites, and there is a lot of misleading information out there. One thing we do know to be absolutely true is that CCSVI surgery is a risky procedure.

When are we going to have the information we need to know whether CCSVI surgery is a real possibility to help MS patients have better lives?

Until there is a follow-up to Dr. Zamboni's study via large clinical studies, says Dr. Fox, there is no way to know for sure whether CCSVI surgery really is hope…or just hype.

It's understandably difficult for MS patients to be patient…but for now, that's the strategy that seems to make sense.

Living Better with Multiple Sclerosis: Symptoms and Solutions

Annette Funicello (1942-2013) was the star of the popular 1950s television series *The Mickey Mouse Club*. She also starred in the motion pictures *Babes in Toyland* and *The Shaggy Dog*, as well as several beach party movies with Frankie Avalon. Ms. Funicello was the recipient of numerous awards in recognition of her professional accomplishments and her efforts to raise public awareness about MS.

This article was originally published in *Bottom Line/Health* (then called *Health Confidential*) in 1994.

Seven years ago, I was diagnosed with multiple sclerosis—an often debilitating neuro-logical disorder that causes vision problems, muscle weakness and poor coordination.

At the time, I knew nothing about the illness—and I decided to keep it that way. For several years, I avoided thinking and talking about MS—and kept my diagnosis a secret from everyone but my mother, husband and children. I didn't even tell my father. I thought I could beat MS on my own and no one would ever have to know.

Looking back, I can see that my refusal to learn about my illness and my need to hide it were attempts to fend off fear. Unfortunately, the ignorance and secrecy only fueled my anxiety.

Since then, I've found far more effective ways of coping with MS…and with chronic illness in general. *Here's what I wish I'd known earlier…*

• **Educate yourself.** Learn as much as you can about your illness—whether it's MS or another chronic ailment.

There are still many unanswered questions about MS—including what causes it, how best to treat it and what any individual's prognosis will be. *Yet the more I've learned about MS, the more I realize that there is good news…*

1. MS is not fatal, contagious or hereditary. That's why I always use the term *illness* rather than the more frightening word *disease* when speaking about MS.

2. MS is not always progressive. The damaged nerve cells that are characteristic of MS sometimes heal on their own, although we're still not sure under what conditions. Roughly three-quarters of people with MS experience spontaneous remissions during the course of their illness—and, in some cases, complete relief of symptoms. And researchers are getting close to finding a cure.

Sources of information: Your doctor, your local library and nonprofit organizations such as the National Multiple Sclerosis Society. These organizations can put you in touch with support groups and other local resources.

• **Admit you have a problem**—and ask for the help and understanding you need. To convince family and friends that nothing was seriously wrong with me, I became a good liar. When I started having trouble with my balance, for example, I blamed it on tendinitis and a bad knee. Being dishonest with people I cared about sapped my self-esteem.

When you lie, you have to work hard to keep your stories straight. That takes a great deal of energy. It also creates a lot of psychological stress. As someone coping with the symptoms of MS, I certainly didn't need more of that.

I kept my illness secret partly because I didn't want to hurt anyone. But by avoiding people, making excuses and hiding the truth, I suspect I caused them—and myself—even more pain.

I "went public" with my diagnosis in 1992. I wasn't trying to be noble. Reporters from the tabloids had started knocking on neighbors' doors, trying to confirm rumors that my unsteady balance stemmed from a drinking problem. I realized I had to tell the truth—in public—before someone created an ugly story.

Once I did, a huge weight was lifted off my shoulders. There was an outpouring of support from friends and strangers alike. The calls, cards and letters made me realize how much I'd been cheating myself by trying to bear this burden alone.

My family has been wonderful, too. On bad days, when my symptoms flare up, they understand and aren't frightened—and I don't need to hide it.

• **Having MS has changed the way I view other people's disabilities.** I used to feel sorry for wheelchair-bound people and those with other disabilities. Not anymore. I know that I don't want pity...and that people who cope with disability every day are tough. We learn to live with our challenges. We do our best with what we have.

• **Keep busy**—but know your limits. The busier I am, the less time I have to think abut my illness. That helps me avoid the temptation of self-pity.

Since my diagnosis, I've launched several business ventures. More important, I started the Annette Funicello Research Fund for Neurological Diseases, which will help finance research into MS and related illnesses.

As busy as I am, I'm careful not to get overtired. In the beginning, I pushed myself too hard. I thought that by refusing to slow down, I could prove that my illness didn't really exist.

Now I rest when I need to. I hold most of my business meetings at home. When I travel, I keep my schedule as light as possible.

What's important is balance. Resting doesn't mean retiring from life.

• **Find ways to cope that work for you.** While I would not presume to tell anyone else how to deal with a chronic illness, I think that sharing information is important. So here are three things I've discovered that help me. Maybe they'll help you or someone close to you, too.

1. Stay cool. Because heat exacerbates MS symptoms, it's important to keep body temperature down—especially in summer. My favorite way to keep cool is to suck on crushed ice.

2. Elevate the legs. I've found that 20 minutes of lying down with a pillow under my knees and lower legs seems to make walking easier. I might do this several times a day.

3. Follow a healthy lifestyle. I firmly believe that anything that reduces stress helps fight illness. I feel much better now that I've given up smoking and drinking alcohol. I've also noticed that my symptoms are less bothersome when I eat a low-fat diet.

• **Stay optimistic.** I've tried more than two dozen treatments for MS, from acupuncture to vitamins to various prescription drugs. I discuss everything with my doctor and make sure I understand the risks and side effects of each treatment I try.

I must say that I'm very skeptical of "fad" treatments such as hyperbaric chambers...removing fillings from the teeth...chelation therapy. I keep my spirits up by making the most of my good days and by remembering how many people are working to solve the puzzle of MS. I take one day at a time, and if one treatment doesn't work, I go on to the next.

So far, nothing has led to a remission. Although that's a little discouraging, I haven't stopped fighting—far from it.

I've always been religious, and my faith has been a great help. I know that my illness has a purpose, even though I don't yet know what that purpose might be.

I take comfort in knowing that the prayers of many loved ones are behind me. I keep a smile on my face—and I never give up hope.

MS May Be Slowed by a Cholesterol-Lowering Med

In a recent finding, high doses of the statin drug *simvastatin* slowed brain atrophy in some patients with advanced multiple sclerosis (MS). A very early Phase II trial found that some MS patients who were given 80 milligrams (mg) of simvastatin a day for two years had less neural degeneration.

Patricia K. Coyle, MD, professor of neurology and director of the Multiple Sclerosis Comprehensive Care Center, Stony Brook University Medical Center, East Setauket, New York.

New Help for Multiple Sclerosis Patients

An injection of *botulinum toxin* (Botox) lessened arm tremors by two points (on a 10-point scale), reducing moderate tremor to mild. It also improved patients' ability to write and draw by one point.

Study of MS patients by researchers at The Royal Melbourne Hospital and University of Melbourne, both in Australia, published in *Neurology*.

Marijuana for MS— Does It Help or Do Users Just Mind Less?

Moses Rodriguez, MD, a neurologist at Mayo Clinic in Rochester, Minnesota, professor of immunology and neurology at the Mayo Clinic College of Medicine.

Does marijuana reduce the debilitating physical symptoms of multiple sclerosis (MS)—or does it just help patients care a little less about them? If you or a loved one suffers from MS, this could be a very important question.

It's widely accepted that marijuana has some therapeutic value for MS-related symptoms, including for painful muscle spasticity. In fact, clinical studies have demonstrated that when two of marijuana's active ingredients, 9-tetrahydrocannabinol (THC) and cannabidiol (CBD), are isolated and then combined into a drug, they can reduce muscle spasticity with only minor psychotropic effects. Sativex, a pharmaceutical formulation of marijuana that is approved for neuropathic pain in MS patients in Canada but not in the US, contains both ingredients.

Yet for many, the intoxicating effects of marijuana's ingredients are troubling.

With the hope of making a case for FDA approval here, researchers at the Global Neuroscience Initiative Foundation in Los Angeles selected six recent randomized controlled trials involving a total of 481 patients with MS who took oral preparations of combination THC and CBD extracts. The findings are interesting—according to the admittedly subjective reports of the patients, the extracts relieved spasticity...but when several objective measures of spasticity (including a mobility index and patients' "walk time") were examined, no significant improvements were evident. And, though the combination dose was thought to keep people from getting high, patients in each of the six trials experienced adverse effects in the form of intoxication and sedation. The study was published in the online journal *BMC Neurology*.

185

GOOD STUFF OR NOT?

So—is marijuana helpful for MS patients? The answer, according to Moses Rodriguez, MD, a neurologist at the Mayo Clinic College of Medicine in Rochester, Minnesota, and a nationally recognized MS expert, is yes and no. Dr. Rodriguez said that although many MS patients (including some of his own) report that marijuana is effective in alleviating spasticity, he said that there are no standards regulating how it should be used and "the data proving its efficacy is weak and its side effects are worrisome."

One challenge, he explained, is that scientists still don't understand why marijuana helps. "We know that it works on receptors in the brain, but marijuana does not have a direct effect on the muscles, so it is difficult to break away the drug's general well-being effects from its anti-spasticity effects," he said. He also pointed out that little is known about marijuana's systemic and long-term effects on MS patients, which is of potential concern. Therefore, Dr. Rodriguez remains "very cautious" about recommending marijuana to his patients, "especially when other agents are available on the market that can effectively control spasticity, such as *baclofen* and *tizanidine*," he said. (*Note*: There is also little data on long-term effects of these drugs and they, too, have side effects.) The National Multiple Sclerosis Society takes a similar stance—it does not recommend medical marijuana, citing "insufficient evidence of a clear benefit compared with existing therapies and issues of side effects, systemic effects and long-term effects."

Dr. Rodriguez believes that there may come a day when new marijuana agents will be manufactured that offer the anti-spasticity effects without the side effects. Until then, he recommends staying with FDA-approved drugs for MS-related spasticity.

Cough Syrup as a Treatment for MS

Wenbin Deng, PhD, associate professor of neuroscience, department of biochemistry and molecular medicine, University of California-Davis School of Medicine.

Multiple sclerosis is one of the most common incurable autoimmune diseases and can be a cause for despair. More than 400,000 Americans cope with a vast array of symptoms that create moderate problems for some—such as blurry vision and poor coordination—and deeply debilitating symptoms for others, such as muscle weakness, numbness and difficulty moving that can even lead to paralysis. After so many decades of intense research, one would hope that truly effective treatments might be around the corner.

Something that sounds unlikely involves a study showing that the active ingredient in an over-the-counter (OTC) cough medicine—yes, a common drugstore cough syrup—might actually offer a long-awaited breakthrough.

A SAFE MEDICINE FOR THE LONG TERM?

First, some background. Typically, a fatty sheath (known as myelin) surrounds the nerves that network throughout the body. But multiple sclerosis spurs the immune system into a haywire process, causing it to attack itself and impair the myelin in the brain and spinal cord, initiating the symptoms that are the hallmark of the disease. Tests led by Wenbin Deng, PhD, of the University of California-Davis School of Medicine, found that the drug contained in most cough medicines, *dextromethorphan*, greatly cut the loss of this fatty sheath in mice with laboratory-induced MS. The same drug also minimized the development of paralysis among mice during flare-ups of the disease.

Fortunately, dextromethorphan happens to be a very safe drug—"essentially not toxic at all when used at low doses," said Dr. Deng, an associate professor of neuroscience. It contains low-dose, morphinelike agents known as morphinans that have a very low risk of being addictive. "The wonderful thing," Dr. Deng continued, "is that this is something we could safely use in MS patients for the long term, since it has been proven safe over the past 50 years in OTC cough medicine."

Dr. Deng said that a chance meeting with MS patients in North Carolina a few years ago spurred the idea of testing dextromethorphan as an MS treatment. A community of MS patients there had already been using certain OTC medications to control their symptoms, he said, just as people with a wide variety of ailments try all kinds of scientifically unproven remedies. But in this case, the buzz about dextromethorphan seemed unusually positive for a simple OTC medicine. Dr. Deng began to wonder what the results might be in a more controlled setting.

Dr. Deng's study, which was published recently in *Neurobiology of Disease*, found that low doses were most effective—high dosages did not offer any benefit. Dr. Deng was careful to caution me that animal studies are only the first step in figuring out whether his results will eventually hold true for humans. The next step is conducting preclinical studies to determine what doses might work best in human MS patients. After that, randomized, clinical trials would test the drug's effects versus those of a placebo.

Until further research on this topic takes place, this is a case where each patient has to make a personal decision in consultation with his/her doctors.

Old Drug Helps MS

Phenytoin, a drug long used for epilepsy, may help prevent optical nerve damage in those with optic neuritis, a common early symptom of MS.

The Lancet Neurology.

Ever Feel "Spaced Out"?

Lara Jehi, MD, a neurologist who specializes in treating epilepsy in adults. She is associate director of clinical research at the Cleveland Clinic Epilepsy Center and has published 62 papers on epilepsy in medical journals, including the *Journal of Neurosurgery.*

The room suddenly looks different…or you "space out" for 30 seconds or longer, staring vacantly into space unaware of your surroundings…or black out and fall to the floor. You may even smell, see or hear something that isn't there.

Do not ignore it. You could be having an epileptic seizure—a hallmark of epilepsy, a widely misunderstood and life-threatening condition that affects one of every 26 people in their lifetimes.

Most people associate epilepsy with lost consciousness, convulsing limbs and twitching—but these generalized tonic-clonic seizures (once known as "grand mal" seizures) are actually less common than more subtle partial seizure episodes, such as those described above.

That's especially true in adults. While epilepsy often starts in childhood, risk progressively increases starting at about age 55.

Why it goes undetected: Because adult-onset seizures are rarely dramatic, most doctors don't think of epilepsy very often—if at all—when evaluating their older patients.

IS IT EPILEPSY?

Many things can cause a seizure—for example, acute infection, fever, low blood sugar, poisoning and medication side effects. What generally makes it epilepsy is repetition—the same experience, reflecting the same abnormal brain activity, unprovoked by outside stimulus, over and over.

Why does it happen? Much of the time, epilepsy in older adults is the result of more generalized brain disease. Stroke is responsible in one-third of the cases with an identifiable cause. When there's an underlying cause, such as stroke, a single seizure can be labeled epilepsy (see next page).

Alzheimer's and Parkinson's disease account for a total of 11% of cases. Head trauma is responsible for 2% of epilepsy in older adults. Tumors—including metastases of cancer originating elsewhere—also may be involved. But often, no underlying cause can be found.

GETTING THE RIGHT DIAGNOSIS

If you think that you may have had a seizure, discuss this with your internist, who may refer you to a neurologist. Diagnosing epilepsy is not always easy. An electroencephalogram (EEG), a test that records electrical activity in the brain, may show abnormal brain activity only when a seizure is occurring, and brain scans, such as an MRI, can look normal.

That's why it takes an expert to identify epilepsy based on the patient's description of the episodes and other aspects of a person's medical history, such as stroke.

Important update: Traditionally, the diagnosis of epilepsy has required at least two seizures. But the International League Against Epilepsy, a prestigious group of researchers and clinicians, recently broadened the definition to include a single seizure when tests and/or history suggest a high risk for recurrence.

Examples: An MRI shows evidence of a prior stroke…or an EEG finds brain wave patterns typical of epilepsy.

Treatment is essential: Epilepsy is a life-threatening condition that requires treatment. With untreated epilepsy, abnormal brain activity can actually stop the heart—a complication that occurs in roughly 1% of epilepsy patients each year.

A diagnosis of epilepsy should prompt further investigation—the seizures may be the first warning of another serious brain condition. For example, a study in *The Lancet* found that the risk for stroke nearly tripled among older adults who had started having seizures without prior strokes, suggesting undetected brain artery disease.

THE BEST MEDICATION

Medication is effective in quelling seizures two-thirds of the time. In older people, epilepsy is more likely to respond to drug treatment, often at a lower dose than a younger person would require. But some side effects of commonly used medications, such as sedation,

bone loss and difficulty concentrating, can be particularly problematic in older adults. Also, most older adults take medication for other chronic medical problems, which can interact with certain antiepileptic drugs.

What often works best: Several of the newer antiseizure medications—*lamotrigine* (Lamictal), *gabapentin* (Neurontin) and *levetiracetam* (Keppra)—appear to be as effective as tried-and-true standbys like *phenytoin* (Dilantin) in older patients, but with fewer side effects and less interaction with other prescriptions. Side effects can include liver problems, thinning hair, dizziness and loss of balance. Medication is usually taken for at least two years.

Note: People with epilepsy can drive as long as they have not experienced seizures within a certain amount of time (which varies by state).

WHEN TO CONSIDER SURGERY

When seizures persist despite medication, surgery should be considered. The most effective procedure, resective surgery, removes the usually tiny segment of the brain where abnormal activity originates.

A study presented at the 2013 annual meeting of the American Epilepsy Society found good results in nine out of 10 patients ages 60 to 74 (one patient died of a brain tumor) who received resective surgery—seven becoming seizure free—with no postoperative complications.

Breakthrough treatment: When the part of the brain responsible for seizures can't be removed—it is too large or too close to critical structures or multiple brain areas are involved—a device can be permanently implanted to modify brain activity electrically. One device, approved by the FDA, functions as a kind of pacemaker for the brain. The Neuropace RNS System detects seizure activity as it starts and produces a mild shock to abort the episode.

In a trial of nearly 200 people whose partial seizures couldn't be controlled with medication, the device reduced episode frequency by more than half, after two years of use. There is a small risk for brain bleeding and infection.

Millions of Americans Will Have a Sudden Seizure

Gholam Motamedi, MD, professor of neurology, director of clinical neurophysiology and director of the epilepsy program at Georgetown University Hospital in Washington, DC.

There are many misconceptions about seizures. For example, many people believe that seizures always are due to epilepsy. Not true. Up to 10% of Americans will have a single seizure at some time in their lives and never have another one. A patient has to have two unprovoked seizures (seizures without a known cause) before neurologists diagnose epilepsy—a condition that affects about 1% of the population.

Another myth is that seizures are always dangerous. In fact, the vast majority of people recover normally after seizures. But a seizure can be a sign of a serious illness, including a brain tumor.

WHAT'S A SEIZURE?

Seizures occur when groups of brain cells discharge sudden bursts of unusual electrical activity. A partial (also called focal) seizure originates from a relatively small number of cells in a particular part of the brain. A generalized seizure involves abnormal electrical activity throughout the brain.

Only the most severe seizures, known as tonic-clonic (or grand mal), are likely to cause the dramatic symptoms that most people associate with seizures, such as a loss of consciousness, whole-body shaking, a loss of bladder control and/or biting of the tongue.

As many as one in 200 patients with severe epilepsy will die from Sudden Unexpected Death in Epilepsy (SUDEP). This usually occurs in patients with other medical conditions who are taking multiple drugs. It's possible that the electrical disturbances that cause seizures also affect electrical control of the heart.

Most seizures, however, are more subtle. Patients may notice unusual smells or tastes. They might stare into space, smack their lips or pick at their clothing. Some patients experience nothing more than a minute or two of confusion and disorientation.

CAUSES

The late senator Edward Kennedy was hospitalized after having a seizure. Neurologists discovered that he had a brain tumor.

Patients who have experienced brain injuries or suffered a stroke will sometimes have seizures. Seizures also are common in alcoholics who stop drinking, even for short periods, though if the patient stays off alcohol, the seizures usually will cease.

For most patients who experience seizures, there is no known cause. The seizures are probably triggered by disorders at the cellular level that can't yet be detected with magnetic resonance imaging (MRI) or other tests.

DIAGNOSING A SEIZURE

Anyone who has a seizure should see a doctor promptly to rule out any medical problems, including stroke.

Be sure to call 911 if someone has a seizure that lasts more than 10 minutes. A prolonged seizure, known as status epilepticus, may be caused by a dangerous infection (such as meningitis) or other underlying diseases, though it's often caused by a patient forgetting to take his/her medications. Prolonged seizures may be life-threatening in some cases.

Adults who experience a new onset of seizures usually are given an MRI to rule out tumors and other brain abnormalities. They also will be given an electroencephalogram (EEG) to record electrical activity in the brain.

Patients with epilepsy usually exhibit "spikes," sharp discharges of electricity in the brain that are present even when they're not having seizures. In some cases, patients may be monitored (via electrodes on the scalp) for one to 10 days, either in the hospital or with a mobile EEG unit.

TREATMENT

Only about 10% to 30% of otherwise healthy patients who have a single seizure will have a second one. If a patient's EEG and MRI are normal, treatment probably won't be required.

Among patients who have had two or more seizures, however, the risk for subsequent

189

seizures rises to 70% or more. Most of these patients require treatment for epilepsy. *Best options...*

• **Medication.** About two-thirds of patients with epilepsy become seizure-free on medications that inhibit abnormal electrical activity in the brain. These include prescription drugs, such as *carbamazepine* (Tegretol) and *phenytoin* (Dilantin), as well as other drugs.

Possible side effects: Fatigue and/or dizziness. Less often, the drugs may impair speech or coordination.

It's a bad sign when patients don't respond satisfactorily to the initial drug therapy. About 50% of patients become seizure-free on the first medication. Among those who don't, only about 15% will be seizure-free after switching to a second drug or multiple-drug therapy. Those who still don't respond are unlikely to be helped significantly with higher doses and/or different drugs.

Recent finding: Researchers at the University of Alabama at Birmingham Epilepsy Center analyzed eight years of insurance data from more than 30,000 epileptics and found that those who didn't take their prescribed seizure medication regularly—who started and stopped the drug—were three times more likely to die than epileptics who maintained their medication regimens. They also had more hospitalizations, car accidents and broken bones. The results were published in *Neurology*.

• **Surgery.** Brain surgery is recommended for patients who don't achieve adequate seizure control with medications. Up to 80% of patients who have surgery become seizure-free. Most of the remaining 20% show significant improvement.

Surgery is most commonly done in patients with certain types of epilepsy, in which the abnormal brain cells are located in a single area and are relatively easy to remove.

Most cases involve temporal lobe epilepsy, in which an abnormal clump of tissue is present in either the right or left temporal lobes, located in the area of the brain above the ears. The procedure, called temporal lobe resection, is done under general anesthetic. Most patients stay in the hospital for two to four days after the surgery. Risks include some degree of per-

manent language and/or motor difficulties depending on the location of the surgery.

• **High-fat diet.** A very high-fat diet (known as a ketogenic diet) appears to reduce seizures in children. A study published in *The Lancet Neurology* found that 38% of children on the diet had about a 50% reduction in seizures, compared with 6% in a control group.

It's not known why a high-fat diet helps control seizures. It's a difficult diet to follow, because patients must eat about four parts fat to each part combined protein and carbohydrates. Researchers are investigating a modified form of the diet for adults.

Could You or a Loved One Have Epilepsy?

Lara Jehi, MD, an epileptologist (a neurologist who specializes in treating epilepsy) and clinical neurophysiologist at the Epilepsy Center at the Cleveland Clinic and research director of the clinic's Epilepsy Outcome Program. She is a recipient of the Young Investigator Award from the American Epilepsy Society and has published several medical journal articles and book chapters on epilepsy.

I f you experience occasional confusion—so-called "senior moments"—or times when you "zone out" by staring into space, your doctor may suspect a heart problem or early-stage Alzheimer's disease. But one possible cause that is often overlooked is epilepsy.

Epilepsy is widely known to strike younger adults, but researchers estimate that one out of every 20 people over age 65 has the condition. Many experts believe the true number is even higher because data count only people who have had obvious seizures, which don't necessarily occur in older adults with epilepsy.

What you need to know...

EPILEPSY IN OLDER ADULTS

Epilepsy is caused by abnormal electrical activity in the brain. In younger people, this tends to express itself in very noticeable movements, such as full-body fidgeting, jerking movements or uncontrollable shaking.

In older adults, the abnormal brain activity typically produces a much milder physical response. The reason isn't known, but researchers theorize that as the brain ages, connections between its regions weaken, so the spread of electrical activity—which is what produces seizures—becomes less pronounced.

When epilepsy begins later in life, it typically results from a health problem that alters brain function. Cerebrovascular disease (reduced blood flow to the brain)—which can result in a stroke—causes one-third of new epilepsy cases in older adults. Other conditions that can lead to epilepsy include head injury...a brain tumor...infectious diseases, such as meningitis and encephalitis (both of which cause inflammation in the brain)...and excessive drinking (which damages parts of the brain where seizures are likely to arise).

WHAT ARE THE RED FLAGS?

Besides occasional confusion and staring spells, signs of epilepsy in an older adult include...

• **Uncontrollable twitching of a specific body part.**

• **Numbness or tingling on one side of the body (typically in the arm).**

• **Dropping things for no apparent reason.**

• **Falling or passing out due to a brief loss of consciousness.**

In some cases, symptoms are so mild that family members describe an older person with epilepsy simply as being "a little out of it" or "not acting himself."

Important tip-off: Each episode typically involves the same sensation in the same part of the body. Symptoms often occur for a few minutes then go away, only to return later. They may recur many times in a day or appear as rarely as once a week or even once a month.

GETTING A CORRECT DIAGNOSIS

Untreated epilepsy is dangerous because it puts the person at serious risk for brain damage (shrinkage in the area of the brain where the seizures originate) from continued attacks, as well as driving mishaps, falls and other epilepsy-related injuries.

If epilepsy is suspected, the patient should see an epileptologist (a neurologist who specializes in the treatment of epilepsy) or a general neurologist.* The brain's electrical activity will be recorded with an electroencephalograph (EEG), a device that uses small, adhesive sensors (electrodes) that are placed on a person's scalp. The procedure is noninvasive and painless. If the EEG shows abnormal brain activity that is characteristic of epilepsy, the diagnosis is made.

BEST MEDICATIONS

Antiseizure medication is the first step in treating epilepsy. Older adults are typically prescribed one of three antiseizure medications—*levetiracetam* (Keppra), *lamotrigine* (Lamictal) or *gabapentin* (Neurontin).

Levetiracetam's primary side effects are depression or anxiety...lamotrigine can cause a skin rash...and gabapentin is generally safe but has to be taken at high doses in order to be effective. In people who respond to one of these drugs, symptoms are usually eliminated within two months.

Latest development: The antiseizure drug *pregabalin* (Lyrica) was recently approved by the FDA for the treatment of partial onset seizures, the most common form of epilepsy in adults. Pregabalin now must be used in combination with other epilepsy medication, but it shows promise as a primary drug treatment. Its side effects include depression and anxiety.

Caution: The FDA has reported that the drugs mentioned above and other antiseizure drugs have been linked to increased risk for suicidal thoughts and behavior and advises that patients who take these medications should pay close attention to changes in mood.

THE SURGICAL OPTION

If medication does not relieve epilepsy symptoms, surgery is considered. The procedure, which involves removal of the part of the brain from which the seizure originates, effectively relieves epilepsy symptoms about 70% of the time. The surgery typically requires a hospital stay of three to five days, often fol-

*To find an epileptologist near you, contact the Epilepsy Foundation of America, 800-332-1000, Epilepsy.com.

lowed by a week or two of rehabilitation to help the patient regain strength and balance. Normal activities usually can be resumed within six weeks.

If surgery isn't possible—for example, the brain location where the seizure originates may be too close to an area vital for a basic function, such as speech or mobility—then vagus nerve stimulation may be recommended.

With this procedure, an electrical wire is wrapped around the vagus nerve (a large nerve that stretches from the side of the neck into the brain) and connected to a small lithium battery that is implanted under the skin, where it sends regular electrical impulses through the nerve.

For reasons that aren't completely clear, this form of stimulation disrupts epileptic episodes.

The downside: In about 50% of cases, this procedure reduces—but does not eliminate—the frequency of epileptic attacks.

WHAT IS EPILEPSY?

Epilepsy is caused by abnormal electrical activity in the brain. Symptoms vary widely, depending on a number of factors, including the area of the brain that is affected and a person's age. In older adults, epilepsy often is mistaken for some other condition, such as stroke or Alzheimer's disease.

A Medical Marijuana Milestone

Preliminary results of Phase 3 clinical trial of Epidiolex, sponsored by GW Pharmaceuticals, London, UK., *The New York Times,* CNN.

Medical marijuana is moving slowly but surely into the medical mainstream.

The latest news: Epidiolex, an experimental drug made by GW Pharmaceuticals from a purified marijuana extract, reduces seizures by 39% in children with a rare form of epilepsy, Dravet syndrome (severe myoclonic epilepsy of infancy), according to a prelimi-

nary report. If it's approved by the FDA, it would be the first marijuana-derived US-approved medicine.

The key ingredient—cannabidiol (CBD). Unlike its more famous cousin tetrahydrocannabinol (THC), it doesn't produce a high, but it has raised many hopes in the epilepsy community. The marijuana compound became famous a few years ago when CNN's Sanjay Gupta, MD, told the story of Charlotte Figi, a girl with Dravet syndrome whose seizures went from 300 a week to one after she started being treated with CBD-rich marijuana. Charlotte's Web, a CBD-rich hemp oil produced by a company in Colorado, is now sold for therapeutic purposes for epilepsy that doesn't respond to medications. Because it's so low in THC that it actually qualifies as hemp oil, it can be sold without a prescription and by mail.

For now, many patients prefer the whole-plant extract approach to the purified pharmaceutical. That may change, at least for some patients and doctors, as prescription drugs come onto the market.

But one thing is clear—the age of medical marijuana is evolving rapidly.

Brain Wave Therapy for Pain, Epilepsy and More

Celeste De Bease, PhD, medical psychologist and bioneurofeedback therapist, based in Bala Cynwyd, Pennsylvania.

People with epilepsy, Parkinson's disease, attention deficit disorder (ADD) or addictions may be able to learn how to "think themselves better" by altering their brain waves to improve their symptoms. A relatively new form of treatment called neurotherapy (also known as neurofeedback) is similar to biofeedback but has a unique focus on controlling brain wave activity rather than skin temperature, heart rate, breathing and muscle tension.

Neurotherapy is now used with a wide scope of health issues, including not only those listed above but also autism, chronic pain, posttraumatic stress disorder, depression and anxiety. *Medical psychologist and bioneurofeedback therapist Celeste De Bease, PhD, explains how...*

HIGH-TECH MIND-BODY MEDICINE

According to Dr. De Bease, many neurological problems involve disordered brain waves. Neurofeedback helps patients learn to set them right.

The brain produces brain waves at varying electrical frequencies measured in hertz (cycles per second). (Just to compare, the current used for household electricity is 60 Hz here in the US.) *Brain wave electrical frequencies include...*

• **Delta**—1 to 3 Hz and the slowest of all, is mostly seen during sleep.

• **Theta**—4 to 7 Hz, a state of deep relaxation that can bring bursts of creative insight. It occurs during daydreaming and advanced meditation.

• **Alpha**—8 to 13 Hz, a pleasurable, relaxed state associated with being calm and lucid. it occurs in some forms of meditation and sometimes with dream sleep.

• **Beta**—14 to 30 Hz, is the frequency produced during normal waking activities, when you are processing information for daily living, problem solving and the like.

• **High Beta**—any Beta over 21 Hz, these waves show that the brain is in its racing mode associated with anxiety and tension.

Many patients with neurological problems tend toward either under- or over-arousal of the brain. Neurofeedback teaches methods to gain control by using video display (like a video game) images that correspond to different brain waves. Working with the therapist, people can learn ways to produce faster or slower waves. Even children can do this.

MIND CONTROL?

Dr. De Bease explained that people with ADD or depression, or who suffer from mental fog and lethargic thinking in general, benefit from learning how to speed up their brain waves—those who need to slow them down to calm over-arousal include people with com-

pulsions, autism, posttraumatic stress disorder, chronic-pain disorders, epilepsy and insomnia. Parkinson's disease patients can benefit from slower brain waves that relax their nervous systems and contribute to better motor functioning.

Neurofeedback technology is continuing to evolve, Dr. De Bease said. Where there used to be just a few approaches, therapists now have many well-researched training protocols to work with, and their techniques become more customized as the science and training are refined. For instance, placement of electrodes varies depending on the issue being addressed—for people with ADD, Dr. De Bease said that she places electrodes on the scalp directly above the frontal cortex, which controls the function of paying attention.

PRACTICAL ADVICE

The goal of neurotherapy is to recognize how it feels to operate in the desired brain wave activity range and to then learn how to get there at will. Effective training typically takes 10 or more sessions, depending on the problem. Prices vary by area and may range from $50 to more than $100/session. Some health insurance plans cover neurofeedback for some conditions, but usually only after you get a diagnosis and prescription from your doctor.

Dr. De Bease calls neurotherapy "a powerful technique," but cautions that it is crucial to find a Biofeedback Certified Professional (BCP) who is well-trained specifically in this technique, especially in light of the fact that many who call themselves qualified have completed just a weekend training program. Look for a practitioner who is certified by the Biofeedback Certification International Alliance (BCIA.org). This means that, among other credentials, the practitioner has had 25 hours of practice mentored by a BCIA-approved practitioner and 100 patient/client sessions reviewed and approved by BCIA.

Neurofeedback can benefit healthy people, too. Dr. De Bease said she works primarily with medical conditions but knows many therapists who focus on performance enhancement, which includes training athletes, business professionals and even members of the military in the use of neurofeedback. Certainly this is a therapy worth looking into—it's noninvasive and drug-free, not terribly expensive, and may help with many conditions.

Epilepsy Breakthroughs...

A Brain Pacemaker for Epilepsy

Patients with epilepsy who don't respond to drugs may improve with a "brain pacemaker," an implanted or noninvasive belt-worn device that delivers electrical signals to the trigeminal nerve in the head. More than half of the patients in a small study who used the device had a 50% or more reduction in seizures. The system is also being developed for depression, ADHD, PTSD and traumatic brain injury.

Ivanhoe.com, Neurosigma.com

Head Off Epilepsy

The main ingredient in many dandruff shampoos, zinc pyrithione, calms overstimulated nerve cells in the head, making it a possible treatment for seizures. More research is needed.

John Hopkins Medical Institutions.

Tree Treatment for Epilepsy?

The sticky resins from conifer trees (such as pines, junipers and firs) contain substances that may reduce the electrical excitability of nerve cells and could lead to new epilepsy treatments.

Scientific Reports.

3-D TV Health Danger

3-D TV poses health risks. The makers of 3-D televisions, such as Samsung, have warned that people with certain serious medical conditions, such as epilepsy or a family history of stroke, as well as people who are tired or under the influence of alcohol should not watch 3-D television or movies. 3-D can trigger an epileptic seizure or stroke and can lead to headaches, migraines and nausea.

Melvin Schrier, OD, retired optometrist and vision consultant, Rancho Palos Verdes, California.

Epilepsy Linked to Migraines

People who have three or more close relatives with the seizure disorder had more than twice the risk for migraine headaches with aura—headaches with additional symptoms such as nausea and/or sensitivity to sound or light. The genetic link may explain why antiseizure drugs help prevent migraines or lessen their severity in people prone to migraines.

Melodie R. Winawer, MD, associate professor of neurology, Columbia University, New York City, and leader of a study of 730 epilepsy patients, published in *Epilepsia*.

Uncontrollable Emotional Outbursts...

Marc E. Agronin, MD, vice president, behavioral health and clinical research, Miami Jewish Health Systems and author of *How We Age*. MarcAgronin.com

Uncontrollable laughter or crying can sometimes be due to a disorder known as pseudobulbar affect (PBA). It is typically associated with neurological conditions such as stroke, multiple sclerosis (MS), Alzheimer's disease, Parkinson's disease, traumatic brain injury, brain tumors and amyotrophic lateral sclerosis (ALS). These conditions can affect the frontal lobe of the brain that keeps emotions under control. People with PBA may have dozens of episodes of uncontrollable laughter or crying during the day, which can be extremely distressing and embarrassing.

These sudden bouts of emotion are sometimes not connected to surrounding events or the person's true feelings and can be completely inappropriate, such as laughing during a funeral. Emotions can also quickly switch, for example, from laughter to sobbing.

A medication called Nuedexta (*dextromethorphan* and *quinidine*) has been FDA-approved for the treatment of PBA. Side effects can include changes in heart rhythm, so it may not be appropriate for people with certain types of heart disease.

Uncontrollable emotional outbursts can also reflect an underlying psychiatric condition, such as bipolar disorder, especially if they are associated with symptoms of severe depression, mania or psychosis.

Anyone who displays erratic bouts of emotion should be evaluated by a neurologist to determine the underlying cause of the episodes.

ALS Breakthrough... Thanks to the Ice Bucket

Paper titled "New gene variants present in three percent of all ALS patients: Largest-ever study of inherited ALS identifies new ALS gene, NEK1" by researchers at University of Massachusetts Medical School et al. published in *Nature Genetics*.

Remember the Ice Bucket Challenge in the summer of 2014?

Every time you turned around, social media was showing someone dumping a bucket of icy water over his or her head—or coming up with a quirky way to "take the challenge"—in order to raise funds to find a cure for amyotrophic lateral sclerosis (ALS), aka Lou Gehrig's disease.

Now it may bring us closer to a cure.

Ice Bucket donations paid for the largest-ever study of ALS, a progressive neurodegenerative disease that affects the brain and spinal cord and frequently leads to paralysis and death as quickly as two years from diagnosis. It often runs in families.

Result: A breakthrough discovery of a new gene called NEK1, which is involved in many neuron functions. Some variants of the gene

are prone to loss of function. The researchers found a significant association between this genetic abnormality and increased risk for familial ALS. While only a small percentage of people with ALS have the familial kind, the researchers believe that NEK1 may also be involved in nonfamilial ALS.

While there isn't a cure—yet—understanding more about NEK1 is an important step toward developing treatment for this devastating disease.

All that ice, dumped on all those shivering heads and shoulders, made it possible.

Pseudo-Seizure

At a major US hospital, more than one-third of patients in an epilepsy unit were recently found to have psychogenic nonepileptic seizures. These occur in patients with normal brain activity, but who lack effective coping mechanisms for stress.

Johns Hopkins Medicine.

Hope for ALS

The only FDA-approved drug for treating amyotrophic lateral sclerosis (ALS) isn't very effective.

What's new: In animal research, the heart drug *digoxin* stopped the destruction of nerve cells that can lead to paralysis and death. More research is needed.

Nature Neuroscience.

Vegetables Can Prevent Lou Gehrig's Disease

In a recent finding, people who ate foods with the most carotenoids were 25% less likely to develop the muscle-paralyzing disease amyotrophic lateral sclerosis (ALS) than people who ate the least. The most beneficial carotenoids were beta-carotene, found in carrots, squash and sweet potatoes...and lutein, in dark green vegetables, such as kale and spinach. Aim for nine servings daily.

Kathryn C. Fitzgerald, a doctoral student in the department of nutrition, Harvard School of Public Health, Boston, and leader of a study published online in *Annals of Neurology.*

Natural Comforts for ALS

Thomas Kruzel, ND, naturopathic physician, Rockwood Natural Medicine Clinic, Scottsdale, Arizona.

A re there any self-care strategies that might help alleviate the symptoms of amyotrophic lateral sclerosis (ALS)?

ALS, also known as Lou Gehrig's disease, is a rare neurodegenerative disorder that affects nerve cells in the brain and spinal cord. It's a progressive disease and results in total paralysis. But, no two ALS patients will progress at the same rate.

Patients with ALS should take a daily multivitamin and mineral supplement without iron that includes B-complex, C, D and E vitamins...and calcium and magnesium to help strengthen the immune system as well as muscle and nerve function.

The progression of muscle weakness, cramping and spasms can be eased with the homeopathic remedies Magnesium phosphoricum, Cuprum metallicum, Plumbum metallicum or nux vomica (follow label instructions for dosage). Alternating hot and cold compresses to areas with muscle cramps will help increase blood flow and reduce pain. Acupuncture can also help relieve symptoms.

CHAPTER 7

Stroke Risks, Prevention and Recovery

Stroke: You Can Do Much More to Protect Yourself

No one likes to think about having a stroke. But maybe you should.

The grim reality: Stroke strikes nearly 795,000 Americans each year and is the leading cause of disability.

Now for the remarkable part: About 80% of strokes can be prevented. You may think that you've heard it all when it comes to preventing strokes—it's about controlling your blood pressure, eating a good diet and getting some exercise, right? Actually, that's only part of what you can be doing to protect yourself. *Surprising recent findings on stroke—and the latest advice on how to avoid it...*

•**Even "low" high blood pressure is a red flag.** High blood pressure—a reading of 140/90 mmHg or higher—is widely known to increase one's odds of having a stroke. But even slight elevations in blood pressure may also be a problem.

An important recent study that looked at data from more than half a million patients found that those with blood pressure readings that were just slightly higher than a normal reading of 120/80 mmHg were more likely to have a stroke.

Any increase in blood pressure is worrisome. In fact, the risk for a stroke or heart attack doubles for each 20-point rise in systolic (the top number) pressure above 115/75 mmHg—and for each 10-point rise in diastolic (the bottom number) pressure.

My advice: Don't wait for your doctor to recommend treatment if your blood pressure is even a few points higher than normal. Tell him/her that you are concerned. Lifestyle changes—such as getting adequate exercise, avoid-

Ralph L. Sacco, MD, chairman of neurology, the Olemberg Family Chair in Neurological Disorders and the Miller Professor of Neurology, Epidemiology and Public Health, Human Genetics and Neurosurgery at the Miller School of Medicine at the University of Miami.

197

ing excess alcohol and maintaining a healthful diet—often reverse slightly elevated blood pressure. Blood pressure consistently above 140/90 mmHg generally requires medication.

•**Sleep can be dangerous.** People who are sleep deprived—generally defined as getting less than six hours of sleep per night—are at increased risk for stroke.

What most people don't realize is that getting too much sleep is also a problem. When researchers at the University of Cambridge tracked the sleep habits of nearly 10,000 people over a 10-year period, they found that those who slept more than eight hours a night were 46% more likely to have a stroke than those who slept six to eight hours.

It is possible that people who spend less/more time sleeping have other, unrecognized conditions that affect both sleep and stroke risk.

Example: Sleep apnea, a breathing disorder that interferes with sleep, causes an increase in blood pressure that can lead to stroke. Meanwhile, sleeping too much can be a symptom of depression—another stroke risk factor.

My advice: See a doctor if you tend to wake up unrefreshed…are a loud snorer…or often snort or thrash while you sleep. You may have sleep apnea. If you sleep too much, also talk to your doctor to see if you are suffering from depression or some other condition that may increase your stroke risk.

What's the sweet spot for nightly shut-eye? When it comes to stroke risk, it's six to eight hours per night.

•**What you drink matters, too.** A Mediterranean-style diet—plenty of whole grains, legumes, nuts, fish, produce and olive oil—is perhaps the best diet going when it comes to minimizing stroke risk. A recent study concluded that about 30% of strokes could be prevented if people simply switched to this diet.

But there's more you can do. Research has found that people who drank six cups of green or black tea a day were 42% less likely to have strokes than people who did not drink tea. With three daily cups, risk dropped by 21%.

The antioxidant epigallocatechin gallate or the amino acid L-theanine may be responsible.

•**Emotional stress shouldn't be pooh-poohed.** If you're prone to angry outbursts, don't assume it's no big deal. Emotional stress triggers the release of cortisol, adrenaline and other so-called stress hormones that can increase blood pressure and heart rate, leading to stroke.

In one study, about 30% of stroke patients had heightened negative emotions (such as anger) in the two hours preceding the stroke.

My advice: Don't ignore your mental health—especially anger (it's often a sign of depression, a potent stroke risk factor). If you're suffering from "negative" emotions, exercise regularly, try relaxation strategies (such as meditation) and don't hesitate to get professional help.

•**Be alert for subtle signs of stroke.** The acronym "FAST" helps people identify signs of stroke. "F" stands for facial drooping—does one side of the face droop or is it numb? Is the person's smile uneven? "A" stands for arm weakness—ask the person to raise both arms. Does one arm drift downward? "S" stands for speech difficulty—is speech slurred? Is the person unable to speak or hard to understand? Can he/she repeat a simple sentence such as, "The sky is blue" correctly? "T" stands for time—if a person shows any of these symptoms (even if they go away), call 911 immediately. Note the time so that you know when symptoms first appeared.

But stroke can also cause one symptom that isn't widely known—a loss of touch sensation. This can occur if a stroke causes injury to the parts of the brain that detect touch. If you suddenly can't "feel" your fingers or toes—or have trouble with simple tasks such as buttoning a shirt—you could be having a stroke. You might notice that you can't feel temperatures or that you can't feel it when your feet touch the floor.

It's never normal to lose your sense of touch for an unknown reason—or to have unexpected difficulty seeing, hearing and/or speaking. Get to an emergency room!

Also important: If you think you're having a stroke, don't waste time calling your regular doctor. Call an ambulance, and ask to be taken to the nearest hospital with a primary stroke center. You'll get much better care than you would at a regular hospital emergency room.

A meta-analysis found that there were 21% fewer deaths among patients treated at stroke centers, and the surviving patients had faster recoveries and fewer stroke-related complications.

My advice: If you have any stroke risk factors, including high blood pressure, diabetes or elevated cholesterol, find out now which hospitals in your area have stroke centers. To find one near you, go to Hospitalmaps.heart.org.

Could a Jolt to the Neck Cause a Stroke?

Rebecca Gottesman, MD, associate professor of neurology and epidemiology at The Johns Hopkins University School of Medicine and director of clinical research at Johns Hopkins Bayview Neurology, both in Baltimore.

Most strokes occur due to years of high blood pressure…or when the gradual buildup of fatty substances (plaque) in the arteries cuts off blood flow to the brain.

An unusual and little-recognized trigger: Some people get strokes from simply moving the neck in an extreme way or holding it in an odd position. This sort of neck movement might occur during a car accident, for example—but it might also be caused by normal activities such as riding a roller coaster, craning your neck to paint a ceiling or leaning back to have your hair shampooed at a hair salon (the so-called "beauty parlor syndrome").

The culprit in such strokes is a vertebral artery dissection (VAD), a tear in the innermost or middle layer of the three-layered vertebral artery wall, which can disrupt blood flow to the brain. Sometimes, the damage is minor and the artery repairs itself without difficulty. In other cases, however, the arterial injury leads to a stroke.

Recent development: The American Heart Association (AHA) issued a warning that neck manipulation (used, for example, during certain chiropractic or physical therapy treatments) has been linked to stroke due to such arterial injuries. While no direct cause-and-effect relationship has been found, the AHA now advises health-care practitioners to inform their patients of the association before performing neck manipulation.

WHEN AN ARTERY SHREDS

The right and left vertebral arteries run up the back of the neck and into the skull, carrying blood to the brain. A stroke-inducing arterial tear can result from virtually any sudden and/or extreme movement that turns or stretches the neck excessively. But in many cases, people with VAD can recall nothing more unusual than a sneeze or vigorous sexual activity in the preceding days, and sometimes there is nothing to blame it on.

Why the cause can be elusive: Some people are apparently more vulnerable to VAD than others. It is more common in those with known connective tissue disorders such as Marfan's syndrome or fibromuscular dysplasia. Also, some studies have found that artery walls in people who have suffered dissections look subtly abnormal under the microscope, suggesting a congenital abnormality.

But practically speaking, there is no way to predict who will get a VAD or what will cause it. There are warning signs, though. And if you've already suffered a VAD, there are steps you can take to help prevent another one.

RED FLAGS FOR VAD

Each year, approximately 4,500 Americans suffer VAD. The condition is a leading cause of stroke in adults under age 45. VAD also can occur, though less commonly, in older adults. Of course, the best course is to spot a VAD early—before it can cause a stroke.

Recent finding: An analysis of 75 studies involving nearly 2,000 people diagnosed with VAD found that dizziness or vertigo was the most common symptom, reported by 58% of sufferers, with headache (51%) and neck pain (46%) close behind.

The trouble is that dizziness, headache and neck pain are extremely common and can be caused by many different conditions. And you can't run to the doctor to check out every headache or dizzy spell.

When to be concerned: If you have a headache that is more severe than usual...suffer extreme dizziness...have neck pain that is unusual for you...or if any of these symptoms occur at the same time or last longer than a day. Call or visit your doctor without delay.

When to be very concerned: If you develop symptoms such as double vision, difficulty walking, speaking or swallowing, and/or weakness on one side of your face or body, particularly if they occur with dizziness, neck pain or headache. These could be signs that a stroke or transient ischemic attack (TIA), a temporary blockage of brain circulation, is occurring.

A sudden and severe "thunderclap" headache (the kind that people describe as "the worst headache of my life") may indicate that a brain hemorrhage is imminent or has happened.

Prompt emergency care in these situations could mean the difference between complete recovery and disability or death.

PREVENTING AN ARTERIAL TEAR

If you have ever had an episode of VAD, you are at increased risk for another. This doesn't mean that you should stop all exercise or keep your neck in a brace, but you may want to pass on activities that could easily lead to a neck injury, such as mountain biking and skydiving.

Also, if you've had a VAD, avoid any situations where your neck is stretched out for prolonged periods—for example, try to avoid hyperextending your neck at an extreme angle backward while getting your hair shampooed or styled. Don't give up yoga, but skip postures that stress your neck. If you receive chiropractic care, it's safest for manipulations to be performed below neck level.

DIAGNOSING AND TREATING AN ARTERIAL TEAR

If your doctor suspects that you've suffered a vertebral artery dissection (VAD), he/she will probably order a CT scan or MRI. Treatment for a VAD usually includes a drug to keep clots from forming, most commonly *warfarin* (Coumadin). If you have a VAD, it's common to take the drug for three to six months. If symptoms persist, your doctor may recommend that a stent or coil be surgically placed in the damaged artery.

Precautions: While VAD is less likely to cause a stroke once you begin taking an anticoagulant, anticlotting drugs themselves carry the risk of bleeding. Your doctor should advise you what activities to avoid during this time— this usually includes anything that could cause head injury. Patients on oral anticoagulants also should have their blood levels checked regularly and need to maintain a regular diet in order to keep their blood thin enough while they are taking this medication.

Better Stroke Prevention

In a study of 451 patients at high risk for stroke, those who took medication to lower cholesterol, blood pressure and clotting were 9% less likely to have a stroke within three years than those who took the same drugs and had stent surgery in the brain to open narrowed arteries.

Possible reason: Complications from surgery in small brain arteries can lead to stroke.

Colin Derdeyn, MD, director, Stroke and Cerebrovascular Center, Washington University School of Medicine, St. Louis, Missouri.

Uncommon Stroke Risks You Need to Know

Louis R. Caplan, MD, senior neurologist at Beth Israel Deaconess Medical Center and a professor of neurology at Harvard Medical School, both in Boston. He has written or edited more than 40 books, including *Stroke (What Do I Do Now?)* and *Navigating the Complexities of Stroke.*

Steven R. Messé, MD, assistant professor of neurology and director of the vascular neurology fellowship at the Hospital of the University of Pennsylvania in Philadelphia. Board-certified in neurology and vascular neurology, he has published scientific papers in *Stroke, Neurology* and the *Journal of Neurology, Neurosurgery and Psychiatry.*

What if there were more to preventing a stroke than keeping your blood pressure under control...getting regular exercise…watching your body weight…and not smoking? Researchers are now discovering that there is.

New thinking: While most stroke sufferers say that "it just came out of the blue," an increasing body of evidence shows that these potentially devastating "brain attacks" can be caused by conditions that you might ordinarily think are completely unrelated.

Once you're aware of these "hidden" risk factors—and take the necessary steps to prevent or control them—you can improve your odds of never having a stroke. *Recently discovered stroke risk factors…*

INFLAMMATORY BOWEL DISEASE

Both Crohn's disease and ulcerative colitis can severely damage the large or small intestine. But that is not the only risk. Among patients who have either one of these conditions, known as inflammatory bowel disease (IBD), stroke is the third most common cause of death, according to some estimates.

During flare-ups, patients with IBD have elevated blood levels of substances that trigger clots—the cause of most strokes. A Harvard study, for example, found that many IBD patients have high levels of C-reactive protein (CRP), an inflammatory marker that has been linked to atherosclerotic lesions, damaged areas in blood vessels that can lead to stroke-causing clots in the brain.

If you have IBD: Ask your doctor what you can do to reduce your risk for blood clots and inflammation. Some patients with IBD can't take aspirin or other anticlotting drugs because these medications frequently cause intestinal bleeding. Instead of aspirin, you might be advised to take an autoimmune medication such as *azathioprine* (Azasan, Imuran), which suppresses the immune system and reduces inflammation. During flare-ups, some patients are given steroids to further reduce inflammation.

Side effects, including nausea and vomiting with azathioprine use and weight gain and increased blood pressure with steroid use, usually can be minimized by taking the lowest possible dose.

Some physicians recommend omega-3 fish oil supplements for IBD, which are less likely to cause side effects. Ask your doctor whether these supplements (and what dose) are right for you.

Important: Strokes tend to occur in IBD patients when inflammation is most severe. To check inflammatory markers, CRP levels and erythrocyte sedimentation rate (ESR) can be measured. Tests for clotting include fibrinogen and d-dimer. The results of these tests will help determine the course of the patient's IBD treatment.

MIGRAINES

Migraine headaches accompanied by auras (characterized by the appearance of flashing lights or other visual disturbances) are actually a greater risk factor for stroke than obesity, smoking or diabetes (see below), according to a startling study presented at the American Academy of Neurology's annual meeting in 2013.

When researchers use MRIs to examine blood vessels in the brain, they find more tiny areas of arterial damage in patients who have migraines with auras than in those who don't get migraines. (Research shows that there is no link between stroke and migraines that aren't accompanied by auras.)

If you have migraines with auras: Reduce your risk by controlling other stroke risk factors—don't smoke…lose weight if you're overweight…and control cholesterol levels.

Also: Women under age 50 who have migraines (with or without auras) may be advised to not use combined-hormone forms of birth control pills—they slightly increase risk for stroke. In addition, patients who have migraines with auras should not take beta-blockers, such as *propranolol* (Inderal), or the triptan drugs, such as *sumatriptan* (Imitrex), commonly used for migraine headaches. These drugs can also increase stroke risk. For frequent migraines with auras, I often prescribe the blood pressure drug *verapamil* (Calan) and a daily 325-mg aspirin. Ask your doctor for advice.

RHEUMATOID ARTHRITIS

Rheumatoid arthritis, unlike the common "wear-and-tear" variety (osteoarthritis), is an autoimmune disease that not only causes inflammation in the joints but may also trigger it in the heart, blood vessels and other parts of the body.

Arterial inflammation increases the risk for blood clots, heart attack and stroke. In fact, patients with severe rheumatoid arthritis were almost twice as likely to have a stroke as those without the disease, according to a study published in *Arthritis Care & Research*.

If you have rheumatoid arthritis: Work with your rheumatologist to manage flare-ups and reduce systemic inflammation. Your doctor will probably recommend that you take one or more anti-inflammatory painkillers, such as *ibuprofen* (Motrin). In addition, he/she might prescribe a disease-modifying antirheumatic drug (DMARD), such as *methotrexate* (Trexall), to slow the progression of the disease—and the increased risk for stroke. Fish oil also may be prescribed to reduce joint tenderness.

Strokes tend to occur in rheumatoid arthritis patients when inflammation is peaking. Ask your doctor if you should have the inflammation tests (CRP and ESR) mentioned in the IBD section.

DIABETES

If you have diabetes or diabetes risk factors—such as obesity, a sedentary lifestyle or a family history of diabetes—protect yourself. People with diabetes are up to four times more likely to have a stroke than those without it.

High blood sugar in people with diabetes damages blood vessels throughout the body, including in the brain. The damage can lead to both ischemic (clot-related) and hemorrhagic (bleeding) strokes.

If you have diabetes: Work closely with your doctor. Patients who achieve good glucose control with oral medications and/or insulin are much less likely to suffer from vascular damage.

Also important: Lose weight if you need to. Weight loss combined with exercise helps your body metabolize blood sugar more ef-

ficiently. In those with mild diabetes, weight loss combined with exercise may restore normal blood sugar levels...and can reduce complications and the need for medications in those with more serious diabetes.

CLOTTING DISORDERS

Any condition that affects the blood's normal clotting functions can increase risk for stroke.

Examples: Thrombocytosis (excessive platelets in the blood)...an elevated hematocrit (higher-than-normal percentage of red blood cells)...or Factor V Leiden (an inherited tendency to form blood clots). Clotting tests (fibrinogen and d-dimer) are recommended for these disorders.

If you have a clotting disorder: Ask your doctor what you can do to protect yourself from stroke.

Example: If you have an elevated hematocrit, your doctor might advise you to drink more fluids.

This is particularly important for older adults, who tend to drink less later in the day because they don't want to get up at night to urinate. I recommend that these patients drink approximately 80 ounces of noncaffeine-containing fluids during the day, stopping by 7 pm. People who don't take in enough fluids can develop "thick" blood that impedes circulation—and increases the risk for clots.

CHIROPRACTIC ADJUSTMENT

Because chiropractic adjustments to the neck often involve physical manipulation of the cervical spine (neck region), neurologists and chiropractors have long debated whether such movements can lead to a rare form of ischemic stroke known as vertebrobasilar artery (VBA) stroke, which can be triggered by a tear in the vertebral arteries that run along the neck bones.

Latest research: A study of 818 people found that those under age 45 who had suffered VBA strokes and were hospitalized for that type of stroke were three times more likely to have seen a chiropractor or a primary care physician before the hospitalization than people without VBA strokes. In people over age 45, VBA stroke was associated with visits to primary care practitioners.

The researchers speculated that the visits to both practitioners occurred when people had symptoms of a VBA tear, such as neck pain or stiffness, but had not yet had a VBA stroke.

Self-defense: It is unlikely that a chiropractic adjustment of the neck will greatly increase your risk for a stroke. But since all medical treatments have some risks, you'll need to decide whether the benefits of a chiropractic manipulation of the neck outweigh the likely small risk for stroke.

Warning: You can cause a VBA tear by bending your head backward over a sink while having your hair washed at a hair salon. If you've had a previous stroke or TIA, do not put your head in this position. If you have no history of stroke, make sure your neck is resting comfortably and securely on a towel and not on the sink itself.

Fight Killer Blood Clots— Reduce Your Risk with These Nondrug Approaches

Decker Weiss, NMD, a naturopathic medical doctor who specializes in integrative cardiology. He is founder and owner of Weiss Natural Medicine, in Scottsdale, Arizona, DrDeckerWeiss.com, and author of *The Weiss Method: A Natural Program for Reversing Heart Disease and Preventing Heart Attacks.*

Millions of Americans take anticlotting medications, or "blood thinners," including aspirin and *warfarin* (Coumadin), to prevent clots and reduce the risk for such conditions as heart attack and stroke.

These drugs are extremely effective. Daily aspirin, for example, can reduce the risk for a first heart attack by 44%, according to data from the Physicians' Health Study.

The downside: Even at low doses, every anticlotting agent can cause bleeding—often from the stomach, gums or intestines—as a side effect. Sometimes, gastrointestinal bleed-

ing can occur even without causing noticeable symptoms.

In addition, warfarin, one of the leading blood thinners, doubles the risk for intracerebral hemorrhage (bleeding in the brain).

NATURAL BLOOD THINNERS

The good news is that certain herbs and other supplements can be used for their anti-clotting properties—and may have a reduced risk for side effects, such as bleeding.

This approach is not intended to replace medications—patients with a high risk for clotting need to take such drugs. Under a doctor's supervision, these supplements can be combined with blood-thinning medications to boost the drugs' effectiveness and potentially allow you to take a lower dose, thus reducing the risk for bleeding.

Those with only a slight risk for clots (due to family history, for example) may want to consider using natural anticoagulants alone, under a doctor's supervision, to promote better circulation.

Bonus: Natural blood thinners usually have anti-inflammatory properties. This is important because most chronic diseases, including heart disease, rheumatoid arthritis and stroke, are caused in part by inflammation.

The supplements below can be taken alone or in combination, depending on the degree of protection that's required.

Some of these supplements may interact with prescription medications, so consult a doctor who is knowledgeable about supplement use.* *Best choices…*

• **Fish oil.** Studies of large populations show that people who eat a lot of cold-water fish, such as salmon and mackerel, tend to have lower heart attack death rates than people who don't eat fish.

The omega-3 fatty acids in cold-water fish are strong anticlotting agents. Fish oil is thought to inhibit platelet aggregation (clumping), part of the clotting process. One report, published in *The Annals of Pharmacotherapy,*

---

*To find a doctor who has experience treating patients with supplements, consult the American Association of Naturopathic Physicians, 866-538-2267, Naturopathic.org.

found that taking fish oil along with warfarin caused an increase in anticlotting activity.

Typical dose: Depending on other risk factors, such as elevated cholesterol and high blood pressure, one tablet twice daily of Vectomega's Whole Food Omega-3 DHA/EPA Complex—it provides 292 mg of omega-3s (DHA and EPA balanced) in a phospholipid peptide complex, in which the fish oil is bound to peptides to increase absorbability. Or one teaspoon twice daily of Nordic Naturals' Ultimate Omega Liquid, which provides 1,626 mg of EPA and 1,126 mg of DHA.

• **Ginger and curcumin.** Ginger reduces levels of fibrinogen, a precursor to fibrin, a protein that is a major component of blood clots. Curcumin has only modest effects on coagulation but is a stronger anti-inflammatory agent. That's why I advise patients to take these herbs together. Studies have shown that both ginger and curcumin can reduce inflammation in the body. An Australian study found that substances in ginger inhibited the activity of arachidonic acid, part of the chemical sequence involved in clotting. In the study, ginger compounds were more effective than aspirin at blocking platelet activity.

Typical dose: Twice daily, 50 mg to 100 mg of ginger and one or two 375-mg capsules of curcumin.

Good products: Gaia Herbs' Ginger Supreme Phyto-Caps and EuroPharma's CuraMed curcumin complex.

• **Nattokinase.** Extracted from soybeans, nattokinase is an enzyme that helps prevent clot formation—it also makes platelets less likely to clump together. Unlike warfarin, which only prevents clots, nattokinase appears to break down clots that already have formed.

Typical dose: Depending on other risk factors, one to two capsules or tablets (2,000 fibrin units per 100 mg) twice daily.

Important: I recommend taking nattokinase between meals. The anticlotting properties are strongest when it is taken without food.

• **Vinpocetine.** This supplement is extracted from periwinkle. It's extremely important to take vinpocetine under a doctor's supervision. Vinpocetine is the most potent natural substance for preventing clots—and, like prescription anticlotting agents, it can cause internal bleeding in some patients. For this reason, I recommend it mainly for high-risk patients who are unable to take warfarin because of side effects and/or complications.

Typical dose: 2 mg total—in divided doses twice daily. Higher doses (5 mg total in divided doses) might be needed, but don't increase from the starting dose without talking with your doctor. Should be taken without food.

• **Ginkgo.** The extract from the dried leaves of the ginkgo biloba tree has traditionally been used to treat intermittent claudication, leg pain caused by insufficient blood flow, as well as cognitive impairments (such as memory problems) due to poor blood circulation in the brain.

Ginkgo is effective at reducing clots and also acts as a vasodilator that helps improve blood flow to the brain, heart and other parts of the body. I don't recommend it as often as other anticoagulants because it has little effect on inflammation. If you use ginkgo, ask your doctor about combining it with curcumin or other anti-inflammatory herbs/supplements.

Typical dose: About 40 mg, three times daily.

• **Garlic.** Studies have shown that patients who take garlic supplements have a lower risk for clots. Use only those products that list a high allicin content—the main active ingredient in garlic. This can be found frequently in fresh garlic supplements.

Typical dose: The optimal dose for garlic hasn't been definitively established. However, some studies indicate that you need at least 180 mg of allicin twice daily.

Good brand: Allimax.

Important: In general, natural therapies should be started at low doses that are slowly increased, under a doctor's supervision, over time. I recommend that the supplements described in this article be used at least twice daily to ensure that adequate levels of the therapeutic compounds are maintained in the body.

Is It a Migraine, Low Blood Sugar, a Seizure... or a Stroke?

Edward Jauch, MD, professor and director, division of emergency medicine, professor department of neurosciences, comprehensive stroke program, and director, acute stroke trials, Medical University of South Carolina, Charleston.

They're called stroke mimics. The symptoms are similar to a stroke—slurred speech, a weakness on one side of your body and confusion—but what you're experiencing is actually low blood sugar, a migraine or another condition. If you know you have diabetes, suffer from migraines, have a seizure disorder or other conditions, you may be tempted to ignore possible stroke symptoms.

That's a big mistake.

Reason: When you're having a stroke, minutes—even seconds—count. Getting emergency treatment with blood clot–dissolving medications—typically tissue plasminogen activator (tPA)—or other therapies can mean the difference between life and death and can dramatically affect recovery. Edward Jauch, MD, director of the division of emergency medicine at the Medical University of South Carolina, explained more about stroke mimics...

MIMIC #1: **Low Blood Sugar (Hypoglycemia).**

When blood sugar dips too low, a common problem for people who take medication for diabetes, the symptoms mimic a stroke—confusion, feeling dizzy or light-headed, slurred speech and/or muscle weakness.

Clues that it may be hypoglycemia, not stroke: Symptoms may build up slowly, rather than occur suddenly, as they do with a stroke. If you do a finger prick and discover your blood sugar is low, and if symptoms resolve after eating a glucose tablet or drinking a half cup of fruit juice, it's likely not a stroke.

But if you have any doubts, call 911. Be sure to tell the EMS professionals that the patient is a diabetic so they can rule out hypoglycemia with a finger-prick test—and maybe save a trip to the ER. It's actually standard practice to test everyone's glucose right away, whether or not they have diabetes, but it's not always followed, says Dr. Jauch.

MIMIC #2: **Hemiplegic Migraine.**

You may remember when the newscaster Serene Branson frighteningly lost her speech during a live broadcast, and everyone thought she had had a stroke. Well, it turned out to be a hemiplegic migraine. This type of migraine can cause loss of speech, weakness and other strokelike symptoms.

Clues that it may be a migraine, not a stroke...

• **You know you get migraines,** the pain is familiar, and an aura precedes the symptoms.

• **The headache comes on gradually,** over several minutes or longer, intensifies to a peak and tends to be throbbing or a dull ache.

• **You have known triggers such as stress,** caffeine, foods, weather changes, etc.

• **You have visual disturbances** such as seeing flashing lights or wavy lines.

Signs that it may be a stroke, not a migraine...

• **You're older than 50, and you've never had a migraine.** Migraines don't tend to develop after age 50.

• **The headache comes on suddenly and is the worst headache of your life.**

• **You have visual disturbances that involve loss of part of your visual field**—you may bump into things because you don't see them, for example.

As always, when in doubt, call 911. It's particularly important for people who get migraines frequently to pay attention to possible stroke symptoms. "There's a small increased risk for stroke in people who have migraines, but we are still researching if treatment of a migraine reduces stroke risk," says Dr. Jauch.

MIMIC #3: **A Seizure.**

Some seizures leave people with neurological symptoms such as difficulty speaking or a weakness in one or more limbs often on one side of the body, known as Todd's paralysis. "When you have a seizure, your brain turns off, just like when you shut down a computer," Dr. Jauch explains. "When you turn the computer back on, it takes a while to boot up. Your brain, too, may take some time to get back to normal."

Clues that it may be a seizure…

•**The patient has a history of seizures,** a bite mark on the side of the tongue—or confusion that gradually improves.

•**Typically symptoms subside with time**…from a few minutes to a few hours.

Clues that it may be a stroke: If there is confusion, it is persistent and doesn't improve.

If you're concerned that it's a stroke, time isn't on your side. EMS guidelines state that the ER team should consider stroke if someone has a seizure and has symptoms of neurological deficits, such as weakness, numbness or language issues, particularly if the patient doesn't have a history of seizures. Sometimes, seizures are symptoms of a stroke.

MIMIC #4: **Bell's Palsy.**

Bell's palsy causes facial drooping, but it's not because of a stroke. It's typically caused by a viral infection such as shingles or the flu or Lyme disease that leads to an inflammation or infection in the facial nerve (called the seventh cranial nerve). It can also cause your eyelid to droop, drooling, dryness of the eye or mouth or excessive tearing in one eye. Though this is easy for the pros to diagnose, patients often confuse it with a stroke.

Clues that it may be Bell's palsy…

•**It typically causes significant facial distortion including the forehead.** Facial symptoms are your only symptoms.

Clues that it may be a stroke…

•**You're older than 60, when Bell's palsy becomes less common.**

•**You have other stroke symptoms, not just facial droop.**

Not sure? You know what to do—call 911.

MIMIC #5: **A Brain Tumor.**

Brain tumors can also cause symptoms that mimic stroke, such as headache, confusion, nausea, weakness and disturbance in the way you walk.

Clues that it's a brain tumor rather than a stroke: Symptoms are headaches that are worse in the morning, when coughing, exercising or changing position.

Both are serious ailments, of course, so these symptoms, whatever the cause, require immediate attention. For any of these unexplained symptoms, you would likely be given a CT scan, which would pick up the tumor versus signs of a stroke.

WHAT HAPPENS IF I THINK IT'S A STROKE AND IT'S NOT?

Stroke mimics confuse even health-care professionals. In one study, about 20% of the time when neurologists thought patients were having a stroke, the cause was a different condition. The result can be getting a CT scan and treatment when it's not needed, with all the anxiety that entails. But the risk for harm is much lower than having a stroke and not getting it promptly treated.

Here's what you can do: Help health-care professionals by giving them the right information. Let them know if the symptoms came on suddenly (common in strokes) or more gradually (uncommon), and let them know when the symptoms began or when the person was last known to be normal. If the patient has diabetes or is subject to frequent migraines or has a seizure disorder, tell the EMS professionals right away. Also let them know if the person takes any form of regular medications. It'll help them sort things out quicker.

HOW TO SPEED UP STROKE TREATMENT

Everyone should know the classic signs of a stroke, made easy to remember with the acronym, FAST…

Face drooping. One side of the face may droop or become numb. Ask the person to smile, and check to see if the smile is uneven.

Arm weakness. One arm only may be weak or numb. Ask the person to raise both arms, and check to see if one arm drifts downward.

Speech problems. Speech may be slurred, or the person may have trouble speaking or being understood. Ask the person to repeat a simple sentence, such as "The sun is shining."

Time. Act quickly! If you think you or someone you're with is having a stroke, call 911 immediately. "We know that if you use the ambulance, you will get to the hospital faster, you see a doctor faster, you get a CT scan faster, you're more likely to get tPA, and you're more likely to get it faster." After calling 911, check the time so that the first responders know when symptoms started. When the ambulance arrives—and again when you get to the ER— say the word stroke if you think that's what you or the patient is having. Don't just say, "my arm is numb" or "I'm dizzy." Says Dr. Jauch, "The sooner someone says, 'I think I'm having a stroke,' the sooner health-care providers can start the proven system called the Stroke Chain of Survival."

Few Women Understand Their Unique Stroke Risks

Few women understand their unique risk factors for stroke. Only 11% of those surveyed knew that being pregnant, having lupus or migraine headaches or taking oral contraception or hormone replacement therapy are stroke risk factors specific to women. And only 10% knew that hiccups combined with atypical chest pain can be an early warning sign of stroke. Some risk factors, such as high blood pressure and smoking, are the same for both men and women.

National survey of 1,000 women by The Ohio State University Wexner Medical Center, Columbus.

Think You Know Your True Risk for Heart Attack and Stroke?

James Ehrlich, MD, a clinical associate professor of endocrinology at the University of Colorado, Denver. He is a coauthor of *The Physician's Guide to Coronary Imaging*, a multimedia CD (available to physicians only).

You may think that you are at low risk for a heart attack because the heart tests that your doctor has ordered had "negative" results. The standard blood test that you received may show that your cholesterol and triglyceride levels are fine. And you may have even received a clean bill of health after taking a cardiac stress test (exercising on a treadmill while heart rhythms are electronically monitored).

Surprising fact: Those two standard heart tests miss many high-risk individuals with early heart disease. For example, a study published in the *Journal of the American College of Cardiology* found that 95% of women who had heart attacks at age 65 or younger were considered low risk.

For the greatest protection: In addition to the standard heart tests, all adults should consider receiving the highly accurate heart tests described in this article, which are not regularly ordered by most physicians but serve as stronger predictors of cardiovascular disease.

Why don't more doctors have conversations with their patients about these important tests? Many physicians closely adhere to the guidelines of the government's Preventive Services Task Force, whose evidence-based recommendations tend to include tests that are less sophisticated and less expensive.

But if your primary care physician or cardiologist does not mention these tests, ask him/her which ones might be right for you. The results will provide the best possible information for your doctor to create a customized medical and lifestyle regimen that can help prevent heart attacks and strokes.

CORONARY CALCIUM CT SCAN

This radiological imaging test—also called a CT heart scan—detects and quantifies calcified plaque, a marker for atherosclerosis (fatty buildup in the arteries). This test is up to 10 times more predictive of future heart problems than a cholesterol test and can detect early heart disease that often goes undetected by a stress test.

My advice: Men over age 35 and women over age 40 with one to two risk factors for cardiovascular disease are good candidates for screening with a heart scan. Risk factors include being overweight…having hypertension, diabetes (or prediabetes), high LDL "bad" cholesterol, low HDL "good" cholesterol, elevated triglycerides, a family history of heart disease…and/or smoking.

Risks: Cardiac CT tests expose patients to ionizing radiation (the same type used in X-rays), which has been linked to an increased risk for cancer. Heart scans, such as electron-beam CT scans and late-generation spiral CT scans, now are performed at lower radiation doses—the equivalent of 10 to 25 chest X-rays is typical. These CT scans use faster speeds than standard CT scans to produce the image, are accurate and expose you to less radiation.

Cost and coverage: $150 to $500 and may be covered by insurance.

CAROTID TEST

An ultrasound test of the carotid (neck) arteries leading to the brain does not involve radiation and measures two important conditions that help predict cardiovascular disease—the dangerous presence of plaque and the thickness of the two inner layers of each artery (the intima and media).

The carotid test is a stronger predictor of a future stroke than coronary calcium and a moderate predictor of heart attack risk.

My advice: I recommend this test for men over age 35 and women over age 40 with one to two risk factors such as hypertension and/or a family history of heart disease or stroke. People with such risk factors as high cholesterol and type 2 diabetes also may benefit from the test.

Results: If there is any noticeable plaque or the thickness of the intima/media is in the top 25% for people of your age, sex and ethnicity, you are at a higher than desirable cardiovascular risk and should pay close attention to all risk factors—especially hypertension.

Cost and coverage: $100 to $500 and often is covered by insurance.

ADVANCED LIPOPROTEIN ANALYSIS

Advanced lipoprotein analysis includes blood tests that measure hidden risk factors such as…

• **Lp(a),** a dangerous particle that often is elevated in families with a history of premature heart attacks.

• **ApoB/ApoAI,** a ratio of dangerous particles to protective particles.

My advice: This analysis is especially useful for people with heart disease that occurs in the absence of risk factors or who have a family history of premature heart disease (heart attack before age 55 in a father or brother and before age 65 in a mother or sister, for example). Those with type 2 diabetes (or prediabetes) or "metabolic syndrome"—often with a bulging waistline, hypertension, low HDL, elevated triglycerides and/or elevated blood sugar—also are good candidates.

Cost and coverage: Varies widely from as little as $40 to as much as $400—often covered by insurance.

However, not all labs perform these tests.

Labs that perform advanced lipoprotein analysis: Boston Heart Lab (BostonHeartLab.com)…LabCorp (LabCorp.com)…and SpectraCell (SpectraCell.com).

OTHER BIOMARKERS

• **Lp-PLA2 (PLAC test).** This blood test, which measures inflammation in blood vessels themselves, is a powerful predictor of the most common type of stroke (ischemic stroke). The test is more specific for vascular disease than the commonly ordered test for C-reactive protein (which is elevated with any type of inflammation in the body).

Cost and coverage: About $50 to $200 and may be covered by insurance.

•**BNP or NT-proBNP (B-type natriuretic peptide).** This is an early indicator of a weakening heart muscle (even before overt heart failure) and an excellent test for managing patients with heart failure. The test can also be used to help predict risk for heart attack.

Cost and coverage: About $50 to $250 and may be covered by insurance.

ASPIRIN RESISTANCE TESTING

Aspirin helps stop blood components called platelets from sticking together, which reduces the risk for an artery-plugging blood clot. A daily "baby" aspirin (81 mg) or higher doses usually are prescribed for anyone who has had a heart attack or stroke...or for someone who is at risk for either condition.

However, 25% of people are aspirin resistant—the drug doesn't effectively prevent platelet "stickiness."

Aspirin resistance testing measures a urinary metabolite (11-dehydrothromboxane B2), which is high if you are aspirin resistant.

Who should be tested: Anyone taking aspirin to treat or prevent cardiovascular disease.

Cost and coverage: $30 to $150 and often covered by insurance.

Good news: Recent research published in the *Journal of the American College of Cardiology* shows that supplementing the diet with omega-3 fatty acids can overcome aspirin resistance.

SOBERING STATISTICS

About 84 million American adults have cardiovascular disease. This may include narrowed, blocked arteries (coronary artery disease)...irregular heartbeats (arrhythmia)...and/or a weakened heart muscle (heart failure).

Every year, 1.5 million of those Americans have heart attacks and 500,000 of them die. Another 800,000 have strokes, 130,000 of whom die.

Artery Inflammation: Six Simple, Lifesaving Tests

Bradley Bale, MD, medical director, Grace Clinic Heart Health Program, Lubbock, Texas, and cofounder, Heart Attack & Stroke Prevention Center, Spokane. He is coauthor, with Amy Doneen, ARNP, and Lisa Collier Cool, of *Beat the Heart Attack Gene: The Revolutionary Plan to Prevent Heart Disease, Stroke and Diabetes.*

A fire could be smoldering inside your arteries...a type of fire that could erupt at any moment, triggering a heart attack or stroke. In fact, the fire could be building right this minute and you wouldn't even know it. That's because the usual things doctors look at when gauging cardiovascular risk—cholesterol, blood pressure, blood sugar, weight—can all appear to be fine even when your arteries are dangerously hot.

What does work to detect hot arteries? A set of six simple, inexpensive and readily available blood and urine tests.

Problem: Few doctors order these tests, and few patients know enough to ask for them. Without the warnings these tests provide, patients often have no way of knowing just how great their risk is for heart attack or stroke and whether or not their preventive treatments are working—until it's too late. *Here's how to protect yourself...*

THE BODY'S ARMY ON ATTACK

Hot arteries are not actually hot (as in very warm)—instead, in this case "hot" refers to the effects of chronic inflammation. Why call them hot, then? Chronic arterial inflammation can put you on the fast track to developing vascular disease by speeding up the aging of your arteries. It's so dangerous to the arterial lining that it's worse than having high LDL cholesterol. And if your arteries are already clogged with plaque—which acts as kindling for a heart attack or stroke—inflammation is what lights the match.

Inflammation in the body isn't always bad, of course. In fact, it's an important aspect of healing. When something in your body is under attack, the immune system sends in troops of white blood cells to repair and fight

209

off the attacker, and temporary inflammation results. That's why when you cut yourself, for example, you'll see swelling at the site of the injury—it's a sign that your white blood cells are at work for your benefit.

But: When an attack against your body persists (for instance, as occurs when you have an ongoing infection of the gums), your white blood cells continue to drive inflammation. When it turns chronic, inflammation becomes highly damaging to many tissues, including the arteries.

Normally, the endothelium (lining of the arteries) serves as a protective barrier between blood and the deeper layers of the arterial wall. However, when that lining is inflamed, it can't function well and it gets sticky, almost like flypaper, trapping white blood cells on their way through the body. The inflamed endothelium becomes leaky, too, allowing LDL "bad" cholesterol to penetrate into the wall of the artery. The white blood cells then gobble up the cholesterol, forming fatty streaks that ultimately turn into plaque, a condition called atherosclerosis. Then when the plaque itself becomes inflamed, it can rupture, tearing through the endothelium into the channel of the artery where blood flows. This material triggers the formation of a blood clot—a clot that could end up blocking blood flow to the heart or brain.

THE 6-PART FIRE PANEL

Just as firefighters have ways of determining whether a blaze is hiding within the walls of a building, certain tests can reveal whether inflammation is lurking within the walls of your arteries. I use a set of six tests that I call the "fire panel." Each reveals different risk factors and, for several of the tests, too-high scores can have more than one cause—so it's important to get all six tests, not just one or two.

The fire panel can identify people at risk for developing atherosclerosis...reveal whether patients who already have atherosclerosis have dangerously hot arteries that could lead to a heart attack or stroke...and evaluate patients who have survived a heart attack or stroke to see whether their current treatments are working to reduce the inflammation that threatens their lives. Your individual test results will help determine your most appropriate course of treatment.

I recommend that all adults have this panel of tests done at least every 12 months—or every three to six months for patients at high risk for heart attack or stroke. All of these tests are readily available...are inexpensive and usually covered by insurance...and can be ordered by your regular doctor. *Here are the six tests...*

• **F2 Isoprostanes.** My nickname for this blood test is the "lifestyle lie detector" because it reveals whether or not patients are practicing heart-healthy habits. The test, which measures a biomarker of oxidative stress, helps determine how fast your body's cells are oxidizing, or breaking down. According to one study, people who have the highest levels of F2 isoprostanes are nine times more likely to have blockages in their coronary arteries than people with the lowest levels.

The score you want: A normal score is less than 0.86 ng/L...an optimal score is less than 0.25 ng/L.

• **Fibrinogen.** An abnormally high level of this sticky, fibrous protein in your blood can contribute to the formation of clots...it's also a marker of inflammation. One study divided people into four groups (quartiles) based on their fibrinogen levels and found that stroke risk rose by nearly 50% for each quartile. High fibrinogen is particularly dangerous for people who also have high blood pressure because both conditions damage the blood vessel lining and make it easier for plaque to burrow inside.

Normal range: 440 mg/dL or lower.

• **High-Sensitivity C-Reactive Protein (hs-CRP).** Your liver produces C-reactive protein, and the amount of it in your blood rises when there is inflammation in your body—so an elevated hs-CRP level generally is considered a precursor to cardiovascular disease. The large-scale Harvard Women's Health Study cited this test as being more accurate than cholesterol in predicting risk for cardiovascular disease... while another study of women found that those with high scores were up to four times more likely to have a heart attack or stroke than women with lower scores. A high hs-CRP score is especially worrisome for a person with a large waist. Excess belly fat often is a sign of insulin resistance (in which cells don't readily accept insulin), a condition that further magnifies heart attack and stroke risk.

The score you're aiming for: Under 1.0 mg/L is normal...0.5 mg/L is optimal.

•**Microalbumin/Creatinine Urine Ratio (MACR).** This test looks for albumin in the urine. Albumin is a large protein molecule that circulates in the blood and shouldn't spill from capillaries in the kidneys into the urine, so its presence suggests dysfunction of the endothelium. Though this test provides valuable information about arterial wall health, doctors rarely use it for this purpose.

Important: New evidence shows that MACR levels that have traditionally been considered "normal" can signal increased risk for cardiovascular events.

Optimal ratios, according to the latest research: 7.5 or lower for women and 4.0 or lower for men.

•**Lipoprotein-Associated Phospholipase A-2 (Lp-PLA2).** This enzyme in the blood is attached to LDL cholesterol and rises when artery walls become inflamed. Recent research suggests that it plays a key role in the atherosclerosis disease process, contributing to the formation of plaque as well as to the plaque's vulnerability to rupture, Dr. Bale said. People with periodontal (gum) disease are especially likely to have elevated Lp-PLA2 scores—chronic inflammation can start in unhealthy gums and, from there, spread to the arteries.

Normal range: Less than 200 ng/mL.

•**Myeloperoxidase (MPO).** This immune system enzyme normally is found at elevated levels only at the site of an infection. When it is elevated in the bloodstream, it must be assumed that it's due to significant inflammation in the artery walls and leaking through the endothelium. This is a very bad sign. "MPO produces numerous oxidants that make all cholesterol compounds, including HDL 'good' cholesterol, more inflammatory. If your blood levels of MPO are high, HDL goes rogue and joins the gang of inflammatory thugs. It also interacts with another substance in the blood-stream to produce an acid that can eat holes in blood vessel walls. Smokers are particularly prone to high MPO levels.

Normal range: Less than 420 pmol/L.

HOW TO PUT OUT THE FIRES

While the "fire panel" tests above may seem exotic, the solution to the hot artery problem, for most of us, is not. That's because the best way to combat chronic inflammation is simply to maintain a healthful lifestyle. You just have to do it! *Key factors include...*

•**Following a heart-healthy Mediterranean-style diet.**

•**Managing stress.**

•**Getting plenty of exercise.**

•**Guarding against insulin resistance.**

•**Taking good care of your teeth and gums.**

•**Not smoking.**

In some cases, lifestyle changes alone are enough to quell the flames of chronic inflammation and to put your arteries on the road to recovery. In other cases, patients also need medication such as statins and/or dietary supplements such as niacin and fish oil. Either way, the good news is that once you shut the inflammation off, the body has a chance to heal whatever disease and damage has occurred—so you're no longer on the fast track to a heart attack or stroke.

Double Whammy for Heart Attack and Stroke

A combination drug prevents heart attack and stroke better than a statin alone. Vytorin, which contains the statin *simvastatin* plus *ezetimibe*, a drug that prevents the body from absorbing cholesterol, brought down levels of LDL (bad) cholesterol more than simvastatin did on its own. Vytorin had no more side effects than taking a statin alone. Patients who took Vytorin had 6.4% reduced risk for cardiac events. Vytorin should be considered when a statin alone leaves the patient with LDL greater than 70 mg/dL or when the patient cannot take a full dose of a statin because of a side effect.

Robert M. Califf, MD, commissioner of the Food and Drug Administration, and former vice-chancellor for clinical and translational research and director of the Duke Translational Medicine Institute, Durham, North Carolina. He led a study presented at a recent meeting of the American Heart Association.

More Magnesium, Please!

Roger Bonomo, MD, neurologist in private practice, stroke specialist and former director, Stroke Center, Lenox Hill Hospital, New York City.

Consuming an additional 100 mg of magnesium a day may reduce your risk for stroke by 9%. And magnesium isn't an expensive drug with side effects—it's a natural mineral that's already in many of the foods we eat. Most of us, especially those of us at high risk for stroke, high blood pressure or diabetes—would benefit from eating more magnesium-rich foods, such as...

- **Pumpkin seeds** (191 mg per ¼ cup)
- **Almonds** (160 mg per 2 oz.)
- **Spinach** (156 mg per cup)
- **Cashews** (148 mg per 2 oz.)
- **White beans** (134 mg per cup)
- **Artichokes** (97 mg per one large artichoke)
- **Brown rice** (84 mg per cup)
- **Shrimp** (39 mg per 4 oz.)

You can also supercharge your cooking with magnesium if you use oat bran (221 mg per cup) and buckwheat flour (301 mg per cup).

Should anyone be concerned about overdosing on magnesium? "It's hard to eat too much magnesium," he said. "If we do, our kidneys excrete the extra through urine, so only those with kidney failure need to make sure they don't consume too much."

Coffee Reduces Stroke Risk

Drinking one or more cups of caffeinated or decaffeinated coffee daily was associated with a 22% to 25% reduction in stroke risk.

Theory: Coffee beans contain antioxidants and other disease-fighting chemicals that may reduce inflammation and improve insulin activity, which lowers blood glucose levels and reduces stroke risk.

Susanna C. Larsson, PhD, a nutritional epidemiologist, Institute of Environmental Medicine, Karolinska Institute, Stockholm, Sweden, and lead researcher of a study of 34,670 women, published in *Stroke*.

How Much Tea Cuts Stroke Risk?

A recent analysis of nine studies involving nearly 195,000 adults found that for each additional three cups of black or green tea consumed daily, stroke risk dropped by 21%.

Theory: The antioxidant epigallocatechin gallate or the amino acid theanine, both found in tea, may have anti-inflammatory effects that protect the heart and brain. (Processing for decaffeinated tea may remove these ingredients.)

Lenore Arab, PhD, professor of medicine and biological chemistry, David Geffen School of Medicine, University of California, Los Angeles.

Optimism Prevents Strokes

Each "unit increase" in optimism—the general expectation that more good than bad will happen in the future—reduced stroke risk by 9% over the next two years in a recent study. And each unit increase in sense of purpose reduced heart attack risk by 27% over the same period.

Possible reason: People with purpose and a positive outlook may take better care of themselves.

The late Christopher Peterson, PhD, professor of psychology, University of Michigan, Ann Arbor, and coauthor of two studies published in *Stroke*.

How Art Safeguards Your Brain Against Stroke

Ercole Vellone, Dr, RN, an assistant professor of nursing science in the School of Nursing at University of Rome "Tor Vergata" in Italy, and lead author of a study on stroke presented at a recent meeting of the Council on Cardiovascular Nursing and Allied Professions of the European Society of Cardiology.

As we stroll through a favorite museum, listen to some great music or splurge on theater tickets, we could be benefiting our brains—in a way that is far more significant and surprising than the simple fun such activities provide. Why? Because when it comes to recovering from stroke, a recent study suggests, art lovers enjoy an important advantage. This is big news, given that stroke is the leading cause of disability and the number-three cause of death among adults in the Western world.

Researchers asked 192 stroke survivors whether they liked or did not like art, such as painting, music and theater. Of the participants, 105 said that they did like the arts…the other 87 had no particular interest in art (the clinical condition of both groups was similar).

Findings: After adjusting for participants' prestroke health status, researchers found that, regardless of the gravity of the strokes, patients who regarded art as an "integrated part of their former lifestyle" tended to…

- **Have more energy.**
- **Experience less difficulty walking.**
- **Feel calmer, happier, less depressed and less anxious.**
- **Have better memory.**
- **Show superior communication abilities** (such as speaking, comprehension and correctly naming people and objects).

- **Have better general health.**

Why art is smart: Researchers suggested that art may create long-term changes to the brain that help it recover after a trauma such as a stroke.

Not a lifelong lover of the arts? It is unclear whether nurturing a new appreciation for art later in life—or even after a stroke has already occurred—also has recovery benefits. But it might! So why not take yourself to a play, concert or gallery more often? Your brain may someday be the better for it.

Dietary Fiber Cuts Stroke Risk

For every 7 grams (g) of fiber daily, the risk for a first-time stroke decreased by 7%, in a recent analysis. One serving of whole-wheat pasta or two servings of fruits and vegetables contain about 7 g of fiber. Other top fiber sources include brown rice, spelt, quinoa and other whole-grain foods…almonds and other nuts…lentils and other dried beans.

Recommended daily fiber intake: People age 50 or younger, 38 g (men) and 25 g (women)…over age 50, 30 g (men) and 21 g (women).

Victoria J. Burley, PhD, associate professor in nutritional epidemiology at University of Leeds, England, and coauthor of an analysis of eight studies, published in *Stroke*.

Animal Protein for Stroke Prevention

Xinfeng Liu, MD, PhD, professor and chairman, department of neurology, Jinling Hospital, Nanjing University School of Medicine, China. His study was published in *Neurology*.

You already know what not to eat to protect yourself from stroke, so you stay away from foods that are high in salt and artery-clogging fats. And you probably know that you should be eating lots of fruits, vegetables and whole grains for their fiber and healthful antioxidants. But there's another nutrient that you need for stroke protection. Protein—yes, protein. And here's the surprise—although nuts, beans and grains are all protein sources known for helping heart health, the results of a recent study suggest that a certain kind of animal protein may be the best for stroke protection.

You're probably thinking that makes no sense. Many studies have shown that protein-rich diets, particularly diets in which the protein mostly comes from animals, are not beneficial for stroke prevention. At the same time, other studies have shown that protein-rich diets can reduce stroke risk.

Researchers from China who tried to make sense of conflicting studies about protein and stroke risk found that people whose diets included a moderate to moderately high amount of protein—particularly animal protein (up to 2.19 ounces per day compared with the average US recommended amount of 1.6 to 2 ounces of protein from any source)—were less likely to have a stroke than people who included only a little bit of protein in their diets. In looking at a group of studies that, in total, included 254,489 people, the researchers discovered that people who ate the most protein from any source had a 20% lower risk of stroke compared with those who consumed the least protein. Also, interestingly, the more protein eaten from any source, the lower the risk of stroke. That is, for every 0.7 ounces more of protein (moderately) consumed, stroke risk dropped by 26%.

In studies that specifically looked at either animal protein or vegetable protein, the researchers discovered that eating more, rather than less, animal protein reduced risk by 29% and eating more, rather than less, vegetable protein reduced risk by 12%. The range between high and low consumption in the studies on vegetable protein wasn't that wide, though, which may be why a larger difference in stroke risk reduction wasn't seen in them.

THE BEST SOURCE OF PROTEIN

Here's the most valuable takeaway from the meta-study—the greatest benefit for stroke protection, by far, seemed to come from getting animal protein from fish.

When the Chinese researchers looked more closely at the individual scientific studies, they noticed something striking about cultural and regional differences that put the puzzle about protein and stroke risk all together for them. Studies from Japan—a country in which fish consumption is particularly high—showed that people who ate the most protein had half the stroke risk of people who ate the least. And a research paper from Sweden—another country big on fish-eating—showed that stroke risk was reduced by 26% in higher consumers of protein. Compare these risk numbers to the one pooled from four studies from the United States, whose residents, on average, get the least amount of their protein from fish. Stroke risk reduction from higher protein consumption was only 9%.

How does protein reduce stroke risk? One theory is that it does so by lowering blood pressure, a well-known risk factor for stroke. Red meat, poultry, fish and dairy all contain L-arginine, an amino acid that our bodies convert to nitric oxide. Nitric oxide causes blood vessels to open wider, which improves blood flow and reduces blood pressure. But this good effect might be countered by the types of fat (and cholesterol) in red meat and dairy. This is why fish, which contains other heart-healthy nutrients such as omega-3 fatty acids, looks like the better choice.

This study makes a strong case that fish should be our main source of protein. The Mediterranean diet—a diet high in whole grains, vegetables, olive oil, fish and fruit and low in red meat—is beneficial for stroke reduction. So, if you're already fortifying your diet with vegetables and protein and especially substituting fish for red meat, you're doing it right. If not, consider making this heart-healthy change now.

Most Important Meal

Did you know that eating breakfast may lower stroke risk? People who never ate breakfast had a higher risk for hemorrhagic (bleeding in the brain) strokes than people who ate breakfast daily.

Possible reason: High blood pressure is a major risk factor for hemorrhagic stroke. Eating breakfast is associated with a drop in blood pressure.

Study of 82,772 people led by researchers at Osaka University Graduate School of Medicine, Japan, published in *Stroke*.

A Grapefruit a Day Helps Keep Stroke Away

Kathryn M. Rexrode, MD, MPH, physician, division of preventive medicine, Brigham and Women's Hospital, and assistant professor of medicine, Harvard Medical School, both in Boston.

Mmm, citrus. There's nothing like a refreshing orange, a tangy tangerine or a sweet pink grapefruit. It really does taste like sunshine.

But these juicy fruits aren't just delicious—they may actually help you ward off a stroke, according to recent research.

And you may be surprised to hear that it's not because of the vitamin C…

HONING IN ON FLAVONOIDS

A zillion studies have shown the health benefits of eating fruit, including studies that have shown that people who eat five or more servings of fruits and vegetables have a 25% lower risk for stroke (both ischemic and hemorrhagic) compared with those who eat three or fewer servings. Researchers have suspected that flavonoids, antioxidant compounds found in many fruits and vegetables, are one key to their power since they reduce inflammation and improve blood vessel function.

But there are six different types of flavonoids found in foods, and each has a subtly different chemical structure. Given the variety, researchers from England, Italy and the US wanted to learn which specific flavonoids and which fruits or vegetables, in particular, are most beneficial for preventing stroke.

One of the authors—Kathryn M. Rexrode, MD, MPH, a physician in the division of preventive medicine at Brigham and Women's Hospital and assistant professor of medicine at Harvard Medical School, both in Boston—explained more about the study…

THE FLAVONOID THAT CAME OUT ON TOP

The researchers used information from 70,000 women who were followed for 14 years as part of the Nurses' Health Study. Every two years, the participants completed questionnaires that covered their medical histories and lifestyles. And every four years, the women completed food questionnaires, which asked how much of certain foods and drinks they consumed and how often they consumed them.

The women's diets were analyzed for the six different types of flavonoids, and their medical histories were reviewed for the number and type of strokes that the women had. What they found was that high consumption—more than about 63 milligrams per day of a certain subclass of flavonoids called flavanones (the amount found in about one to two servings of citrus per day)—was associated with a 19% reduced risk for ischemic stroke (the type caused by a clot, not by a bleed), compared with low flavanone consumption (under 13.7 milligrams per day). And this was after adjusting for other stroke risk factors, such as smoking, age, body mass index and others. The other five flavonoids studied reduced stroke risk, too, but not by as much (only by 4% to 13%).

Dr. Rexrode said that one reason that the flavanones may have been associated with decreased risk for ischemic stroke is that flavanones may inhibit platelet function and clotting factors. The researchers didn't study whether citrus affected risk for hemorrhagic stroke, but Dr. Rexrode said that it's unlikely that eating citrus would lead to an increased risk for hemorrhagic stroke. She said that it takes a relatively small amount of clotting to cause an ischemic stroke, but, on the other hand, it takes a relatively large amount of excessive bleeding to cause a hemorrhagic stroke.

Although this study, which was published in *Stroke*, looked only at women, Dr. Rexrode said that there is no reason to think that these findings wouldn't apply to men, too.

PICK YOUR CITRUS

Dr. Rexrode said that you can get all the flavanones you need (about 63 milligrams) from eating one or two servings of citrus each day. Whole fruits are always better than juices or smoothies, she said, because the bulk of the flavanones are found in the inner membranes of the fruit and the pith or white part of the fruit. The pith is generally removed when the fruit is juiced or cleaned for smoothies.

The USDA provides information about the amount of flavanones in every 100 grams of edible fruit, so to save you the trouble of weighing your fruits, here are estimates of the flavanone content for some common citruses...

• **Grapefruit** (one-half of a four-inch diameter) 47 milligrams

• **Orange** (25⁄8 inch diameter) 42 milligrams

• **Tangerine** (2½ inch diameter) 18 milligrams

Dr. Rexrode doesn't recommend supplements—she said sticking to whole fruit is best. And don't overdo it on citrus, or else your stomach or teeth might suffer from the acid. Just a serving or two a day is all you need!

Tomato Sauce Reduces Stroke Risk

Recent finding: People with the highest blood levels of the antioxidant lycopene had 55% lower risk for stroke than people with the lowest levels. Lycopene is found in tomatoes, red peppers, carrots, papaya and watermelon. It is even more concentrated in cooked tomato products, such as tomato sauce.

Rafael Alexander Ortiz, MD, chief, Neuro-Endovascular Surgery and Interventional Neuroradiology, Lenox Hill Hospital, New York City.

New Stroke Fighter: Red Peppers

Eating red peppers and other vitamin C–rich fruits and veggies may reduce your risk for intracerebral hemorrhagic stroke (a blood vessel rupture in the brain). And what's so great about red peppers? At 190 mg per cup, they contain three times more vitamin C than an orange. Other good sources of vitamin C— broccoli and strawberries. Researchers believe that this vitamin may reduce stroke risk by regulating blood pressure and strengthening collagen, which promotes healthy blood vessels.

Stéphane Vannier, MD, neurologist, Pontchaillou University Hospital, Rennes, France, from research presented at the annual meeting of the American Academy of Neurology.

Tasty Treat to Stop Stroke

In one study, people who ate one serving of chocolate a week were 22% less likely to have a stroke than those who ate no chocolate. In another study, people who ate 50 grams (1.75 ounces) of chocolate per week were 46% less likely to die following a stroke than those who ate no chocolate.

Possible reason: Chocolate is a rich source of antioxidants that may protect against stroke.

Sarah Sahib, researcher at McMaster University, Hamilton, Ontario, Canada, lead author of an analysis of studies on chocolate and stroke.

Olive Oil Can Keep Strokes Away

People who consistently added olive oil to their food in cooking and salad dressings were 41% less likely to suffer from an ischemic stroke than people who did not use olive oil, a recent study found. An ischemic stroke, in which blood flow to a part of the brain is blocked, is the most common kind of stroke.

Cécilia Samieri, PhD, researcher, department of epidemiology, Université Bordeaux Segalen, France, and leader of two studies on olive oil consumption and stroke risk, published in *Neurology*.

Women, Reduce Stroke Risk with Potassium

Sylvia Wassertheil-Smoller, PhD, Dorothy and William Manealoff Foundation and Molly Rosen Chair in Social Medicine Emerita, department of epidemiology and population health, Albert Einstein College of Medicine in Brooklyn. Her study was published in *Stroke*.

Bananas are rich in it, dried fruits such as raisins, prunes and apricots are, too. Potatoes, white beans and tomato sauce are great sources as well. You may have guessed the nutrient—potassium. And what does getting enough potassium do besides help your muscles move and regulate your blood pressure and heartbeat? It's crucial to heart health, especially for postmenopausal women. And a recent study showed that postmenopausal women who consumed more potassium were less likely to have strokes.

In this study, women who consumed the most potassium (at least 3,194 milligrams [mg] per day) were 12% less likely to suffer any type of stroke than women who consumed the least potassium (less than 1,926 mg per day). And they were 16% less likely to suffer an ischemic stroke, the most common type, caused when a blood clot blocks oxygen and nutrients to the brain. For women who kept their blood pressure and weight in check and knew to bulk up on potassium, protection against ischemic stroke was more than doubled (a 27% to 30% lower risk) compared with women who consumed a minimum of dietary potassium. That is a huge risk reduction.

Incidentally, even the high-range number for potassium intake mentioned above—around 3,200 mg per day—may be considered on the low side. The World Health Organization recommends 3,510 mg...while the US Department of Agriculture (USDA) recommends 4,700 mg a day. But the sad fact is that most postmenopausal women are nowhere near that goal. In one recent study, the average daily intake of potassium among the 90,000-plus participants was only 2,611 mg—that's barely more than half the daily amount that the USDA says we need!

ARE YOU GETTING ENOUGH?

The irony is that potassium is found in nearly all food groups, especially fruits, vegetables, dairy products and fish and seafood. You can make every meal—breakfast, lunch and dinner—potassium-rich. *See for yourself...*

• **Breakfast or snack time.** A banana provides 422 mg of potassium. A cup of cantaloupe, 430 mg. Eight ounces of yogurt gives you up to 579 mg. Toss in a cup of strawberries and you get 255 mg more. Prune juice packs 707 mg in a cup (a cup of stewed prunes, 796 mg). And a cup of orange juice will provide 496 mg. Dried apricots or peaches are sweet and tasty sources of potassium, too, delivering between 378 mg and 398 mg per quarter cup.

• **Lunch and dinner.** A small baked potato, including the skin, has 738 mg of potassium, a medium sweet potato with skin, 542 mg. Tomato products are great sources of potassium...one-half cup of tomato sauce provides 405 mg. All types of beans, especially white beans (595 mg per half-cup) are excellent sources, too. And a cup of cooked spinach packs 840 mg. Fish and seafood are also great. For example, three ounces of yellowfin tuna provides 484 mg of potassium.

That's just a small sampling, but you can see how having a deliciously varied diet of healthful foods can provide all the potassium you need for heart health and stroke risk reduction. For more information on the potassium content of foods, check out this cheat sheet of low-calorie, high-potassium foods from the University of Massachusetts School of Medicine...UMassMed.edu/uploadedfiles/SourcesDietaryPotassium.pdf

DO YOU NEED A SUPPLEMENT?

The benefits of potassium come from dietary intake. Supplements do not seem to have the same beneficial effect, said Sylvia

217

Wassertheil-Smoller, PhD, who participated in the study on potassium and stroke risk in postmenopausal women. Dr. Wassertheil-Smoller is chair of social medicine at Albert Einstein College of Medicine in Brooklyn, New York. She and other experts agree that having too much potassium in the blood can be dangerous to the heart. So check with your doctor before taking a potassium supplement. If a potassium supplement is recommended to you, your doctor should monitor your blood potassium levels to make sure they do not go higher than what is healthy and normal.

Overactive Thyroid Linked to Stroke

A diagnosis of hyperthyroidism, or overactive thyroid, before age 45 increases stroke risk by 44%.

Possible connection: Hyperthyroidism is linked to atrial fibrillation, a heart rhythm disorder that is associated with elevated stroke risk.

To cut stroke risk: Follow a low-fat, high-fiber diet, and exercise regularly. Don't smoke. Have blood pressure, blood sugar and cholesterol levels measured at least once a year.

Brian Silver, MD, associate professor of neurology, Warren Alpert Medical School, Brown University, Providence, Rhode Island.

Antioxidants Protect Against Stroke

Researchers from the University of Parma in Italy have found that people whose diets were high in antioxidants had a 59% lower risk for ischemic stroke, the most common type of stroke, than people whose diets were low in antioxidants.

Food sources consumed: Fruits, vegetables, coffee, dark chocolate, red wine, whole-grain cereals and nuts.

D. Del Rio, et al., "Total Antioxidant Capacity of the Diet Is Associated with Lower Risk of Ischemic Stroke in a Large Italian Cohort," *Journal of Nutrition* (2011).

Vitamin Protection from Stroke Damage?

Chandan K. Sen, PhD, professor in the department of surgery and associate dean, College of Medicine, The Ohio State University, Columbus.

Surely, by now, people are well-aware that when it comes to surviving stroke, time is of the essence. The sooner patients get treated, the more likely their brains will be spared significant damage. Is it worth considering, then, if you're at high risk for stroke, that taking a supplement might offer your brain protection ahead of time? According to the results of a recent study from The Ohio State University in Columbus, such a day may be close at hand.

NOT JUST ANY VITAMIN E

The study, funded by the National Institutes of Health, looked into whether taking a natural form of vitamin E called tocotrienols (more on that in a minute) might prepare the brain to react better after an ischemic stroke (a stroke caused by a blood clot). Most strokes (87%) are ischemic. The report, an animal study, used dogs because their brains more closely resemble those of humans than do those of commonly studied animals, such as mice and rats. For 10 weeks, researchers gave one group of dogs 200 mg a day of tocotrienols and the other group a placebo. Then, while the animals were under anesthesia, they induced strokes in both groups by blocking the middle cerebral artery in their brains for one hour. Next, researchers conducted imaging studies of the animals' brains both one hour after and 24 hours after the induced strokes to learn what changes had taken place. *What they discovered...*

• **More blood flow.** In the vitamin E group, minor blood vessels (collateral vessels) that are a normal part of the brain's circulatory system became larger in the area of the blockage, enabling more blood flow to continue in that area and protect the brain. This did not happen to the same extent in the control group.

• **Less tissue damage.** Twenty-four hours after the strokes, brain lesions that indicate tissue damage were 80% smaller in the vitamin E group compared with those in the placebo group.

• **Less nerve damage.** In the vitamin E group after 24 hours, the brain's internal communication network—a crisscrossing of nerves—remained relatively intact at the location of the stroke...while in the placebo group, the network showed major disruptions.

WAKING UP SLEEPING ARTERIES

The senior author of the study, Chandan K. Sen, PhD, professor in the department of surgery, has been researching tocotrienol vitamin E and its effect on the brain for more than a decade. He says that the brain contains collateral vessels that normally remain dormant. When a person has a stroke, those collateral vessels enlarge and join together to improve blood flow in the affected part of the brain. Researchers found that the tocotrienol vitamin E essentially helped "wake up" these previously inactive arteries more effectively at the time of the trauma to the brain.

Dr. Sen and his group have a clinical trial under way using tocotrienol vitamin E in a group of people who are at an increased risk for stroke. The participants in this trial are taking 400 mg daily of tocotrienol E to see if the vitamin helps prevent stroke or, in cases when stroke occurs, if it helps reduce damage to the brain, as it did with the dogs. When asked for a recommendation, Dr. Sen said that he would like to wait for the outcomes of the clinical trial. But people at a high risk for stroke may want to talk to their doctors about taking natural Vitamin E as we wait for the clinical trial to be completed.

READ THE LABEL

There are two categories of natural vitamin E—tocotrienols (which were used in the st

and tocopherols. Both types include four subtypes called alpha, beta, delta and gamma. In his research, Dr. Sen uses a mix of natural vitamin E that's rich in alpha-tocotrienol. If your doctor advises you to start taking natural vitamin E to help prevent stroke, Dr. Sen says to look for a supplement in a health-food store or online that contains a high percentage of alpha-tocotrienol. You may notice that many vitamin E supplements contain some tocopherols, as well. This is fine, so long as the tocopherol is natural and not synthetic. Check the label, and if it includes the words synthetic alpha tocopherol—or "dl" instead of "d," the natural form—return the bottle to the shelf and look for all-natural E.

Folic Acid Cuts Stroke Risk

According to a large study, supplements of the B vitamin decrease incidence of a first stroke in people with high blood pressure by 21%. People with normal blood pressure are likely to benefit, too. A standard daily multivitamin should provide adequate folic acid.

Better: Getting the vitamin from food, especially broccoli, beans (cooked from dried) and dark, leafy greens.

Also: Enriched grain products.

Meir Stampfer, MD, DrPH, professor of medicine at Harvard Medical School, Boston, and coauthor of an editorial published in *JAMA*.

MRI Can Identify Yo
Stroke Risk

Atrial-fibrilla identified with a cardiac for str from the common heart-rhythm MRI rial fibrillation (A-fib) already have higher risk for stroke.

Recent finding: A-fib patients with a specific alteration in the function of the heart's left atrium have slower blood flow and are at even higher risk for blood clots and future stroke.

Hiroshi Ashikaga, MD, PhD, assistant professor of medicine and biomedical engineering at Johns Hopkins University School of Medicine, Baltimore.

Shingles Increases Stroke Risk

Having shingles anywhere on the body increases the risk of having a stroke over the next 12 months by about 30%. Having eye-related (ocular) shingles increases the risk by more than 400%. People who have had shingles should take extra care to reduce stroke risk. Exercise regularly...maintain a healthy, low-salt, low-fat diet...don't smoke...and, if necessary, take medication to control blood pressure and cholesterol.

Daniel T. Lackland, DrPH, professor of epidemiology, department of neurosciences, Medical University of South Carolina, Charleston, and spokesperson for the American Stroke Association. StrokeAssociation.org.

Sinus Infections May Raise Odds of Stroke

People who were diagnosed with a sinus infection ones without are likely to have a stroke than

Possible reason sinuses.
may put pressure on blamed sinus tissue sal sprays may help reduce Saline nasal your doctor for details.

Study by researchers at Taipei Medical Ask Taiwan, published in *American Journal of Rhi & Allergy.*

Cold Weather and Stroke

A study of nearly 300,000 adults with atrial fibrillation (AFib) found that their risk for an ischemic stroke was nearly 20% higher in winter than in summer.

Theory: Cold weather promotes the formation of blood clots that can travel to the brain.

If you have AFib: Dress warmly and talk to your doctor about other ways to control your risk for stroke during the colder months, such as making sure that your dose of any medication you may be taking (for example, a blood thinner) is adequate.

Tze-Fan Chao, MD, cardiologist, Taipei Veterans General Hospital, Taiwan.

Keep It Down!

Ongoing and lengthy exposure to everyday noises, such as cell phone rings or traffic, increases heart rate and decreases heart rate variability—two risk factors for cardiac problems and stroke.

Self-defense: Take deep breaths to ease your body's response to noise. Block out loud noises with earplugs, sound-blocking headphones and/or white noise.

Seth Goldbarg, MD, electrophysiologist, New York-Presbyterian/Queens Hospital, Flushing, New York, writing in *Prevention.*

The Dangers of Too Much... and Too Little...Sleep

Study of nearly 10,000 people, ages 42 to 81, over 10 years by researchers at Cambridge Institute of Public Health, University of Cambridge, UK, published in *Neurology.*

Megan Ruiter, PhD, professor, psychology, The University of Alabama at Birmingham.

Sleeping more than eight hours a night linked to stroke. It is unclear if over-causes cardiovascular concerns that can lead to stroke or if it is an indicator of other health issues. Oversleeping has also been linked to diabetes, obesity and other health problems.

TOO LITTLE SLEEP RAISES STROKE RISK

Adults with normal body weight who regularly slept less than six hours per night were four times more likely to have a stroke than those who slept seven or eight hours a night. Researchers monitored stroke symptoms (such as weakness on one side of the body) for three years in 5,666 people (age 45 and older) with no history of stroke or sleep apnea.

Theory: Poor sleep triggers more established stroke risk factors, such as high blood pressure and high cholesterol.

If you regularly sleep less than six hours per night: Talk to your doctor.

Do All Painkillers Raise Stroke Risk?

Harlan Krumholz, MD, professor of cardiology at Yale School of Medicine, New Haven, Connecticut, and author of *The Expert Guide to Beating Heart Disease: What You Absolutely Must Know.*

Several years ago, lots of people were horrified to learn that certain prescription painkillers—Vioxx and Bextra, in particular—were dangerous and put them at significant risk for cardiovascular problems. Not only were these people rightfully outraged at having been misled about the safety of the drugs they were taking, they were outraged as well at the prospect of having to endure more of the pain they were trying to escape. Many ended up taking other, more well-known, over-the-counter brands of nonsteroidal anti-inflammatory drugs (NSAIDs), such as Advil, Motrin, Aleve and others. Now a recent study delivers yet more painful news—it seems that these drugs also carry stroke risks.

A group of researchers at the University Bern conducted a meta-analysis of m

30 randomized trials with a combined total of 116,429 patients taking placebo or NSAIDs. The researchers found abundant evidence of a heightened risk for cardiovascular events and found that taking drugs containing *ibuprofen*, including brand names such as Motrin, Advil and Nuprin, and those containing *naproxen* (such as the brand Aleve and a few others) raises the likelihood of suffering a stroke.

These are everyday drugs that sit in most of America's medicine cabinets right now. So, even though this finding is based on a "study of studies" rather than a customized clinical trial that is the gold standard, it's an important one—as many people take these drugs often and without giving it much thought.

Harlan Krumholz, MD, professor of cardiology at Yale School of Medicine and author of the book *The Expert Guide to Beating Heart Disease: What You Absolutely Must Know*, explained that the reason NSAIDs carry cardiovascular risk is that these drugs "disturb the balance of the blood's clotting system, and some of them tend to cause clot formation." He cautions that everyone who takes NSAIDs is at some risk for heart problems from them. "In particular, people with heart disease should avoid using these medications," Dr. Krumholz said.

Since there is also some risk (albeit small) associated with products containing *acetaminophen* (such as Tylenol), Dr. Krumholz said that for people with heart issues, aspirin is probably the safest pain reliever. It is, after all, recommended for this group as protection against future heart attacks.

Overlooked Stroke Risk

People with most stress, depression, anger, hostility were up to twice as likely suffer a stroke or transient ischemic (TIA), also known as a "mini-stroke," those with the lowest levels of those traits, according to a recent 11-year study.

Why: Chronic psychological problems are just as significant as traditional stroke risk factors, such as smoking and high blood pressure.

Susan Everson-Rose, PhD, MPH, associate professor of medicine, University of Minnesota, Minneapolis.

A Single Drink Doubles Your Stroke Risk

Stroke risk is doubled in the hour after you have just one alcoholic drink. The heightened risk for ischemic stroke goes away within three hours.

Theory: Alcohol may temporarily raise blood pressure or affect the blood's ability to clot.

Self-defense: Avoid consuming multiple drinks in a short time because this may cause a sharp increase in stroke risk. One drink is defined as 12 ounces of beer, four ounces of wine, 1.5 ounces of 80-proof spirits or one ounce of 100-proof spirits.

Murray A. Mittleman, MD, DrPH, director of the Cardiovascular Epidemiology Research Unit, Beth Israel Deaconess Medical Center, Harvard Medical School, Boston, and leader of a study published in *Stroke*.

Blood Test for Stroke Risk

Recent finding: A 33-study analysis involving about 280,000 adults showed that those
with a ... marker for glomerular filtration rate (GFR)—a
risk for stroke.ey disease—had a 43% higher
those with healthy rates.

Theory: Impaired kidney function may
cause clotting, thereby ... stroke risk.

If you have, or are at risking stroke risk.
ease (due to family history, **judney dis-**
Ask your doctor how often you sho... **le):**
your GFR measured.

Jeffrey Saver, MD, professor of neurology, director
of the Stroke Unit, UCLA.

How to Survive the Worst Type of Stroke

Edward C. Jauch, MD, director of the division of emergency medicine at the Medical University of South Carolina in Charleston, where he is also a professor in the department of neurosciences, the associate vice-chair for research in the department of medicine and director of Acute Stroke Trials, ongoing clinical research into the optimal treatment approaches for stroke.

If someone asked you for a quick definition of a stroke, you would probably say that it is caused by a blood clot...and requires quick treatment with a clot-dissolving drug. These points are true for the most common strokes, called ischemic strokes, but there's another type of stroke that doesn't get nearly as much attention.

The "other" stroke: A hemorrhagic, or bleeding, stroke is entirely different from an ischemic stroke—and usually more devastating. Fortunately, recent research has uncovered potentially lifesaving advice for people who suffer this type of stroke. *The facts you (and your loved ones) need...*

THE GRIM STATISTICS

Up to 20% of the nearly 800,000 new or recurrent strokes that occur each year in the US are hemorrhagic strokes, but they account for 40% of stroke deaths.

What makes these strokes so dangerous? Hemorrhagic strokes result from bleeding into or around the brain, a catastrophic event that damages brain tissue. In addition, as the pooled blood degrades, it releases iron from red blood cells. Iron is toxic for brain tissue.

WORST HEADACHE OF YOUR LIFE

While most people can identify the main symptoms of an ischemic stroke (for example, facial drooping...numbness or weakness on one side of the body...and/or trouble speaking), the red flags for hemorrhagic stroke are not as well known.

With hemorrhagic strokes, a sudden, intense headache is usually the main symptom. S...imes mild headaches can be a warning ...days or weeks before this type of

Important: Headache sometimes occurs with an ischemic stroke, but it's usually accompanied by other symptoms, such as those described above. With a hemorrhagic stroke, additional symptoms may include nausea, vomiting and/or loss of consciousness. Symptoms can overlap, however, with both types of stroke, and only an imaging test can tell the difference.

If you have a severe headache that's unusual for you: Call 911. This is particularly true if you have stroke risk factors such as smoking, high blood pressure or diabetes.

A lifesaving recent finding: For people suffering a subarachnoid hemorrhage (a type of hemorrhagic stroke described below), treatment at a comprehensive stroke center was associated with a 27% reduced risk for death, compared with care at a hospital that did not provide specialized stroke care. Comprehensive stroke centers have specialists who are trained to deal with these strokes and 24-hour access to a neurosurgeon (if needed).

For the nearest comprehensive stroke center: Go to the National Stroke Association website, Stroke.org/emergency-stroke-center-locations. A family member can ask the ambulance driver to take you there.

HOW BLEEDING STROKES OCCUR

There are two main types of hemorrhagic stroke…

• **Subarachnoid hemorrhage.** About half of hemorrhagic strokes occur in the subarachnoid space, between the inner and middle layers of tissue that cover the brain.

What happens: Most subarachnoid hemorrhages are caused by a ruptured aneurysm, a bulge in an artery wall that tends to develop after age 40, due to years of high blood pressure. It can also be congenital (present at birth). An aneurysm that doesn't bleed isn't necessarily a problem—you can have one for decades and not know it unless it shows up during an imaging test for some other condition.

But once an aneurysm "bursts" and bleeds, you will likely have a "thunderclap" headache that gets progressively worse—and may be followed by a brief loss of consciousn[ess]. You may also have blurred vision o[r]

vision and/or pain behind and above one eye. Permanent brain damage or death can occur within hours or even minutes. Get to an ER.

Next steps: This type of stroke can be quickly identified with a CT scan or an MRI, and with magnetic resonance angiography (MRA) and/or cerebral angiography (a catheter is used to inject a dye, which illuminates blood vessels in the brain). *Once the damaged artery is identified, there are two main choices…*

• Clipping, the traditional approach, is done under general anesthesia. A surgeon creates an opening in the skull (craniotomy), locates the aneurysm and seals it off with a titanium clip that remains on the artery permanently.

• Endovascular coiling is a newer approach. With this minimally invasive technique, there is no incision in the skull. A tiny catheter is inserted into an artery in the groin, then threaded through the vascular system (with the aid of a special type of X-ray) until it's inside the aneurysm. Then, a flexible platinum coil is placed within the aneurysm to stop the bleeding.

Which technique is better? It depends on the location and size of the aneurysm, as well as the overall health of the patient. One large study found that the risk for disability or death in patients who were treated with coils was almost 27% lower than in those who were clipped. However, the study found a greater risk for the brain to bleed again with coils versus clipping.

• **Intracerebral hemorrhage.** Intracerebral hemorrhages cause bleeding within the brain. They're often caused by decades of high blood pressure, which can damage small blood vessels. They can also be caused by excessive doses of blood thinners taken for cardiovascular disease…or bleeding disorder such as hemophilia).

Along with a severe headache, symptoms might include weakness, paralysis, a loss of speech or vision and mental confusion. Headache with this type of stroke are more common with this type of stroke than with ischemic stroke, but only a CT scan or MRI provide an accurate diagnosis.

In some cases, surgery or endoscopic drainage may be helpful to remove blood that's causing excess pressure. *Next steps…*

• Lower systolic (top number) blood pressure to below 140. This will reduce brain bleeding.

• Reverse the medication's effects in patients with strokes that are caused by blood thinners. This can be done, for example, by giving an intravenous solution that contains clotting factors, platelets or other products that help blood clot.

Survivors of hemorrhagic stroke should receive rehabilitation care to aid their recovery.

Breakthroughs in Stroke Recovery

Murray Flaster, MD, PhD, an associate professor of neurology and neurological surgery and director of Loyola Outpatient Clinics at Loyola University Chicago Stritch School of Medicine, where he specializes in vascular neurology and neurological intensive care.

Physician scientists have now discovered that a series of surprisingly simple treatments—performed in the first 24 to 48 hours after a stroke—can prevent additional brain damage and help reduce the risk for disability and complications, including cognitive impairments.

Important: The recommendations described in this article apply only to patients who have had an ischemic stroke (caused by a blood clot). Almost 90% of all strokes are ischemic. Unless it's otherwise noted, these recommendations do not apply to patients who have suffered a hemorrhagic (bleeding) stroke.

The most important treatments following stro... :

• **Mai... or raise blood pressure.** It sounds cou... tuitive because high blood pressure is one... because main risk factors for stroke—and ... st stroke patients have a spike in blood ... of about 20 points. But studies have sh... at higher-than-normal blood pressure can ... recover faster, with less brain dama...tients

Giving blood pressure–lowering dru... the hospital can cause a decrease in cerebr... perfusion pressure (a measurement of blood flow to the brain) that can increase damage.

Recommended: As a general rule, your blood pressure should not be lowered immediately after a stroke, even if you have existing hypertension. As long as your blood pressure reading is below 220/120 (normal is about 120/80), it should be left alone.

In some patients, particularly those with a blockage in a major blood vessel, it might be advisable to actively raise blood pressure with a vasopressive medication, such as *phenylephrine* (Neo-Synephrine).

Exceptions: Blood pressure may still need to be lowered in patients who have had a hemorrhagic stroke (caused by bleeding in the brain) or in those who are taking clot-dissolving drugs. Raising blood pressure in patients who are actively bleeding or at risk for bleeding can potentially cause more bleeding.

• **Reduce body temperature.** Fever is common in stroke patients due to infection or the stroke itself, with up to 25% having a temperature of 100.4°F or higher within 48 hours after being admitted to the hospital. A fever is dangerous because it increases the metabolic demands of damaged brain tissue—energy that should go toward healing. It also triggers the release of inflammatory substances that can cause additional damage.

Recommended: *Acetaminophen* (Tylenol) and hydration. Cooling blankets may be used for fever above 101°F. An experimental treatment called therapeutic hypothermia involves rapidly lowering body temperature with a cooled saline solution given intravenously.

• **Rehydrate.** Dehydration is common in stroke patients because fever and other complications can reduce the body's fluids. If you've had a stroke and are dehydrated, your risk of forming additional blood clots is increased by fivefold.

Reason: Dehydration reduces the volume of blood in the body. This, in turn, reduces blood pressure and increases the tendency of blood to clot.

Recommended: Intravenous (IV) saline solution for at least 24 to 48 hours.

• **Lower the bed.** When the head of the ... ...sed, the increased elevation can de... ...l blood flow, particularly when the stroke affects the middle cerebral artery, which is common in ischemic stroke.

Important finding: Studies suggest that lowering the head of the bed from 30 degrees to 15 degrees increases blood flow through the middle cerebral artery by 12%. There's an additional 8% increase when the bed is flat.

The trade-off: Many patients aren't comfortable when the bed is completely flat. They also have more trouble swallowing, which increases the risk that they'll get pneumonia after inhaling (aspirating) foreign material from the mouth. Therefore, the head of the bed should initially be elevated to about 15 degrees. If the patient doesn't improve, the bed can be lowered.

• **Use an insulin drip.** It's common for stroke patients to have high blood sugar because of preexisting diabetes or prediabetes. In addition, the stroke itself can temporarily raise blood sugar (in fact, any major stressor in the body can raise blood glucose levels). High blood sugar, or hyperglycemia, is associated with a 2.7-fold increase in poor outcomes following stroke. Poor outcomes could include language difficulties, paralysis, cognitive impairments, etc.

Recommended: Stroke patients should be tested for hyperglycemia immediately after arriving in the hospital emergency department and then as frequently as needed. If blood sugar is higher than 155 mg/dL, insulin should be administered intravenously.

Important: To help prevent stroke-related complications that are worsened by elevated blood sugar, these patients should not be given saline that contains glucose—even if they could benefit nutritionally from the additional sugar.

• **Give a statin quickly.** Stroke patients routinely have their cholesterol tested in the hospital.

Recommended: There's no need to wait for the results before giving patients a cholesterol-lowering statin drug, such as *atorvastatin* (Lipitor) or *pravastatin* (Pravachol).

Reason: Even if your cholesterol is normal, statins reduce the inflammatory brain damage that's caused by stroke. Giving these medica-

tions quickly can help patients recover more promptly. Continuing statin therapy (if you have high cholesterol and are already taking a statin) can help prevent a subsequent stroke.

• **Start activity early.** Hospitalized patients who are physically active to any degree—even if it is just sitting up in bed—improve more quickly and have fewer complications than those who are initially immobile.

Other benefits: Physical activity also reduces the risk for pneumonia, deep-vein thrombosis, pulmonary embolism and bedsores.

Recommended: Some form of activity within hours after having a stroke if the patient is neurologically stable. We encourage patients to spend as little time in bed as possible even if their mobility is impaired and to do as much as they can tolerate.

Important: Activity should always be carefully guided by nurses, therapists or other members of the hospital team to avoid injury.

Let's Bust a Myth About Stroke Recovery

The National Stroke Association. Stroke.org
Health Insider research.

One of the most discouraging myths about stroke is the *recovery window.* That's the common idea that whatever gains you make after a few months or a year are all you can expect.

Wrong. Disproven.

Study after study has shown that it's simply not true, yet the myth persists. And that's bad because it makes people stop trying to improve—and live with more disability than they need to. According to the National Stroke Association, although the early days after a stroke are a crucial time for treatment and rehabilitation, it's never too late to make improvements after a stroke.

That's good news for the 6.5 million Americans who are stroke survivors. The Association, as part of its Come Back Strong campaign, has launched a free app, available for both Apple and Android devices, for stroke survivors—and caregivers. The app makes it easy to track medications, improve rehab techniques through video instruction and find a support group and important contact information, including for your own doctors, for emergencies. Google Come Back Strong App.

DIY Test to Prevent Second Stroke

About 25% to 35% of stroke survivors experience atrial fibrillation (AF)—a type of irregular heartbeat that is associated with increased stroke risk. Patients and their relatives can be trained to detect an irregular rhythm by taking a wrist pulse. If an irregularity is detected and AF confirmed, physicians may prescribe medication or other treatment to decrease stroke risk.

Bernd Kallmünzer, MD, a neurologist with the stroke unit at University Medical Center, Erlangen, Germany. He is lead author of a study of 256 stroke patients, published in *Neurology*.

Two-Pill Treatment Cuts Stroke Risk by One-Third After a TIA

S. Claiborne Johnston, MD, PhD, dean, Dell Medical School, The University of Texas at Austin. His study published in *The New England Journal of Medicine*.

Most individuals who've had an ischemic attack (TIA) emerge without permanent damage. But 10% to 20% of TIA patients go on to have a full-blown stroke within 90 days.

Breakthrough: Now there's a way to reduce that risk by one-third. It involves adding a second type of pill to the standard pill

that TIA patients take. But to work best, the dual treatment should begin right away after a TIA.

DYNAMIC DRUG DUO

The vast majority of strokes are ischemic strokes, the type caused by a blood clot. That's why it's standard for TIA patients to start taking a daily aspirin, because aspirin is known to help prevent clots. Aspirin's benefits in this regard, though, are rather modest. So researchers set out to determine whether adding the anticoagulant drug *clopidogrel* (Plavix) would help. Like aspirin, clopidogrel works by preventing platelets (a type of blood cell) from collecting and forming clots. Clopidogrel is not risk-free—it can cause significant bleeding—but researchers wanted to see whether its benefits outweighed its risks for TIA patients.

The recent study included 5,170 people who had had a TIA or a similar kind of ministroke called an acute minor ischemic stroke within the previous 24 hours. All patients received aspirin right away. The first dose ranged from 75 milligrams (mg) to 300 mg, depending on their doctors' decisions, then the dose was dropped to 75 mg from day two onward.

Patients were randomly divided into two groups. In one group, patients received daily aspirin plus a placebo through day 90. In the other group, patients received clopidogrel at a dose of 300 mg on day one and 75 mg on days two through 90, plus daily aspirin for 21 days. In this dual-therapy group, aspirin was discontinued after 21 days to minimize the risk for bleeding.

Here's what happened over the course of the 90 days...

•**Stroke occurred in 12% of patients in the aspirin-only group,** but in only 8% of the patients in the clopidogrel-plus-aspirin group—meaning that the likelihood of suffering a stroke was one-third lower in the clopidogrel-plus-aspirin group.

•**Fatal or disabling stroke occurred in 7% of aspirin-only users...**but in only 5% of clopidogrel-plus-aspirin users.

•**Hemorrhagic stroke (the type caused by bleeding rather than a clot) occurred at** an identical rate of 0.3% in both groups... and other severe bleeding events (such as bleeding that required surgery or transfusion) occurred at an identical rate of 0.2% in both groups. This was important—because it meant that adding the 90-day clopidogrel therapy to the 21-day aspirin therapy did not increase patients' risk for hemorrhagic stroke or other severe bleeding problems. The rate of mild bleeding events (such as bruising or oozing from puncture sites) was slightly higher among the clopidogrel-plus-aspirin users.

TIMING MATTERS BIG TIME

Because this study was conducted in China, some experts would like to see the results confirmed before the two-pill therapy becomes the standard of care in the US. It's also worth noting that, because the study follow-up period lasted 90 days, it's not known whether any participants went on to have strokes later—but remember, the riskiest period for stroke occurs right after a TIA. That's why the researchers said that starting treatment with clopidogrel-plus-aspirin as soon as possible after TIA symptoms appear is likely to produce the greatest benefit. Note that doctors generally recommend that TIA patients stay on antiplatelet therapy indefinitely.

What to watch for: The most typical warning signs of a TIA are exactly the same as those of a stroke—sudden numbness or weakness of the face, arm or leg, especially on one side of the body...sudden confusion or trouble speaking or understanding speech...sudden loss of balance or coordination or difficulty with walking...sudden problems with vision in one or both eyes...and/or a sudden, severe headache with no known cause.

As soon as symptoms appear: Seek emergency medical help without delay! If it turns out that you are having a TIA, ask your doctor whether the dual clopidogrel-plus-aspirin therapy is right for you. Remember, the sooner you get started on the treatment, the better your chances of avoiding a full-blown stroke.

Exciting New Treatment for Stroke Victims

Randolph S. Marshall, MD, chief, stroke division, The Neurological Institute of New York at Columbia University Medical Center in New York City.

Imagine looking at a wall clock and seeing only the right half of the face...or hearing only sounds that come from your right. Not seeing or responding to stimuli on the left side is a fact of life for about 50% of stroke patients due to a brain condition called hemispatial neglect ("hemineglect"). Only about half of hemineglect patients go on to recover without treatment, and recovery can take days to years, depending on the severity of the stroke. Now a recent study brings good news...it reveals that applying magnetic stimulation daily for just two weeks to certain areas of the brain may jump-start recovery and help stroke survivors see, hear and respond normally.

This technique, called continuous theta-burst stimulation or TBS, was developed about 15 years ago primarily to treat depression. But if future research confirms the recent findings, it could soon be used to treat stroke victims, too. Researchers at the Santa Lucia Foundation in Rome performed the study, which was published in *Neurology*.

REBALANCING THE BRAIN

When a stroke affects the right side of the brain, it causes hyperactivity on the left side of the brain, and this is what leads to an inability to see, hear and/or respond to stimuli on the left. Hemineglect can technically occur on either side of the brain, but because of the brain's anatomy, the sensory deficit most often occurs on the left.

The traditional treatment for hemineglect consists of mental rehab tasks, for example, matching objects on a computer screen, completing paper-and-pencil tasks to improve visual scanning (for example, the ability to find a friend in a crowded restaurant) and doing physical therapy exercises (such as repetitive movements of the arm or leg) to improve motor skills. Researchers wanted to investigate whether several weeks of TBS therapy would promote faster and longer-term recovery.

A STIMULATING STUDY

Twenty patients who had had strokes causing hemineglect participated in the four-week study. Five days a week, all participants took part in standard mental and physical rehab sessions. For the first two weeks of the study, though, on weekday mornings, all patients had 15 minutes of either "real" or "sham" TBS sessions. Then, to measure whether participants had improvement in their ability to perceive stimuli that take place on their left sides, researchers gave participants the Behavioral Inattention Test (BIT), which covered such tasks as drawing, dialing a phone and reading a menu.

The results: Researchers found that test scores for those who received real TBS treatment improved by 16% immediately following the two weeks of therapy, revealing that perception and response to left-side stimuli had improved. After four weeks, TBS patients showed a 23% improvement in test scores, indicating that TBS benefits continued after treatment had ended—and grew. On the other hand, participants receiving sham TBS showed no clinically significant improvements in test scores after two or four weeks.

A TREATMENT OF THE FUTURE

Randolph S. Marshall, MD, chief of the stroke division at The Neurological Institute of New York at Columbia University Medical Center in New York City and coauthor of the accompanying editorial in the journal, said that this study showed the longest-lasting effect of TBS thus far and that once patients with hemineglect start to improve, the improvement usually continues. No one knows exactly how TBS works in the brain, but Dr. Marshall said it seems to make neuron firing less frequent and thus calms the overexcitability in the brain.

Psychiatrists who administer TBS for depression conduct treatments in their offices and clinics, but for now, TBS for hemineglect is taking place only for research at some teaching hospitals, said Dr. Marshall. So you can't even ask for it off-label right now, un-

fortunately. More research will help discover how to maximize the treatment's effectiveness, figure out which patients are most likely to benefit from it and identify potential side effects—and it will help persuade insurance companies to cover the cost. (TBS sessions for depression run from about $200 to $300 each.) Dr. Marshall anticipates that within a few years, the country's network of specialized stroke centers will have doctors trained and ready to put TBS therapy into practice.

After a Stroke, the Patient's Blood Sugar Should Be Monitored Carefully

Hyperglycemia—high blood sugar—has been linked to poorer outcomes after a stroke. The patient's temperature should remain between 95.9°F and 99.5°F. For each 1° Celsius (approximately 1.8° Fahrenheit) increase in body temperature, risk for death or severe disability more than doubles. The patient should lie flat for 24 hours. Sitting upright decreases blood flow to the brain. If the person has difficulty breathing when lying prone, keep the head of his/her bed at the lowest elevation that he can tolerate.

Study of stroke patients by researchers at Loyola University Medical Center, Maywood, Illinois, published in *MedLink Neurology*.

Treatment Improves Stroke Recovery

Research on stent retrievers was halted early because patients showed such significant benefit—including a 70% increase in functional independence 90 days after a stroke.

How the retrievers are used: The stent is inserted into an artery in the groin and guided to the brain clot. The stent grabs the clot and is pulled out. Side effects may include bleeding in the brain—but the benefits outweigh the risks.

Igor Rybinnik, MD, medical director of the Comprehensive Stroke Center at Robert Wood Johnson University Hospital, Rahway, New Jersey.

Reduce Poststroke Disability

According to a preliminary study, 42% of female patients who received IV uric acid in addition to the usual treatment, the clot-busting drug tPA, were relatively free of disability three months after a stroke compared with 29% of women given tPa and no uric acid. Little difference was found among men.

Theory: Men tend to have higher blood levels of uric acid.

Ángel Chamorro, MD, PhD, director of the Comprehensive Stroke Center, Hospital Clinic, University of Barcelona, Spain, and senior author of a study of 411 patients, published in *Stroke*.

Bed Position Important

Better stroke recovery depends on bed position. Doctors must evaluate the type of stroke and initial progress of the patient to decide what bed position in the first 24 to 48 hours is best for recovery. Sitting upright can harm some patients by decreasing blood flow to the brain. For those patients, lying flat can improve blood flow. But if a stroke increases brain swelling, sitting upright can improve blood drainage and make damage from the swelling less likely. Ask your doctor which position is best for you.

Murray Flaster, MD, PhD, a neurologist and stroke specialist at Loyola University Medical Center, Maywood, Illinois. He reported on stroke-care issues in *MedLink Neurology*.

Do-It-Yourself Stroke Rehab? Surprising Findings...

Pamela Woods Duncan, PhD, PT, professor of physical therapy, Duke University School of Medicine, Durham, North Carolina.

While many people survive strokes and manage to keep their own "selves" very much intact, for others the remnant physical or mental damage of the stroke goes on and on. Careers and relationships suffer when a formerly vibrant, independent person is transformed into one who is in need of assistance for everything from driving to dialing the phone to showering and dressing.

Since 1995, survival rates for stroke patients have been boosted by nearly 30%—but, sadly, many of those patients have remained deeply impaired. They have trouble walking and they are at high risk for falls. Innovative therapies have been developed for physical therapy to aid in recovery. While helpful, much of this technology is expensive to develop, costly to purchase and must be administered by a trained specialist as part of a structured exercise program, putting it out of reach for many patients.

Now a study from Duke University has taken the results of patients doing intensive, center-based rehab with high-tech equipment and compared them with the results of people who work at home with a visiting physical therapist. The researchers also investigated whether rehab started long after a stroke—as much as six months later—still can be helpful.

EXCITING, UNEXPECTED RESULTS

The study examined the progress of 408 stroke survivors, all of whom had their strokes either two months or six months earlier. Some of the patients who had suffered strokes six months previously were wait-listed to begin therapy at a center and so had not received any rehab. All of the patients were divided into three groups. Those who had strokes two months previously either underwent therapy in a center for high-tech rehab (group one)...or had home-based rehab with a therapist (group two), emphasizing progressive strength, balance and walking exercises. The third group

229

of patients—those who were wait-listed—also started the high-tech program. Rehab for all groups took place in three weekly sessions over 12 weeks.

Pamela Woods Duncan, PhD, PT, professor of physical therapy at Duke University School of Medicine explained that the goal of the study was to determine how well patients functioned one year after a stroke with different therapy protocols—and that the research yielded two excellent findings.

First, while the researchers had anticipated that high-tech rehab would be more effective, much to their surprise that was not the case. "Using technology was not superior to working with patients at home in function, balance and walking exercises," Dr. Duncan said.

Furthermore, the study put to rest the belief that only early rehab works. The results were the same in all three groups including the late starters—52% of all patients showed significant improvement, walking well in the home and walking more in their communities.

ON YOUR OWN?

Stroke patients absolutely need rehabilitation and regular exercise, Dr. Duncan said, but added that it would be a grave mistake to misinterpret these findings to mean that stroke patients can do well simply by exercising on their own at home. Stroke patients need careful cardiovascular monitoring and a trained therapist to design and conduct a program that is in keeping with their progress. Safety is an issue, especially early on in rehab when the risk of falling is high—so using professional therapists, at least initially, is critical. That said, in-home therapy uses less expensive equipment (such as elastic bands), requires less training for therapists and needs fewer clinical staff members than in-patient care. And, physical therapy for stroke patients is not just a 12-week endeavor—it must be a lifelong habit in order to keep the muscles strong and supple. Developing an at-home therapy plan that can be administered by family members can be cost-effective and also very helpful at maintaining and even continuing to improve the physical function of the patient.

New Device Reduces Stroke Risk

The Enroute Transcarotid Neuroprotection System (TNS) provides a way for doctors to access neck arteries through an incision in the neck, rather than through the groin. The system is for patients with narrowed carotid arteries who have twisted blood vessels that don't allow access via the groin. Enroute TNS has been approved by the FDA for people undergoing procedures to restore normal blood flow in neck arteries.

William Maisel, MD, MPH, chief scientist and deputy center director for science, Center for Devices and Radiological Health, US Food and Drug Administration, Silver Spring, Maryland.

Better Than Stents

Aggressive nonsurgical treatment prevents stroke recurrence more effectively than stents.

Recent finding: People at high risk for a second stroke who received anticlotting medications and intense management of cardiovascular risks (blood pressure and cholesterol) and who strictly adhered to a lifestyle-modification program (diet and exercise) had fewer incidences of stroke recurrence than patients who received this treatment in addition to receiving a stent.

Colin P. Derdeyn, MD, professor of radiology, neurology and neurological surgery at Washington University School of Medicine in St. Louis and lead author of a study published in *The Lancet.*

PT and Stroke Recovery

Even a year after surviving a severe stroke, intense physical therapy helps patients recover a surprising amount of arm function.

Recent study: 39 patients (a year or more post-stroke) who did physical therapy involving exercises, electrical stimulation and/or a robotic device five hours a day, five days a week for 12 weeks doubled or nearly doubled their ability to do everyday activities, such as placing the affected arm into a sweater sleeve.

Janis Daly, PhD, professor of neurology, University of Florida College of Medicine, Gainesville.

Yoga Boosts Balance Long After a Stroke

Arlene A. Schmid, PhD, OTR (occupational therapist registered), an assistant professor in the department of occupational therapy at Indiana University and a rehabilitation research scientist at Roudebush VA Medical Center, both in Indianapolis. She is lead author of a study on yoga and balance published in *Stroke*.

Many people think of yoga as exercise for the limber-limbed young. So you may be happily surprised to learn that yoga can help stroke survivors improve their balance and become more active—even if they start practicing yoga long after their strokes occurred.

This news from a small but encouraging study is important because stroke victims often are left with long-term balance problems that contribute to disability and increase the risk for potentially fatal falls. What's more, the study results challenge the discouraging yet common notion that significant improvement in motor skills is unlikely when more than six months have passed since a patient's stroke.

Study scoop: Participants included 47 adults, average age 63, who had suffered strokes anywhere from six months to more than 11 years earlier. All had finished their stroke rehabilitation programs…could stand on their own or with a device…and continued to receive usual medical care throughout the study. For eight weeks, one group of participants attended twice-weekly hour-long group classes involving modified yoga postures, breathing techniques and meditation, with classes growing more challenging over time. A second "yoga-plus" group took the same yoga classes and also received an audio recording of yoga/relaxation techniques to use

three times weekly at home. A third group, which served as a control, received no yoga instruction. All participants completed tests of balance, independence and quality of life at the start and end of the study.

Results: No significant changes were seen in the control group. In contrast, members of both the yoga and yoga-plus groups experienced significant improvement in their ability to balance and raised their scores on tests of independence and quality of life. Yoga participants also felt less afraid of falling and reported attempting more challenging activities because of their improved balance—for instance, they talked about walking through a grocery store instead of using a motorized scooter…being able to take a shower…and feeling inspired to visit friends. (Comparing the two yoga groups, the addition of the audio recording did not change the results significantly, though the yoga-plus people did report enjoying listening to it.)

How does yoga work its magic? Researchers suggested that yoga's mind-body connection may make it more therapeutic than traditional exercise…and that yoga is especially effective in improving poststroke function because it promotes coordination of complex movements, balance, strengthening and breathing.

Stroke patients: Ask your doctor or occupational therapist whether yoga is appropriate for you. If so, request a referral to a registered yoga therapist who is experienced in working with stroke survivors.

Singing Gives Speech Back to Mute Stroke Patients

Study titled "Melodic intonation therapy: back to basics for future research," published in *Frontiers in Neurology*.

For hundreds of years, scientists, physicians and others have observed that many people who cannot speak well or even speak at all—folks who have had a stroke, for instance—can still sing perfectly well. So this concept is being applied to a specific type of stroke rehabilitation therapy that can help you or a loved one make a comeback if stroke robs you of the ability to speak. The technique may also help people who have other serious neurologic problems that take away their voices. *Here's how this marvelous speech-restoring technique, called melodic intonation therapy, works its magic…*

AT A LOSS FOR WORDS

Mute is what we call the inability to speak. The technical terms are apraxia of speech (AOS), in which people know what they want to say (and what it means) but can't say it because a brain glitch makes their speech muscles uncooperative…and aphasia, in which people have trouble (to greater or lesser degree) understanding language or even the concept of speech because of damage to the main language centers in the left half of their brains. Aphasia and AOS often happen at the same time because of a stroke.

It's often difficult for doctors to know whether a mute stroke patient is suffering from aphasia or only AOS, but, either way, a technique called melodic intonation therapy, or MIT, can help the patient get his or her voice back by "remodeling" the brain. Although MIT has long been used to help patients with aphasia speak, its greater success might be its impact on AOS. This idea comes from a review of the scientific literature, which showed that MIT works better in patients who have a sense of grammar—such as adult patients with known AOS due to stroke—than in patients whose stroke has strongly affected their ability to understand language.

This means MIT can help people other than stroke patients—including, for example, people with Parkinson's, palsy or other serious neurologic diseases that affect their muscles rather than their cognitive ability to recognize language. If you have faced a speech challenge with little success from other therapies, MIT could be a game changer for you.

FROM SONG TO SPEECH

MIT is a technique that uses a patient's ability to sing—which is often preserved even

when the ability to speak is gone—to get him or her to be able to speak again. In this way, it is similar to music therapy used for people who stutter (and also for children who are mute because of AOS), but MIT aims to get the right part of the brain to take on new tasks and grow in new ways to compensate for the left part damaged by a stroke.

How it's done: First, patients listen to and hum along with a therapist. This leads to singing common phrases in unison with the therapist, such as "Good morning," "How are you?" or "Please pass the salt." The phrases are sung in an exaggerated manner—as if performing on a Broadway stage. As the patient sings the phrases, he or she uses the left hand (which, unlike the right hand, is generally unaffected when a stroke strikes the left side of the brain) to tap out the rhythm. This helps stimulate new language pathways in the right brain to make up for the damaged parts in the left.

The stroke patient goes on to practice singing phrases unaccompanied by the therapist and practices longer, more complex phrases. Eventually, the singing is phased out, leaving the patient with a new way to speak. In other words, the patient can stop singing the notes…and keep saying the words.

WHO BENEFITS MOST

Depending on the type and extent of stroke injury a person has, he or she may be able to return to near normal speech or simply be helped to communicate basic needs. *Generally, though, MIT works best in a stroke patient—or anyone—who can…*

• **Understand words spoken by others** but has great difficulty or an inability to repeat words spoken by others.

• **Clearly sing along to well-known songs** but make only nonsense words or mere syllables when he or she tries to speak.

• **Pay attention and have the motivation to want to speak again.**

So if someone close to you has a stroke that leaves him or her without speech or unable to sensibly say words or sentences—or if that person is you—don't assume the silence can't be broken. Ask the neurologist or other health practitioner who is arranging rehabilitation about including MIT in that care. And because MIT may be particularly effective in people who lose the ability to speak because of palsy and other neurodegenerative disorders, such patients or their loved ones ought to inquire about trying MIT instead of traditional music therapy. It could be a breakthrough that transforms the quality of life.

Vision Rehab: Helping Stroke Patients to See Again

Krystel R. Huxlin, PhD, a neuroscientist and professor of ophthalmology at the Flaum Eye Institute at the University of Rochester School of Medicine and Dentistry in New York. Her research on visual retraining for stroke patients has been published in *The Journal of Neuroscience.*

NovaVision.com

When you think of all the devastating consequences of stroke, visual impairment may not be one of the first to come to mind...yet about 20% to 25% of stroke victims are left with vision problems. These visual deficits were once thought to be permanent—but now a promising new therapy is helping train the brain to see better again. Software used for this therapy is now FDA approved and commercially available. Interested patients may also be able to benefit by participating in ongoing research studies.

Krystel R. Huxlin, PhD, a professor of ophthalmology at the Flaum Eye Institute at the University of Rochester School of Medicine and Dentistry, is a researcher at the forefront of the development of the technique. She explained that stroke patients who suffer damage to a part of the brain called the primary visual cortex typically are blind in one-quarter to one-half of their normal visual field.

Reason: The primary visual cortex acts as a gateway for the transfer of information between the eyes and the other brain areas that process visual information. If that gateway is damaged by stroke, patients may have prob-

lems with most everyday activities, including reading, driving and even walking.

HOW VISION RETRAINING WORKS

To address the problem, Dr. Huxlin explained, her team first runs tests to map a patient's blind field and understand his or her exact visual impairments. Then, the visual retraining software is customized to address that patient's needs.

On a home computer, the patient uses the specialized software to do targeted visual exercises for about an hour at least five days per week. Dr. Huxlin's patients train for a minimum of three months—and most choose to continue much longer because their blind field continues to shrink and results are so rewarding.

During each training session, the patient fixes her gaze on a small black square in the middle of the screen. Every few seconds, a group of about 100 small dots appears within a circle on the screen that is somewhere in her damaged visual field. The dots appear to move as a group to the left or right, then disappear after half a second. The patient decides which way the dots are moving, indicating her choice with the keyboard. A chime signals whether she has chosen correctly, providing feedback that speeds up learning.

At first, most patients cannot actually see the dots, but nonetheless their brains are able to sense that the dots are moving, Dr. Huxlin said. With practice, a patient's brain eventually recovers the ability to consciously perceive the dots and discern the direction of their movement in the retrained blind field location. Then, the researchers move the dots to another spot in her blind field so the brain can start relearning how to see the new area.

Secret to success: The therapy exploits a phenomenon called blindsight, in which a stroke patient's eyes are able to take in visual information but the damaged brain cannot make sense of it to create conscious vision. "The training drives whatever spared visual circuitry the person still has, making it work harder, so eventually that visual information is brought into consciousness," said Dr. Huxlin. The 17 patients she has studied so far who trained as prescribed all had significantly improved vision. The improvement seems to be permanent—and some patients have even been able to regain a driver's license.

WHO CAN BENEFIT

Visual retraining potentially can benefit patients whose strokes were recent and those whose strokes occurred several years ago, Dr. Huxlin said, provided they are not totally blind. Patients also must be able to complete basic tasks, such as using a computer, fixating points on the screen precisely, pressing keys and following instructions.

A version of computer-based, at-home visual retraining or vision restoration theray (VRT) is available from the company NovaVision. NovaVision has the only FDA-approved VRT program in the US, according to its website, NovaVision.com.

Software from Dr. Huxlin's specific research is currently not available commercially. But stroke survivors interested in participating in Dr. Huxlin's ongoing research can e-mail her at khuxlin@ur.rochester.edu to see if they meet the criteria for study enrollment and, if so, they will be put on a waiting list.

Also helpful: Dr. Huxlin said that, in addition to visual retraining, stroke sufferers can help compensate for vision loss by staying as physically active as possible—for instance, by playing sports such as golf or tennis or by regularly taking walks around the neighborhood or a park. "Those kinds of activities force you to make up for visual deficits by moving your head and eyes more. This pushes your visual system to be more actively engaged—to search for and find the information you need to extract from your environment in order to function," she explained. For patients unable to engage in sports or walk outside, playing action video games would be a reasonable alternative, she added.

Bottom line: For stroke survivors, the future has never looked brighter.

Can Stroking Prevent Stroke?

Melissa Faith Davis, BS, and Christopher Car Lay, BS, graduate student researchers, dynamic brain reorganization, department of neurobiology and behavior, University of California-Irvine.

An astonishingly simple, easy-to-do intervention may help stroke victims—perhaps even slowing or stopping the resulting destruction of brain tissue that causes disability. What is it? Gentle stroking, light touch, soft music or other forms of sensory stimulation…it's really that basic!

This intriguing discovery involved tickling the whiskers of rats while they were having strokes, and it falls into the "really surprising" category because the benefit was far more dramatic than what researchers expected.

How did tickling stop a stroke? Imaging revealed that the sensory stimulation provided by stroking the whisker prompted the blocked blood to find new pathways into the cerebral cortex, the part of the brain affected by the stroke.

There are some caveats: This worked only when the whiskers were tickled within an hour or two of the onset of the stroke—if more than three hours had passed since the stroke began, it actually made the stroke worse. This time limit is consistent with what happens when strokes in people are treated with tPA (tissue plasminogen activator), Davis pointed out. And it's not yet known whether this sort of stimulation would be safe for a person who has had a hemorrhagic stroke (caused by a broken blood vessel in the brain rather than a blockage, which accounts for about 15% of all strokes) since it might increase bleeding or have another as yet unknown neurological effect.

HOW DOES THIS HELP HUMANS?

Early stroke symptoms generally provide information about the part of the brain that is being affected—whether the visual center, auditory or motor control. So if a person has suffered a stroke in the auditory cortex (where sound is recognized), it may be that playing music will bring more blood to that part of the brain, possibly rescuing it from blood deprivation and potential damage. This is as yet theoretical, but the research team is already studying the practical applications. The day may not be far off when instead of keeping a stroke patient quiet, as is currently the standard practice, health-care professionals will instead lightly pat the person's hands and face…sing…play cartoons…or provide other forms of sensory stimulation to keep fresh blood flowing in the victim's brain.

An Epilepsy Drug May Be the Answer to Stroke Survival

Mark S. Shapiro, PhD, professor, and Sonya M. Bierbower, PhD, postdoctoral fellow, department of physiology, University of Texas Health Science Center, San Antonio. Their study was published in *The Journal of Neuroscience.*

Fast action is needed to survive a stroke. Once brain cells die due to lack of oxygen during an ischemic stroke (a stroke caused by a blood clot), there's no saving them, and reactive oxygen species released by the dying cells injure nearby brain tissue. A quick dose of the clot buster tPA can come to the rescue, but it has to be given within the first four hours after a stroke, and its use is limited because its blood-thinning effects are so powerful. It is not an option for patients who have high blood pressure, a history of bleeding or weak blood vessels. But a drug used to treat another serious health condition that works in an entirely different way may allow many more people to survive strokes with minimal disability.

SOOTHES BRAIN CELLS

The drug is *retigabine* (also called *ezogabine*, brand name Potiga), an antiseizure drug for certain forms of epilepsy. Retigabine treats epilepsy by reducing the electrical activity of nerve cells that are out of control because of excessive electrical firing during an epileptic

seizure. The researchers theorized that retigabine may reduce damage to the brain in stroke patients by decreasing the excitability of the dying nerve cells and preventing the cells from firing when they really should be preserving their strength.

The researchers are not entirely sure that the drug will have the same effect in people as it did in mice, but retigabine has been on the market and used in humans since 2011 for treating epilepsy. Although the drug isn't currently FDA-approved to treat ischemic strokes, doctors can use the drug off-label for conditions other than epilepsy and may consider doing so if evidence mounts about retigabine's lifesaving potential. Like all drugs, it can cause side effects, which can include mild and temporary imbalance, drowsiness or confusion, vision loss, and pain or difficulty urinating. Whereas the drug is used on a daily basis in patients with epilepsy, it would be used, like tPA, as a one-time emergency medication in stroke patients and so any side effects would not persist longer than a day or two. However, the research suggests that the prevention of brain damage would be permanent. Thus the benefits will need to be weighed against risks as research about the drug for stroke patients continues.

In the meantime, researchers are planning clinical trials of the drug for stroke patients that will likely compare its effectiveness and safety to tPA. If you know that you are at high risk for stroke, you may want to speak with your doctor about participating in a clinical trial of retigabine and also discuss what emergency-care plan is in place for you should you have a stroke.

Better Stroke Recovery

Forty-eight stroke survivors underwent conventional gait rehabilitation. Half of them also had 20 sessions of electromechanical robotic gait training. With this therapy, an electromechanical device moves a patient's feet and is controlled by a physical therapist who progressively increases the patient's weight load and walking pace. Among the most severely impaired, five times more patients who received robotic therapy were able to walk unassisted after two years. Robotic therapy made little difference among the less severely impaired.

Giovanni Morone, MD, physiatry specialist, Santa Lucia Foundation, Institute for Research Hospitalization and Health Care, Rome, Italy.

Magnets May Help Stroke Patients

In a procedure called repetitive transcranial magnetic stimulation, electromagnets are strategically placed on a stroke patient's head. The magnets deliver tiny electric currents to the area of the brain affected by the stroke, reducing muscle weakness and improving overall motor function.

Recent finding: Patients given this treatment in addition to physical therapy showed significant improvement in motor function, compared with those who did not receive brain stimulation. Study participants had strokes between one and 36 months before starting this treatment.

Anwar Etribi, PhD, emeritus professor of neurology, Ain Shams University, Cairo, Egypt, and leader of a study published in *European Journal of Neurology*.

Can Antidepressants Help With Stroke Recovery?

Robert Robinson, MD, Penningroth professor and head of psychiatry, Carver College of Medicine, The University of Iowa, Iowa City. Dr. Robinson is internationally recognized as an expert in the study of poststroke depression.

Scientists keep working to try to make further improvements in stroke prevention and rehabilitation. Recently, they have come up with a novel way to speed recovery…and extend progress. Would you believe it's as simple as taking a short course of antidepressants?

ENCOURAGING NEW BRAIN CELLS TO GROW

Recent research shows that poststroke depression slowed recovery and made patients more likely to die. The much better news is that additional research has discovered antidepressants improve recovery both in stroke patients who are depressed—and also in those who are not.

The Modified Rankin Scale, a measure of physical and motor disability, is used to evaluate stroke and brain injuries. Study participants who took an antidepressant improved 1 to 1.5 categories, on average, over the placebo group when measured on the scale. For example, in some instances, people who initially could not manage daily activities such as dressing or feeding themselves were once again able to do so without help. Other patients who were unable to walk without assistance or were bedridden were able to walk independently or with assistance.

The placebo group also improved for several months, but their progress then leveled off. The antidepressant group continued to make progress for at least nine additional months after they had stopped taking the medication. It's possible that improvements lasted even longer, but the study ended at one year.

Other research demonstrates that antidepressants encourage cognitive recovery and, perhaps most impressively, nearly double your chances of survival six to nine years poststroke, according to researchers. Although scientists don't know exactly how antidepressants work this particular magic, it's likely that they block inflammation. When you have a stroke, your body releases inflammatory proteins that block cellular growth. By inhibiting the release of these proteins, antidepressants encourage the growth of new cells and allow your brain to recover more rapidly from its injury.

Study results were published online in the *American Journal of Geriatric Psychiatry*.

HEALING CONTINUES AFTER MEDICATION STOPS

The idea that antidepressants might benefit early recovery from stroke has been around for a number of years. But one major question left unanswered by previous studies was, "Does the effect last after the medication stops?" What the recent study demonstrates is that not only does the beneficial effect last, but the improvement in physical recovery continues to increase even after the patients stop taking the medication.

Researchers continue to confirm the valuable role that antidepressants can play in stroke recovery. Meanwhile, if you or a loved one suffers a stroke, it seems logical to ask your doctor whether a short course (at least) of an antidepressant makes sense.

To locate a stroke rehabilitation center near you, contact the Commission on Accreditation of Rehabilitation Facilities (888-281-6531, carf.org/advancedProviderSearch.aspx).

Incredible Eggs!

Eating up to one egg each day cut stroke risk by 12%—without increasing risk for heart disease—a new study of more than 300,000 adults has found.

Theory: Eggs are rich in antioxidants (shown to reduce inflammation) and protein—both of which help lower blood pressure, an important risk factor for stroke.

Important: The new Dietary Guidelines for Americans eliminates restrictions on dietary cholesterol and notes that eggs are an inexpensive source of important nutrients.

Dominik D. Alexander, PhD, MSPH, principal epidemiologist, EpidStat Institute, Ann Arbor, Michigan.

Carotid Artery Blockage

One of your carotid arteries has a complete blockage, but your doctor said surgery to clear it is too risky. Is this dangerous?

When a carotid artery is 100% blocked and is discovered while testing for another health condition, typically no procedure would be recommended. If the blockage has not already caused a stroke, it is unlikely to do so in the future, and if other arteries are clear, they can continue supplying blood to the brain. Surgery can be risky because there's a chance that a small clot or piece of plaque could break loose and travel to the brain, causing a stroke.

In lieu of surgery, your doctor may recommend medication—aspirin or clopidogrel (Plavix), for example—and lifestyle changes. If you begin having symptoms such as dizziness, blurred vision, weakness, and/or numbness, it might make sense to have a procedure to treat it, such as a carotid endarterectomy (surgical removal of plaque) or the insertion of a stent to hold the artery open. All these options should be discussed with your doctor.

Deepak L. Bhatt, MD, MPH, executive director of interventional cardiovascular programs, Brigham and Women's Hospital, Boston.

Brain Bleed Danger

Smoking increases the risk for brain hemorrhages. New study results show that female smokers are at a much greater risk for bleeding in the lining of the brain than nonsmokers. Women who smoked 21 to 30 cigarettes a day were 8.35 times more likely to have a subarachnoid hemorrhage than nonsmokers. While the risk increased for men, it was not as great—men who smoked the same number of cigarettes a day were 2.76 times more likely to have a brain hemorrhage than nonsmokers.

Analysis of data on 65,521 adults, average age of 45, who had taken part in a Finnish national survey beginning in 1972 and who were followed up for an average of 21 years, led by researchers at University of Helsinki, Finland, and published in *Stroke*.

PART 2

Make a Healthy Brain

CHAPTER 8

Brain Fitness

Best Workouts to Keep Your Brain "Buff"

We all want to keep our brains in top shape. But are crossword puzzles, online classes and the other such activities that we've been hearing about for years the best ways to do that? Not really.

Now: To improve memory and preserve overall cognitive function, the latest research reveals that it takes more than quiet puzzle-solving and streaming lectures.

Even more intriguing: Some activities that we once thought were time wasters may actually help build intellectual capacity and other cognitive functions.

Cynthia R. Green, PhD, a psychologist and a leading brain trainer explained more about the most effective ways to keep your brain "buff"…

A HEALTHY BRAIN

The most important steps to keep your brain performing at optimal levels are lifestyle choices…

• **Getting aerobic exercise (at least 150 minutes per week).**

• **Maintaining a healthy body weight.**

• **Not smoking.**

• **Eating a diet that emphasizes fruits and vegetables and is low in refined sugar and white flour**—two of the biggest dietary threats to brain health that have recently been identified by researchers.

Additional benefits are possible with regular brain workouts. In the past, experts thought that nearly any game or activity that challeng-

---

Cynthia R. Green, PhD, a practicing clinical psychologist and the founder and president of Memory Arts, LLC, a brain-health and memory fitness consulting service in Montclair, New Jersey, TotalBrainHealth.com. She is also founding director of the Memory Enhancement Program at the Icahn School of Medicine at Mount Sinai in New York City. She is author of *Your Best Brain Ever: A Complete Guide & Workout.*

es you to think would improve your general brain functioning.

What research now tells us: An increasing body of evidence shows that improved memory requires something more—you need to work against a clock. Games with a time limit force you to think quickly and with agility. These are the factors that lead to improved memory and mental focus. Among Dr. Green's favorite brain workouts—aim for at least 30 minutes daily of any combination of the activities below...

BRAINY COMPUTER GAMES

Specialized brain-training computer programs (such as Lumosity, Fit Brains and CogniFit) are no longer the darlings of the health community. Formerly marketed as a fun way to reduce one's risk for dementia, recent evidence has not supported that claim.

These programs do provide, however, a variety of activities that may help improve intellectual performance, attention, memory and mental flexibility. Lumosity and other programs are a good option for people who enjoy a regimented brain workout, including such activities as remembering sequences and ignoring distractions. Monthly prices range from $4.99 to $19.95.

Other options to consider trying...

• **Action video games.** These games were once considered "brain-numbing" activities that kept players from developing intellectual and social skills. Recent research, however, shows that action video games can promote mental focus, flexible thinking, and decision-making and problem-solving skills. Because these games are timed, they also require quick responses from the players.

Good choices: *World of Warcraft*, *The Elder Scrolls* and *Guild Wars*, all of which involve role-playing by assuming the identity of various characters to battle foes and complete quests, often with other virtual players. These games are available in DVD format for Mac or PC and with an online subscription for virtual play.

Caveat: An hour or two can be a brain booster, but don't overdo it. Too much role-playing takes you away from real-life interactions.

• **Free brain-boosting computer game for a cause.** At FreeRice.com, you can answer fun and challenging questions in such subjects as English vocabulary, foreign languages, math and humanities. With each correct answer, the United Nations World Food Programme donates 10 grains of rice to a Third World country. To date, players have "earned" a total of nearly 100 billion grains of rice—enough to create more than 10 million meals.

To increase the challenge: Set a timer so that you must work against the clock.

APPS FOR YOUR BRAIN

If you'd prefer to use an "app"—a software application that you can use on a smartphone or similar electronic device—there are several good options. *Among the best fun/challenging apps (free on Android and Apple)...*

• **Words with Friends.** This ever-popular game allows you to play a Scrabble-like game against your friends who have also downloaded the app on an electronic device. The game provides even more benefits if it's used with the time-clock feature.

• **Word Streak with Friends** (formerly Scramble with Friends) is a timed find-a-word game. You can play on your own or with friends.

• **Elevate** was named Apple's Best App of 2014. It provides a structured game environment that feels more like a test, focusing on reading, writing and math skills, than a game. Still, this timed app will give Apple users a good brain challenge.

TECH-FREE OPTIONS

If you'd rather not stare at the screen of a computer or some other electronic device for your brain workout, here are some good options...

• **Tech-free games.** SET is a fast-paced card game that tests your visual perception skills. Players race to find a set of three matching cards (based on color, shape, number or shading) from an array of cards placed on a table.

Bonus: This game can be played by one player or as many people as can fit around the table. The winner of dozens of "Best Game" awards, including the high-IQ group Mensa's

Select award, SET is fun for kids and adults alike.

Another good choice: Boggle, which challenges you to create words from a given set of letter cubes within a three-minute period. It can be played by two or more people.

• **Drumming.** Playing any musical instrument requires attention and a keen sense of timing. Basic drumming is a great activity for beginner musicians (especially if you don't have the finger dexterity for piano or guitar).

Even better: Join a drumming circle, which provides the extra challenge of matching your timing and rhythm to the rest of the drummers, along with opportunities for socialization.

Bonus: Research has demonstrated that some forms, such as African djembe drumming, count as a low- to moderate-intensity activity that may reduce blood pressure, which helps protect the brain from blood vessel damage.

• **Meditation.** This practice improves cognitive function and sensory processing and promotes mental focus. Meditating for about 30 minutes daily has also been linked to greater blood flow to the brain and increased gray matter (associated with positive emotions, memory and decision-making). The benefits have even been seen among some people with early-stage neurodegenerative diseases, such as Alzheimer's disease.

A good way to get started: Begin with a simple "mindful eating" exercise—spend the first five minutes of each meal really focusing on what you're eating. Don't talk, read the paper or watch TV...just savor the food. Eventually, you'll want to expand this level of attention to other parts of your day. Such mindfulness habits are a good complement to a regular meditation practice.

• **Coloring.** If you have kids or grandkids, don't just send them off with their crayons. Color with them.

Even better: Get one of the new breed of coloring books with complex designs for adults. While there hasn't been specific research addressing the brain benefits of coloring, this form of play has been shown to reduce stress in children, and it is thought to boost creativity and have a meditative quality.

You can find coloring books made for adults at bookstores and art-supply stores.

Are Brain Games Bogus?

Cynthia R. Green, PhD, clinical psychologist, and founder and president, Memory Arts, LLC, a brain-health and memory fitness consulting service, Montclair, New Jersey. She is also founding director of The Memory Enhancement Program at Mount Sinai School of Medicine in New York City. She is author of *Your Best Brain Ever: A Complete Guide & Workout.* TotalBrainHealth.com

Lumosity makes online brain games. It also made false advertising claims for years, according to the Federal Trade Commission (FTC). "Lumosity preyed on consumers' fears about age-related cognitive decline, suggesting its games could stave off memory loss, dementia and even Alzheimer's disease," according to the FTC. "But Lumosity simply did not have the science to back up its ads." In a settlement, the company agreed to nix the ads and refund $2 million to its one million paying subscribers.

Lumosity's brain games are fun to play, with their addictive inducements to click to test your ability to, for example, match colors or words ever more quickly, and they do sharpen skills such as speed, attention and memory while you play them. But the evidence has been lacking that they lead to real-life changes in how your brain functions in the real world—especially changes that could lead to preventing cognitive decline.

Perhaps what is most shameful, is that the years touting online training as just the "quick fix" that would keep our brains young has masked the real science of what brain fitness is all about, namely engaging in lifestyle behaviors that have been tied to staying sharp.

The Lumosity debacle does not mean that the online brain-training movement is (or should be) dead. Brain games have their place. Games that pit your cognitive skills against the clock do help you hone your attention and memory skills and mental flexibility. Lumosity's games fit into that category—but you can just as easily get them from video games or free apps on your smartphone.

The cognitive science behind brain games continues to evolve, so their potential can't be dismissed. There is promising work in using brain games to prevent, and even treat, depression, for example. A new medical field is emerging that uses neurofeedback—devices that let you see how your brain reacts in real time to your thoughts and emotions—to treat post-traumatic stress disorder (PTSD) and other attention and anxiety disorders.

Someday, new research may well discover that brain games slow down cognitive decline in aging. Or not. Brain games do no harm, and they sharpen certain cognitive skills, so go ahead and play them if you enjoy them. Just don't expect miracles.

In the meantime, it's best to focus on what we know is key to preserving brain health throughout life—regular exercise, a heart-healthy diet, a strong social network and continuing intellectual stimulation. Real brain health science lies in how we live.

How a Harvard Brain Specialist Keeps Her Own Brain Healthy

Marie Pasinski, MD, a memory specialist and neurologist who is on the faculty of Harvard Medical School and a staff neurologist at Massachusetts General Hospital, both in Boston. She is author, with Liz Neporent, of *Chicken Soup for the Soul: Boost Your Brain Power!*

Scientists used to believe that memory and other mental abilities inevitably declined with age. Not anymore. We now know that the brain has the ability to form new neurons and create new neural pathways throughout life. This means that your ability to remember and learn actually can get better as you age.

It doesn't take hard work—or complicated mental "workouts"—to improve mental agility. Here's what Marie Pasinski, MD, a memory

specialist at Harvard Medical School, does to keep her own brain healthy...

HANG OUT WITH FRIENDS

Close relationships are good for the brain. We have found that people who have supportive friends (or spouses) and rich social networks have better cognitive function and lower rates of dementia than those who spend more time alone.

When I take a break during my workday to go for a walk, I like to find someone to go with me. Exercising with friends is ideal because you can catch up on one another's lives while you get in shape.

It's not entirely clear why friendships are so important. One reason is purely mental—the brain is stimulated when you share ideas with other people. Mental stimulation increases the number of neurons and the connections among neurons. Social engagement lowers levels of stress hormones, which appear to be toxic to the neurons in the hippocampus—the brain's memory center. It also appears to lower blood pressure and reduce the risk for stroke.

Spend as much time as you can with people you care about—getting together with one close friend can be just as beneficial as hanging out with a group. Meeting new people is beneficial because it adds an extra jolt of stimulation. You can broaden your social network by volunteering or joining community groups.

DON'T LIVE ON AUTOPILOT

Routine is seductive. People like going to the same restaurants or taking the same route to work. The problem with routine is that it literally creates mental ruts—the brain uses only preexisting pathways and neural connections to complete familiar tasks. It stops growing and improving.

By embracing new experiences, you stimulate your brain to create neurons and forge additional neural pathways. This happens every time you extend your scope of experience and think in new ways. The more you challenge your brain—even when the "challenge" is as simple as looking at unfamiliar scenery—the more its functions improve.

For me, writing is a new experience. I can't spell to save my life. My worst course in college was English 101. When a friend suggested that I write a book about memory, I immediately dismissed the idea. Then, a few weeks later, I learned that Harvard was offering a course on publishing. I decided to take it. Now I've completed two books.

For me, shifting attention from medicine to writing was a radical change. But any change, even a small one, can help boost memory and thinking. If you take a new route to work, you will see different buildings. You will have to think about where you're going. This alone is enough to stimulate the brain's circuitry.

WORK BOTH SIDES OF THE BRAIN

A lot of my patients love to do crossword or other puzzles. They enjoy the challenge, and they've heard that mental activities improve memory. They're right—but only up to a point.

The improvements that you get from mental challenges quickly level off as you gain expertise.

Better: In addition to taking on new challenges, do things that work the underused side of your brain. If you're an accountant who crunches numbers all day, you're drawing heavily on the logical left side of the brain. Take up a hobby that works the right side, the imaginative side, such as painting or making pottery.

For me, playing the piano is a creative and welcome distraction from my work in medicine. I tried to learn to play when I was young, but my teacher was awful! I took it up again later in life. This time, I got to choose my own teacher, who has since become a close friend.

HAVE FUN

People who enjoy what they're doing get a mental boost. "Forcing" yourself to do things that aren't fun won't be anywhere near as good for your brain as activities that you genuinely enjoy. Also, enjoyment triggers the release of dopamine, a neurotransmitter that enhances learning and retention of new material.

I often ask patients to describe some of the things that they would like to do but have never done. Some would like to learn a new language. Others want to take up a new hobby, such as bird-watching or playing a sport. Ideally, whatever you choose will be both unfamiliar and fun.

I've tried all sorts of things in recent years, from joining Facebook and taking improv classes to competing in triathlons and gardening.

MOVE!

I do something physical every day. I enjoy biking, running, swimming, tennis and skiing. I also take jazz-dance classes.

Exercise triggers the release of brain-derived neurotrophic factor, a growth factor that promotes the formation of new synapses in the brain—the connections among brain cells that are critical for memory and other cognitive functions.

Exercise also increases the size of the brain. In one study, nonexercisers were given MRI scans to measure their brain volume. Then they were instructed to walk for 60 minutes, three days a week. After six months, they were given another MRI. The scans showed that they had an increase in the size of the prefrontal cortex, the part of the brain that is involved in reasoning, problem-solving and other "executive" functions.

Exercise also increases the size of the hippocampus, the area of the brain that is closely involved with memory. It improves circulation and helps prevent hypertension and other conditions that increase the risk for dementia.

Even if you don't enjoy "formal" exercise, you can get similar benefits just by moving more. I spend a lot of time at my computer, but I take a break every hour or so just to move around.

EAT BRAIN FOOD

A Mediterranean-style diet, with relatively little red meat and lots of fish, vegetables and whole grains, is the best diet for brain health. People who follow this diet have less atherosclerosis, hypertension and diabetes, conditions that cause inflammation and other brain changes that impair thinking and memory. *Fish and olive oil, two staples of the Mediterranean diet, are particularly good for the brain…*

• **Fish and omega-3s.** About two-thirds of the brain consists of fat. When you eat salmon, sardines or other cold-water fish, the omega-3s from the fish are incorporated into brain tissue. A study published in *American Journal of Clinical Nutrition*, which looked at more than 2,000 men and women ages 70 to 74, found that those who ate, on average, one-third of an ounce or more of fish daily did better on cognitive tests than those who ate less.

I try to eat fish at least a few days a week. If you're not fond of fish, you can get some of the same benefits from eggs or milk that is fortified with omega-3s. Other less potent sources of omega-3s include walnuts, pumpkin seeds and soybeans. You also can take fish-oil supplements. The usual dose is 1,000 milligrams (mg) to 2,000 mg daily. Because the supplements can have a blood-thinning effect and/or interact with some medications, check with your doctor before taking them.

• **Olive oil.** It's a healthy fat that reduces inflammation, improves cholesterol and helps reduce the risk for stroke. I use it for cooking almost every day. People who use olive oil regularly tend to have lower rates of dementia and better cognitive function.

How Healthy Is Your Brain?

Sandra Bond Chapman, PhD, a cognitive neuroscientist who is the founder and chief director of the Center for BrainHealth and the Dee Wyly Distinguished University Chair, both at The University of Texas at Dallas. She is coauthor, with Shelly Kirkland, of *Make Your Brain Smarter: Increase Your Brain's Creativity, Energy, and Focus.* CenterForBrainHealth.org

For most people over age 40, glitches in memory are high on their lists of health concerns. Whether it's lost keys, forgotten names or other "senior moments," we fear each is a sign of a deteriorating brain.

What science now tells us: Memory is not necessarily the most important measure of brain health. And no matter what your age, there are ways to improve the mind. However, many of the popular beliefs about improving mental performance are outdated and incorrect.

Most common myths...

MYTH #1: **Brain health steadily declines with age.** Scientists used to believe that people were born with all of the neurons (brain cells) that they'd ever have and that the ability to form new brain connections ended in adolescence.

It's now known that the brain is the most modifiable part of the body. It's constantly being changed by how we use it, and the changes can be measured within just hours. That's why you can be confounded by, say, a new cell phone in the morning and then be using it proficiently by the end of the day.

While you are focused on new learning—such as writing an original report or preparing new recipes—neural activity increases and promotes the development of new neurons. But if these neurons are not put to proper use, they die.

As you age, your ability to think more broadly and deeply can continue to grow if your brain is exercised properly—thanks to the functions of your frontal lobes, the part of your brain that sits just behind and above your eyes in your skull. Even though brain health is tied to all parts of the brain, the majority of the heavy lifting is directed through the frontal lobe networks. The frontal lobes are responsible for decision making, judgment, planning and other "executive" functions. (To get an idea of how effectively you're engaging your frontal lobes in everyday life, see box on the next page.)

My advice: Engage your frontal lobes by being curious and creative and by solving problems whenever you can. Challenge your brain by thinking deeply and extracting meaning from information you are given.

Example: Think back to a favorite book that you read several years ago, and come up with five to eight different take-home messages that are applicable to different contexts.

Better yet: Read it again, and then come up with the list.

MYTH #2: **A good memory indicates mental robustness.** Surprisingly, memory skills do not correspond to everyday-life performance as much as frontal lobe functioning.

How Fit Are Your Frontal Lobes?		
Are you challenging your brain in your everyday life?		
Ask yourself...		
Do you have the same dinner guests repeatedly?	*or*	Do you invite unexpected guests to vary the conversation?
Do you express the same ideas repeatedly to convey your position on timely issues?	*or*	Do you continually try to see things from new perspectives when discussing a timely topic?
Do you resist new technology such as a new cell phone?	*or*	Do you stay open to moving from old to new technology?
Do your e-mails sound the same? Do you send cards following predictable traditions?	*or*	Do you think of creative ideas and unique timing to convey personal messages?
If the left column describes you more accurately, you may need to more actively engage your frontal lobes.		

This means that you can have an excellent memory but not be very innovative, insightful, creative or mentally productive.

My advice: Don't worry when you can't remember everything. Although we tend to note what we forget, we rarely take stock of all the things we do remember.

A brain that gets too occupied with remembering everything works less efficiently and becomes stressed, overwhelmed and bogged down in the details. If something is important in your life—it could be your work, a hobby or even a weekly card game—you'll remember the details that really matter.

Do not worry about, say, occasional forgotten names or unimportant tasks. But when forgetting regularly interferes with your performance, it may be a sign that something more than benign memory glitches is taking over. Many things can impair memory—not enough sleep, some medications, such as antidepressants and blood pressure drugs, and stress. Memory issues do not always mean Alzheimer's disease. See your doctor if you're concerned about your memory.

MYTH #3: **Multitasking gives your brain a good workout.** Again, not true. When you multitask, the brain has to call on different regions to handle the load. It works inefficiently because the communication isn't synchronized. When you "overuse" your brain in this way, the frontal lobes become fatigued.

This slows efficiency and decreases performance.

My advice: Whatever you're doing, focus on that and nothing else for at least 15 minutes. Put a "do not disturb" sign on the door. Turn off your phones, and don't check your e-mail. You'll think more clearly in those 15 minutes than someone who multitasks for an hour.

MYTH #4: **People with a high IQ have the most brainpower.** Today's IQ tests are based on measurements that were developed more than a century ago. They mainly emphasize such skills as knowledge, memory and speed in ability to perform mathematical equations—all of which were much more important in the days before computers and the Internet.

What's more important is knowing how to use knowledge in novel ways and bringing together facts from disparate areas to create original ideas. As Einstein said, "Imagination is more important than knowledge. Knowledge is limited. Imagination encircles the world."

My advice: Whenever you're confronted with a problem, stop and think deeply about the knowledge you already have. Connecting it and generating original ideas is crucial to brain health.

MYTH #5: **Unrelenting mental work boosts brain capacity.** It's true that high achievers can put in long hours and consider lots of information when they try to solve vexing problems. But they also know when to stop looking at more information—and they reach that point earlier than most people do.

Productivity and achievement are not linked to how many hours are worked and how much information is accessed. In fact, decreasing exposure allows your frontal lobes to be deployed to focus on key data, and, even more importantly, to know what information to ignore.

Using knowledge to support a novel approach is essential to enhancing integrated reasoning and deeper-level thinking.

Example: Instead of taking copious notes on specific points made in a meeting, boil down the discussion to key issues, new decisions and possibilities.

My advice: Keep your key frontal lobe operations finely tuned by blocking, discarding and ignoring less relevant tasks and information. Consolidating facts and options into big ideas and perspectives is necessary to cultivate creative thinking and problem solving.

Best Way to Fight Memory Loss

The combination of computer use and exercise is better than mental or physical activity alone. The exact reason is not yet known, but it may be that physical activity improves blood flow to the brain and therefore delivers more nutrients...while mental activity works at the molecular level to boost synaptic activities.

Yonas E. Geda, MD, MSc, a neuropsychiatrist at Mayo Clinic, Scottsdale, Arizona, and leader of a study of 926 people, ages 70 to 93, published in *Mayo Clinic Proceedings.*

Are You Shrinking Your Brain?

Daniel G. Amen, MD, a brain-imaging specialist, is the founder, CEO and medical director of the Amen Clinics and author of several books, including *Use Your Brain to Change Your Age: Secrets to Look, Feel, and Think Younger Every Day.*

When scientists talk about memory and learning, the hippocampus, a small, seahorse-shaped structure located deep inside the brain, gets most of the credit for these vital cognitive functions.

What you don't hear much about: The prefrontal cortex (PFC), a much larger part of the brain located just behind and slightly beneath the forehead. Known as the "executive" part of the brain because it controls judgment, insights and impulse control, the PFC is just as important when it comes to staying sharp

mentally, learning new information and controlling processes involved in memory.

Unfortunately, millions of Americans don't follow simple lifestyle habits that promote optimal functioning of the PFC.

Result: Lapses in judgment (such as making risky maneuvers when driving)...disorganized thinking (including an inability to prioritize tasks)...shorter attention spans (resulting in difficulty with reading and other activities that require focus)...and impairments in learning and memory.

IMPROVE YOUR BRAIN—LIVE LONGER

The PFC needs good "fuel" to thrive. That's why people with healthful habits tend to have a larger PFC than those who don't take good care of themselves. As a result, they're more likely to live longer (because their judgment about risks is better), and they're less likely to develop Alzheimer's disease.

Important finding: A 2007 study of Catholic nuns and priests found that those who had the most self-discipline were 89% less likely to develop Alzheimer's disease. Self-discipline is one of the traits that is enhanced when you have a robust PFC.

POWER UP YOUR "WIRING"

To protect your PFC—and other key parts of the brain...

• **Rethink your alcohol intake.** Millions of Americans drink a glass or two of red wine a day because it's good for the heart. But the cardio-protective properties of alcohol—it raises HDL "good" cholesterol and reduces clots, thus reducing the risk for a heart attack—may be offset by the damage it can do to the brain. Alcohol decreases the size and functioning of the PFC. What's more, even moderate drinking (two drinks daily for men and one for women) can impair brain circulation.

My advice: If your doctor agrees that you can forgo the cardiovascular benefits of drinking wine, limit your intake to no more than two or three alcoholic beverages per week.

• **"Water" your brain.** The brain is 80% water. People who don't drink enough water or who drink a lot of dehydrating liquids, such as alcohol or caffeinated coffee or tea, often have impairments in cognition and judgment, which can occur when the PFC is damaged.

My advice: Drink plenty of water—eight glasses (64 ounces) of water every day is typically sufficient. If you like, add a splash of lemon or lime juice for flavor.

• **Slow down on the omega-6s.** Most Americans get far too many inflammation-promoting omega-6 essential fatty acids in their diets—primarily from cooking oils (such as corn and vegetable), fatty red meats and processed foods—that are harmful to the brain. That's why a plant-based, anti-inflammatory diet is among the most effective ways to reduce damage to the PFC and other areas of the brain.

My advice: Eat lots of greens—including salads—along with vegetables, fruit, whole grains and legumes. Approximately three servings of lean protein daily will help balance blood sugar and keep you feeling sharp. Also, eat at least three servings weekly of cold-water fish such as salmon, mackerel and sardines. The omega-3s in these fish have potent anti-inflammatory effects. Fish oil supplements (1 g to 3 g daily) are also helpful. Check with your doctor first if you use a blood thinner.

Aim to change your diet so that your intake of omega-6 fatty acids is no more than three times higher than your intake of omega-3s.

Good rule of thumb: A plant-based diet that's high in fish provides the ideal 3:1 (or lower) ratio of omega-6s to omega-3s.

• **Try green tea and rhodiola.** Distractibility, disorganization and poor impulse control are commonly associated with children who may be suffering from attention-deficit/hyperactivity disorder (ADHD), but many adults (who may or may not have ADHD) also struggle with such symptoms.

Often linked to low activity in the PFC, these symptoms can be reversed, in part, with green tea and rhodiola, a plant-based supplement frequently used as an energy booster. In one study, researchers at my clinic did brain scans before and after giving patients green tea and rhodiola. Two months later, scans showed a significant increase in circulation in the PFC.

How it helps: Green tea appears to benefit the PFC by increasing the availability of dopamine, a brain chemical that controls the brain's reward and pleasure centers. It also helps regulate emotional responses, such as the motivation to take positive actions. Rhodiola is an "adaptogen," a substance that normalizes the body's functions by boosting blood flow to the brain and raising dopamine and serotonin levels.

My advice: Take 200 mg of rhodiola and drink two to three cups of green tea daily (avoid drinking it in the evening since the tea's caffeine can interfere with sleep…or drink decaffeinated green tea).

• **Keep your BMI in check.** People who are overweight—with a body mass index (BMI) of 25 or higher—have less circulation in the PFC than those of normal weights. Excess body weight is associated with atherosclerosis, diabetes and other conditions that impede circulation throughout the body.

Danger: A high BMI can cause the brain to shrink. Research has shown that people who are obese typically have about 8% less brain tissue than normal-weight adults.

My advice: At least once a year, check your BMI by using an online calculator, such as the National Heart, Lung and Blood Institute's nhlbi.nih.gov/health/educational/lose_wt/bmi tools.htm. A BMI of 18.5 to 24.9 is considered normal. If your BMI is 25 or higher, you need to lose weight.

• **Don't ignore sleep problems.** An estimated 18 million Americans have sleep apnea, a condition in which breathing intermittently stops during sleep. Unfortunately, the condition is undiagnosed in most of these people.

Why does this matter? Scans on patients with sleep apnea show brain changes that resemble early Alzheimer's disease. Poor sleep decreases blood flow to the PFC and other parts of the brain. Snoring, daytime fatigue and morning headaches are common symptoms of sleep apnea. Your doctor may recommend tests in a sleep laboratory.

My advice: If you're overweight, sleep apnea can often be reduced or even eliminated with weight loss. Many patients also benefit from continuous positive airway pressure (CPAP) units, which help keep the airways open during sleep.

Also important: Avoid sleepless nights. Patients with chronic insomnia have a higher risk for cognitive declines than people who sleep well. To prevent insomnia, follow the tried-and-true strategies—relax in a warm bath before bed…reduce arousal by not watching TV or using a computer in the hour before bedtime…and go to bed and wake up at the same times every day.

Also helpful: Melatonin. The standard dose of this sleep hormone supplement is 1 mg to 6 mg taken a half hour before bed. Start with the lower dose and increase it over a period of weeks, if necessary.

Check with your doctor first if you take an antidepressant, blood pressure medication, blood thinner, steroid or nonsteroidal anti-inflammatory drug—melatonin may interact with these medications.

Meditate for a Bigger Brain

Compared with nonmeditators, people who had meditated between 10 and 90 minutes a day for five to 46 years had significantly greater brain volume in some regions linked to emotion, according to brain scans.

Theory: Meditation may promote better nerve connections or larger cells in certain brain regions—which may explain many meditators' emotional stability and mental focus.

Eileen Luders, PhD, associate professor, department of neurology, Brain Mapping Center, University of California, Los Angeles, and lead author of a study of 44 people.

Don't Let Your Brain Shrink

Exercise prevents brain shrinkage. People who have the APOE epsilon4 allele (e4 gene) are at increased risk for Alzheimer's disease.

Recent finding: After 18 months, the brain scans of people with the e4 gene who exercised moderately a few times a week showed dramatically less shrinkage in the hippocampus—which is associated with Alzheimer's—compared with people with the gene who were not physically active.

Stephen Rao, PhD, a professor and director of Schey Center for Cognitive Neuroimaging, Cleveland Clinic, and leader of a study of 97 people, published in *Frontiers in Aging Neuroscience*.

Best New Brain Boosters— Your Brain Can Improve at Any Age

Sandra Bond Chapman, PhD, a cognitive neuroscientist, founder and chief director of the Center for Brain-Health and the Dee Wyly Distinguished University Chair at The University of Texas at Dallas. She is coauthor, with Shelly Kirkland, of *Make Your Brain Smarter: Increase Your Brain's Creativity, Energy, and Focus*. BrainHealth. UTDallas.edu

Expecting crossword puzzles or any particular activity to give your brain a full workout is a bit like expecting bicep curls to tone your entire body. Our bodies need specific types of exercise to optimize results—and so do our brains.

Newest thinking: One of the most effective ways to maintain (or even improve) your brainpower is to tailor specific workouts to your age.

One of the country's leading neuroscientists, Sandra Bond Chapman, PhD, spoke about the best ways to stay mentally sharp…

DON'T DWELL ON YOUR MEMORY

When I talk to people about mental fitness, they almost always say that their main goal is to improve their memory. But virtually everyone is surprised to learn that the ability to remember facts has almost nothing to do with brain efficiency.

The ability to understand big ideas, extrapolate meaning and make sound decisions in real-life contexts is far more vital to effective brain performance than maintaining a repository of data. Unnecessary memorization wastes brain energy, depleting reserves better served for higher-order thinking. Fortunately, increasing higher-order thinking ability may naturally help improve your memory.

MENTAL FITNESS FOR LIFE

What exactly can you do to improve your mental fitness? Here are some regimens that are geared toward the changes your brain is undergoing as it ages.

AGES 46 TO 65

Beginning in one's mid-40s, it's common to start losing the capacity to quickly process new information and store and retrieve data (such as a person's name). However, most people in the 46-to-65 age group are more adept at sorting through information efficiently and accurately discerning critical points to more quickly weigh facts than younger counterparts.

Best brain-boosting strategies if you're age 46 to 65…

•**Narrow your focus.** Multitasking isn't recommended for anyone, but particularly not for people in this age group. As you age, the capacity to rapidly switch from task to task (as occurs with multitasking) slows, adding to brain fatigue and reducing efficiency.

To keep the mind sharp: Pick one job—such as answering e-mails or planning a report—and take your time doing it. Making an effort to create meaningful responses and original content not only increases work quality and productivity but also flexes your brain.

•**Synthesize.** Not every detail is important, so don't let yourself get lost in a sea of information.

To keep the mind sharp: Gather enough information for the task at hand, then focus mainly on the key meanings. Applying internally generated novel ideas to affect an outcome boosts brain health.

Note: Don't feel insecure because your grasp of details may not be what it used to be. This can be a strength—it means that you're more likely to see the bigger picture.

AGES 66 AND OLDER

You may notice increasing incidences of memory glitches, but it is probably not as dramatic as you think. People tend to notice when they forget a few minor details, such as the name of the movie they saw last month. They don't consider the tens of thousands of details that they didn't forget.*

Try to nourish your brain by putting accumulated knowledge and wisdom to work. Deep thinking and disciplined use of brainpower helps fine-tune brain resources for optimal performance.

Best brain-boosting strategies if you're age 66 or older…

•**Get off autopilot.** At this age, you are especially at risk for slipping into autopilot—a dangerous state, since a bored brain is going backward.

To keep the mind sharp: Continue to push yourself to learn something new, especially if it's related to technology, which can help build new connections in the brain. You will feel energized as you go from being a novice to an expert in an area of interest.

•**Stay challenged.** The problem with crossword puzzles and other brain teasers is that they get easier with practice. People who do crosswords get better mainly at crosswords, and the gains generally don't translate into other high-level mental areas.

To keep the mind sharp: Take on real challenges that you are motivated to master. Forcing yourself to learn a new language just to exercise your brain will not produce the same far-reaching cognitive benefits as honing a foreign language for practical use, such as for a trip. The brain expands and develops new pathways when it's pushed to explore unfamiliar areas.

FORTIFYING YOUNGER BRAINS

Adults who are under age 45 tend to be very comfortable with collecting facts—but they often are less confident than they could be when dealing with abstract concepts and making

*If problems with memory or decision-making begin to interfere with daily life, such as completing household tasks, consult your doctor.

decisions. *How people in this age group can improve their brain performance...*

• **Don't get distracted.** Younger adults have a tremendous ability to memorize, but they're typically poor at choosing what they need to remember. Most people will function just fine if they ignore about 50% of the information that comes their way.

Helpful: Focus on accomplishing your top two or three priorities for the day without letting distractions, such as constant text, e-mail and social-media alerts, disrupt your progress.

• **Zoom out.** When every fact in the world is a click away, our brains often get stuck regurgitating facts and blindly following directions.

Helpful: When you're reading for knowledge (not for entertainment), skim the material quickly...find the takeaway message...and then condense it to a succinct thought. Translating new information into your own words increases comprehension and helps you achieve new perspectives that can inspire your brain to generate new ideas and solutions.

Surprising Brain Booster

Paul Nussbaum, PhD, clinical neuropsychologist and president of the Brain Health Center, Wexford, Pennsylvania. PaulNussbaum.com

S ome people love to travel. But if you're someone who needs a good reason to pack your bags, here's one to consider: Your brain will love it if you hit the road!

Here's why: The brain's ability to grow, known as plasticity, never stops. When you take in new sights and information—walking unfamiliar streets, admiring the scenery and listening to (and speaking) unfamiliar languages—the brain forms new neurons and connections. It literally gets bigger and more vibrant, explains Paul Nussbaum, PhD, a clinical neuropsychologist and president of the Brain Health Center, in Wexford, Pennsylvania.

You may also get a boost in creativity. Research that looked at fashion executives found that those who had lived abroad created products that were consistently more creative than those produced by their stay-at-home peers.

Of course, not everyone has the time (or the cash or inclination) for exotic vacations. That's OK. Your brain will also be happy with a stimulating "staycation."

The trick: Do anything that isn't routine. Go on weekend road trips. Visit that museum you've always been meaning to see. Introduce yourself to someone whom you've been tempted to talk to but never did.

But if you can travel, go ahead and book those tickets. Even when the trip is over, you'll hopefully have photos to remind you of your adventures and memories to share with others. Remembering stimulates the same neurochemistry as the experience itself. Your brain wants to be stimulated, and reliving your travels is yet another great way to do it.

Better Brain-Building Activities

R etired adults age 75 and older who held demanding jobs that required strategic thinking, verbal skills and some advanced-level education scored higher on cognitive tests over an eight-year period than adults whose jobs did not.

Explanation: These skills use areas of the brain that build a cognitive reserve, which helps protect memory and thinking abilities.

Even if you didn't have this type of job, you can still develop cognitive skills after retirement by doing volunteer work that involves organization and planning.

Francisca S. Then, PhD, research fellow, Institute for Social Medicine, Occupational Health and Public Health, University of Leipzig, Germany.

Fight Dementia By Learning a Second Language

In a study of people with dementia, bilingual people developed dementia about five years later than people who spoke just one language.

Possible reason: Switching from one language to another in the course of routine communication helps to stimulate the brain.

Study of the medical records of 648 people, average age 66, by researchers at University of Edinburgh, Scotland, and Nizam's Institute of Medical Sciences, Hyderabad, India, published in *Neurology*.

Challenge Your Brain

A reader asks: My husband wants to buy a Ping-Pong table because he thinks it would be good "brain exercise." Is he correct?

It depends. Two things would make it "brain exercise"—if he's learning something new, and if it provides aerobic exercise. The first condition involves developing new branches and connections between brain cells (neurons), as well as reinforcing established neural pathways. Aerobic exercise provides more oxygen to the brain, thereby increasing mental energy. If he is already an accomplished Ping-Pong player, then condition one would not apply (unless he learns to play with his nondominant hand). If he plays competitively and/or vigorously, he will reap the benefits of the second condition. Additionally, recent research shows that social interaction boosts brain power. So if having the table increases time spent with family and friends, that's a bonus for the brain.

Answer from Pierce J. Howard, PhD, managing director, research and development, Center for Applied Cognitive Studies, Charlotte, North Carolina.

How Google Exercises Your Brain

Gary Small, MD, director of the Longevity Center at the Jane & Terry Semel Institute for Neuroscience & Human Behavior, University of California, Los Angeles. He is also coauthor of many books, including *iBrain*.

Can you use the Internet to better your brain? Yes, say researchers at University of California at Los Angeles who conducted a study called "Your Brain on Google." The research team, led by Gary Small, MD, of UCLA's Longevity Center, explored whether searching the Internet stimulates areas of the brain that control decision making, complex reasoning and vision. The researchers discovered it does, but only for those who use Google or other search engines in a certain way.

NET-NET...

The study included 24 people aged 55 to 76. Half the subjects (the "Net Naïve" group) had little or no experience in searching the Internet, while the other half (the "Net Savvy" group) were skilled computer users who regularly use the Internet. This age group was chosen because researchers postulated that age-related brain changes are associated with declines in cognitive abilities, such as processing speed and working memory, and that routine computer use might have an impact—negative or positive. Both groups were asked to perform two tasks. First, to read text on a computer screen, and second to use Google to search the web. The reading material and research topics were interesting and similar in content (for instance, the benefits of drinking coffee, planning a trip to the Galapagos Islands, how to choose a car, etc.).

Meanwhile, as the subjects worked on their computers, researchers scanned their brains with a functional magnetic resonance imaging (fMRI) device to ascertain which parts were active. During the text-reading phase, these fMRI scans revealed similar activity for both groups in the regions that control language, reading, memory and vision. But there were very dissimilar results when the two groups performed Web searches. When the Net Naïve group searched the Internet, their brain activity was similar to what they had experienced while reading...in contrast, the Net Savvy group produced activity in areas of the brain that control decision making and complex reasoning. Previous studies have shown that this type of brain activity is important for everyday cognitive tasks.

ENGAGING CONTENT

This result shows that the Internet is itself "brain stimulation," said Dr. Small. He explained that this may be especially helpful as people age because, compared with reading, Web searches require making more decisions. For instance, searchers must decide which information to pursue and which to ignore. Dr. Small says the Net Naïve group may show less brain stimulation than the Net Savvy group because of their inexperience with the Internet. When this group was given some training their brains showed similar patterns of activity to those who were adept at Internet use.

So, if you haven't been very involved with using your computer to research topics of interest, give it a try—it's great mental exercise.

Log On to Facebook to Boost Brain Function

Researchers divided 42 older healthy adults (ages 68 to 91) into three groups—one was taught to use Facebook, another to use a simple online diary and the third received no training.

Outcome: After eight weeks, the Facebook group had a 25% boost in brain function, including working memory (required for learning and reasoning), while the other groups saw no change.

Theory: Learning a new skill that involves complex functions as well as a strong social component helps to stave off cognitive decline.

Janelle Wohltmann, researcher, department of psychology, The University of Arizona, Tucson.

Learn a Word a Day and Other Fun Ways to Add Healthy Years to Your Life

The late Robert N. Butler, MD, president and chief executive officer of the International Longevity Center-USA. He also was professor of geriatrics at Brookdale Department of Geriatrics and Adult Development at Mount Sinai Medical Center in New York City. He wrote *The Longevity Prescription: The 8 Proven Keys to a Long, Healthy Life* and won the 1976 Pulitzer Prize for his book *Why Survive? Being Old in America.*

We all know that eating right and exercising can boost our chances of a long, healthy life. But sometimes it seems as if the changes we have to make to live a healthier life are simply too overwhelming. The good news is that just a few little changes can have a significant impact on our health. *Here, the little changes that can make a big difference...*

●**Learn a word a day.** Pick a word out of the paper or dictionary every day. Or have a word e-mailed to you daily (Dictionary.Reference.com/wordoftheday). Put it on an index card, and drill yourself. This type of cognitive calisthenic keeps your brain sharp.

The brain continues to regenerate nerve cells throughout life. This process, known as neurogenesis, helps older adults to improve memory and other cognitive functions as they age.

Example: A 2006 study published in *The Journal of the American Medical Association* compared two groups of older adults. Those in one group were given training in memory, reasoning and mental processing. After just 10 sessions of 60 to 75 minutes each, the participants had immediate and long-lasting improvements, compared with those who didn't get the training.

If learning a word a day doesn't appeal to you, pick an activity that you enjoy and find mentally challenging.

Examples: Reading history books, learning chess or memorizing poems. When the activity starts getting easier, move on to harder challenges.

People who do this can regain as much as two decades of memory power. In other words, someone who starts at age 70 could achieve the memory of the average 50-year-old.

• **Make social connections.** Go on a cruise. Take a bus tour. Go to a reunion. All of these are great ways to connect with people. Why bother? Because emotional connections add years to your life.

Example: Studies published in the last 10 years show that people in happy marriages have less heart disease and live longer than those in unhappy relationships or who are divorced or widowed. Being happily married at age 50 is a better predictor of good health at age 80 than having low cholesterol.

The same benefits occur when people maintain any close relationship—with friends, children or even pets. People who are emotionally bonded with others suffer less depression. They also tend to have less stress and lower levels of disease-causing stress hormones. And inviting new people into your life can help you cope with the dislocations—due to death, divorce, retirement, etc.—that occur over time.

Emotional connections don't just happen—people have to work at them. Think of the friendships that are important to you. If you are like most people, maybe a few of these relationships are active, but others have gone dormant for a variety of reasons. Ask yourself why some relationships have lapsed and what you can do to revive them. If you have lost touch with someone special, send an e-mail or pick up the phone.

We all have "relationship opportunities" that we can take advantage of. Talk to the stranger next to you at a concert or a sports event. If you volunteer, invite one of your coworkers for coffee.

• **Take a nap.** It's a myth that older people need less sleep than younger adults. They often do sleep less, but this is mainly because they're more likely to have physical issues, such as arthritis or the need to use the bathroom at night, that interfere with restful sleep.

People who don't get enough sleep often have declines in immune function, which can increase the risk for cancer as well as infections. They also have a higher risk for hypertension and possibly prediabetes.

A short nap—no more than 20 to 30 minutes—can make up for a bad night's sleep. But beware of excessive napping. A long nap or more than one short nap per day can ruin a good night's sleep. Napping late in the day, say, after 3:00, also can interfere with a night's sleep.

• **Climb the stairs.** It takes very little time but is a great way to get your heart and lungs working. Most exercise guidelines recommend at least 20 to 30 minutes of exercise most days of the week. That much exercise, or more, is clearly beneficial, but short amounts of activity can have a significant impact.

In a study of 5,000 people over age 70, all the participants had some physical limitations, but those who got even minimal exercise (defined as the equivalent of walking a mile at least once a week) were 55% less likely to develop more serious physical limitations (defined as severe joint pain or muscle weakness) that could compromise independence.

• **Watch the birds.** For many people, contact with the natural world has a restorative effect. A few minutes observing birds at a feeder or watching a sunset can restore our equilibrium. The natural world has a pace that reminds us that life does not have to be lived in a rush.

Taking a few moments to destress is worth doing because an estimated 60% of all doctor visits are for stress-related disorders.

Connecting with nature also can boost our performance. A study at Kansas State University gave 90 women a five-minute typing assignment. The researchers found that those who worked with a bouquet of flowers nearby outperformed those with no flowers.

• **See a funny movie.** A good guffaw is more complicated than most people imagine. Laughter involves 15 facial muscles, along with the lungs, larynx and epiglottis. It even seems to protect against heart disease.

A study at Loma Linda University School of Medicine found that volunteers who watched a humorous video had reduced levels of the stress hormones cortisol and epinephrine. These and other stress-related chemicals have been linked with increased inflammation and an elevated risk for heart disease and many other conditions.

Use Your Brain When You Exercise

Physical-mental exercise slows cognitive decline.

Recent study: Among adults over age 60 with mild cognitive impairment, those who spent a half-hour doing stimulating tasks that worked the body and the mind three times a week (examples include mowing the lawn in a specific pattern or finding items in an unfamiliar supermarket) showed greater improvement in memory and problem-solving skills than those who did only mental exercise.

Explanation: This kind of exercise may stimulate the growth and functioning of new brain cells, slowing cognitive decline.

Lawla Law, PhD, assistant professor, Tung Wah College, Kowloon, Hong Kong.

Cell Phone Games Are Great for Your Brain

Games on your cell phone are better for your brain than crossword or sudoku puzzles.

Reason: They have a timing component.

As you age, your brain faces more challenges with short-term memory and the cognitive tasks of paying attention and juggling multiple abilities. It's important to challenge these skills, and playing games against a clock provides a better brain workout than puzzles and board games.

Cynthia R. Green, PhD, president, Memory Arts, LLC, Montclair, New Jersey. TotalBrainHealth.com

More Physical Activity, Less Risk for Alzheimer's Disease

People in the lowest 10% for physical activity were more than twice as likely to develop Alzheimer's disease as people in the highest 10%.

Possible reason: Physical activity may increase the size of blood vessels and the number of neurons in the brain. Any type of movement—not just formal exercise—makes a difference.

Study of 716 people by researchers at Rush University Medical Center, Chicago, published in *Neurology*.

What's the Best Brain Exercise?

Laura D. Baker, PhD, associate professor, department of psychiatry and behavioral sciences, University of Washington School of Medicine, Seattle.

Arthur E. Kramer, PhD, professor of psychology, division of visual cognition and human performance, director, Beekman Institute for Advanced Science and Technology at University of Illinois at Urbana-Champaign, and director of the University's Biomedical Imaging Center.

Why is everyone so excited about trading real activities for virtual ones?

Apparently, these electronic and video games are fun and useful. Studies have shown how video games can improve hand-eye coordination and sharpen mental functions, such as decision making. But can such games—even ones that require players to be physically active—ever be a legitimate substitute for actual exercise and sports, where physical exertion is combined with split-second reactions?

According to two brain and behavior researchers, Laura D. Baker, PhD, at University of Washington School of Medicine, and Arthur F. Kramer, PhD, director of the Beekman Institute for Advanced Science and Technology at the University of Illinois at Urbana-Champaign, there are a number of studies that examine how such physical exercise benefits the mind.

For instance, Dr. Baker and her colleagues recently completed a study showing that six months of aerobic exercise improved cognitive functions (including attention, speed of processing information and the ability to switch quickly from one task to another) of aging people (average age 70) with mild memory problems. The researchers noted that other studies have shown this to be true for people of other ages as well, including young adults and older ones who have no memory challenges. Meanwhile, Dr. Kramer and his research team have conducted exercise studies demonstrating that aerobic fitness improves memory in preadolescent children.

REAL MIND-BODY BENEFITS?

Can physical exercise improve any of the same mental functions associated with video games—hand-eye coordination, decision making, multitasking and memory? "One would think so," Dr. Kramer said, noting that this is one of the questions being explored in current research. So far the results are preliminary, he said, but all point in the direction of "yes."

To illustrate, he described one of his recent studies examining how multitasking affects cognition. Researchers recruited college students to walk across a "virtual street" while listening to an iPod or talking on a cell phone. It turned out that those who were most adept at crossing the street safely while using these devices had one thing in common—they were athletes. Dr. Kramer said that further studies will examine whether this is due to natural selection (perhaps people who are better at multitasking are the ones likely to engage in sports) or the result of the sports they play. But, he said, previous research indicates that it's likely the latter—fitness training, including playing a sport, helps sharpen your ability to multitask.

Another study is looking specifically at blood circulation and the brain. It's commonly known that physical activity boosts circulation, delivering more nutrients to the brain. Dr. Baker said that researchers are now examining how aging slows this process, causing the accumulation of what she calls "gunk" in the blood vessels. She noted that exercise might be a way to clean up the vessels to improve blood flow.

How? Dr. Baker explained that the capillaries that branch from the main arteries in the brain's frontal lobes are longer than in other brain regions, which means that the frontal lobes provide more potential places for debris buildup as we grow older. Multitasking ability is compromised for all of us as we age, she said, adding that research appears to support the theory that aerobic exercise increases flow and reduces some of the buildup. Moreover, Dr. Baker said, physical exercise increases sensitivity to insulin, an effect that enables the brain to make better use of its natural fuel, glucose.

AEROBIC EXERCISE SHARPENS MEMORY

Aerobic exercise also appears to benefit the hippocampus, said Dr. Kramer, referring to the part of the brain involved with memory, especially memory that involves remembering associations, such as someone's name, face, etc. "In the real world, this means that aerobic exercise is likely to help in such tasks as cooking a seven-course meal (which requires a good memory) or driving in an unfamiliar environment (requiring an accurate sense of space)." Dr. Kramer also pointed out that aerobic exercise stimulates the release of endorphins, which helps create a sense of well-being.

Both experts emphasized that any activity that gets the heart and lungs working harder is likely to increase your brain power—bicycling, swimming, ice skating, tennis, basketball, racketball, walking, jogging, running and even some types of dancing. Dr. Baker's advice couldn't be simpler: "Find an activity you love and do it often."

Theoretical conclusion? Playing video games is better for your brain than, say, sitting passively on the couch in front of a TV set. But when it comes to brain-building and overall benefit, video and electronic games are outclassed by vigorous physical exercise!

Aerobic Workouts Protect Your Memory

In a recent finding, older women at risk for dementia were able to increase the size of their hippocampus, the area of the brain connected to verbal memory and learning, by doing regular aerobic workouts.

Study of 86 women, ages 70 to 80, by researchers at University of British Columbia, Vancouver, published online in *British Journal of Sports Medicine*.

The Ultimate Brainpower Workout: If You Exercise the Right Way, You Can Reduce Your Risk for Alzheimer's by Up to 50%

John J. Ratey, MD, an associate clinical professor of psychiatry at Harvard Medical School and a psychiatrist at the Beth Israel-Deaconess Massachusetts Mental Health Center, both in Boston. An adjunct professor at the National Taiwan Sports University, he is author, with Eric Hagerman, of *Spark: The Revolutionary New Science of Exercise and the Brain*. JohnRatey.com

We have known for a long time that exercise helps keep our bodies fit.

Now: More and more evidence shows that exercise also promotes brain fitness. For example, a study recently published in *Archives of Neurology* showed that moderate-intensity exercise reduced the odds of developing mild cognitive impairment, which often precedes Alzheimer's disease, by 30% to 40% in the 1,324 study participants (median age 80).

But what type of exercise does the best job of strengthening the brain, and how much is needed for optimal effect?

What you need to know...

THE AGING BRAIN

After age 40, we lose about 5% of our brain cells (neurons) per decade—a process that often accelerates in those who are age 70 and older.

Since the average person has hundreds of billions of neurons, his/her cognitive reserves—that is, the brain's healthy cells that help compensate for damage by recruiting other brain areas to assist with tasks—may be sufficient to maintain mental agility…but not always.

The risk: Millions of Americans who are middle-aged and older start to "slip" in their mental capacities. Even if they have no signs of dementia, it may be harder for them to remember words, names or people than it once was. Or they may struggle to learn new information or take longer to think through problems and find solutions.

Why does this gradual mental decline affect some people much more than others?

Age-related loss of neurons, which affects all of us as we grow older, is just one factor. There's also a decline in dopamine, a neurotransmitter that controls motivation and motor function. This decline interferes with the electrical signals in the brain that allow the remaining neurons to communicate, which is necessary for memory, speech and other key brain functions.

STRONGER BODY, BIGGER BRAIN

Scientists now know that the brain has plasticity, the ability to form new neurons and connections between neurons. This process can increase the brain's ability to take in information, process it and remember it.

What few people realize: Researchers have now identified a molecule—brain-derived neurotrophic factor (BDNF)—that's largely responsible for plasticity, and its levels increase dramatically with exercise. In animal studies at the University of California, Irvine, mice that exercised regularly were found to have BDNF levels that were about four times higher than those in sedentary mice. Many researchers think that humans show a similar increase.

The BDNF molecule could explain, in part, why people who exercise tend to have less memory loss, are less prone to anxiety and depression, and have up to a 50% lower risk of developing Alzheimer's disease or other forms of dementia than those who are sedentary.

Best exercises for the brain...

THE AEROBIC FORMULA

For overall fitness, the Centers for Disease Control and Prevention recommends doing some form of aerobic exercise, such as walking, for 30 minutes at least five days a week. But that's not enough for brain fitness.

Walking at an easy pace might increase your heart rate to about 50% of its maximum. But this has little effect on the brain. For optimal brain benefits, you need to exercise hard enough so that your heart is pumping at 70% to 75% of its maximum rate.* Many treadmills have built-in heart-rate monitors, and heart-rate monitors that you wear are available at most pharmacies.

Good brands of heart-rate monitors: Garmin, Polar and Timex.

Important finding: One study published in *Archives of Neurology* found that people who walked or jogged on a treadmill for 35 minutes at a moderate intensity had improvements in cognitive flexibility (the ability to think flexibly and creatively, rather than merely repeating information) after just one session.

My advice: Exercise at a moderate intensity for 45 minutes to an hour, six days a week.

Remember, a moderate-intensity aerobic workout means elevating your heart rate to 70% to 75% of its maximum capacity. At this rate, you will most likely break a sweat and/or have difficulty carrying on a conversation. You can achieve this by jogging, bicycling, swimming or walking briskly—and then pushing yourself harder when the exercise starts to feel easy.

Example: Once you're comfortable walking for 45 minutes to an hour at the pace described above, increase the intensity by

*To calculate your maximum heart rate, subtract your age from 220. The goal is to exercise at an intensity that raises your pulse to 70% to 75% of your maximum heart rate. The average 65-year-old man, for example, will need to raise his heart rate to about 108 to 116 beats per minute.

walking faster, swinging your arms or holding hand weights.

If a moderate intensity is too much for you, exercising at 60% of your maximum heart rate has also been shown to offer some improvement in cognitive health.

CROSS TRAINING

To add variety to your aerobic exercise regimen, try some form of cross training. It combines different forms of exercise to target various parts of the body. Circuit training, in which you move quickly from one exercise machine to the next without pausing, is one form of cross training. Another is swimming followed by fast walking.

Cross training is useful because it generally results in a prolonged elevation in heart rate, the critical factor for generating BDNF. Cross training is desirable because it challenges not only your aerobic capacity and strength but also calls upon parts of the brain that govern coordination, planning, etc.

My advice: Whenever possible, incorporate some form of cross training into your regular workouts. In addition, balance exercises are a good way to round out your regimen. Try to work balance exercises, such as tai chi or even any fast-paced form of dancing, into your schedule once or twice a week. These exercises are especially good because they increase your heart rate and require you to think about what you're doing.

Bonus: The social interaction that occurs in tai chi or dance classes and other group activities increases serotonin, a neurotransmitter that reduces anxiety and depression, both of which can impair cognitive functions.

THE POWER OF MOOD WORKOUTS

Research shows that the hippocampus (the brain's memory center) is 15% smaller in depressed individuals than in those without depression. Exercise may be one of the most effective ways to reverse depression—perhaps because it influences the same neurochemicals that are affected by antidepressants.

My advice: If you suffer from depression, be sure to follow the exercise guidelines described above. This may allow you to reduce or even eliminate antidepressant medication.

DON'T FORGET MENTAL WORKOUTS

Many different studies have shown that higher levels of education are associated with a decreased risk for dementia. But it doesn't matter where you went to school—or even if you went to school. The key factor is continued learning.

Like physical activity, mental workouts increase the number of connections between neurons that enhance memory and cognitive functions.

Perform mental workouts as often as possible.

Good choices: Try vocabulary quizzes, read books on subject matters you're not already familiar with or do any activity that requires you to push yourself intellectually.

Brain-Saving Workouts

Animals that ran a little over one-third mile a week were less likely to develop infection-induced memory loss, a common cause of dementia in older adults who have suffered a bacterial infection or undergone surgery.

Journal of Neuroscience.

Yoga Improves Brain Power More Than Aerobic Exercise

Edward McAuley, PhD, professor, University of Illinois at Urbana-Champaign, Urbana, Illinois. This study was published in *Journal of Physical Activity & Health.*

A good workout can help your brain as much as your body, you've no doubt heard. That's one reason why so many people go for a run when they want to clear their heads. But did you know that, when it comes to boosting your mental prowess, you're probably better off striking a yoga pose than hitting the track or treadmill? A recent study shows why…

Participants included 30 adults who did not regularly practice yoga or any similar type of mind-body based exercise (such as tai chi). Each came to the study center on three separate days and took tests designed to measure various aspects of cognitive function.

On one day, they did no exercise prior to taking the tests. On another day, they did 20 minutes of yoga poses, focusing on their breathing and ending with a brief seated meditation, then immediately took the cognitive tests. And on yet another day, they ran on a treadmill for 20 minutes (getting their heart rates up to 60% to 70% of maximum) and then took the same cognitive tests.

The results were surprising—because the participants scored significantly higher after doing yoga than after an aerobic workout or after no exercise. *Specifically…*

• **One test measured inhibitory control,** the ability to ignore irrelevant information and maintain focus on relevant items. On a computer screen, the participants saw numerous rows of arrows facing left or right and had to press the arrow on the keyboard that corresponded to the direction of the arrows in a certain "target" position.

Results: The average score for correct responses after yoga was 90%…but just 83% after running, which was about the same as after no exercise.

• **Another test looked at working memory (which is responsible for creating and storing memories and retrieving information),** with the participants having to remember ever-changing sequences of shapes and respond as quickly as possible.

Results: The average score was 87% after yoga…but just 77% after running and 78% after no exercise. Response time also was faster after yoga—an average of 0.55 seconds, compared with 0.64 seconds after running and 0.60 seconds after no exercise.

Explanation: The researchers offered several possible reasons why yoga boosts brain power. Other studies have shown that yoga improves mood, and better mood is associated with better cognitive function. Yoga also reduces the anxiety that can get in the way of tasks that require full attention. In addition, yoga's emphasis on body awareness and breath control may help enhance the ability to concentrate.

Some questions remain, of course. This study did not demonstrate how long the mental performance-enhancing benefits of yoga might last, given that the participants took their cognitive tests within five minutes after finishing their yoga sessions. And the participants in this study were all women, so we can't say for sure whether men would benefit similarly (though it makes sense that they would).

Still, provided you have your doctor's go-ahead to do yoga, there's certainly no harm—and potentially much to be gained—in doing some yoga poses whenever you feel in need of a brain boost or are about to tackle some challenging mental task.

For inspiration and pose illustrations: Check out the *Yoga Journal* website, Yoga Journal.com

Don't Quit Getting Fit!

Brain benefits of exercise diminish quickly if you stop being active. When runners stopped exercising, they had much less blood flow in their brains within 10 days.

Bottom line: If you take a break from regular physical activity, don't wait too long to resume it.

J. Carson Smith, PhD, is associate professor of kinesiology and director, kinesiology undergraduate honors program, University of Maryland School of Public Health, College Park, and leader of a study of competitive master athletes, published in *Frontiers in Aging Neuroscience*.

CHAPTER 9

Brain Food and Supplements

The Groundbreaking Alzheimer's Prevention Diet

As head of the renowned Alzheimer's Prevention Clinic at Weill Cornell Medicine and NewYork-Presbyterian, Richard S. Isaacson, MD, is on top of the latest research on Alzheimer's disease. Groundbreaking studies show that proper diet can make a real difference not only in slowing the progression of the disease but also in preventing it.

Here, Dr. Isaacson explains how we can change our eating habits to fight Alzheimer's. His recommendations are not specifically designed for weight loss, but most overweight people who follow this eating plan will lose weight—important because obesity more than triples the risk for Alzheimer's.

FEWER CALORIES

The Okinawa Centenarian Study (an ongoing study of centenarians in the Japanese prefecture of Okinawa) found that these long-lived people typically consume fewer calories (up to 1,900 calories a day) than the average American (up to 2,600 calories).

Lowering calorie intake appears to reduce beta-amyloid, particles of protein that form brain plaques—the hallmark of Alzheimer's disease. A 2012 study at the Mayo Clinic found that people who overate had twice the risk for memory loss...and those who consumed more than 2,142 calories a day were more likely to have cognitive impairment.

I generally advise my patients to try to have fewer than 2,100 calories a day. I can't give an exact number because calorie requirements depend on body type, activity level, etc. Many of my patients tend to consume less than

Richard S. Isaacson, MD, director of the Alzheimer's Prevention Clinic, Weill Cornell Memory Disorders Program at Weill Cornell Medicine and NewYork-Presbyterian, New York City. He is coauthor of *The Alzheimer's Prevention & Treatment Diet: Using Nutrition to Combat the Effects of Alzheimer's Disease.*

1,800 calories a day, which may be even more protective.

Bonus: Calorie restriction also lowers insulin, body fat, inflammation and blood pressure, all of which can reduce the risk for cognitive impairment. It even improves neurogenesis, the formation of new brain cells.

LESS CARBS, MORE KETONES

Glucose from the breakdown of carbohydrates is the fuel that keeps the body running. But you don't need a lot of carbs. Ketones, another source of fuel, are healthier for the brain.

When you restrict carbohydrates, the body manufactures ketones from stored fat. On occasion, a "ketogenic diet" is recommended for some patients with Alzheimer's disease because ketones produce fewer wastes and put less stress on damaged brain cells. There's some evidence that this diet improves mild cognitive impairment symptoms (and theoretically may slow further damage).

We previously found in our clinic that patients consumed an average of 278 grams of carbohydrates daily before their first visits. We recommend reducing that slowly over the nine weeks of the diet plan to 100 to 120 grams of carbohydrates daily. (One sweet potato has about 23 grams.) The USDA SuperTracker website (SuperTracker.USDA.gov) gives carbohydrate amounts and other nutritional information for specific foods. Eat healthful carbohydrates such as beans and whole grains in moderation. Unlike refined carbs, they are high in fiber and can help to reduce insulin resistance and improve blood sugar control—which reduces risk for Alzheimer's.

FASTING

Some trendy diets recommend extreme fasts. With the Alzheimer's prevention diet, you'll fast—but mainly when you wouldn't be eating anyway, during sleep!

Several times a week, you'll go without food (particularly carbohydrates) for more than 12 hours. After 12 hours, the body starts making ketones. This type of fast, known as time-restricted eating, reduces inflammation, improves metabolic efficiency and improves insulin levels, insulin sensitivity and brain health.

How to do it: Eat an early supper—say, at about 5 pm. You won't eat again until after 5 am the next day. Your eventual goal will be to fast for 12 to 14 hours five nights a week.

MORE PROTEIN

The Institute of Medicine recommends getting 10% to 35% of calories from protein—go for the higher end. On a 2,000-calorie diet, that's about 175 grams. (Five ounces of cooked salmon has about 36 grams of protein.)

The amino acids in protein are important for memory and other brain functions. Protein-rich foods often are high in B vitamins, including folic acid and vitamins B-6 and B-12. The Bs are critical because they reduce homocysteine, an amino acid linked to poor brain performance and an increased Alzheimer's risk.

Which protein: Chicken, fish, nuts, legumes and eggs all are good choices. I recommend limiting red meat to one weekly serving because of potential associated health risks, including an increased risk for certain cancers...and because too much saturated fat (see below) can be a problem.

Helpful: Aim for four to eight eggs a week. They're high in selenium, lutein, zeaxanthin and other brain-healthy antioxidants.

LIMIT SATURATED FAT

A large study found that people who eat a lot of foods high in saturated fat—rich desserts, red meat, fast food, etc.—may be up to 2.4 times more likely to develop Alzheimer's disease.

Saturated fat limits the body's ability to "clear" beta-amyloid deposits from the brain. It also raises cholesterol and increases the risk for cardiovascular diseases—and what's bad for the heart also is bad for the brain.

Consuming some saturated fat is healthful—it's only in excess that it causes problems. The American Heart Association advises limiting it to about 5% to 6% of total calories. I recommend a little more—up to 10% of your daily calories. On a 2,000-calorie diet, the upper limit would be about 20 grams. (One ounce of cheese can have as much as eight grams.)

FISH, TURMERIC AND COCOA

Studies have shown that a few specific foods can fight Alzheimer's...

• **Fish.** A UCLA study found that adults who regularly ate foods high in omega-3 fatty acids (the healthful fats in fish) had a lower risk for mental decline. Other research has shown that low blood levels of DHA (a type of omega-3) are linked to smaller brain volume and lower scores on cognitive tests.

My advice: Eat one serving of fatty fish (such as wild salmon, mackerel and sardines) at least twice a week. (For more on fish and the brain, see the next two articles.)

• **Turmeric.** In India, where people use the spice turmeric frequently, the risk for Alzheimer's is lower than in the US. This doesn't prove that turmeric is responsible (genetic factors, for example, also could be involved), but other evidence suggests that it's protective. Turmeric contains the compound curcumin, which has potent antioxidant and anti-inflammatory effects.

My advice: Use the spice in recipes—don't depend on supplements—because curcumin is fat-soluble and absorption is enhanced by the fat in foods.

• **Cocoa.** The flavanols in cocoa improve memory and other cognitive functions. They also have been linked to reduced blood pressure and improved insulin resistance.

My advice: Buy chocolate bars or cocoa powder that lists purified cocoa flavanols on the label.

Does Fish Protect the Brain—or Poison It With Mercury?

Study titled "Association of Seafood Consumption, Brain Mercury Level, and APOE-ε4 Status with Brain Neuropathology in Older Adults" by researchers at Rush University Medical Center, Chicago, Missouri University Researcher Reactor, Columbia, and Wageningen University, the Netherlands, published in *JAMA*.

When it comes to preventing dementia, eating seafood is a double-edged sword. On the one hand, it's high in mercury, a neurotoxin. Bad for the brain. On the other hand, it's high in omega-3 fatty acids, which support nerve functioning. Good for the brain.

So what happens to people who eat seafood regularly, compared with those who eat little or none? They're less likely to get dementia. All those omega-3s protect the brain even with the extra mercury.

This is something of a breakthrough finding. While earlier population studies had suggested that the cardiovascular and other benefits of eating seafood outweighed the risks of consuming contaminants, doubts remained. In a recent study, researchers at Rush University Medical Center in Chicago looked at what you might call hard evidence—autopsies of 286 men and women (average age 90). They had already been studying these people when they were alive, so they knew how much seafood they were eating, and now they could look directly at their body tissues and inside their brains to see if there was accumulation of mercury—and neurological evidence of Alzheimer's disease.

The surprise answer was that while the seafood eaters did have higher levels of mercury, there was no increased incidence of Alzheimer's. That's true even for those who had the highest levels of mercury.

While mercury didn't harm, however, seafood protected those at the highest risk. These are the estimated about one-quarter of the population who carry a gene variant (apolipoprotein E4) that triples Alzheimer's risk. Seafood didn't protect everyone, but in this group, those who ate seafood regularly, compared with those who rarely or never ate it, were 47% less likely to show the brain pathology that defines Alzheimer's disease.

Bottom line: By all means, choose seafood lowest in mercury—good choices include catfish, clams, flounder, salmon, sardines, scallops, shrimp, squid and light (not albacore) tuna. But don't let worry about mercury stop you from getting the brain-protective benefits of seafood.

The Truth About Brain Food…and Supplements That Keep Your Memory Intact

Mark A. Stengler, NMD, a naturopathic medical doctor and leading authority on the practice of alternative and integrated medicine. Dr. Stengler is author of the *Health Revelations* newsletter, author of *The Natural Physician's Healing Therapies*, founder and medical director of the Stengler Center for Integrative Medicine in Encinitas, California, and served as an associate clinical professor at the National College of Natural Medicine in Portland, Oregon. MarkStengler.com

The sooner you get started with a brain-protecting regimen, the more you will benefit.

For optimal brain function, your diet should be well-balanced with carbohydrates (40%), protein (30%) and fats (30%). You can accomplish this by eating meals that include whole grains, fruits and vegetables (for complex carbohydrates)…fish, poultry, lean meats, legumes, nuts and seeds (for protein)…and fish oil, olive oil, avocados, almonds, walnuts and ground flaxseed (for fats). Steer clear of dairy products and packaged and processed foods, such as cookies, white bread and pasta, which are packed with simple carbohydrates that wreak havoc on glucose levels, contributing to diabetes, stroke/vascular disease and dementia.

THE VALUE OF FISH

Fish provides docosahexaenoic acid (DHA) and eicosapentaenoic acid (EPA), the most plentiful fatty acids in the brain. DHA, an omega-3 fatty acid, is found in abundance in cold-water fish such as mackerel, sardines, salmon and herring. You also can get it from fish-oil supplements, egg yolks, DHA-enriched eggs and some algae supplements, such as Neuromins, a product that is available at most health-food stores. Foods such as walnuts… leafy, green vegetables…and supplements including flaxseed and hemp oil contain alpha-linolenic acid, an omega-3 fatty acid that can be converted by the body into DHA and EPA.

How essential is DHA to memory? It has been known for some years that people have a higher risk of Alzheimer's if they have low blood levels of DHA. A study in *Archives of Neurology* revealed that people who ate fish one to three times a month had a 40% lower risk of Alzheimer's than those who never ate fish. Those who consumed fish once a week or more had a 60% lower risk. Fish may be baked, broiled or grilled.

It also makes sense to take a fish-oil supplement daily. I suggest 1,000 mg of combined DHA and EPA. Good brands are Nordic Naturals (800-662-2544, NordicNaturals.com) and Carlson Laboratories (888-234-5656, Carlson Labs.com), both available at health-food stores.

Caution: Fish oil can thin blood, so check with your doctor before using it if you take blood-thinning medications such as *warfarin* (Coumadin).

GLA IS ESSENTIAL

Omega-6s make up another class of essential fatty acids that are necessary for good brain function. Omega-6 is found in vegetable oils, including safflower, sunflower and corn oils. Most American diets contain too much of these oils due to consumption of packaged and fried foods. However, the most important omega-6 fatty acid is linoleic acid, which is converted in the body to gamma-linolenic acid (GLA). This essential fatty acid plays a big role in the formation of healthy brain-cell membranes, the part of the cell that stores information. Taking borage oil or evening primrose oil are healthful ways to increase GLA intake—hempseed and hempseed oil also are good sources. Another way to get GLA in the diet is by consuming flaxseed (with water to prevent constipation) or flaxseed oil.

THE EUROPEAN CURE

For years, European doctors have recommended a supplement called L-alpha-glyceryl-phosphorylcholine (GPC) to promote mental acuity (the ability to respond quickly and appropriately to mental challenges). GPC actually is used by the brain more effectively than PC to form acetylcholine—but it costs twice as much and is less widely available in the US. A good GPC supplement by Source Naturals is sold in some health-food stores under the brand name Alpha GPC (to find a retailer, go to SourceNaturals.com). Take two 300-mg capsules twice daily for the first four weeks, then two 300-mg capsules once daily as a maintenance dosage. Side effects are rare, but take GPC with a meal if it seems to interfere with your digestion.

PS: BE SURE TO GET MORE

Phosphatidylserine (PS) is a fat that the brain needs to preserve the key brain chemicals serotonin and dopamine. It also has been shown to reduce levels of the stress hormone cortisol. PS is found in fish, soy and leafy, green vegetables. As we age, PS levels in the body start to decline, so most people need to take a supplement once they're past age 50.

A normal daily diet has about 70 mg of PS. You need about four times that much if you have memory problems. Nearly anyone can benefit from a 300-mg daily supplement of PS. You're likely to notice improvements in mental alertness after four to eight weeks. A small percentage of people have digestive upset, such as bloating and diarrhea, but you can reduce the dosage if this is a problem. PS is available at health-food stores and pharmacies. Make sure you buy a product that lists "phosphatidylserine" on the label. (Some supplements contain "phosphorylated serine," a nutrient complex that doesn't provide the same benefits as PS.) A high-quality PS supplement is made by Jarrow Formulas (to find a retailer, call 800-726-0886 or go to Jarrow.com).

HELP FROM ALC

When taken as a supplement, a nutrient known as acetyl-L-carnitine (ALC) has been shown to improve cognitive function and memory in older adults. Researchers also have found that ALC slows the progression of early-stage Alzheimer's disease. By improving communication between the two main hemispheres of the brain, ALC helps enhance the interplay of creative and cognitive brain activity.

For people with mild memory problems, I recommend taking 500 mg of ALC daily on an empty stomach. For those with more severe problems such as dementia, I suggest the same dose three times daily. Cut back if you have digestive upset. Most health-food stores

carry a reliable ALC formula produced by Now Foods (888-669-3663, NowCatalog.com).

ADD ANTIOXIDANTS

In all likelihood, Alzheimer's disease and other types of dementia are related to excessive damage by free radicals (normal by-products of metabolism that can destroy cells, organs and tissues). Free radicals irreversibly injure our cells and contribute to accelerated aging, but studies have shown that this damage can be warded off by getting enough antioxidant nutrients to help guard our brain-cell membranes.

There's ample evidence that a daily dose of 2,000 international units (IU) of the powerful antioxidant vitamin E can slow the decline of cognitive function in people who have moderate to severe Alzheimer's disease. There have been controversial vitamin E studies that seemed to show a link to worsening chronic disease. However, I don't have much confidence in those studies because they were performed on unhealthy people. When it comes to Alzheimer's, results of vitamin E studies have been quite good.

All fresh fruits, vegetables and other plant foods provide multiple naturally occurring antioxidants. Juices are an especially concentrated source of antioxidants. In fact, a study of nearly 2,000 Japanese Americans found that those who reported drinking fruit and vegetable juices at least three times a week had a 75% lower risk of developing dementia than those who drank juices less than once a week. The most nutritious fruit juices include cranberry, pomegranate, apple and blueberry. I also like mixed vegetable juices containing any combination of spinach, celery, lettuce, parsley, watercress, carrot and tomato.

If there is a strong family history of dementia or you have beginning signs of it, take up to 2,000 IU of vitamin E daily. Green tea also is an excellent source of antioxidants. I recommend drinking two to four cups of green tea daily and eight ounces of fresh juice.

The Diet That Cuts Your Alzheimer's Risk in Half

Martha Clare Morris, ScD, professor and director of the Section of Nutrition and Nutritional Epidemiology at Rush University, Chicago, where she is assistant provost for community research. She specializes in dietary and other preventable risk factors in the development of Alzheimer's disease and other chronic diseases in older adults.

Some of the same diets that are good for cardiovascular health also are good for the brain. But there's a new diet—combining the best aspects of other diets—that is so effective it reduces the risk for Alzheimer's disease even in those who don't give the diet their best effort.

The MIND diet blends components from DASH (a blood pressure–lowering diet) and the popular Mediterranean diet, with an extra emphasis on berries, leafy greens and a few other brain-healthy foods.

How good is it? People who carefully followed the diet were about 53% less likely to develop Alzheimer's disease in subsequent years. Those who approached it more casually didn't do quite as well but still reduced their risk considerably, by about 35%.

BLENDED BENEFITS

The MIND diet was developed by researchers at Rush University who examined years of studies to identify specific foods and nutrients that seemed to be particularly good—or bad—for long-term brain health. The MIND (it stands for Mediterranean-DASH Intervention for Neurodegenerative Delay) diet is a hybrid plan that incorporates the "best of the best."

In a study in the journal *Alzheimer's & Dementia*, the researchers followed more than 900 participants. None had dementia when the study started. The participants filled out food questionnaires and had repeated neurological tests over a period averaging more than four years.

Some participants followed the MIND diet. Others followed the older DASH diet or the Mediterranean diet. All three diets reduced the risk for Alzheimer's disease. But only the MIND diet did so even when the participants followed the plan only "moderately well."

This is an important distinction because few people are perfect about sticking to diets. Most cheat now and then and eat more unhealthy foods than they should.

The MIND diet specifies "brain-healthy" food groups and five groups that need to be limited, either eaten in moderation or preferably not at all.

WHAT TO EAT

• **More leafy greens.** Kale really is a superfood for the brain. So are spinach, chard, beet greens and other dark, leafy greens. The Mediterranean and DASH diets advise people to eat more vegetables, but they don't specify which ones.

The MIND diet specifically recommends one serving of greens a day, in addition to one other vegetable. Previous research has shown that a vegetable-rich diet can help prevent cognitive decline, but two of the larger studies found that leafy greens were singularly protective.

• **Lots of nuts.** The diet calls for eating nuts five times a week. Nuts are high in vitamin E and monounsaturated and polyunsaturated fats—all good for brain health.

The study didn't look at which nuts were more likely to be beneficial. Eating a variety is probably a good idea because you'll get a varied mix of protective nutrients and antioxidants. Raw or roasted nuts are fine (as long as they're not roasted in fat and highly salted). If you are allergic to nuts, seeds such as sunflower and pumpkin seeds are good sources of these nutrients as well.

• **Berries.** These are the only fruits that are specifically included in the MIND diet. Other fruits are undoubtedly good for you, but none has been shown in studies to promote cognitive health. Berries, on the other hand, have been shown to slow age-related cognitive decline. In laboratory studies, a berry-rich diet improves memory and protects against abnormal changes in the brain. Blueberries seem to be particularly potent. Eat berries at least twice a week.

•**Beans and whole grains.** These fiber-rich and folate-rich foods provide high levels of protein with much less saturated fat than you would get from an equivalent helping of meat. The MIND diet calls for three daily servings of whole grains and three weekly servings of beans.

•**Include fish and poultry—but you don't need to go overboard.** Seafood is a key component of the Mediterranean diet, and some proponents recommend eating it four times a week or more. The MIND diet calls for only one weekly serving, although more is OK. A once-a-week fish meal is enough for brain health.

There is no data to specify the number of poultry servings needed for brain health, but we recommend two servings a week.

•**A glass of wine.** People who drink no wine—or those who drink too much—are more likely to suffer cognitive declines than those who drink just a little.

Recommended: One glass a day. Red wine, in particular, is high in flavonoids and polyphenols that may be protective for the brain.

FOODS TO LIMIT

•**Limit red meat, cheese, butter and margarine**—along with fast food, fried food and pastries and other sweets. The usual suspects, in other words.

All of these food groups increase the risk for Alzheimer's disease, probably because of their high levels of saturated fat (or, in the case of some margarines, trans fats). Saturated fat has been linked to higher cholesterol, more systemic inflammation and possibly a disruption of the blood-brain barrier that may allow harmful substances into the brain.

However, most nutritionists acknowlege the importance of letting people enjoy some treats and not being so restrictive that they give up eating healthfully altogether.

Try to follow these recommendations...

Red meat: No more than three servings a week.

Butter and margarine: Less than one tablespoon daily. Cook with olive oil instead.

Cheese: Less than one serving a week.

Pastries and sweets: Yes, you can enjoy some treats, but limit yourself to five servings or fewer a week.

Fried or fast food: Less than one serving a week.

Additional Studies Show Mediterranean Diet Fights Alzheimer's

Nikolaos Scarmeas, MD, associate professor of clinical neurology, Columbia University Medical Center, New York City, and lead author of a study of 2,258 elderly patients.

Yian Gu, PhD, assistant professor, neuropsychology, Columbia University College of Physicians & Surgeons, New York City.

The Mediterranean diet reduces Alzheimer's risk. Elderly patients who strictly followed the diet were 40% less likely to develop the disease than similar patients who did not.

Theory: The diet—which is high in monounsaturated fats (such as olive oil), produce, fish and legumes and low in meat and dairy—is associated with lower rates of cardiovascular disease and inflammation, both of which increase risk of Alzheimer's.

EATING THE RIGHT FIVE FOODS CAN POSTPONE BRAIN AGING BY FIVE YEARS

Recent study: Adults age 65 and older who frequently ate at least five foods from the Mediterranean diet (such as fish, vegetables, fruit, whole grains, legumes and olive oil) and consumed moderate amounts of wine and low amounts of dairy, meat and poultry were found to have larger brain volumes than those who didn't eat this way. The difference in brain volume was comparable to about five fewer years of brain aging.

Theory: The Mediterranean diet may help slow the loss of brain cells during aging.

Good and Easy...Eating the Mediterranean Way

Wendy Kohatsu, MD, assistant clinical professor of family medicine at the University of California, San Francisco, and director of the Integrative Medicine Fellowship at the Santa Rosa Family Medicine Residency Program in Santa Rosa, California. Dr. Kohatsu is also a graduate of the Oregon Culinary Institute.

There is abundant scientific evidence on the health benefits of the so-called Mediterranean diet, which promotes the traditional eating habits of long-lived people in such countries as Greece and Italy.

Landmark research: Among the most compelling evidence is one long-term European study of healthy men and women ages 70 to 90.

It found that following the Mediterranean diet as part of an overall healthful lifestyle, including regular exercise, was associated with a more than 50% lower rate of death from all causes over a decade. Numerous studies have associated this type of eating with reduced risk for heart disease, cancer, cognitive decline, diabetes and obesity.

But many Americans are reluctant to try the Mediterranean diet for fear that it will be difficult or costly to follow because it emphasizes such foods as omega-3–rich fish, vegetables and nuts.

Surprising findings: Mediterranean eating does not increase food costs, according to a recent study—and this style of eating need not be complicated.

Below, Wendy Kohatsu, MD, an assistant clinical professor of family medicine at the University of California, San Francisco, and a chef who conducts cooking demonstrations for patients and doctors, explains the best ways to incorporate Mediterranean eating into your daily diet...

EASY WAYS TO GET STARTED

To effectively tap into the Mediterranean diet's powerful health benefits, it's important to know exactly which foods should be eaten—and in what quantities.

Start by getting four to five daily servings of whole grains (one serving equals one-half cup of cooked quinoa, brown rice or whole-wheat pasta, for example, or one slice of whole-wheat bread) and two to three daily servings of low- or nonfat dairy products (such as yogurt, cottage cheese or milk), which are an important source of bone-protecting calcium. *In addition, be sure to consume...*

•**Oily fish.** This high-quality protein contains abundant omega-3 fatty acids, which help fight the inflammation that plays a role in cardiovascular disease, Alzheimer's disease and asthma.

Best choices: Follow the acronym SMASH—salmon (wild)...mackerel (Spanish, not king, which tends to have higher levels of mercury)...anchovies...sardines...and herring.

How much: Three ounces (the size of a deck of cards), twice a week.

Chef's secret: Drain canned sardines (the large size), grill briefly, sprinkle with fresh lemon juice and chopped parsley.

Beware: Some fish—such as shark, swordfish, golden bass (tilefish), king mackerel and albacore tuna—can be high in mercury. Avoid these. If you eat tuna, choose the "light" version, which contains less mercury than albacore tuna does.

If you don't like fish: Take a fish oil supplement (1,000 mg daily). Choose a brand that guarantees that no lead or mercury is present.

My favorite brands: Carlson's and Nordic Naturals.

Vegetarians can get omega-3s from flaxseed, walnuts and other nonfish sources. However, nonfish food sources of omega-3s are largely in the form of alpha-linolenic acid (ALA), which is not as potent as the more biologically powerful fatty acids found in fish. Algae-derived docosahexaenoic acid (DHA) capsules contain the omega-3s found in fish. The recommended dose of DHA capsules is 1,000 mg daily.

What most people don't know: A small but important study shows that eating oily fish with beans, such as lentils and chickpeas (also known as garbanzo beans), improves absorption of the iron found in beans.

• **Olive oil.** Olive oil contains about 77% healthful monounsaturated fats. Olive oil is also high in sterols, plant extracts that help reduce LDL "bad" cholesterol and increase HDL "good" cholesterol.

Best choice: Look for extra-virgin (or "first-press") olive oil. ("Extra virgin" means that the oil is derived from the first pressing of the olives.)

How much: Use olive oil as your primary fat—in salad dressings, marinades and sautées. To minimize your total daily intake of fat, do not exceed 18 g to 20 g of saturated fat and 0 g of trans fat from all food sources.

Chef's secret: If you dislike the "grassy" taste of some extra-virgin olive oils, look for Spanish and Moroccan versions, which tend to be more mellow. One good choice is olive oil made from the arbequina olive, which has a buttery taste.

What most people don't know: Nutrients in extra-virgin olive oil may offer some pain-relieving qualities over the long term.

• **Nuts.** Like extra-virgin olive oil, nuts are high in healthful monounsaturated fats. In fact, a recent Spanish study found that a Mediterranean diet that included walnuts significantly lowered risk for heart disease.

What kinds: Besides walnuts, best choices include almonds and peanuts. Choose plain raw nuts—not salted or honey-roasted.

How much: One-quarter cup daily.

Beware: A quarter cup of nuts contains about 200 calories. Eat only a small handful daily—for example, about 23 almonds or 35 peanuts. If you're allergic to nuts, try pumpkin, sunflower or sesame seeds instead.

Chef's secret: Store nuts in your freezer to prevent them from going rancid.

• **Fruits and vegetables.** Many of the most healthful vegetables—including those of the brassica family, such as cabbage, kale, broccoli and cauliflower—originated in the Mediterranean area.

What kinds: Choose brightly colored fruit, such as citrus and berries, and vegetables,

such as spinach, watercress, beets, carrots and broccoli.

How much: Five to nine servings daily. (A serving is one-half cup of cooked vegetables, one cup of leafy greens, one medium orange or one-half cup of berries.)

Contrary to popular belief, frozen vegetables, which are often far less costly than fresh produce, are just as nutritious—if not more so because they're frozen at their peak level of freshness and don't spoil in the freezer.

Chef's secret: Cooking tomatoes in olive oil concentrates the tomatoes' levels of lycopene, a powerful antioxidant that has been associated with a decreased risk for prostate, lung and stomach cancers.

The Way We Eat May Be "Making Us Crazy"

Russell B. Marz, ND, LAc, assistant professor of nutrition, National University of Natural Medicine, Portland, Oregon, and medical director of the Tabor Hill Clinic in Portland, Oregon.
Mental Health Foundation. MentalHealth.org.uk

Poor diet gets a hunk of the blame for rising rates of mental illness, according to recent research from the UK. "Feeding Minds," a report by the British Mental Health Foundation, describes how eating habits have devolved over the past 60 years. The recent report emphasizes the link between diet and mental health, saying "the evidence indicates that food plays an important contributing role in the development, management and prevention of specific mental health problems, such as depression, schizophrenia, attention deficit hyperactivity disorder, and Alzheimer's disease."

Bad habits—like skipping breakfast, grabbing a fast-food burger for lunch and popping a frozen pizza into the microwave and calling it "dinner"—have become a way of life, in large part because people are busy. This kind of food may fill the stomach, but not the body's nutritional needs. The "Feeding Minds" report found that British people now eat 34% fewer vegetables and 59% less fish than 60 years ago. Fast and processed foods are almost always low in critical brain-supporting components such as vitamins, minerals and essential fatty acids, and are loaded with refined carbohydrates, saturated fats and additives—a recipe for irritability, mood swings and worse. Another factor is that industrial farming has altered our food at the most basic level. Changes in feed have increased body fat composition of certain animals and farmed fish we eat—as a result we now often take in a far higher ratio of omega-6 fatty acids to omega-3s, a shift that has been linked with depression as well as deficits in memory and focus.

Food allergens are yet another contributor to mental health issues, including mood and attention problems. According to Russell B. Marz, ND, an assistant professor of nutrition at the National University of Natural Medicine in Portland, Oregon, the growing use of genetically modified high fructose corn syrup in many foods and beverages has been suspected not only in increasing rates of obesity and diabetes, but also serious food allergies.

POOR DIET & MENTAL HEALTH

These changes add up to neurological challenges such as slower brain function and chronic inflammation. *Poor diet has been linked with mental health in a number of conditions...*

- **ADHD** (Attention Deficit Hyperactivity Disorder). Studies show that people with ADHD are low in certain types of omega-3 fatty acids, like DHA.
- **Anxiety.** Nervousness and anxiety are associated with a lack of folic acid, niacinamide, pyridoxine, magnesium and calcium.
- **Dementia and Alzheimer's disease.** Research has linked Alzheimer's with an increased level of homocysteine, an amino acid metabolite associated with decreased levels of folate, B-12 and pyridoxine.
- **Depression.** Depression is linked to low fish consumption, as well as deficiencies in B vitamins, vitamin C, folic acid, magnesium, selenium and zinc.
- **Irritability.** A lack of vitamin B-6 (pyridoxine), magnesium and selenium is commonly found in people who are irritable.
- **Poor memory and concentration.** Lapses in memory and concentration may be linked to a lack of B-12 and other B vitamins, omega-3 fatty acids and zinc.
- **Schizophrenia.** Evidence suggests that people with this disorder have low levels of polyunsaturated fatty acids or antioxidant enzymes in the brain...and low levels of EPA (eicosapentaenoic acid).

EAT YOUR WAY TO MIND-BODY HEALTH

With growing evidence of the link between mental health and diet, it's yet one more compelling reason, if indeed anyone still needs one, to follow a healthy diet. Fortunately the same whole foods that nourish the body also nourish the mind.

- **Avoid additives,** preservatives and pesticides. Pesticides and other chemicals can aggravate problems like depression by impairing the absorption of vital nutrients such as pyridoxine, cautions Dr. Marz. When possible, buy free-range, antibiotic-free meat and local produce that is in season and organically grown. The fewer chemicals, the better for your health. If you purchase non-organic fruits and vegetables, wash and peel them to reduce chemical residues.
- **Include protein in every meal.** Protein is the body's source of essential amino acids, required to produce neurotransmitters such as serotonin (which stabilizes mood and promotes sleep) and dopamine (which imparts energy and mental focus). If you lack sufficient amino acids, you cannot manufacture enough of these chemicals. Protein also helps stabilize blood glucose levels and prevent mood swings. Good sources include fish, eggs, skinless chicken and lean meats. Seafood or animal protein is the best source of vitamin B-12, but if you're over 50 you may have trouble absorbing this nutrient and require a supplement.
- **Eat fish such as salmon or halibut two or three times a week,** as they are excellent sources of the omega-3 fatty acids eicosapentaenoic acid (EPA) and docosahexaenoic acid

(DHA). Seventy percent of the brain is composed of fat (if you exclude the water), making essential fatty acids (omega-3 and omega-6) a must for optimal brain function. Research from the Framingham Heart Study shows that people who ate fish more than two times a week halved their risk of Alzheimer's. Another option is to take a daily fish oil supplement of combined DHA and EPA.

•**Go nuts.** Eat a handful of nuts and/or seeds daily. Walnuts, cashews, peanuts and sunflower and pumpkin seeds are rich sources of magnesium and zinc. Walnuts, pumpkin seeds, flax and hemp seeds are also good sources of omega-3 fatty acids. One mice study showed that a diet high in almonds may lower the risk of or prevent Alzheimer's disease.

• **Eat lots of fresh produce**—five to 13 servings a day, according to US guidelines. Leafy green veggies such as spinach and kale are rich in folic acid, which supports concentration and memory…citrus fruits, peppers and strawberries are excellent sources of vitamin C…broccoli, Brussels sprouts and cabbage are sources of magnesium. In Dr. Marz's opinion, including more nutrient- and fiber-rich foods in your diet is even more important than including protein.

• **Stay hydrated.** About 50% to 65% of your body weight consists of water, which carries vital nutrients into cells and ushers waste products out. This seemingly simple advice constitutes a cornerstone of health.

• **If you drink alcohol, do so in moderation only.** A study in the October 2008 issue of the *Archives of Neurology* notes that alcohol causes shrinkage of the brain. The more you drink, the more your brain shrinks. It's best to drink alcoholic beverages with your meal and choose organic red wines and unprocessed darker beers that contain higher phenolic levels. Experts generally advise against more than one alcoholic beverage a day for women and two for men.

ONE PIECE OF THE PUZZLE

Of course, a good diet is not a panacea for mental problems any more than a bad diet is the sole cause. Serious diseases such as depression and schizophrenia obviously require expert medical treatment. That said, diet is one piece of the puzzle, and a healthful diet is a must for optimal health overall.

Note: You can download a free copy of the "Feeding Minds" report—complete with recipes and nutritional advice—at the website of the British Mental Health Foundation, Mental Health.org.uk.

Can French Fries Cause Alzheimer's?

Richard M. LoPachin, PhD, neurochemist and director of research, department of anesthesiology, Montefiore Medical Center, Albert Einstein College of Medicine, Bronx, New York.

Researchers have an abundance of theories on what causes Alzheimer's disease, but it's been challenging to nail down the scientific proof. Though the central cause has been elusive, one thing that all these researchers agree on is that early in the disease process, nerve endings in the brain get destroyed. Now some recent research reported in the *Journal of Neurochemistry* has unearthed one potential agent of destruction—a group of toxic chemicals called type-2 alkenes that damage nerve endings when they accumulate in the brain. The brain itself produces some of these neurotoxicants naturally, but others come from our environment.

A DANGEROUS PATH

Richard M. LoPachin, PhD, a neurochemist and director of research in the department of anesthesiology at Montefiore Medical Center, Bronx, New York, and a researcher in Alzheimer's disease, said that years ago, he did animal studies demonstrating that type 2-alkenes destroy nerve endings in the brain. Other studies have found an excess of these neurotoxicants in the brains of Alzheimer's patients. The recent research suggests that the damage originates when some of the brain's mitochondria (the power-producers that exist in all cells) become dysfunctional, creating free radicals that ultimately generate the type 2-alkenes. Some people may be genetically predisposed to this type of mitochondria failure, and in these folks, the destruction is "a low-grade event that accumulates damage over many years," Dr. LoPachin said. It seems that such damage can be sped up with exposure to type-2 alkenes that we eat or breathe.

For instance, we know that people who smoke are at higher risk for Alzheimer's—Dr. LoPachin said that he believes it is the type-2 alkenes in tobacco that cause this higher risk and noted that these neurotoxicants exist in other places, too, including in auto exhaust, industrial pollution and smoke from burning organic material, including fireplaces and coal stoves. As to those french fries, Dr. LoPachin explained that potatoes have a certain amino acid (asparagine) that reacts with potatoes' natural sugar at high temperatures to produce dangerous type-2 alkenes.

NO MORE FRIES?

Does this mean that you have to forever avoid fireplaces and french fries? Well, it's not a bad idea (especially the fries)—but fortunately research has identified natural compounds that are quite helpful in partially protecting the brain against type-2 alkenes.

In particular, Dr. LoPachin says that curcumin (found in the spice turmeric and in curries that use it)…resveratrol (in red wine and grape skins)…and phloretin (apple skins) are strong neuroprotectors, but he adds that these are only a few among thousands of other protective phytopolyphenols in various fruits and vegetables. Researchers are working to isolate some of these compounds for potential use as therapeutic agents, but Dr. LoPachin advises getting phytopolyphenols in their natural state by eating them in foods, where they are accompanied by other helpful cofactors and offer greater bioavailability.

Once again it seems that the real secret to minimizing the risk for dire health problems is quite simple—eat lots and lots of fruits and vegetables!

7 Foods That Make You Smarter

Daniel G. Amen, MD, and Tana Amen, BSN. Dr. Amen is medical director of Amen Clinics, Inc. He is a clinical neuroscientist, psychiatrist, brain-imaging specialist and author of *Use Your Brain to Change Your Age*. His wife, Tana Amen, is a nutritional and fitness expert. AmenClinics.com

We all know that we need to eat right to keep our minds sharp. But some foods really pack a punch when it comes to memory, learning and other cognitive abilities. *Here, one of America's top brain specialists reveals the seven super brain boosters…*

1. Coconut water. It's high in potassium, a mineral that is critical for brain health. Potassium causes nerve cells to "fire" at the right speed. People who don't get enough potassium tend to have a slower rate of brain activity and may experience confusion and slower reaction times.

Potassium is particularly important if you eat a lot of salt. The body needs to maintain a proper sodium-potassium balance. You should consume roughly twice as much potassium as sodium.

A medium-sized banana has more potassium (about 450 mg) than coconut water (about 250 mg per eight-ounce serving), but bananas also are higher on the glycemic index, a measure of how quickly the food is converted into glucose. The brain works more efficiently when sugars enter the bloodstream gradually rather than "spiking." Coconut water achieves this more readily than bananas.

Recommended: About one cup of coconut water daily. It has a light taste and is low in calories. If you want, you can add it to smoothies or mix it with milk and pour it over breakfast cereals.

2. Blueberries. Sure, blueberries are good for you, but you may not realize just how super rich in inflammation-fighting antioxidants they are. Their oxygen radical absorbance capacity (ORAC, a measure of a food's antioxidant ability) is 2,400, compared with 670 for cherries and 483 for pink grapefruit.

Studies at Tufts University showed that animals that had blueberries added to their diet performed better on cognitive tests than those given a standard diet. They also had increased cell growth in the hippocampus, the part of the brain associated with memory.

Recommended: One-half cup daily. If you don't like blueberries, opt for strawberries or acai berries (a purple, slightly tart berry available in many health-food stores).

Or try Concord grape juice. Researchers from the University of Cincinnati tested Concord grape juice versus a placebo beverage on 21 volunteers, average age 76, suffering from mild cognitive impairment. After 16 weeks, those in the grape-juice group scored better on tests of memory than those drinking the placebo. Also, MRI testing showed greater activation in key parts of the brain, suggesting increased blood flow.

3. Sardines. Salmon often is touted as a healthy fish that is high in omega-3 fatty acids, fats that protect the brain as well as the heart and arteries. Sardines are even better. They also contain generous amounts of omega-3s, but because of their small size, they accumulate lower levels of mercury and other toxins than larger fish.

The membranes that surround brain cells require omega-3s for the efficient transmission of signals. A Danish study that looked at the diets of more than 5,000 adults found that those who ate the most fish were more likely to maintain their memory than those who ate the least. Other research has shown that people who eat fish as little as once a week can lower their risk for dementia.

Recommended: At least two to three servings of fish a week. If you prefer salmon to sardines, be sure to buy wild salmon. It contains more omega-3s than farm-raised fish.

Also helpful: Avocados. They're among the best plant sources of omega-3s.

4. Walnuts. All nuts are good for the brain (as long as they're not roasted in oil and covered with salt). Like fish, nuts are rich in omega-3 fatty acids. They're also loaded with vitamin E, which, in some studies, has been shown to slow the progression of Alzheimer's disease.

In addition, nuts reduce LDL "bad"cholesterol (important for preventing stroke). Walnuts are particularly good because they have very high levels of omega-3s. Macadamia nuts are another good choice.

Bonus: The Adventist Health Study, conducted by researchers at Loma Linda University, found that people who ate nuts five or more times a week were about half as likely to have a heart attack as those who rarely ate nuts.

Recommended: About one-quarter cup daily. Nuts are higher in calories than most plant foods, so you don't want to eat too many.

5. Sweet potatoes. They are another low-glycemic food that causes only small fluctuations in blood sugar. This can help you maintain energy and concentration throughout the day. We routinely advise patients to eat sweet potatoes because they satisfy a craving for carbohydrates, and they're also high in beta-carotene and other important antioxidants that keep the brain sharp.

One sweet potato (when you eat the skin) provides more fiber than a bowl of oatmeal. Dietary fiber lowers cholesterol and improves brain circulation.

Recommended: Eat sweet potatoes two to three times a week. If you don't like sweet potatoes, eat yellow squash or spaghetti squash.

6. Green tea. It contains the potent antioxidant epigallocatechin gallate that protects brain cells from free radicals caused by air pollution, toxins, a high-fat diet, etc. Green tea also contains compounds that increase levels of dopamine in the brain. Dopamine is a neurotransmitter that stimulates the brain's reward and pleasure centers and makes you more motivated to make positive lifestyle choices.

Bonus: A double-blind study that looked at patients with mild cognitive impairment found that an amino acid in green tea, L-theanine, improved concentration and energy and reduced anxiety.

Recommended: Two cups daily.

7. Turmeric. The bright yellow color indicates high levels of antioxidants. People who use this spice several times a week have significant reductions in C-reactive protein, a substance that indicates inflammation in the brain and/or other tissues.

A study that looked at more than 1,000 elderly people found that those who ate curry—which includes generous amounts of turmeric—regularly did better on mental-status evaluations than those who rarely or never ate it. All spices with bright, deep colors are high in neuroprotective antioxidants.

Examples: Both ginger and cinnamon appear to have brain-protective properties similar to those of turmeric. And sage improves memory.

Recommended: Add one-quarter teaspoon to one-half teaspoon of any of these spices to your food every day.

Brain Food for the Sexes

Daniel G. Amen, MD, a brain-imaging specialist who is founder, CEO and medical director of Amen Clinics. Based in Newport Beach, California, he is author of numerous books, including *Unleash the Power of the Female Brain.* AmenClinics.com

---

Women and men need different foods. The reason? They have very different brains.

We did a study of 46,000 brain scans involving about 26,000 patients. Using a brain-imaging test called SPECT (single photon emission computed tomography), we found clear differences between male and female brains.

In general: Women's brains are more active than men's brains. Much of this activity is in the region known as the prefrontal cortex, which controls judgment, impulse control and organization. Women also produce less serotonin than men. Serotonin is the neurotransmitter that makes you less worried and more relaxed, so women are more prone to anxiety and depression.

Men, on the other hand, produce less dopamine. Dopamine is involved with focus and impulse control, so men are more likely to be impulsive and have trouble concentrating.

BEST FOODS FOR WOMEN

Foods that increase serotonin are critical for women. *When their serotonin levels rise, women naturally experience less anxiety and are less likely to get upset…*

• **Chickpeas.** Also known as garbanzo beans, chickpeas increase the brain's production of serotonin. Other carbohydrates do the same thing, but chickpeas are better because they're high in nutrients and fiber, with about 12 grams of fiber per one-cup serving. Fiber slows the body's absorption of sugars…prevents sharp spikes in insulin…and helps the brain work at optimal levels.

• **Sweet potatoes.** They're my favorite starch because they taste good, are high in vitamin C and fiber and don't raise blood sugar/insulin as quickly as white potatoes. They're a "smart" carbohydrate that causes a gradual increase in serotonin.

• **Blueberries.** They're called "brain berries" for a reason. Blueberries are a concentrated source of flavonoids and other antioxidants that reduce brain inflammation. This is important for good mood and memory. Studies have shown that people who eat blueberries may have less risk for dementia-related cognitive declines.

You will get some of the same benefits with other berries, including strawberries, but blueberries are a better choice for brain function.

• **Dark chocolate.** It is one of the healthiest foods that you can eat. Chocolate increases levels of nitric oxide, a molecule that dilates arteries throughout the body, including those in the brain. One study found that women who ate the most chocolate had greater improvements in verbal fluency and other mental functions than those who ate the least. Chocolate also can improve your mood and energy levels. Because it's high in antioxidants, it reduces the "oxidative stress" that can impair memory and other brain functions.

I recommend dark chocolate with natural sweeteners. My company, Amen Clinics, makes a Brain on Joy Bar with dark chocolate and coconut.

BEST FOODS FOR MEN

Men naturally gravitate to high-protein foods. The protein increases dopamine and provides fuel for a man's greater muscle mass. *The trick for men is choosing healthier protein sources...*

• **Salmon.** Between 15% and 20% of the brain's cerebral cortex consists of docosahexaenoic acid (DHA), one of the omega-3 fatty acids found in salmon and other fatty fish such as tuna, trout, sardines, herring and mackerel. Men who don't eat fish are more likely to have brain inflammation that can impair the transmission of nerve signals.

A study published in *Alzheimer's & Dementia: The Journal of the Alzheimer's Association* found that elderly adults who got more DHA had improvements in memory and learning. The study focused on supplements, but you can get plenty of DHA and other omega-3s by eating fatty fish more often.

• **Eggs.** They are not the dietary danger that people once thought. Recent research has shown that people who eat a few eggs a week—or even as many as one a day—are no more likely to develop heart disease or have a stroke than those who don't eat eggs.

Eggs are an excellent source of protein, inexpensive and easy to prepare. They also are high in vitamin B-12, which can reduce age-related brain shrinkage and improve cognitive function.

• **Sesame seeds and Brazil nuts.** In addition to increasing dopamine, they contain antioxidants that protect brain cells. Like other nuts and seeds, they're high in protein and monounsaturated fats that reduce LDL "bad" cholesterol.

Nuts and seeds are good for the heart as well as the brain. The landmark Adventist Health Study, conducted by researchers at Loma Linda University, found that people who ate nuts five or more times a week were only about half as likely to have a heart attack as those who rarely ate them.

Eat Your Way to a Better Memory

Oranges are a great source of folate, which boosts recall and information processing. Aim for one medium-sized orange per day. Black beans are rich in fiber and vitamin B-1, which helps memory by synthesizing acetylcholine, a neurotransmitter that is crucial for memory. Aim for one-half cup a day. Sage improves recall for up to four hours after consumption. Add one teaspoon of sage-infused olive oil to canned or homemade soup, or use it in a meat marinade.

Natural Health.

Foods That Fight Memory Loss

Rhoda Au, PhD, professor of neurology, Boston University School of Medicine, and director of neuropsychology, Framingham Heart Study.

There's a way to potentially prevent Alzheimer's—a disease that we know frustratingly little about—and it's not some exotic, expensive or potentially dangerous drug. It's actually an affordable, natural component that's found in everyday foods. A recent study confirms an association between dietary choline, an amino acid found in eggs and some other foods, and better cognitive performance.

BRAIN BOOSTER

Researchers, from Boston University School of Medicine, investigated the dietary habits of 744 women and 647 men ranging from 36 to 83 years of age. Participants filled out questionnaires about their diets, first in the early 1900s and then between 1998 and 2001. The researchers also did MRI brain scans to see if there were any tell-tale lesions in the white matter areas called *white-matter hyperintensities* (WMH). WMH in the brain is considered a marker of vascular disease and is strongly associated with cognitive impairments that precede Alzheimer's disease.

The results: First, this study demonstrated that people who were more recently eating the most choline performed better on tests of verbal and visual memory, compared with those who had the lowest choline intake. Researchers also found that those who had eaten the highest amounts of choline years earlier were more likely to have little or no WMH. In other words, eating lots of choline may make your memory sharper, and it also may reduce the risk for damage to the brain and even Alzheimer's disease.

HOW THE NUTRIENT PROTECTS YOUR NOGGIN

Study coauthor Rhoda Au, PhD, professor of neurology at Boston University emphasized that this specific research is an observational study, so it doesn't prove cause and effect, but it does show a link between choline and memory. Why? Choline's crucial contribution to cognition, said Dr. Au, may be as a building block for a neurotransmitter called acetylcholine, which is known to help transmit information between neurons faster.

DIET "DOS"

How much choline do you need each day? The recommendation from the Institute of Medicine for men is a daily intake of 550 mg and for women, 425 mg. *The richest food sources are...*

- **3.5 ounces of beef liver**—430 mg
- **One large egg**—126 mg
- **3.5 ounces of salmon**—91 mg
- **3.5 ounces (just under one-half cup) of broccoli, Brussels sprouts, cauliflower or navy beans**—approximately 40 mg.

Other sources of choline include cod, almonds, tofu, milk and peanut butter.

Supplements of choline are available, but high doses (more than 3,500 mg per day for adults over age 18, according to Institute of Medicine) can cause symptoms like vomiting and excessive sweating. So if you want to take a supplement, talk to your doctor first—discuss how much you eat in your diet already so you can figure out whether (and what amount of) a supplement is necessary.

Nutrients That Prevent Dementia

Gabriele Nagel, MD, MPH, an epidemiologist and professor of medicine, and Christine von Arnim, MD, a neurologist and professor of medicine, both at the University of Ulm, Germany. They are leading authors of a study published in *Journal of Alzheimer's Disease.*

You've probably heard that pirates and sailors of yore stocked up on vitamin C-rich citrus fruits to prevent scurvy.

But it's possible that those seafaring men also kept their minds sharper for longer (assuming that they went easy on the rum).

Yes, it turns out that we can learn a thing or two from Blackbeard and the like!

A recent study found that senior citizens who consume plenty of vitamin C—plus another easy-to-find nutrient—may be less likely to develop dementia with age.

BRAIN-BOOSTING VITAMINS

Here's how this research came about. A group of German scientists knew that oxidative stress—which restricts the use of oxygen in the body, causing cells to break down—plays an important role in the aging process, where all of our body's systems (including the neurological system) begin to slowly break down. Dementia occurs when the brain degenerates more aggressively than normal. So the researchers, according to Gabriele Nagel, MD, MPH, the study's lead author, wanted to see whether antioxidants, vitamins that can fight off the damage caused by oxidative stress, might help prevent brain degeneration.

For the study, Dr. Nagel and her colleague Christine von Arnim, MD, analyzed data on more than 1,500 men and women between the ages of 65 and 90—some had mild dementia and some were healthy.

When researchers analyzed their blood samples, they noticed a trend: People with dementia had significantly lower blood levels of vitamin C and another antioxidant, beta-carotene, than people without dementia. And this held true after controlling for body mass index, education levels, smoking status, alcohol consumption and current dietary supplement use. The researchers also tested the blood for concentrations of several other antioxidants, including coenzyme Q10, lycopene and vitamin E—but they found no similar connection between those other antioxidants and a reduced dementia risk.

ASSESSING ANTIOXIDANTS

So does this mean that eating more foods containing vitamin C and beta-carotene helps prevent dementia? It's a possibility, although that's not what this study proved. It showed only an association, meaning that some other relationship could have caused the results—for example, it's possible that people with dementia tend to consume less of those particular antioxidants.

On the other hand, vitamin C and beta-carotene are not (of course) exotic and dangerous substances...they're healthful nutrients found naturally in certain wholesome foods...so if we want to think of this dementia study as another reason to eat these foods, there's no harm done!

STOCK UP ON "C" AND BETA-CAROTENE

Beta-carotene is found in high amounts in (as you know) carrots—but also in sweet potatoes, kale, winter squash, cabbage and pumpkins. Good sources of vitamin C include not only citrus fruits but also spinach, strawberries, kiwi, bell peppers, broccoli, cauliflower and Brussels sprouts—and that's certainly better eating than you'd find on any pirate ship!

Why Vegetarians Have It All Wrong

Terry Wahls, MD, an internist and a clinical professor of medicine at the University of Iowa Carver College of Medicine in Iowa City. She is author of *The Wahls Protocol: A Radical New Way to Treat All Chronic Autoimmune Conditions Using Paleo Principles* and founder of The Wahls Foundation, which educates the public and health-care practitioners on the benefits of integrative treatment for multiple sclerosis and other chronic diseases.

A diet rich in fruits and vegetables and whole grains, but with little or no meat, has long been touted as the best way to lower your risk for heart disease, prevent weight gain and reduce risk for certain cancers.

But as a medical doctor with progressive multiple sclerosis (MS), I believe that meat (grass-fed beef...organic chicken, pork and lamb...and wild game and fish) has played a critical role in my recovery—and that meat can help protect against other autoimmune diseases, Parkinson's disease, Alzheimer's disease and early cognitive impairment.

HOW MEAT BENEFITS THE BRAIN

•**Meat provides vitamin B-12.** A diet without meat raises your risk for vitamin B-12 deficiency. If your body doesn't get enough B-12, you can develop neurological symptoms such as problems with balance and co-ordination, difficulties with decision-making and cognitive decline. Vitamin B-12 is found naturally only in animal foods such as clams, liver, salmon and beef. A synthetic form is often added to cereals and nutritional yeast, but I recommend avoiding gluten because many people are sensitive to it. Alternatively, you could take a B-12 supplement, but I prefer natural food sources, which supply additional vitamins and nutrients.

•**Meat is the best source of complete proteins.** Protein is essential to make, repair and maintain the structure of all the cells in our bodies, including cells in the brain. The amino acids found in protein help the brain produce crucial neurotransmitters that regulate mood and maintain and repair brain cells. If you don't have enough protein to do this, brain function deteriorates.

Meat contains all of the essential amino acids your body needs to manufacture protein. To get a complete protein from a nonmeat source, you would have to combine a grain and a legume, for example.

•**Certain meats provide omega-3 fatty acids.** Cell membranes throughout the body, including in the brain, rely on essential fatty acids to stay healthy. The brain is especially dependent on the omega-3 fatty acids docosahexaenoic acid (DHA) and eicosapentaenoic acid (EPA) that are found in fish such as sardines, herring and anchovies (the fish I prefer to eat because small fish have less risk for heavy metal and plastic contamination) as well as organic chicken and grass-fed beef. These omega-3s help preserve the integrity of cell membranes in the brain and stave off neurological problems like mood disorders and cognitive decline.

While you can get alpha linolenic acid (ALA), another omega-3, from plant sources, your body can convert only small amounts of ALA into DHA and EPA. DHA and EPA supplements are available, but numerous studies have shown that foods high in omega-3s are more beneficial to brain health than supplements.

THE BEST MEAT FOR YOUR BRAIN

Most grass-fed beef, organic chicken and wild game and fish are beneficial for brain health, but organ meats (particularly heart, liver and tongue) provide the most nutrition. Organ meats are chock-full of vitamins A and B and essential nutrients such as creatine, carnitine and coenzyme Q10 (CoQ10). There are a variety of ways to add organ meats to your meals and make them more palatable. *To get the most nutrition from meat…*

• **Start with heart.** Beef and bison heart taste a lot like steak, especially if you serve them up with mushrooms. Just don't overcook organ meat, or it will be dry and tough. Cooking it to medium rare also helps the meat retain vitamins.

• **Disguise liver.** If you don't like the taste of liver, purée small raw pieces of it in a blender with water to make a slurry. Add this mixture to soups, stews or chili, and let the food simmer a few minutes.

• **Try sausage or liver pâté.** Your local butcher can make a sausage out of ground liver and some other ground meat, such as pork or chicken. Start with a ratio of one part liver to six parts ground meat, and work up to a ratio of one to three. If you don't like the taste of liver, ask the butcher to add spices to conceal it.

• **Make a bone broth.** Put the carcass of a chicken or beef or pork knuckle bones into a pot. Add one tablespoon of vinegar per one quart of water, and toss in one whole onion and carrot and a few cloves of garlic. Let the broth simmer for at least six hours, then strain out the bone, vegetables and foam. Use the broth as a stock for soup or drink it.

• **Consider an organ meat supplement.** If you just can't stomach the idea of eating organ meat, consider taking a supplement.

Good choice: Organ Delight from Dr. Ron's Ultra-Pure (DrRons.com).

THE WAHLS PROTOCOL

Keep in mind that I'm not advocating a meat-only diet. In fact, the Wahls Protocol diet (the eating plan I developed to combat my own MS) starts by recommending six to nine cups a day (depending on your size and gender) of vegetables, fruits and berries (get twice as many veggies as fruits and berries).

In particular, I prefer green, leafy vegetables…sulfur-rich vegetables in the cabbage and onion families…deeply colored vegetables such as yams, beets, peppers and tomatoes… and brightly colored berries such as raspberries, strawberries and cranberries.

For meat, I recommend six to 12 ounces a day (depending on your size and gender) for disease treatment and prevention.

My regimen also incorporates a CoQ10 supplement, a spirulina or chlorella algae supplement and green tea—which is high in quercetin, an antioxidant with anti-inflammatory properties.

Why Sardines Are So Healthy

Karen Collins, MS, RDN, registered dietitian nutritionist, syndicated columnist and nutrition adviser to the American Institute for Cancer Research. She was an expert reviewer for the Institute's international report, *Food, Nutrition, Physical Activity and the Prevention of Cancer: A Global Perspective.* KarenCollinsNutrition.com

What makes sardines the sea's superfood? Canned sardines have more omega-3 fatty acids than most fish. And because they're a small fish that's low on the food chain, they contain less mercury than many other fish. They're also inexpensive and are a sustainable source of protein. So why do Americans eat only minnow-size amounts?

Sardines are an oily fish, and oily fish can taste a little…well, fishy. You might prefer sardines that are lightly smoked or sardines nestled in mustard or tomato sauce.

Here, more on the health benefits of sardines…

Great for omega-3s: A recent report from the USDA concluded that 80% to 90% of Americans eat less than eight ounces of fish a week, the minimum recommended amount. This means that you're probably not getting enough omega-3s, beneficial fats that have been shown to reduce the risk for heart disease and that may protect against cancer, depression, rheumatoid arthritis and other serious conditions.

All cold-water fish provide omega-3s, but sardines are among the best. A four-ounce serving of sardines has about 1.1 to 1.6 grams. That's right up there with salmon (1.2 to 2.4 g depending on the salmon) and much higher than cod (0.2 g) or the most common types of tuna (0.3 g).

Your body needs these important types of fats. A study published in *Neurology* found that people who ate fish three or more times a week were about 26% less likely to have silent infarcts, damaged brain areas that can lead to dementia and stroke. Omega-3s have been found to reduce heart irregularities (arrhythmias) that can be deadly and even may provide some blood pressure control help. Some experts speculate that the anti-inflammatory effects of omega-3s could help prevent some cancers…and eating more fish can help people eat less red meat or processed meat, important for decreasing the risk for colorectal cancer.

Other health benefits: Sardines are high in protein, vitamin D and selenium—and sardines with bones give an extra shot of calcium. A three-ounce serving of bones-in sardines has as much calcium as a glass of milk.

Less mercury: Some people avoid seafood altogether because they're worried about mercury, a contaminant found in virtually all fish, including farmed fish.

Good news: Sardines are among the lowest-mercury fish in the sea. They do contain trace amounts, but that might be offset by their high selenium content. The research isn't conclusive, but it's possible that a high-selenium diet could reduce the risks of mercury, either by "binding up" the mineral or by reducing its oxidative effects.

The health benefits of sardines and other fish more than outweigh the potential downsides of mercury—so much so that the EPA's and FDA's recently revised guidelines encourage pregnant women and young children (who are particularly susceptible to mercury) to eat eight to 12 ounces of low-mercury fish a week.

The New "Brain Food"

Want your brain to be as sharp as someone's a decade younger? Eat more spinach and kale. A 10-year study of more than 950 older adults found that those who ate just one or two servings of leafy greens per day had the cognitive abilities of people 11 years younger.

Why it works: The lutein and vitamin K in the greens protect cognitive function.

Important: If you take the blood thinner *warfarin*, work with your doctor to modify your dosage if you increase your intake of leafy greens.

Martha Clare Morris, ScD, director of nutrition and nutritional epidemiology, Rush University, Chicago.

Move Over Spinach… Slice Up These Three Super Greens

Mark A. Stengler, NMD, licensed naturopathic medical doctor in private practice, Stengler Center for Integrative Medicine, Encinitas, California…author of many books, including *The Natural Physician's Healing Therapies* and coauthor of *Prescription for Natural Cures*.

It seems to me that everyone cooks with spinach because it is easy to do. But other dark green leafy vegetables are some of the most healthful and delicious foods around. So why don't we eat more of them? Brimming with nutrients, kale and mustard greens are cruciferous vegetables full of anti-inflammatory antioxidants and indole-3-carbinol, a chemical believed to block the growth of some cancer cells. And Swiss chard has lots of calcium plus abundant amounts of beta-carotene.

Despite these health benefits, many people are put off by these unfamiliar greens. I find that once people know how to cook kale, mustard greens and Swiss chard, they discover them to be both tasty and easy to serve. Nevia No, the owner of Bodhitree Farm in Burlington County, New Jersey, sells these greens and others at farmers' markets in New York City. Her vegetables are a favorite among Manhattan

chefs…and she often can be found providing cooking demonstrations to show how easy it is to release the flavors of these greens.

The Most Nutritious Vegetable Is Watercress!

This cruciferous vegetable scored 100 after being rated on 16 key nutrients and fiber by the CDC.

Other vegetables on the honor roll: Chinese cabbage, chard, beet greens, spinach,

HOW THE GREENS STACK UP…

To select the freshest produce…choose greens with leaves that look firm and perky. Avoid bunches with limp, wilted or faded leaves. While all of these greens can be eaten raw, fresh greens are most flavorful when cooked for just a short time—about five to six minutes.

	FLAVOR	NUTRITION	WAYS TO COOK	QUICK RECIPE
KALE	Sweet with a nutty undertone.	Contains vitamins A and C, calcium, magnesium and iron.	Sauté or steam, boil, braise with broth. Add to soups and stews. Add raw to salads.	**For hearty bruschetta,** sauté 1 cup steamed kale in olive oil with 3 finely chopped garlic cloves. Add 1 can rinsed cannellini beans, partially mashing them, and $\frac{1}{8}$ tsp ground black pepper. Serve spooned onto toasted slices of whole-wheat Italian bread.
SWISS CHARD	White-stemmed is sweetest … red-stemmed is most earthy tasting.	Contains vitamin A, calcium, phosphorus, magnesium and iron. High in sodium. Use caution if following a restricted sodium diet.	Sauté. Braise with broth, add to soups and stews.	**For easy chunky soup,** place 3 cups vegetable broth, 4 cups chopped chard, 1 can rinsed canned chickpeas, $\frac{1}{2}$ cup each frozen corn and cut green beans, a small chopped red onion and chopped garlic in a deep pot. Simmer 15 minutes, uncovered. Serve with grated Parmesan cheese.
MUSTARD GREENS	A peppery, radishlike bite.	Contains vitamins A and C, potassium, calcium, phosphorus and magnesium.	Sauté, steam, slow-cook southern-style with preservative-free chicken or turkey sausage. Add raw to salads in thin shreds.	**For Asian-style greens,** sauté $\frac{1}{2}$ cup chopped onion and 1 cup sliced carrots for 3 minutes. Add $\frac{1}{2}$ cup chicken broth and 1 Tbsp soy sauce, and simmer until crisp-tender, 5 minutes. Mix in 2 cups steamed mustard greens and 1 tsp roasted sesame oil.

chicory, leaf lettuce, parsley, romaine lettuce, collards and turnip greens.

Study of the nutrient density of 47 fruits and vegetables by researchers at Centers for Disease Control and Prevention, Atlanta.

Seeds for Brain Health

Flaxseeds, sunflower seeds, sesame seeds and pumpkin seeds all contain high levels of polyunsaturated oils, as well as protein, vitamins and minerals—including magnesium, which is especially important for brain health.

Best: Nibble seeds instead of other snacks, or add them to salads. There is no need to measure them precisely—about three to four tablespoons a day is ideal.

Larry McCleary, MD, a retired pediatric neurosurgeon in Incline Village, Nevada, and author of *The Brain Trust Program.*

Health Benefits from Dark Chocolate for Your Brain

Bill Gottlieb, CHC, founder and president of Good For You Health Coaching, author of several books including *Health-Defense: How to Stay Vibrantly Healthy in a Toxic World* and *The Every-Other-Day Diet: The Diet That Lets You Eat All You Want (Half the Time) and Keep the Weight Off*, with Krista Varady, PhD. BillGottliebHealth.com

You may already know that dark chocolate is good for you, in particular for your heart. More than 300 scientific studies have established the power of dark chocolate to prevent and reverse heart disease. Dark chocolate is uniquely rich in cocoa flavanols—powerful anti-inflammatory and antioxidant compounds such as epicatechin that are a nutritional tonic for arteries. Green tea, red wine, grapes, coffee and apples also are rich sources of flavanols—but ounce for ounce, dark chocolate contains more than any other food.

Good news: Consuming dark chocolate boosts blood flow to the brain, supplying brain cells (neurons) with more oxygen and glucose. And those well-nourished neurons also perform better. Studies show that ingesting flavanol-rich dark chocolate improves "working memory" (short-term memory used to process information) and attentiveness and decreases mental fatigue.

Recent developments: In a study from Harvard Medical School, one month of consuming dark chocolate improved brain blood flow and mental performance in older people (average age 73) who had poor blood flow to the brain and structural damage to the white matter of the brain, which relays messages between neurons.

In another study, dark chocolate improved the mental functioning of people with mild cognitive impairment—the stage of mental decline before dementia.

WHICH CHOCOLATE IS BEST?

Nearly every client in my health-coaching practice gets a recommendation to consume a daily dose of about 400 milligrams (mg) of cocoa flavanols—the amount used in many of the studies that show a therapeutic effect.

Important: Higher doses don't produce better results.

And the healthiest way to get those flavanols is with unsweetened cocoa powder that delivers all the flavanols of dark chocolate without burdening your daily diet with extra calories and sugar. (Using cocoa powder also helps you control your intake—it's notoriously easy to consume an entire three-ounce bar of chocolate even though your optimal daily "dose" is only one ounce.)

Red flag: Do not use "Dutch" cocoa powder, which is treated with an alkalizing agent for a richer color and milder taste—a process that strips cocoa of 98% of its epicatechin.

My advice: Mix one tablespoon of unsweetened cocoa powder in an eight-to-12-ounce mug of hot water or milk (nondairy milks such as coconut, almond, soy and rice milk are delicious alternatives) and add a no-calorie natural sweetener, such as stevia.

Good products: I recommend CocoaVia, the powder developed by Mars, Incoporated. The Mars Center for Cocoa Health Science has conducted extensive scientific research on cocoa flavanols for two decades, and one "stick" of its powder reliably delivers 375 mg of cocoa flavanols, standardized for epicatechin. You can mix it with cold or warm milk, coffee drinks, smoothies, yogurt or oatmeal. Another high-quality cocoa powder is CocoaWell from Reservage. (*Note*: CocoaVia does process its products with alkali, but it's not a concern because the powder is reliably standardized to deliver a high, therapeutic dose of coca flavanols.)

Dark chocolate bars don't reliably deliver a therapeutic dose of cocoa flavanols. But if you prefer to eat dark chocolate, look for a bar with 70% or more cocoa, and consume about one ounce (28 grams) per day. According to a report from ConsumerLab.com, dark chocolate brands with high levels of flavanols (about one-quarter to one-half the amount in the best brands of cocoa powder) include Endangered Species, Ghirardelli and Lindt.

Contrarian View About the Memory and Antioxidant Powers of Chocolate

Leo Galland, MD, director, Foundation for Integrated Medicine, New York City. PillAdvised.com

You've probably read through many articles about how chocolate boosts brain power and helps fight dementia and memory loss, but, sadly, the media hype is overblown. *There certainly is healing power in cocoa, but here's the real story about how you can best benefit from it...*

THE BITTER TRUTH

The most recent study on the benefits of cocoa comes from Columbia University in New York City. Like similar studies before it, the Columbia findings spurred a wave of news reports and press releases exclaiming that hot cocoa and chocolate improve memory. In this small study of 37 people, participants (healthy men and women aged 50 to 69) received either high-dose flavonol cocoa (900 mg per day) or low-dose flavonol cocoa (10 mg per day). Flavonols are a type of flavonoid, an anti-inflammatory compound found in a wide range of fruits, vegetables and other plant-based foods. And 900 mg of flavonol equals nearly a day's worth of flavonoids that a person would get from a typical Western diet—so that's a lot of flavonols packed into an experimental cocoa drink.

Participants' brains were scanned before and after the three-month study period, and they also were given memory and reaction-time tests.

The results: Participants in the high-dose group had memory skills comparable to people who were 20 to 30 years younger, whereas minimal improvement was seen in participants in the low-dose group.

These findings are consistent with several larger and better-designed clinical trials of cocoa flavonols, but the study may have received more hype than it deserved. The same could be said of an earlier study conducted by Harvard researchers, which showed that both high-dose (609 mg) and low-dose (13 mg) cocoa-based flavonol consumption (in the form of a cocoa drink) improved blood flow in the brain. Publication of the Harvard study was also followed by several misleading news reports claiming that two cups of cocoa a day keep dementia away.

The problem: It's hard to apply these lessons to real life.

Commercial brands of chocolate and cocoa are often processed to the point where most, if not all, of the beneficial antioxidants (flavonols and other important flavonoids) are removed.

THE BEST SOURCES OF ANTIOXIDANTS

Although dark and bitter chocolate and green tea and even black tea can provide some nutritional flavonols, the best approach is eating a diet rich in flavonoids in general. Remember, flavonoids are the group of antioxidants that flavonols belong to. Foods rich in flavonoids include colorful fruits (especially apples, citrus and berries), dark leafy green vegetables (such as kale and spinach), asparagus, colorful nightshade vegetables (such as peppers, tomatoes and eggplant) and dark-colored beans (such as adzuki, black beans and red kidney beans).

A diet that includes a rich variety of vegetables, such as an Asian diet, can pack about 4,000 mg of flavonoids a day. The typical meat-and-potatoes Western diet, in contrast, provides an average of only about 1,000 mg of flavonoids per day.

So, while you could get a bit of a day's worth of flavonols from dark or bitter chocolate, an ordinary chocolate bar or a milky cup of cocoa will only give you a sugar rush and extra calories to work off. Get your flavonols—and other flavonoids—instead from a wide variety of fruits and vegetables and from beverages such as green tea.

This Is Your Brain on Good Cocoa

People with impaired blood flow in the brain who drank two cups of flavonol-rich cocoa per day for one month did better on memory tests than similar people who drank flavonol-poor cocoa. Choose chocolate with at least 35% cocoa or cocoa solids.

Study of 60 people led by researchers at Brigham and Women's Hospital, Boston, and the VA Boston Healthcare System, published in *Neurology*.

Boost Cocoa and Dark Chocolate Health Benefits at the Gut Level

John Finley, PhD, professor, food science, Louisiana State University, Baton Rouge. His research was presented at the annual meeting of the American Chemical Society.

Did you know that the "good" probiotic bacteria in your gut microbiome—the symbiotic cosmos of microbes living in your stomach and intestines—absolutely love cocoa? Not only do they eat it up and grow, they use it to boost your body's probiotic potency and provide a heart-healthy anti-inflammatory effect.

Although scientists already knew that antioxidant compounds called flavonols in cocoa beans are what gives dark chocolate (semisweet, bittersweet and unsweetened) its many healthful properties—including the ability to fight inflammation and high blood pressure and regulate insulin and cholesterol—just how these flavonols in cocoa work had been a mystery. But this mystery was recently solved thanks to a team of food scientists from Louisiana State University in Baton Rouge.

The team studied how flavonols in cocoa—which in and of themselves are too large to be absorbed by the gut—are transformed during human digestion. They did this by simulating the human gastrointestinal tract in test tubes. First, they "digested" unsweetened cocoa powder by mixing the cocoa with digestive enzymes, just as our stomachs would. What was left over after digestion—a small amount of nondigestible fiber (a prebiotic, or type of common food fiber that probiotics need to promote digestive health) and the flavonols—was then mixed with healthy human feces, which is the best source of normal human gut bacteria. In this way, the researchers could closely investigate how the nondigestible cocoa fiber—the prebiotic—and flavonols interact with "good" probiotic gut bacteria, which have names like those you find on yogurt containers, Lactobacillus and Bifidobacterium.

Over the next 24 hours, the fecal bacteria concoction became increasingly more acidic, which meant that the probiotic bacteria were fermenting the fiber. This fermentation made the large flavonol molecules break down into smaller molecules that could be absorbed, like other nutrients, through the gut into the bloodstream. From there, these antioxidant flavonols could do their job of reducing inflammation in cardiovascular tissue, allowing blood to flow through arteries more smoothly and, thereby, helping to prevent a cardiovascular event, such as stroke.

HOW YOU CAN GET THE MOST FROM COCOA

This study, basically, gives us insight about how cocoa "works" in providing health benefits. Now, if you want to take advantage of this science, you certainly can, but most chocolate bars on the market do not contain enough cocoa solids to really benefit you and are full of sugar and additives besides. But you can claim the antioxidant, anti-inflammatory power of cocoa by enjoying dark chocolate—the purer and higher the cocoa content, the better. *Here's how…*

• **Boost dark chocolate's prebiotic potential by combining it with certain carbohydrate-rich prebiotic foods,** such as bananas or wheat-based foods, like wholegrain breads. (Fibrous vegetables such as raw dandelion greens, asparagus and leeks are also great prebiotic sources, so if you want to get creative with dark chocolate-covered asparagus…lots of luck!)

• **Combine dark chocolate with fruits like pomegranates or acai berries** to boost fermentation processes in your gut and pack a double punch of anti-inflammatory antioxidants from both the fruits and cocoa.

So go ahead and indulge in cocoa with a healthy, gut-health–boosting snack on the side to get the most from the natural probiotic cosmos already living inside you.

Water Helps Your Brain

Drinking water is the easiest thing you can do for your brain, but most people don't drink anywhere near enough.

Fact: About 80% of the brain is comprised of water. If you don't drink enough—or if you drink a lot of dehydrating liquids, such as coffee or alcohol—you're going to struggle to think clearly and you may have memory problems. That's because dehydration increases stress hormones, and stress hormones interfere with cognitive abilities.

Recommended: Drink half your weight in water ounces every day.

Example: If you weigh 150 pounds, you'll want to drink 75 ounces of water a day. Drink more during the warm months or if you exercise regularly and lose water in perspiration.

Daniel G. Amen, MD, and Tana Amen, RN, BSN. Dr. Amen is a brain-imaging specialist and founder, CEO and medical director of the Amen Clinics. Tana Amen is a nutritional and fitness expert. Dr. Amen is author of *Use Your Brain to Change Your Age.* AmenClinics.com

5 Best Brain-Boosting Drinks

David Grotto, RD, a registered dietitian and founder and president of Nutrition Housecall, LLC, a Chicago–based nutrition consulting firm. He is an adviser to *Fitness* magazine and blogs for the Real Life Nutrition community featured on WebMD. He is author of *The Best Things You Can Eat.*

Some of the easiest-to-prepare brain foods—meaning foods that can preserve and even improve your memory and other cognitive functions—are actually delicious drinks.

You probably already know about green tea, which is high in epigallocatechin-3-gallate (EGCG), a potent compound that appears to protect neurons from age-related damage. But the following five drinks are scientifically proven to help your brain, too…

BEET JUICE

Beets are a nutritional powerhouse—and so is the juice. It increases levels of nitric oxide, a blood gas that improves blood flow. How does that help your brain? Your brain needs good blood flow to function optimally.

A recent study looked at brain scans of participants before and after they drank beet juice. The post-beverage scans showed an increase in circulation to the brain's white matter in the frontal lobes—a part of the brain that's often damaged in people with dementia.

You can buy ready-made beet juice at health-food stores, although it's much less expensive to make your own with fresh beets (include the root and greens, which are nutritious as well).

Beet juice has a naturally sweet taste, but you may want to add a little apple juice or another fruit juice—both for flavor and to make the mixture more pourable.

BERRY SMOOTHIES

Acai, a South American fruit that reduces inflammation, is ranked near the top of brain-healthy foods because it dilates blood vessels and increases blood flow.

Its juice has a pleasant taste—something like a cross between raspberry and cocoa—but it's very expensive (typically about $30 or more for a quart).

What I recommend: Blend a variety of everyday frozen berries that have been shown to boost brain health—raspberries, blueberries and strawberries, for example—along with a little acai juice (and a bit of any other fruit juice, if you wish) to make an easy, delicious smoothie.

Why use frozen berries? They retain the nutritional benefit of fresh berries—and they're easy to buy and last a long time in the freezer...they give your smoothie a nice texture, which you can vary by adding more or less juice...and they're less expensive than fresh berries if you buy large bags.

CARROT JUICE

The old adage is that carrots are good for the eyes (indeed they are)—but we now know that carrot juice is absolutely great for the brain. Like other deeply colored vegetables (sweet potatoes, kale, red peppers, etc.), carrots are high in beta-carotene, an antioxidant that reduces inflammation—believed to be a factor in brain deterioration.

If you have tried carrot juice but didn't like the taste (it's surprisingly sweet), that's no problem. It is a very good "base" for multi-vegetable juices. (Some choices that are good for covering up the carrot flavor include kale, spinach and other dark greens.)

COCOA

A Harvard/Brigham and Women's Hospital study found that adults who drank two daily cups of cocoa did better on memory tests than those who didn't drink it.

The flavanols (a class of antioxidants) in cocoa relax the endothelial linings of blood vessels and help reduce blood pressure. High blood pressure is a leading risk factor for dementia. The antioxidants in cocoa also reduce the cell-damaging effects of free radicals—this may improve long-term brain health.

Important: Do not go overboard with sugar, though—sugar is not good for your brain (and the jury is still out on artificial sweeteners).

Here's my advice: Buy a brand of unsweetened cocoa powder that is processed to remain high in flavanols. You don't have to buy an expensive specialty brand to get the brain-protecting effects. Most major brands of cocoa powder have respectable levels of cocoa flavanols. I advise against using milk chocolate or chocolate syrup—they typically have the least amount of flavanols and the most sugar.

At first, make your hot cocoa with your usual amount of sugar...then slowly cut back. You'll grow to appreciate the deep and pleasantly bitter true taste of the cocoa itself as less and less sugar stops masking it. As for using milk or water for your cocoa, that's your choice.

RED WINE

Everyone knows that red wine promotes cardiovascular health (easy does it). What you might not know is that red wine has been linked to a lower risk for dementia.

One reason is that people who drink moderate amounts of red wine—up to two glasses a day for men or one glass for women—have an increase in HDL "good" cholesterol. Research from Columbia University has found that people with the highest levels of HDL were less likely to develop dementia than those with the lowest levels.

Want to supercharge the brain-boosting power of your red wine? Make delicious Sangria! You'll get the wine's benefits and extra antioxidants and other nutrients from the fruit.

Sangria is typically made by steeping pieces of fresh fruit—lemon, orange, apple and just about any other fruit you like—in a rich red wine such as Merlot or Cabernet Sauvignon (or a Spanish red if you want to be autentico) and adding sugar and another liquor, such as brandy or rum.

My advice: Skip the sugar and extra liquor, but go ahead and add some orange juice to dilute the wine a bit and add some sweetness.

Best Juice Machines

Here, a juicer and two blenders that I recommend for quality and affordability…

• **Green Star GS-1000 Juice Extractor** uses a low-speed, low-heat system to preserve nutrients from produce. $420, *Tribestlife.com.*

• **Ninja DUO Blender** has a powerful 1,500-watt motor and six blades to pulverize produce for drinks with lots of pulp. $160, *NinjaKitchen.com.*

• **Vitamix 5200** is a multipurpose blender that also chops and churns veggies and fruits into smoothies. Easy 60-second self-cleaning feature. $449, *Vitamix.com.*

Shinichi Kuriyama, MD, PhD, associate professor of epidemiology, Tohoku University Graduate School of Medicine, Sendai, Japan.

Green Tea Boosts Brain Power

In a recent Japanese study of cognitive function in people age 70 or older, participants who drank two or more cups of green tea daily had a 54% lower prevalence of cognitive decline—measured via memory, attention and language-use tests—than those who drank three cups or less weekly.

Theory: Antioxidants in green tea may reduce the buildup of a type of plaque in the brain that is responsible for memory loss in Alzheimer's disease.

Self-defense: Drink two or more cups of green tea daily to help promote brain health.

Qi Dai, MD, PhD, professor of medicine, division of general internal medicine and public health, Vanderbilt School of Medicine, Nashville, and leader of a study of 1,836 people of Japanese descent, published in *The American Journal of Medicine.*

A Good Reason to Drink Juice!

Fruit juice may lower the risk for Alzheimer's disease.

Recent finding: People who report drinking at least three servings of juice a week are 76% less likely to develop Alzheimer's than those who drink juice less than once a week. The research is preliminary and not conclusive—juice drinkers may lead a more healthful life in general.

Qi Dai, MD, PhD, professor of medicine, Vanderbilt School of Medicine, Nashville, and leader of a study of 1,836 people, published in *The American Journal of Medicine.*

Blueberry Juice for Your Brain

Improve your memory with blueberry juice. Adults with early memory decline who drank two-and-a-half cups of blueberry juice made from frozen wild blueberries daily for 12 weeks showed significant improvement on learning and memory tests, say University of

Cincinnati researchers. To get blueberries' anti-oxidants without too much sugar, mix blueberry juice concentrate (available at health-food stores) with water.

Mark A. Stengler, NMD, licensed naturopathic medical doctor in private practice, Stengler Center for Integrative Medicine, Encinitas, California...author of many books, including *The Natural Physician's Healing Therapies* and coauthor of *Prescription for Natural Cures.* MarkStengler.com

Why a Daily Drink May Help Your Memory

Light-to-moderate drinking in later life may keep memory strong, according to a recent study. Consuming up to one drink a day was associated with better episodic memory—the ability to remember specific events. Episodic memory is the type that usually diminishes in dementia.

Theory: Alcohol may help preserve the hippocampus, a brain area that shrinks in people with dementia.

Faika Zanjani, PhD, associate professor, department of behavioral and community health, University of Maryland School of Public Health, College Park, and leader of a study of 664 people, average age 75 at the end of the study, published in *American Journal of Alzheimer's Disease & Other Dementias.*

Is Coconut Water Good for You?

Mark A. Stengler, NMD, licensed naturopathic medical doctor in private practice, Stengler Center for Integrative Medicine, Encinitas, California...author of many books, including *The Natural Physician's Healing Therapies* and coauthor of *Prescription for Natural Cures.* MarkStengler.com

Many people see coconut water at the grocery store and wonder if it's a healthful alternative to juices, soft drinks or sports drinks. You'll recognize it by brand names such as Zico...Vita Coco...Naked Juice...or O.N.E. The manufacturers claim that it's good for you, but is it? *Let's take a look...*

I often recommend coconut water to my patients who need to boost their potassium intake. In addition to providing potassium, coconut water contains fewer calories and less sugar than sports drinks.

Example: Naked Juice Coconut Water has 44 calories and 8 grams of sugar per cup, while Gatorade G-Natural has 50 calories and 14 grams of sugar per cup.

Coconut water also contains healthful amounts of B vitamins and, most important, cytokinins (plant growth hormones), including kinetin, a potent antioxidant that lab studies have suggested may have anti-aging, anticancer and anti-blood-clotting effects...and zeatin, which is known to improve nerve signal transmission and inhibit formation of the brain plaques associated with Alzheimer's disease.

While I do recommend coconut water to people who need extra potassium—and as an occasional thirst quencher for people who like it—it is best consumed in moderation, not as a substitute for water. People with diabetes should steer clear of coconut water and other drinks that contain sugar—or consume small amounts of coconut water diluted with water. People with chronic kidney disease should avoid coconut water because of its high potassium content.

Coffee: The Good News... and the Bad News

Wilkie A. Wilson, Jr., PhD, a neuropharmacologist and research professor of prevention science at the Social Science Research Institute at Duke University, Durham, North Carolina. Dr. Wilson is coauthor, with Cynthia Kuhn, PhD, and Scott Swartzwelder, PhD, of *Buzzed: The Straight Facts About the Most Used and Abused Drugs from Alcohol to Ecstasy.*

Here's a shocking statistic—90% of Americans need a drug just to get through the day. If they don't get it, many suffer withdrawal symptoms. That may sound like an exaggeration, but think about the caffeine that nearly all American adults get in their coffee, tea, soda, chocolate and aspirin each day. Caffeine is a drug—and a potent one.

HOW CAFFEINE HELPS

An increasing body of evidence shows that caffeine—whether it's from coffee, tea, colas or some other source—has positive health effects. *Key examples…*

• **Less cognitive decline.** In a 2012 study, 124 participants with mild cognitive impairment (which often precedes Alzheimer's disease) had memory tests at the start of the study and again two to four years later. Those who had caffeine levels consistent with three daily cups of coffee did not develop Alzheimer's, while those who developed dementia had caffeine levels that were, on average, 51% lower.

The study did not prove that caffeine is protective. Coffee, for example, contains other chemical compounds that might protect brain cells. But it's possible that the increased alertness from caffeine could make people more likely to pursue social and intellectual activities that improve brain health.

• **Fewer gallstones.** Two important studies found that coffee drinkers were less likely to develop gallstones (20% less likely in women and 40% in men) than people who don't drink coffee. The reason is not yet known, but it's possible that gallbladder contractions triggered by caffeine reduce buildups of stone-forming cholesterol and bile pigments. Drinkers of decaf didn't get the same benefit.

• **Less Parkinson's disease.** Caffeine intake has been linked to lower incidence of Parkinson's disease, and recent research found that symptoms, such as tremors and stiffness, eased in people with Parkinson's who consumed 100 mg to 200 mg of caffeine twice a day (roughly two to four cups of coffee).

• **Headache relief.** A strong cup of coffee or tea can help ward off a migraine by constricting blood vessels in the brain. Caffeine also offsets the widening of blood vessels that occurs during migraines. Not surprisingly, you'll see caffeine listed on the labels of painkillers, including not only Excedrin but also Anacin and Midol.

• **Better workouts.** Caffeine helps mobilize fatty acids for endurance, so it could improve a workout. But be sure to drink water before, during and after exercise because caffeine can cause dehydration.

RESEARCH CONTINUES

Among the benefits, a recent study published in *Heart* reported that drinking three to five cups of coffee a day is associated with less risk for clogged arteries and heart attack. In a study from the University of Texas Science Center in Houston, men who drank two to three cups of coffee per day had a 42% reduced risk for erectile dysfunction. UK researchers found that women who drank three to four cups of coffee a day were 19% less likely to get endometrial cancer, the most common cancer of the female reproductive organs. And researchers from Brigham and Women's Hospital found that drinking about four-and-a-half cups of coffee was associated with less likelihood for tinnitus.

THE NOT-SO-GOOD NEWS

Even though it's almost impossible for an adult to overdose on coffee, tea or other beverages with caffeine, the FDA has warned consumers to avoid any powdered form of caffeine sold on the Internet. One teaspoon of the powder, which was recently linked to the death of a teenager, contained the equivalent of 25 cups of coffee.

You probably know that even "safe" amounts of caffeine, such as that found in a few cups of coffee, can lead to sleep problems (especially when consumed within six hours of bedtime) and can cause unpleasant effects, such as jitteriness, in some people. *Caffeine also may increase risk for…*

• **High blood pressure.** Caffeine from a cup or two of coffee can temporarily increase the heart rate by as much as 10 to 20 beats per minute in sensitive individuals. This isn't a problem in healthy adults but could be dangerous for those with hypertension. An increased heart rate also can trigger heartbeat irregularities (arrhythmias) in some people.

• **Impaired glucose regulation.** Some studies have found that people with type 2 diabetes who consume two to three cups of coffee may have higher-than-expected surges in glucose (blood sugar) after meals. People with diabetes should talk to their doctors about their use of caffeine, especially if they are having trouble regulating blood glucose.

But just to show you how complicated caffeine research can be, a recent study found that coffee consumption reduced risk for type 2 diabetes. Is it the caffeine or something else in the coffee? Research is ongoing.

• **Stress.** Caffeine increases adrenaline, a hormone that's already elevated during times of stress. The effect can be magnified if you happen to drink even more coffee during stressful times.

There's some evidence that caffeine also can trigger panic attacks in people who have had them previously. Even if you don't have a history of panic attacks, large amounts of caffeine (more than 300 mg, or about three cups of coffee) at one time can trigger them.

• **Incontinence.** Caffeine increases urine production, and studies have linked coffee intake to urinary incontinence.

Takeaway for everyone: To minimize your risk for caffeine-related health problems, consider spreading your coffee intake out over several hours or alternate it with decaf or water.

HOW BIG A BUZZ?

Americans get most of their caffeine from coffee, but it's tricky to predict how much you'll actually get. The exact amount depends on the coffee variety, how it's roasted and even how it's prepared. *Some surprising facts…*

• **The inexpensive bulk coffees in supermarkets,** made from robusta beans, can have double the caffeine of the more expensive arabica beans (used in specialty coffees from Costa Rica and Sumatra, for example).

• **Dark-roasted coffees have a strong taste but actually have less caffeine than lighter varieties.**

• **Drip coffee has more caffeine than percolated or coffee made with a French press.** A "cup" of espresso has about the same amount of caffeine as a cup of percolated coffee, but the espresso cup is only about two ounces. The higher concentration causes the caffeine to be absorbed more quickly, giving an "espresso buzz."

For a Quick Memory Booster, Grab a Cup of Joe

Study participants given 200 milligrams (mg) of caffeine in tablet form—the amount of caffeine contained in a strong cup of coffee—performed better on a memory test than people who were not given caffeine. In the test, participants had to identify pictures that were slightly different from ones they had seen the day before.

Study of 160 people, ages 18 to 30, none of whom consumed caffeine on a regular basis, by researchers at Johns Hopkins University, Baltimore, published in *Nature Neuroscience.*

White Wine Is Good for Your Brain

Red wine has more heart-healthy polyphenols, which provide antioxidant protection and ease inflammation, than white wine, but white has more brain-saving compounds called hydroxycinnamates than red.

Caution: Men should have no more than two five-ounce glasses of wine a day…women should have no more than one glass a day.

Men's Health. MensHealth.com

Milk Helps Prevent Alzheimer's

Elderly patients with low levels of vitamin B-12 have twice as much brain shrinkage as those with higher levels. Drinking two glasses of milk (even skim) daily is enough to increase vitamin B-12 to normal levels, which could help slow cognitive decline.

Also: Take up to 500 mcg daily of B-12 supplements.

A. David Smith, FMedSci, professor of pharmacology, Oxford University, Oxford, England.

Olive Oil Helps Your Memory

Saturated fat, such as that found in meat and cheese, contributes to declines in memory and cognition—but monounsaturated fat, like that in olive oil, seems to protect the brain.

Recent study: Women over age 65 who ate the most saturated fat were up to 65% more likely to experience cognitive decline over time than those who ate the least. Women who ate the most monounsaturated fat were 44% less likely to decline in verbal-memory scores and 48% less likely to decline in overall cognition.

Olivia I. Okereke, MD, associate psychiatrist, Brigham and Women's Hospital, Boston, and leader of a study of 6,183 women, published in *Annals of Neurology*.

Beans: The Ultimate Health Food

Jo-Ann Heslin, RD, CDN, a Douglaston, New York–based registered dietitian. She is coauthor of numerous books, including *The Healthy Wholefoods Counter* and two college textbooks on nutrition. A former faculty member of the State University of New York, Downstate Medical Center, in New York City, she was editor of the *Journal of Nutrition for the Elderly* for 23 years.

Beans (in a class of vegetables known as legumes) are the ultimate "combination food," providing maximum nutritional value, including about 15 g of protein and about 13 g of fiber per cup cooked. (A typical serving is one-half cup cooked.)

Compelling scientific evidence: In a landmark study of nearly 800 people (ages 70 and over) from Japan, Sweden, Greece and Australia, the risk for death over a seven-year period dropped by 7% to 8% for each 0.7 ounces (about one-quarter cup cooked) of beans consumed daily.

Bonus: It's especially important to eat beans as we grow older. As we age, our metabolism slows, and we tend to eat less—even though we need more vitamins, minerals and other food-based chemicals to support a weakening immune system...fiber to keep digestion functioning smoothly...and protein to offset the age-related loss of muscle tissue. Beans provide all these benefits—and they're economical and easy to eat for those who have difficulty chewing or swallowing.

BEAN STANDOUTS

More than 100 types of beans are grown worldwide and offer similar basic nutritional advantages. *However, some varieties stand out...*

• **Red beans not only have more antioxidants than blueberries,** but also are a good source of iron (5.2 mg iron per cup cooked).

• **Kidney beans are also rich in antioxidants** and are an especially good source of fiber (13 g fiber per cup cooked).

• **Pinto beans have been shown to reduce markers for heart disease,** including total cholesterol, when one-half cup cooked was consumed daily for eight weeks, according to research published in the *Journal of the American College of Nutrition*.

• **Lima beans are a good source of potassium** and have been shown to reduce blood glucose levels.

• **Navy beans, which also are a rich source of potassium as well as calcium and magnesium,** have been linked to reduced risk for high blood pressure and heart attack.

• **Black beans are another excellent source of antioxidants**—one cup cooked offers the same antioxidant levels as a six-ounce glass of red wine.

• **Garbanzo beans (also known as chickpeas) have been shown to reduce LDL "bad" cholesterol by nearly 5%.**

• **Soybeans have higher-quality protein**— it closely matches that of eggs, meat and milk—and more of it (60% of your daily needs in a single cup) than other types of beans.

Important: Soybeans are the richest source of isoflavones—phytochemicals with estrogen-like properties. Although research findings have been mixed, there is some concern that high intake of isoflavones may promote the growth of precancerous or malignant breast cancer cells. The American Cancer Society recommends that women who are at high risk for breast cancer or with a history of the disease eat no more than moderate amounts of soy foods and avoid isoflavone supplements.

BEST WAYS TO ADD BEANS TO YOUR DIET

Aim for at least three cups of cooked beans (six servings) per week. *For example, you can try…*

•Garbanzo or kidney beans in lettuce salads.

•Navy beans or black beans in soups.

•Roasted soybeans (soy nuts) and edamame (fresh soybeans) as convenient snack foods.

•Three-bean salad containing more dried beans (such as chickpeas and kidney beans) than yellow or green string beans.

For even more variety: Try adzuki beans in rice dishes…anasazi beans in Southwestern soups…and fava beans in stews. These varieties are available at health-food stores and most supermarkets.

NO MORE GAS!

Many people avoid beans because they can cause intestinal gas. To minimize gas, add beans to your diet gradually—start with one-quarter cup on top of a salad, for example…and increase your intake to half-cup and full-cup servings over a period of weeks.

Other gas-control secrets: Get dried beans when they're fresh (otherwise, the beans' natural starches degrade and become more difficult to digest). Look for a "best by" date or buy dried beans at a store where business is brisk. Soak them overnight, then rinse them thoroughly before cooking.

SODIUM-REDUCING TRICKS

The high salt content of canned beans (it's added to preserve texture) is a problem if you're on a low-sodium diet. Canned beans typically contain 300 mg of sodium per one-cup serving. By washing the beans, you can lower the sodium content by 40% or more. Rinsing canned beans thoroughly also helps prevent intestinal gas.

When cooking dried beans, it is not necessary to add salt. However, seasonings, including salt (in moderation), can be added once the beans are cooked. For convenience, freeze serving-sized portions for later use. Frozen cooked beans also are becoming increasingly available at supermarkets and are nearly sodium-free.

10 TOP ANTIOXIDANT FOODS

1. **Red beans**
2. **Wild blueberries**
3. **Red kidney beans**
4. **Pinto beans**
5. **Cultivated blueberries**
6. **Cranberries**
7. **Artichokes**
8. **Blackberries**
9. **Prunes**
10. **Raspberries**

US Department of Agriculture.

Sage for the Brain

Bill Gottlieb, CHC, editor of *Healing Spices: How to Use 50 Everyday and Exotic Spices to Boost Health and Beat Disease*, founder and president of Good For You Health Coaching, former editor in chief of Rodale Books and Prevention Magazine Health Books and author of numerous health books that have sold more than two million copies. BillGottliebHealth.com

The botanical name for sage—Salvia officinalis—comes from the Latin salvare, meaning "to save" or "to cure." *And sage lives up to its name…*

•**Memory problems.** One hour after people took a supplement of sage oil, they had better memory, more focused attention and more alertness, reported researchers in *Journal of Psychopharmacology.* In another study, people who smelled sage had a stronger memory and were in a better mood.

•**Anxiety.** In a study published in *Neuropsychopharmacology,* people who took a supplement of dried sage leaf were less anxious and felt calmer and more content than when they took a placebo.

Why it works: Sage may block the action of cholinesterase, an enzyme that destroys acetylcholine, a brain chemical that plays a role in memory, attention and alertness. Sage also might improve the functioning of cholinergic receptors on brain cells that receive acetylcholine.

How to use sage: Because of its robust flavor, sage is best used in hearty dishes such as pot roast, meat loaf and stuffing. It also goes well with squash, sweet potatoes and apples.

However: The amounts that improve mental and emotional functioning aren't easy to get with diet, so you may want to take a sage leaf supplement. I often recommend the herbal extract from Herb Pharm because it's made from the whole leaf that has been grown organically. Follow the directions on the label.

Curcumin Slows Alzheimer's

Curcumin may prevent and treat Alzheimer's. This antioxidant and anti-inflammatory herb, used in curry powder, improves cognitive functions in Alzheimer's patients and reduces the inflammatory response that may lead to the disease's onset. Add curry to meals, or take a 95% curcumin supplement (daily dosage 250 mg to 500 mg).

Shrikant Mishra, MD, attending physician, neurology, Veterans Affairs, Greater Los Angeles Health Care System.

Turmeric: The Spice That May Prevent Alzheimer's

Mark A. Stengler, NMD, licensed naturopathic medical doctor in private practice, Stengler Center for Integrative Medicine, Encinitas, California...author of many books, including *The Natural Physician's Healing Therapies* and coauthor of *Prescription for Natural Cures.* MarkStengler.com

In India, the smell of turmeric, the bright yellow spice used in curries, fills almost every restaurant and home. Indians eat turmeric because they like it, but rapidly growing evidence indicates that the spice is giving them much more than flavor.

Thousands of years ago, Ayurvedic and traditional Chinese medicine recognized turmeric as a healing agent for everything from flatulence to liver disease. Now modern research demonstrates that properties in this zesty spice may be useful for lowering rates of breast, prostate, lung and colon cancers, and also for treating breast cancer, inflammatory bowel disease, Crohn's disease and possibly cystic fibrosis.

But even newer and especially exciting research concerns the relationship between turmeric and Alzheimer's disease. Nearly 10 years ago, researchers in India became curious about the influence turmeric might have on rates of Alzheimer's. They looked to see how many people over age 65 in a town in India had signs of the disease, versus a similar group of people in a similar-sized Pennsylvania town, where most people eat little—or no—turmeric.

What they found: In India, just 4.7 per 1,000 person-years (a common measure of incidence rate) showed signs of Alzheimer's, compared with a rate of 17.5 per 1,000 person-years in Pennsylvania. In fact, India has among the lowest rates of Alzheimer's disease in the world. Another study, from the National University of Singapore, involved 1,010 people over age 60. Those who reported that they ate curry "often or very often" or even "occasionally" scored higher on mental performance tests than those who rarely or never consumed it.

WHAT IS TURMERIC?

Turmeric is a powder made from the root of the plant Curcuma longa, which grows in southern Asia. The part of the plant that is responsible for healing is the yellow pigment, called curcumin.

When it comes to health-giving properties, curcumin gives twice. It is a potent anti-inflammatory agent, without the potential side effects of anti-inflammatory drugs. These include damage to the lining of the stomach and intestines and a greater risk for kidney and liver problems, heart attack and stroke. Next, curcumin is a powerful antioxidant—it tracks down and reduces free radicals, insidious molecules that otherwise would cause damage in the body. Both of these properties are important when it comes to preventing or slowing the progression of Alzheimer's disease.

In healthy people, immune cells attack and destroy amyloid-beta plaques—a buildup of proteins between neurons in the brain. But in people with Alzheimer's, this immune response is less efficient and allows plaques to form. Plaque triggers inflammation and free radicals, both of which cause cell damage in the brain. Curcumin slows this harmful process in a number of ways—it forms a powerful bond with the amyloid protein that prevents the protein from clumping...it may break down plaques as well, preliminary research demonstrates...and finally, as I noted before, curcumin reduces the oxidative damage and brain inflammation that are linked to Alzheimer's disease.

CHOLESTEROL BLASTER

There is yet more good news about curcumin's power to prevent and even fight Alzheimer's disease. Elevated cholesterol is thought to be involved in the development of Alzheimer's—and studies demonstrate that curcumin reduces cholesterol. In one study, healthy volunteers took 500 mg of curcumin supplements every day for one week.

Result: Reduced levels of total cholesterol and also lipid peroxides (markers of free radical damage to fats).

SPICE UP YOUR DIET

In the meantime, I encourage all my patients, especially those over age 50, to consume one or two teaspoons a day of turmeric. There are many ways to incorporate this spice into your regular diet. You can sprinkle it into egg salad or over vegetables while sautéing... add it to soups or broths...put it on fish or meat...and use it to flavor rice or a creamy vegetable dip. And of course, turmeric adds zing to curries. If you want to make the most healthful curry dishes, it is important to purchase turmeric as a separate spice—lab tests show that many curry powders in this country contain almost no turmeric.

Good brand: Indus Organics (GreatOrganic Spices.com, $5.99 for six ounces).

Those who don't love turmeric—or those who want to get even more of its protective effects—can take curcumin in supplement form. I prescribe 2,000 mg a day for people who have a strong family history of Alzheimer's disease or who show signs of dementia.

Good brands: New Chapter Turmeric force (for store locator, call 800-543-7279, or go to NewChapter.com, $29.95 for 60 400-mg softgels) and Life Extension Super Bio-Curcumin (800-544-4440, LifeExtension.com, $26 for 60 800-mg capsules).

Anyone taking blood-thinning drugs should discuss using turmeric or curcumin supplements with a doctor, because curcumin is a natural blood thinner. Turmeric also can cause gallbladder contractions, so those with a history of gallstones or gallbladder problems also should consult a doctor. There is no risk in mixing curcumin with pharmaceutical drugs for Alzheimer's disease.

Shakespeare's Herb for Better Memory

Ann Kulze, MD, a primary care physician and founder and CEO of Just Wellness, LLC. She is author of *Dr. Ann's 10-Step Diet: A Simple Plan for Permanent Weight Loss and Lifelong Vitality.* DrAnnsWellness.com

---

It turns out that Shakespeare's Ophelia wasn't all that far off when she said that rosemary is for remembrance. According to a study in *Journal of Neurochemistry*, rosemary contains the compound carnosic acid (CA), which helps protect the brain.

This savory herb also contains phytochemicals that can reduce the formation of cancer-causing compounds known as heterocyclic amines (HCAs). HCAs can form when the proteins in meat are heated to high temperatures.

Preliminary research also indicates that rosemary may enhance insulin sensitivity, improving the action and efficiency of insulin in the body, aiding in a healthy metabolism and slowing the aging process.

Suggested uses: I always add one teaspoon of dried rosemary or a tablespoon or two of fresh to a pound of ground meat before grilling burgers. Rosemary also is good in lamb and potato dishes, soups and stews.

Spice It Up! Black Pepper

Mark A. Stengler, NMD, licensed naturopathic medical doctor in private practice, Stengler Center for Integrative Medicine, Encinitas, California...author of many books, including *The Natural Physician's Healing Therapies* and coauthor of *Prescription for Natural Cures.* MarkStengler.com

---

Y ou probably reach for this spice almost daily without giving it much thought. Black pepper comes from the berry (or peppercorn) of the pepper plant Piper nigrum. Cultivated as a spice throughout history, pepper enhances the flavor of most foods without covering or changing it. *It can liven up any type of cuisine—and it also has several health benefits, such as...*

•**Medicinal properties.** Black pepper has long been known to ease heartburn, indigestion, gas, diarrhea and constipation. Piperine, the compound responsible for its pungency, has been shown to have antioxidant and anticarcinogenic properties. In Ayurvedic medicine, black pepper is used to treat colds, breathing and heart problems and diabetes. A recent review of studies conducted at University of Texas MD Anderson Cancer Center determined that frequent dietary use of black pepper may help prevent neurodegenerative diseases, such as Alzheimer's and multiple sclerosis.

•**Nutritional benefits.** Black pepper contains manganese, vitamin K and iron. It also enhances the absorption of selenium, vitamin B and beta-carotene. Every time you sprinkle pepper on food, you get a small benefit. Sprinkle some on a carrot—and you enhance the amount of beta-carotene you absorb.

Ways to use: Black pepper is available ground, crushed or whole. Consider buying organic black pepper to avoid pesticides and toxic metals. For the best flavor, grind whole peppercorns immediately before using. Chances are, you already add a dash of black pepper to omelets and salad dressing, but black pepper also can be added to yogurt-based dishes and as a savory twist to desserts. If you are reducing salt intake, using more pepper is a good alternative way to enhance the flavor of your food.

Maca: The Super Food That Helps with Everything from Memory to Arthritis

Mark A. Stengler, NMD, licensed naturopathic medical doctor in private practice, Stengler Center for Integrative Medicine, Encinitas, California...author of many books, including *The Natural Physician's Healing Therapies* and coauthor of *Prescription for Natural Cures.* MarkStengler.com

---

A n exotic super food you may never have heard of is generating excitement in the world of natural health—a Peruvian root vegetable called maca (*Lepidium meyenii* or *peruvianum*), pronounced MACK-ah.

The root of the maca is shaped like a large radish. It is a cousin to other cruciferous plants, such as cauliflower and brussels sprouts. Peruvians traditionally boil or roast the maca root or grind it into flour for baking. However, despite maca's popular description as a "super food," you won't see it in food form in this country. Instead, the root is dried and ground into a fine powder. It then is distributed primarily in capsules, although you also can buy the powder to blend into beverages or sprinkle on foods.

I began looking into maca for my patients several years ago. In addition to its healthful fiber, complex carbohydrates and protein, maca provides numerous minerals, including calcium, magnesium, phosphorous, potassium, sulfur, iron, zinc, iodine and copper...vitamins B-1, B-2, C and E...nearly 20 amino acids, including linoleic acid, palmitic acid and oleic acid...as well as various plant sterols, which are natural cholesterol-lowering agents. All of these nutrients have been shown to promote health in a multitude of ways.

MACA'S SUPER POWERS

In addition to its documented beneficial effects on the human reproductive system, laboratory tests and animal studies suggest that maca may reduce the risk for…

• **Arthritis**—by promoting cartilage growth.

• **Blood toxicity**—by improving liver function.

• **Diabetes**—by allowing for better control over blood sugar levels and body weight.

• **Digestive health**—by combating ulcers.

• **Fatigue**—by increasing energy and endurance.

• **Heart disease**—by lowering levels of LDL "bad" cholesterol and triglycerides (a type of blood fat).

• **Infertility**—by stimulating production of estrogen and other hormones in women and boosting sperm count in men.

• **Memory and mood**—by enhancing certain brain chemicals.

• **Osteoporosis**—by increasing bone density.

• **Premenstrual syndrome (PMS)**—by regulating hormone levels.

• **Prostate problems**—by reducing prostate enlargement.

THE SAFEST WAY TO START

Maca generally appears to be safe, given its long history of use by Peruvians…but there are a few guidelines to bear in mind. Women who take estrogen to ease menopausal symptoms should talk to their doctors about using maca. They may be able to wean off hormone therapy or at least lower the estrogen dosage under a doctor's supervision.

Breast cancer patients taking *tamoxifen* or other estrogen blockers and women who have had breast cancer must not use maca, because it raises estrogen levels. Women in a family with a strong history of breast cancer should discuss maca use with their doctors first. People who take thyroid medication should be monitored by their doctors because maca may increase thyroid activity. Women who are pregnant or breast-feeding should not take maca, as a general precaution.

Since its long-term effects have not been scientifically studied, I recommend taking a break from maca now and then in order to give the body's cell receptors a break from any hormone stimulation. People who want to try maca to see if it is a "super food" for them should take supplements for three months (six months for women with severe menopausal symptoms), then stop using maca for one or two weeks. They may then continue this regimen as needed for symptom relief.

HOW TO GET YOUR MACA

I recommend organically grown maca products from Natural Health International, or NHI (888-668-3661, NaturalHI.com, available online or through naturopathic doctors).

Cost: About $35 for 120 capsules of 500 mg each. The average dosage of maca supplements is 1,000 mg to 2,000 mg daily, which you can take anytime.

You can also sprinkle maca powder into your favorite foods and drinks. The powder costs about $25/pound and is available online from SuperOrganicFoods.com and iHerb.com. Maca has a slightly nutty flavor and so I recommend mixing it with almond milk.

Other ideas…

• **Sprinkle on cereal (hot or cold).**

• **Mix into your favorite smoothie or protein shake.**

• **Add to yogurt or applesauce,** perhaps with a little cinnamon.

• **Stir into tea**—especially chai blends, as the flavors complement each other.

• **Use in baking**—substitute maca powder for ¼ of the flour in any recipe (any more and it may affect texture or consistency).

Be aware: Maca has a high fiber content and may initially cause gas. I suggest beginning with 1 teaspoon a day, then gradually increasing your intake by one teaspoon every five days, until you find your comfort zone. The optimum dosage is three to six teaspoons per day.

The Most Powerful Brain-Building Nutrients & Herbs

Mao Shing Ni ("Dr. Mao"), PhD, DOM (doctor of oriental medicine), LAc (licensed acupuncturist), chancellor and cofounder of Yo San University in Los Angeles, and codirector of Tao of Wellness, a clinic in Santa Monica, California. He is author of numerous books, including *Second Spring: Dr. Mao's Hundreds of Natural Secrets for Women to Revitalize and Regenerate at Any Age.* TaoOfWellness.com

Cognitive declines can result from hormonal changes and reductions in neurotransmitters, chemicals that help brain cells communicate with each other. Increasing your intake of certain nutrients helps balance hormones and protect neurotransmitters.

Ask your doctor before supplementing, especially if you have a health condition…use medication…or are pregnant or breast-feeding. To reduce the risk for interactions, do not take supplements within 30 minutes of medication…and limit your use of these supplements to any four of the following.

NUTRIENTS YOUR MIND NEEDS

For the foods recommended below, one serving equals four ounces of meat, poultry, fish, or soy products…eight ounces of milk… two ounces of nuts…two eggs (with yolks)… one-half cup of vegetables or fruit…and one cup of leafy greens.

• **Choline.** The neurotransmitter acetylcholine plays a key role in learning and memory. Choline is a precursor to acetylcholine that is produced in the liver. Production of choline declines with age, as does the body's ability to efficiently use the choline that remains.

Brain boost: Eat one or more servings daily of choline-rich broccoli, cauliflower, eggs, kidney beans, navy beans, liver, milk or peanuts.

Supplement option: 1,200 milligrams (mg) daily.

• **DMAE (2-dimethylaminoethanol).** The body uses fatty acids to create brain cells and neurotransmitters. DMAE, a chemical in fatty acids, helps produce acetylcholine.

Brain boost: Have two servings weekly of DMAE-rich anchovies or sardines. If fresh fish is not available, have canned water-packed sardines or anchovies and rinse before eating to reduce salt.

Supplement option: 500 mg twice daily after meals.

• **L-carnitine.** Mitochondria are the engines of cells. The amino acid L-carnitine transports fatty acids to mitochondria for use as fuel and provides nutrients to brain cells.

Brain boost: Have two weekly servings of lamb or poultry, which are rich in L-carnitine.

Supplement option: 500 mg to 1,000 mg before breakfast and again in the afternoon.

• **Vitamin B-12.** This is key to red blood cell formation and nerve cell health. The body's ability to absorb vitamin B-12 diminishes with age—about 10% to 15% of people over age 60 are deficient in it.

Brain boost: Have two servings weekly of beef or lamb…halibut, salmon, sardines or sea bass…eggs…or vitamin B-12–enriched soybean products (miso, tempeh).

Supplement option: 500 micrograms (mcg) to 1,000 mcg daily.

THE MOST HELPFUL HERBS

An easy way to get the benefits of mind-sharpening herbs is to brew them into a tisane, or herbal infusion—more commonly called herbal tea.

To brew: Pour eight ounces of very hot water over one heaping tablespoon of fresh herbs or one teaspoon of dried herbs. Steep for five minutes, strain and drink.

Convenient: To reduce the number of cups needed to meet the daily recommendations below, brew two or more herbs together.

• **Chinese club moss.** This herb contains the chemical huperzine A, which helps conserve acetylcholine.

Brain boost: Drink one to two cups of Chinese club moss tea each day.

Supplement option: 50 mcg of huperzine A twice daily (discontinue if supplements cause gastric upset or hyperactivity).

• **Ginkgo biloba.** This herb increases blood flow to the brain's tiny capillaries and combats DNA damage caused by free radicals.

Caution: Do not use ginkgo if you take blood-thinning medication, such as *warfarin* (Coumadin).

Brain boost: Drink three cups of ginkgo tea daily.

Supplement option: 120 mg daily.

• **Kitchen herbs.** Oregano, peppermint, rosemary and sage have oils that may increase blood flow in the brain and/or support neuro-transmitters, promoting alertness.

Brain boost: Use any or all of these herbs to brew a cup of tea for a pick-me-up in the morning and again in the afternoon.

Also: Use herbs liberally when cooking.

Supplement option: About 150 mg each of any or all of these herbs daily, alone or in combination.

• **Mugwort (wormwood).** This herb improves circulation, aiding delivery of nutrients to brain cells.

Brain boost: Twice a week, drink one cup of mugwort tea…add a half-dozen leaves of fresh mugwort to salad…or sauté leaves with garlic or onions.

Supplement option: 300 mg daily.

Caution: Avoid mugwort during pregnancy—it may stimulate uterine contractions.

• **Green Tea.** Strictly speaking, an herb is a flowering plant whose stem above ground does not become woody. In that sense, the leaf of the Camellia sinensis shrub—otherwise known as tea—is not an herb. Yet green tea (which is less oxidized than black) is so helpful that it must be listed among the top brain boosters.

Along with antioxidant polyphenols, green tea provides the amino acid theanine, which stimulates calming alpha brain waves and improves concentration. Green tea also has been linked to a reduced risk for Alzheimer's disease.

To brew: Pour eight ounces of very hot water over one teaspoon of loose, fresh green tea leaves (or a tea bag if fresh is not available) and steep for three to five minutes. You needn't strain the tea. As you empty your cup, you can add more warm water to the remaining leaves—as long as the water turns green, the tea still contains polyphenols.

Brain boost: Drink three cups of green tea (caffeinated or decaffeinated) daily.

Supplement option: 350 mg of green tea extract daily.

The Vitamin That Sharpens Memory and Other Supplements to Power Up Your Brain

Daniel G. Amen, MD, a brain-imaging specialist and medical director of Amen Clinics, Inc., based in Newport Beach, California. He is author of numerous books, including *Use Your Brain to Change Your Age*. Amen Clinics.com

---

Can supplements help you find your car keys? Some just might. Research shows that taking the right supplements, in combination with a healthy lifestyle, can preserve and improve brain function.

Renowned brain specialist Daniel G. Amen, MD, knows this firsthand. During his studies of single-photon emission computerized tomography (SPECT) imaging, he decided to have some scans done of his own brain. What he found was that years of unhealthy habits—drinking diet soda, eating fast food, not exercising—had caught up with him. He started a healthy brain program, which included brain-building supplements. Now his brain is healthier than it was 20 years earlier.

Here, the best supplements for your brain.

Caution: Most people can safely take all of them daily, but always check with your health-care provider first, particularly if you have any health problems such as high blood pressure or if you are on any medications, including blood thinners.

MEMORY VITAMIN

Americans don't get enough sun, and because of this, about two-thirds of adults don't meet their vitamin D needs through sunshine exposure.

You probably know that vitamin D is essential for bone strength as well as for preventing some cancers, including breast cancer.

What's new: Vitamin D appears to help the immune system remove beta-amyloid, an abnormal protein, from the brain. This is important because beta-amyloid causes the "tangles" that are associated with Alzheimer's disease.

Brain cells use vitamin D for learning, memory and other cognitive functions. It also is an antioxidant that protects neurons from cell-damaging inflammation. A Tufts University study found that elderly adults with optimal levels of vitamin D performed better on cognitive tests and had better brain-processing speeds than those with lower levels.

Recommended: 2,000 international units (IU) of vitamin D daily is a typical dose, but I advise patients to get their blood levels of vitamin D tested before taking supplements. Everyone synthesizes and absorbs vitamin D differently.

MULTIVITAMIN

Most Americans don't eat the recommended five daily servings of fruits and vegetables. A multivitamin, particularly one that includes B vitamins, is good insurance and can help your brain. In a 2010 study, researchers tested the mental performance of 215 participants. The participants then were given either a daily multivitamin or a placebo. When they were retested a month later, those in the vitamin group showed better mental performance than they had in the beginning. There wasn't a change in the control group.

B vitamins nourish the myelin layer that covers brain cells. Studies have shown that adults who don't get enough of these nutrients, particularly vitamins B-6, B-12 and folic acid, tend to have the greatest declines in memory and other cognitive functions.

Recommended: Look for a product with all seven of the major B vitamins.

VINPOCETINE

This vasodilator comes from the periwinkle plant. Unlike many supplements, it's able to cross the blood-brain barrier and improve brain circulation. Studies show that it significantly increases the oxygenation of brain tissue and improves memory, particularly when used in combination with other brain-boosting supplements.

Recommended: 5 milligrams (mg) to 10 mg daily.

GINKGO

When I examine blood flow and activity patterns with SPECT, the "prettiest" brains often are found in people who take ginkgo. This popular herb is among the best-studied supplements. It dilates blood vessels and reduces the "stickiness" of platelets, cell-like structures in blood that increase the risk for clots. Ginkgo contains flavonoids as well as terpenoids, potent antioxidants that prevent damage to brain cells.

There's strong evidence that ginkgo improves memory. It is also thought to help reduce the risk for vascular dementias and, possibly, Alzheimer's disease.

Recommended: 60 mg to 120 mg, twice daily.

ST. JOHN'S WORT

Anxiety, stress and depression cause serious impairments in mental functions. Chronic stress, for example, increases levels of hormones that can damage the hippocampus (the part of the brain involved in memory). People who are depressed tend to sleep poorly and don't take care of themselves. These and other factors can interfere with clear thinking.

The herb St. John's wort is one of the best treatments for depression. It also is used for treating anxiety and stress. It improves mental focus and helps stop your mind from "spinning."

A review of 29 studies involving 5,489 patients, published by *The Cochrane Collaboration* (an organization that analyzes medical research), concluded that St. John's wort was just as effective as prescription antidepressants, while causing fewer side effects.

Recommended: If you feel depressed or anxious, take 900 mg of St. John's wort daily, divided into two doses.

Caution: St. John's wort rarely causes side effects, but it can interact with other medications. Talk to your doctor.

Stop Memory Loss with Doctor-Tested Supplements

Pamela Wartian Smith, MD, MPH, codirector of the master's program in medical sciences at Morsani College of Medicine at University of South Florida. She is author of *What You Must Know About Memory Loss & How You Can Stop It: A Guide to Proven Techniques and Supplements to Maintain, Strengthen, or Regain Memory.* CFHLL.com

---

Mild forgetfulness, known as age-related memory impairment, is a natural part of getting older. By age 75, a person's memory has declined, on average, by about 43%. After age 75, the hippocampus, the part of the brain most closely associated with memory, will eventually atrophy at the rate of 1% to 2% each year.

But you can improve memory with over-the-counter supplements—if you choose the right ones. Here are the supplements I find most effective with my patients. You can take several of these if you choose. You could start with phosphatidylserine and add others depending on your personal needs. For example, if you're taking a medication that depletes CoQ10, you might want to take that supplement. Or if you're under stress, add ashwagandha root. Of course, always check with your doctor before starting any new supplement. To find a practitioner trained in this field, go to Meta bolic-Anti-AgingSpecialist.com.

•**Phosphatidylserine (PS).** Most people haven't heard of it, but PS is one of my first choices for mild memory loss. It's a naturally occurring phospholipid (a molecule that contains two fatty acids) that increases the body's production of acetylcholine and other neurotransmitters. It improves cell-to-cell communication and "nourishes" the brain by improving glucose metabolism.

Studies have shown that healthy people who take PS are more likely to maintain their ability to remember things. For those who have already experienced age-related memory loss, PS can improve memory. It's also thought to improve symptoms caused by some forms of dementia.

Typical dose: 300 mg daily. You're unlikely to notice any side effects.

•**Co-enzyme Q10 (CoQ10).** This is another naturally occurring substance found in many foods (such as fatty fish, meats, nuts, fruits and vegetables) and in nearly all of your body's tissues. CoQ10 increases the production of adenosine triphosphate, a molecule that enhances energy production within cells. It's also a potent antioxidant that reduces cell-damaging inflammation in the brain and other parts of the body.

People with degenerative brain disorders, such as Alzheimer's, tend to have lower levels of CoQ10. Studies suggest that supplemental CoQ10 improves memory by protecting brain cells from oxidative damage.

Important: If you're taking a medication that depletes CoQ10—examples include statins (for lowering cholesterol)…*metformin* (for diabetes)…and beta-blockers (for heart disease and other conditions)—you'll definitely want to take a supplement. I often recommend it for people age 50 and older because the body's production of CoQ10 declines with age. Hard exercise also depletes it.

Typical dose: Between 30 mg and 360 mg daily. Ask your health-care professional how much you need—it will depend on medication use and other factors. Side effects are rare but may include insomnia, agitation and digestive problems such as diarrhea and heartburn.

•**Acetyl-L-carnitine.** A study that looked at people with mild cognitive impairment (an intermediate stage between age-related memory impairment and dementia) found that acetyl-L-carnitine improved memory, attention and even verbal fluency.

Acetyl-L-carnitine (it is derived from an amino acid) is a versatile molecule. It's used by the body to produce acetylcholine, the main neurotransmitter involved in memory. It slows the rate of neurotransmitter decay, increases oxygen availability and helps convert body fat into energy.

Typical dose: 1,000 mg to 2,000 mg daily. Check with your health-care professional before starting acetyl-L-carnitine to see what dose is best for you. If your kidneys are not functioning perfectly, you may need a lower dose. Some people may notice a slight fishy body odor. In my experience, you can prevent this by taking 50 mg to 100 mg of vitamin B-2 at the same time you take acetyl-L-carnitine.

•**Ashwagandha root.** This is an herb that improves the repair and regeneration of brain cells (neurons) and inhibits the body's production of acetylcholinesterase, an enzyme that degrades acetylcholine. It also improves the ability to deal with both physical and emotional stress—both of which have been linked to impaired memory and cognitive decline.

Typical dose: 500 mg to 2,000 mg daily. Start with the lower dose. If after a month you don't notice that your memory and focus have improved, take a little more. GI disturbances are possible but not common.

Warning: Don't take this supplement if you're also taking a prescription medication that has cholinesterase-inhibiting effects, such as *donepezil* (Aricept) or *galantamine* (Razadyne). Ask your health-care professional whether any of your medications have this effect.

•**Ginkgo biloba.** Among the most studied herbal supplements, ginkgo is an antioxidant that protects the hippocampus from age-related atrophy. It's a vasodilator that helps prevent blood clots, improves brain circulation and reduces the risk for vascular dementia, a type of dementia associated with impaired blood flow to the brain. It also increases the effects of serotonin, a neurotransmitter that's involved in mood and learning.

Bonus: In animal studies, ginkgo appears to block the formation of amyloid, the protein that has been linked to Alzheimer's disease. There's strong evidence that ginkgo can stabilize and possibly improve memory.

Typical dose: 60 mg to 120 mg daily. Most people won't have side effects, but ginkgo is a blood thinner that can react with other anticoagulants. If you're taking *warfarin* or another blood thinner (including aspirin and fish oil), be sure to check with your health-care professional before taking ginkgo.

•**Fish oil.** Much of the brain consists of DHA (docosahexaenoic acid), one of the main omega-3 fatty acids. It is essential for brain health. People who take fish-oil supplements have improved brain circulation and a faster transmission of nerve signals.

Studies have found that people who eat a lot of fatty fish have a lower risk for mild cognitive impairment than people who tend to eat little or no fatty fish. One study found that people with age-related memory impairment achieved better scores on memory tests when they took daily DHA supplements.

Typical dose: 2,000 mg daily if you're age 50 or older. Look for a combination supplement that includes equal amounts of DHA and EPA (another omega-3). Fish-oil supplements can increase the effects of blood-thinning medications such as aspirin and warfarin if the dose is above 3,000 mg a day.

•**Huperzine A.** Extracted from a Chinese moss, this is a cholinesterase inhibitor that increases brain levels of acetylcholine. It also protects brain cells from too-high levels of glutamate, another neurotransmitter.

Huperzine A may improve memory and could even help delay symptoms of Alzheimer's disease. A study conducted by the National Institute on Aging found that patients with mild-to-moderate Alzheimer's who took huperzine A had improvements in cognitive functions.

Recommended dose: 400 mcg daily. Don't take it if you're already taking a prescription cholinesterase inhibitor (as discussed in the "Ashwagandha root" section).

The 10 Very Best Foods to Prevent Depression (and Build a Healthier Brain)

Drew Ramsey, MD, psychiatrist, Columbia University Medical Center, and assistant professor, Columbia University College of Physicians and Surgeons, both in New York City. His latest book is *Eat Complete*. DrewRamseyMD.com

Here's a startling statistic—studies show that people who consume a healthy diet are 40% to 50% less likely to develop depression.

What are the absolutely best nutrients—and most nutrient-packed foods—to protect your brain from depression and other ailments?

What protects mood also protects against dementia and other brain-related conditions. The brain is the biggest asset we have, so we should be selecting foods that specifically nourish the brain.

Here's how to build the healthiest brain possible—starting in your kitchen.

NUTRIENTS BRAINS NEED MOST

These key nutrients as the most important...

• **Long-chain omega-3 fatty acids.** There are two major ones. Docosahexaenoic acid (DHA) creates hormones called "neuroprotectins and resolvins" that combat brain inflammation, which is implicated in the development of depression (as well as dementia). Eicosapentaenoic acid (EPA) protects the cardiovascular system, important for a healthy brain.

• **Zinc.** This mineral plays a major role in the development of new brain cells and can boost the efficacy of antidepressant medications.

• **Folate.** Also known as vitamin B-9, folate is needed for good moods and a healthy brain. It helps produce defensin-1, a molecule that protects the brain and increases the concentration of acetylcholine, a neurotransmitter that's crucial to memory and cognition.

• **Iron.** This essential element is a crucial cofactor in the synthesis of mood-regulating neurotransmitters including dopamine and serotonin.

• **Magnesium.** This mineral is required to keep myelin—the insulation of brain cells—healthy. It also increases brain-derived neurotrophic factor (BDNF), which promotes the growth of new neurons and healthy connections among brain cells. A deficiency in magnesium can lead to depression, anxiety, symptoms of ADHD, insomnia and fatigue.

• **Vitamin B-12.** This vitamin, which often is deficient as we age, helps makes neurotransmitters that are key to mood and memory.

• **Vitamin E.** This potent antioxidant vitamin protects polyunsaturated fatty acids in the brain—including DHA. Vitamin E–rich foods, but not supplements, are linked to the prevention of clinical depression as well as slower progression of Alzheimer's disease. One reason may be that most supplements contain only alpha-tocopherol, while other vitamin E compounds, particularly tocotrienols, play important roles in brain function.

• **Dietary fiber.** A high-fiber diet supports healthy gut bacteria (the gut "microbiome"), which growing evidence suggests is key for mental health.

BOOSTING YOUR MOOD AT THE SUPERMARKET

The best brain foods are mostly plant-based, but seafood, wild game and even some organ meats make the top of the list, too...

• **Leafy greens such as kale, mustard greens and collard greens**

• **Bell peppers such as red, green and orange**

• **Cruciferous vegetables such as cauliflower, broccoli and cabbage**

• **Berries such as strawberries, raspberries and blueberries**

• **Nuts such as pecans, walnuts, almonds and cashews**

• **Bivalves such as oysters, clams and mussels**

• **Crustaceans such as crab, lobster and shrimp**

• **Fish such as sardines, salmon and fish roe**

• **Organ meats such as liver, poultry giblets and heart**

• **Game and wild meat such as bison, elk and duck**

Eating these nutrient-dense foods is likely to help prevent and treat mental illness. When someone with depression is treated, the real goal is to prevent that person from ever getting depressed again.

EVERYDAY BRAIN FOODS

Not into eating beef heart? Having a little trouble stocking up on elk? When it comes to meat, wild game may not be widely available, but grass-fed beef, which is higher in omega-3 fatty acids than conventionally raised beef, is stocked in most supermarkets—and may be independently associated with protection from depression.

Other foods that didn't make it to the top of the Brain Food Scale but that still are very good for the brain include eggs (iron, zinc), beans (fiber, magnesium, iron) and fruits and vegetables of all colors (fiber, antioxidants). Plus, small quantities of dark chocolate, which gives you a little dopamine rush. Dopamine, he explains, is a neurotransmitter that provides a feeling of reward.

milk. There are no side effects associated with this dose.

C. Norman Shealy, MD, PhD, founder and CEO of the International Institute of Holistic Medicine. He is author of many books, including *The Healing Remedies Sourcebook*. NormShealy.com

Chromium and Memory

When 26 adults with mild memory loss took a 1,000-mcg chromium picolinate supplement or a placebo daily for 12 weeks, the supplement group performed better on memory tests while the placebo group showed no change.

Theory: This trace mineral reduces insulin resistance, a condition in which the body's cells don't use insulin properly. Too little insulin in the brain may contribute to poor memory.

If you're concerned about your memory: Ask your doctor about taking 400 mcg of chromium picolinate daily.

Caution: This supplement may affect dosage requirements for diabetes medications.

Robert Krikorian, PhD, professor of clinical psychiatry, University of Cincinnati, Ohio.

Lecithin for Poor Memory

Lecithin is the common name for a group of related chemical compounds known as phosphatidylcholine. It's converted in the body into acetylcholine, a neurotransmitter that plays a critical role in many brain functions, including memory. One study found that participants who took two tablespoons of lecithin daily for five weeks had fewer memory lapses and performed better on memory tests than those who took a placebo.

How to use it: Take two heaping tablespoons of the granules twice daily. I put it in water, but it can be mixed in food, juice or

Try Bacopa for Memory Loss

This herbal medicine contains bacosides, compounds that appear to improve the repair, production and signaling of nerve cells. A 12-week study found that people who took 300 mg of Bacopa daily had improvements in memory and information processing.

Typical dose: To help protect your memory, take 300 mg daily. Look for a product that contains 50% bacosides. Take it with food to help avoid stomach upset.

Mark A. Moyad, MD, MPH, director of preventive and alternative medicine at the University of Michigan Medical Center. He is also the author, with Janet Lee, of *The Supplement Handbook*.

CHAPTER 10

Memory Boosters

Best Techniques to Improve Your Memory

Age is the biggest factor for memory loss. We all have memory problems of some sort by age 60, such as momentarily forgetting someone's name, or briefly wondering why we just walked into a room. We can't stop the effects of aging, but we can slow them down.

Using very simple techniques and lifestyle changes—such as reading regularly and playing board games—can have a positive impact on memory retention. Scientific research shows that whenever we push ourselves to solve problems in a new way, we may be strengthening the connections between our brain cells.

MEMORY TECHNIQUES

Some people are so good at memorizing things that they test their talent in competitive matches involving knowledge of trivia or the recall of remarkably large numbers. Scientists have found that those people are no different from the rest of us. There is nothing out of the ordinary in their brain structure nor are there any indications of unusual intelligence. They simply often tap into a memory technique used since antiquity called the Roman Room method.

This method is simple. Visualize yourself walking a familiar route, such as the rooms of your home. Mentally place images of the items to be remembered on specific points on the route. It may be helpful to place items where they may logically be—if you want to remember to buy coffee beans, perhaps they're best mentally placed on the kitchen counter. When you want to recall them, mentally retrace your steps.

Gary Small, MD, professor of psychiatry and bio-behavioral sciences, and director, geriatric psychiatry, University of California, Los Angeles, Longevity Center. Dr. Small is one of the world's leading physician/scientists in the fields of memory and longevity. He is author of *The Memory Bible* and *The Longevity Bible*. DrGarySmall.com

Over time, you can add more objects to the rooms. If one day you want to remember to pick up the newspaper, add it next to the coffee beans on the counter. If it's airline tickets, visualize them taped to the fridge door. You can also extend your route or even add other familiar locations for certain kinds of memory tasks.

The Roman Room method is a very useful technique. Orators back in Ancient Rome would remember lengthy speeches this way, imagining each progression of a speech by mentally walking through rooms where they had placed objects to remind themselves of lines. *Yet since today we have much more clutter coming at us, I also teach my patients an additional memory technique that I call look, snap, connect...*

• **Look reminds us to focus our attention.** The most common explanation for memory loss is that the information never gets into our minds in the first place. Because we are distracted, we don't take in the information or don't allow ourselves to absorb it. Simply reminding ourselves to focus our attention will dramatically boost memory power.

• **Snap stands for creating a mental snapshot or visual image in your mind's eye of the information to be remembered.** For most people, visual images are much easier to remember than other forms of information.

• **Connect means we need to link up the visual images from snap in meaningful ways.** These associations are key to recalling memories when we want them later. When linking your mental images, create a story that has action and detail.

Example: Say that you want to remember five words on your "to do" list: mail, gasoline, grandson, sweater, airline. Come up with a story linking them. For instance, I imagine a grandson knitting a sweater on a plane, then mailing it at the airport, when the plane lands to refuel.

Whatever the story ends up being, having detail, action and, for me, humor, all help to imprint the information.

This linking technique works very well with everyday memory tasks, such as grocery lists or errands to run.

When trying to remember faces and names, create an image either linked to the person whose name you need to remember or a distinguishing feature of his/her face. A redhead named Lucy could be remembered by noting that the red hair reminds you of Lucille Ball. You could remember the last name of a woman named Potvin by imagining that she landscaped her yard with pots full of vines.

MENTAL AEROBICS

It's never too late to improve your memory. Recent studies show that even people in the early stages of Alzheimer's can be taught significant face and name retention under the guidance of a professional. For those of us looking to overcome the common forgetfulness in daily life, we can tackle much of that ourselves by doing activities that involve lateral thinking.

Lateral thinking means that we are trying to solve a problem from many angles instead of tackling it head on. *Here are some mental aerobic exercises to get you started and, hopefully, suggest further how to invoke lateral thinking in your life...*

QUIZ TIME

A lot of memory loss is simply being too busy to absorb what people are saying. These exercises are meant to remind you to slow down, pay attention and consider what is at hand. *In doing so, your memory will improve...*

1. Brush your hair using your nondominant hand. You may find it awkward at first, but over a few days notice how much easier it gets. This and other exercises don't directly help your memory (after all, how often will any of us need to remember to brush with the opposite hand?). What these mental aerobics do is challenge your mind to think differently and examine tasks we often do without thinking, and which lead to our minds getting "flabby."

2. Fill in a grid so that every row, column and two-by-two box contains the numbers 1, 2, 3 and 4.

3. Say "silk" six times. Then answer the following question: *What do cows drink?*

This exercise will help you be more thoughtful about things, which in turn is conducive to better memory.

4. See how many words you can spell from these letters: LIGOBATE.

No letter may be used twice in any given word, and each word must contain the letter L.

5. How many months have 28 days?

6. All of the vowels have been removed from the following saying. The remaining consonants are in the correct sequence, broken into groups of two to five letters. *What is the saying?*

STRK WHLTH RNS HT...

How well did you do? Regardless, this is just a start to remembering more and living better.

Answers to Quiz...

Q2: Across row 1: 1, 2, 3, 4 or 1, 2, 4, 3. Row 2: 4, 3, 1, 2. Row 3: 2, 1, 4, 3 or 2, 1, 3, 4. Row 4: 3, 4, 2, 1.

Q3: Cows drink water. If you said "milk," you need to focus your attention.

Q4: able, agile, ail, alto, bagel, bail, bale, belt, bile, bilge, bleat, blog, boil, bolt, el, gable, Gail, gale, gel, gelato, gilt, glib, gloat, glob, globe, goal, goalie, lab, lag, late, lea, leg, let, lib, lie, lit, lob, lobe, log, loge, lot, oblate, obligate, oblige, ogle, oil, table, tail, tale, teal, tile, toil, toile.

Q5: All of them. (If you say only one month has 28 days, it's an example of not paying attention to the matter at hand—all months have 28 days, after all.)

Q6: Strike while the iron is hot.

Handwriting Is Healthy

Handwriting boosts learning and memory. Physically drawing letters activates a distinct neural pathway that improves reading comprehension and memory of language.

Claudia Aguirre, PhD, neuroscientist and mind-body expert based in the Los Angeles area, writing at HuffingtonPost.com.

Boost Your Memory in Minutes—(and Have Fun Doing It)

Cynthia R. Green, PhD, founder and president of Memory Arts, LLC, a memory fitness and brain-health consulting service in Montclair, New Jersey, and founding director of the Memory Enhancement Program at Mount Sinai School of Medicine in New York City. She is author of Total Memory Workout: 8 Easy Steps to Maximum Memory Fitness. *TotalBrainHealth.com*

We all have heard that the brain, like a muscle, requires regular mental exercise to stay fit. Most people assume that this means hard exercise—learning a new language, attending university classes, etc.

There are easier ways. I recommend fun and simple mental stretch activities that force the brain to look at the world in new ways. These "brain workouts" immediately exercise the brain and help you stay mentally sharp and agile, improving both memory and thinking skills.

Bonus: Similar types of brain workouts can help prevent later-life cognitive declines. A *New England Journal of Medicine* study found that people who spent the most time engaged in mentally stimulating activities, such as playing board games and writing for pleasure, were 63% less likely to develop dementia than those who did the least. *Activities to try...*

• **Tap a tune.** While imagining your favorite song, drum your fingers on a table or desktop to re-create the notes you are hearing in your head. This encourages the brain to coordinate memory, movement and auditory skills.

Expressing yourself this way cross-challenges the brain and causes it to activate different neural networks than the ones it normally uses.

• **Rework a word.** Write down a multisyllable word, such as "resolution," "sufficient" or "beneficence." Then see how many other words you can come up with, using the letters of the original word. This exercise forces you to see familiar things (the original word) in new ways. You can make it harder by giving yourself only two minutes to do the "word search."

Timed activities encourage the use of different mental skills, such as speed, attention and flexibility.

• **Juggle.** Some of the best mental activities also have a physical component. German researchers found that complex motor integration activities, such as juggling, increased the brain's white matter, tissue that is composed of nerve fibers that transmit information to different areas of the brain.

You can learn basic juggling techniques by watching Internet videos.

Helpful: Start with juggling lightweight scarves. They're easier for beginners to juggle than, say, tennis balls.

• **Wear your watch upside down.** Can you tell what time it is when the numbers on your watch are reversed? It's harder than you think. This type of subtle change forces your brain to practice neurobics, activities that engage your attention and involve using one or more of your senses in a new way.

Another example: Using your non-dominant hand to brush your teeth. It takes practice!

• **Doodle.** Doodling does more than keep your hands busy. Using a pen or colored pencils to doodle or draw can change the ways in which you see your environment. It also requires mental focus to look closely at what's around you.

Quick Memory Trick

For an easy trick to help you remember, close your eyes.

Recent research: Adults who closed their eyes after watching videos of crime reenactments had 23% better recall of what they'd seen and heard than those who kept their eyes open.

Explanation: Closing your eyes helps block distractions, improves focus and helps you visualize what you're trying to remember about past events and experiences.

Robert A. Nash, PhD, senior lecturer in psychology, Aston University, Birmingham, UK.

Marilu Henner's Memory Tips

Marilu Henner, health advocate, actress, memory expert and best-selling author of *Total Memory Makeover: Uncover Your Past, Take Charge of Your Future*. Henner is one of only 33 documented people in the world with highly superior autobiographical memory (HSAM), a rare ability that allows her to recall every detail of her life since childhood.

The actress Marilu Henner is one of only a handful of people in the world known to have something called highly superior autobiographical memory (HSAM), an ability that allows her to recall all—yes, all—the details of her life since childhood in vivid detail.

Her book *Total Memory Makeover: Uncover Your Past, Take Charge of Your Future* is truly eye-opening, however, because it has little to do with her having a superior memory—it's about how she has learned to confront painful memories from her past, rather than run away from them.

In other words, it's about something that we all have the power to do!

And you'll find that her unique approach is quite helpful…in fact, it may make many people want to embrace some distressing memories from their past, so they can get over them and move on!

WHAT YOU CAN LEARN FROM YOUR MEMORIES

What Henner has learned is what most psychologists tout—that it's important to quit trying to bury your painful memories and actually face them. Sometimes painful memories make us think of mistakes that we've made, while other times, painful memories evoke a feeling of being wronged or disappointed. But either way, there is almost always something that you can learn—ways to help prevent the same experience from happening again.

REMEMBER THE PAST TO UNLOCK THE FUTURE

The good news is that you don't need to have Henner's incredible ability to be able to retrieve those memories that are still hurting you in your current life. *Here are some of her easy tips on how to dig them up and confront them head on…*

• **Find a "sense-memory object."** The first step to living more happily and successfully today is remembering a painful event clearly. To evoke a strong memory, look at an object from a turning point in your life, such as a photo of yourself drinking too much at a party, or listen to a song that has a strong connection to your past.

• **Think deeply about how that moment made you feel.** For example, if you find that photo of your drunken escapade, focus on how awful that hangover was the next day. Or if you're listening to a song that you and your friends used to listen to while you smoked cigarettes, think about how disgusting your smoker's cough was. Maybe an old poker chip that you keep in a drawer reminds you of the time that you lost thousands playing slots, and it forces you to remember how terrible it felt to argue with your spouse about all the lost money and how embarrassing it was to have to borrow from your in-laws. Perhaps staring at your résumé makes you think of how you interviewed for your dream job but didn't get it—and it crushed your self-esteem. Henner knows a woman who reopened a bottle of perfume that she wore through a failed relationship in order to fully remember how badly that partner treated her.

• **Make a decision to change.** After you've faced the painful memory—really faced it by walking through it mentally in all its gory detail—it will be easier to make the choice to never repeat the kind of mistakes that led you to that moment. In other words, you will find it easier to drink in moderation (or not at all)…to quit smoking…to stop gambling…to get more experience under your belt before applying for another dream job…and to consider your own well-being when choosing a partner.

In her own life, Henner went through a period during which she struggled with food choices and her weight. Because she so vividly remembers how much less healthy and energetic she felt during that time, today she eats better and maintains an optimal weight—and is much happier as a result.

AVOID FUTURE MISTAKES

Since we're all likely to make new kinds of mistakes that we've never made before, Henner suggests keeping a journal. Record events in your life, and more importantly, the emotions and insights that go along with them. Is your relationship with your partner happy or rocky? What's going on at work? How are you filling your spare time? By stepping back to observe and document your life, says Henner, you can see it more objectively and learn to make better choices both now and in the future.

Better Brain Health Found in Bookworms

Memory and thinking tests given to approximately 300 adults revealed that those who participated in reading, writing and similar activities throughout their lives had a 32% lower rate of memory decline than those who did not. Reading helps strengthen circuits in the cerebral cortex, making them more resilient. The brain needs exercise just like other body parts, so keep it in shape at any age with mentally challenging activities, such as reading and/or writing.

Robert Wilson, PhD, senior neuropsychologist, Rush Alzheimer's Disease Center, Chicago.

Leave Your Memory at the Door

Gabriel Radvansky, PhD, professor, department of psychology, University of Notre Dame, Notre Dame, Indiana. He has been researching how memory works for most of his career.

How many times has something like this happened to you? While brushing your teeth, you remember an important phone call that you need to make as soon as you're done. But by the time you have finished brushing, you walk out of the bathroom, grab your coat and car keys and head out the door…totally forgetting all about that call that you really needed to make.

We all do this—quite often, in fact—and it's not because we're getting old and addle-brained. It's actually something that our brains are hard-wired to do! Research from the University of Notre Dame in Indiana, published in *Quarterly Journal of Experimental Psychology*, demonstrates the connection between forgetfulness and walking through doorways.

DOORWAYS DRAIN MEMORY

This study confirms in a "real world" environment what previous research identified in a virtual environment—a phenomenon dubbed the "location-updating effect," showing that the simple act of passing through a doorway as you move from one room to another raises the likelihood that you'll forget what you were just thinking about.

The experiment: A set of volunteers (28 women and 32 men) were split into groups. Group A walked through a series of three rooms. In the first room, they were asked to place six objects (each a different shape and color) into a box and then cover it up and bring it to the next room. In the second room, after they had gone through a doorway, they were given a computer quiz, asking which objects they had put into the box just a few minutes earlier. Group B did the same thing, except they didn't walk through a series of rooms, they walked to different spots within the same room—in other words, they didn't encounter any doorways. The results? Group A—the one that walked through doorways—made 5% more errors on the memory test than Group B.

BOOST YOUR MEMORY

Now, what does this act of walking through doorways mean to our brains? It is an "event boundary" that signals to your brain that your situation has changed. To understand this, think of your mind as being like a filing cabinet. When something changes—whether in time or setting—your brain acknowledges the shift by creating an "event file" as a way of keeping track of your life (without which it

would be a mess!). Walking through a doorway is a signal to your brain to put what you were just thinking about into its own file… which makes information from before the location change not quite as readily available to you as it was earlier. Unfortunately, another experiment that was part of the same study showed that walking back into the original room that you were in doesn't trigger recall.

We should think of this location-updating effect as being beneficial. By creating event boundaries when entering a new space, our minds are getting refreshed, so we're able to focus on the new environment. That's helpful, when your doctor walks through the door to see you, know that she is no longer thinking about the patient that she just saw!

How can we use this information to improve our memory? One idea is to plan around it by leaving sticky notepads in every room—that way, if an idea comes to you, you can write it down immediately so you don't forget it. Another idea is to always have your smartphone handy so that you can leave yourself a voice-mail or send yourself an e-mail or text. And the next time you walk purposefully into a room and instantly forget what brought you there, don't fret. It's probably nothing more than your brain's overly efficient reset button trying to get you ready for what's coming next.

Unclutter Your Mind, Help Your Memory

Researchers from Concordia University in Montreal, Canada, have found that memory loss in older adults is not due to loss of brain function, but rather to the clutter of irrelevant information. To clear out mind clutter, try deep breathing to reduce stressors and mindfulness to bring your full attention to what you're doing.

Karen Li, et al., "The Role of Age and Inhibitory Efficiency in Working Memory Processing and Storage Components," *The Quarterly Journal of Experimental Psychology* (2010).

Multitasking: A Memory Trap

Older adults who were interrupted while viewing an image were less likely to recall the original scene than younger participants.

Reason: Aging impairs the ability to switch between different neural networks.

University of California, San Francisco.

Sharpen Your Memory with Music

Galina Mindlin, MD, PhD, an assistant clinical professor of psychiatry at Columbia University College of Physicians and Surgeons, supervising attending physician in the department of psychiatry and behavioral health at St. Luke's-Roosevelt Hospital Center, and clinical and executive director of the Brain Music Therapy Center, all in New York City. Dr. Mindlin is coauthor of *Your Playlist Can Change Your Life: 10 Proven Ways Your Favorite Music Can Revolutionize Your Health, Memory, Organization, Alertness, and More.* BrainMusicTreatment.com

Imagine yourself giving a toast, making a speech or delivering a big presentation at work—only to forget midway through what you wanted to say. If the mere thought makes you cringe, you'll be intrigued by a book that reveals how to use music to improve your recall. The best part is that whatever type of music appeals most to you is what will be most effective—so you don't have to suffer through music you find boring or annoying.

Because music permeates all areas of the brain, it has a tremendous capacity to deposit any memories you attach to it in assorted locations. This embeds them deeper into your brain and makes it possible to retrieve them from multiple memory banks.

You may remember the buzz back in the 1990s when a small study reported that listening to a Mozart piano sonata produced a temporary improvement in spatial reasoning skills. These modest findings were blown out of proportion in the popular press, which disseminated the exaggerated idea that "Mozart makes you smart." Subsequent research has shown that music can indeed have cognitive benefits, but it's not about Mozart. In fact, my method works with any type of music—country, classical, reggae, rock, rap, pop, opera or whatever—provided you enjoy it. The more you like the music, the more it activates brain networks and functions that amplify and sustain the effects you are working toward, such as increased concentration and alertness.

CHOOSING YOUR MUSIC

So, getting back to memorizing that toast, speech or presentation, here's what you do. *First, create three lists of musical selections...*

1. Calming songs. On this list, include songs that you know from experience make you feel relaxed and balanced because they are associated with pleasurable, peaceful events from your past. For instance, one song might remind you of a blissful solitary stroll in the woods...another might bring back memories of a glorious sunset sail.

Tip: Research shows that songs with a slower tempo of 100 beats per minute (BPM) or less tend to bring on relaxation and calm.

Examples: "New York, New York" sung by Frank Sinatra or "American Pie" by Don McLean.

2. Fast-paced "activating" songs. Activating songs are mentally energizing. They might remind you of a time when you zoomed through a challenging task, celebrated an accomplishment or won a race. Generally, songs that work well in this category have a tempo of 130 BPM or faster—for instance, "Beat It" by Michael Jackson or "Jailhouse Rock" sung by Elvis Presley. Such rhythms tend to boost motivation and endurance.

3. Medium-paced activating songs. Here, select songs that recharge your batteries yet have a slightly slower tempo, typically 100 to 130 BPM. Examples include "Stayin' Alive" by the Bee Gees or the Beatles' "Lady Madonna." These types of songs help your brain lock in whatever you're trying to commit to memory.

Choose half a dozen or more selections for each list.

Reason: Feelings shift from day to day. For example, you might normally feel relaxed by a song you and your husband slow-danced to at your wedding—but if you two just had an argument, that song might upset you today. Assess your current emotions each time you use your playlists, selecting the songs that feel appropriate for the particular moment.

Once you've selected your songs, create your three playlists on your cell phone or record the songs onto CDs or cassettes.

PUTTING YOUR PLAYLISTS TO WORK

Now you're ready to use your music to enhance your ability to memorize whatever it is that you want to commit to memory. *Follow these steps in order...*

•**Listen to one or more calming songs to prepare your brain to be receptive to learning.** As you listen, recall as vividly as possible the relaxing, positive memories associated with each song. Continue listening until you reach that state of relaxed mental alertness.

•**Play fast-paced activating songs to shift your brain into remembering mode.** Again, as you listen, visualize in detail the upbeat memories linked with that music. Continue listening until you feel energized and ready to approach your task.

•**Turn the music off and focus on what you want to remember.** For instance, read your speech aloud from start to finish, moving around or gesturing as you read—the sound of your voice and your physical movements provide additional anchors that help cement the speech in your memory.

•**When you finish rehearsing, listen to one or more mid-tempo activating songs.** This serves as a mental cool-down to further fix the material in your mind.

•**For maximum effect, use this technique daily.** The amount of time you spend depends on the material you're trying to remember, but generally the music portion of the activity takes about 10 to 15 minutes per session.

Key: Remember to have fun with this—it should not be a chore, but instead a source of enjoyment.

Belt Out a Song for Better Health

Michael Miller, MD, a professor of medicine, epidemiology and preventive medicine at the University of Maryland School of Medicine and director of the Center for Preventive Cardiology at the University of Maryland Medical System, both in Baltimore. He is a past president of the American Society of Preventive Cardiology and has been listed among the "Most Influential Physicians" (*USA Today*), "Super Doctors" (*Washington Post Magazine*) and "America's Top Doctors" (Castle Connolly).

O pening our mouths for a bite of the proverbial "apple a day" has its place—but to really keep the doctor away, we should open wide and let out some songs. Why? Because singing has numerous health benefits, recent research shows. And the rewards are ours even if we warble off-key or forget half the lyrics.

Michael Miller, MD, director of the Center for Preventive Cardiology at the University of Maryland Medical System, has researched music's health effects. He pointed out that singing's positive effects are both psychological and physical. *For instance, bursting into song can...*

•**Make you happier and more relaxed.** It boosts production of the feel-good brain chemicals called endorphins...and reduces blood levels of the stress hormone cortisol that is associated with anxiety and depression. Singing also encourages a breathing pattern—with a shorter inhalation and longer exhalation—that promotes relaxation. What's more, songs with personal significance can help you recall positive memories and emotions.

•**Promote cardiovascular health.** Again, endorphins get the credit—because their release causes blood vessels to dilate, allowing blood to flow more easily and reducing blood pressure, Dr. Miller said. For best effect, choose joyful songs, not mournful tunes.

•**Provide aerobic and respiratory benefits.** Singing requires you to take deep breaths. This increases levels of oxygen in the bloodstream, promoting mental alertness...helps clear respiratory tubes and sinuses...and increases your lung capacity.

• **Build strength.** The muscles of your chest, abdomen, back and face all get a workout when you sing your heart out.

How much should you sing? The more the better! *To mix more melody-making into your day...*

• **Think of the world as your stage.** You can croon just about anywhere—not only in the bathroom as you shower, but also in the kitchen while you're cooking, in the car on your way to work or wherever else the urge strikes.

• **Be a songwriter.** Don't worry if you can't remember the words to your favorite songs. Exercise your creativity by making up your own lyrics...or just sing nonsense syllables for the fun of it.

• **Join a musical group.** This has the advantage of assuring that singing becomes part of your regular schedule, and it may lead to new friendships and an increased sense of community. So check out the opportunities with a local musical theater troupe, church choir or amateur band.

• **Try karaoke.** Many karaoke machines for home use are available at electronics stores, mass merchandisers and online. When you're ready to go public, Google "karaoke" plus the name of your town to find local venues that host karaoke nights.

• **Go "caroling"—any time of year.** Who says that door-to-door songfests can occur only during December? Gather up family or friends and spread some melodic merriment throughout your neighborhood. Or take your group to a nearby nursing home to lead a sing-along with the residents—helping to boost their health and mood as well as your own.

Movements That Boost Memory

Teresa Liu-Ambrose, PhD, PT, associate professor, Canada Research Chair in Physical Activity, Mobility, and Cognitive Neuroscience, department of physical therapy, Aging, Mobility, and Cognitive Neuroscience Laboratory, University of British Columbia, and principal investigator, Centre for Hip Health and Mobility and Brain Research Centre, all in Vancouver, Canada. Her study was published in *Archives of Internal Medicine*.

You've probably seen elderly family members and friends slowly lose their memories, and you're determined to do everything that you can to stay sharp.

But if you think that keeping your brain healthy is something that's really difficult or time-consuming, then you will find the following news very exciting.

There's a trick, and it's not hard...nor is it very time-consuming.

The secret lies in strength training, according to Canadian researchers.

A SMARTER WORKOUT

They found that after six months of twice-weekly, hour-long workouts, people who performed strength training had better memory and brain function, compared with those who did moderate to brisk walking and those who did balance, stretching and relaxation movements (the control).

Over the course of the study, the control group showed no improvement on any of the following measures, but check out how much the strength-training group outperformed the aerobic group...

• **The strength-training group showed a 17% improvement in the brain's executive function,** which controls planning, organizing, strategizing and managing time and space, whereas the aerobic group improved just 2%!

• **In terms of associative memory function (the type of memory that links information together,** as in matching an acquaintance's name with his or her face), the aerobic group improved 47%. But that paled in comparison to the improvement made by those in the strength-training group—92%!

• **Brain imaging of the strength-training group members** showed that three regions of their brains associated with cognitive behavior had become more active. Members in the aerobic exercise group, however, did not see any improvements in this area.

We can only speculate as to why strength training came out on top. One reason may be physiological. For example, strength training may reduce systemic inflammation, increase growth factors that promote neuronal growth and maintain insulin sensitivity (conditions such as diabetes increase your risk for dementia). It may also be that during strength training, the exerciser must constantly monitor his or her actions, including breathing properly, counting the number of reps and sets and using correct form. Walking and balance/stretching/relaxation exercises, on the other hand, are more automatic. Since you don't have to pay attention as much while doing them, the moves put fewer demands on the brain.

BUILD MUSCLE—AND BRAIN POWER

To boost your memory and cognitive function, incorporate strength training into your workout schedule. Now, strength training shouldn't replace aerobic exercises or balance/stretching/relaxation exercises—those types of workouts are critical for other reasons, such as improving heart function and flexibility and reducing stress. Instead, strength training should be added to your routine if you don't already do it.

While study subjects performed strength training twice a week, an hour at a time, if that's too much of a time commitment (or if that's too much for you to handle, physically, right now), even adding smaller amounts of strength training to your routine is likely to help your brain a little. *Here's how to get started...*

1. Warm up. To prevent injury or strain, warm up for at least 10 minutes with light aerobic activity that will elevate your heart rate, such as brisk walking, jogging, biking or doing jumping jacks.

2. Build strength. To improve strength in all the major muscle groups, study subjects used dumbbells (starting with two to five pounds), weight lifting machines or body weight resistance (such as push-ups, lunges or squats, for example).

How many exercises you can handle during one workout depends on your level of fitness, so ask a trainer—it's best to start with only a few exercises and then gradually add more as you get stronger. Try performing two sets of each exercise, doing six to eight reps in each set, and resting for one minute in between sets. The trainer can advise you on correct form and provide guidance about when it's time to progress to heavier weights.

3. Cool down. As with the warm-up, slow down your heart rate with at least 10 minutes of light aerobic activity. Then, to prevent stiffness, gently stretch the muscles that you exercised.

And enjoy your brain power!

For a Better Memory, Just Make a Fist

Ruth E. Propper, PhD, associate professor, department of psychology, and director, cerebral lateralization laboratory, Montclair State University, New Jersey. Her study was published in *PLoS One*.

Do you struggle to remember your mental shopping list or forget people's names right after you're introduced? A recent study reveals a "handy" trick that can help—and all you need to be able to do is make a fist.

Background: Previous research has shown that when a person clenches his or her right fist, the frontal lobe on the left side of the brain shows increased activity. Similarly, clenching the left fist activates the right side of the brain.

There is a lot we don't know about how the brain works, but some experts believe that the left frontal lobe is important to encoding (creating) memories, while the right frontal lobe is associated with retrieving (recalling) memories.

So if hand clenching increases activity in different parts of the brain, would clenching the right hand activate the left side of the brain, where memories are encoded…and would clenching the left hand activate the right side of the brain, where memories are recalled?

To test the concept: 51 right-handed people were recruited to participate in the study. (Left-handed people already have superior memories, according to research, so they weren't included in this study.) All of the participants were shown a series of 36 random words, with each word being displayed for five seconds… then later, they were asked to write down as many of the words as they could.

Prior to reading and recalling the words, however, the participants were divided into five groups. In one group, each member was told to tightly squeeze a small rubber ball (to ensure a fist-clenching action) in his right hand for 90 seconds before seeing the words, then squeeze the ball in his left hand for 90 seconds before trying to recall the words. A second group did the opposite (left before reading, right before recalling). Two other groups used their right hands both times…or used their left hands both times. The fifth group didn't clench their fists at all—they simply cupped the ball gently in both hands.

Results: People who were able to recall the most words correctly were those who had squeezed with their right hands before trying to memorize the words and with their left hands before trying to recall the words. These people remembered almost 15% more words, on average, than the second-best performing group, which was the group that did not clench their fists at all. You don't consider a 15% improvement in memory such a big deal? Well, think of it in test-scoring terms—it could be the difference between an A and a C. Curiously, the three groups that did the "wrong" kind of clenching did even worse than the no-clenching group.

Give it a whirl: You don't need a ball. If you want to remember things better, simply clench your right hand for a minute and a half before you try to commit something to memory—a shopping list, a to-do list, a train schedule or the spot at the mall where you parked your

car. Then clench your left hand for a minute and a half before you try to recall that list, train schedule or parking spot number. Just remember to clench right to learn, left to recall (ironically, the "R" and the "L" mnemonics are opposite). Careful—if you swap those, you could wind up recalling less than you would have if you had done no clenching at all.

Six-Minute Memory Booster

Boost your memory in six minutes by simply taking a nap. Napping during the day—for as little as six minutes—brings better performance on memory exercises.

Possible reason: The act of falling asleep might trigger a neurological process that improves memory—even if actual sleep time is minimal.

Olaf Lahl, PhD, researcher, Institute of Experimental Psychology, University of Dusseldorf, Germany.

Visualize to Memorize

Memory aid: Instead of trying to remember a specific thing that you have to do—such as repaying money borrowed from a coworker—visualize a scene in which you actually are doing it.

Example: Imagine taking the money out of your pocket or purse and handing it to the coworker at a specific location, such as the break room. Create the visualization before going to sleep—your brain will strengthen the image overnight, and you will be more likely to do the task the next day.

Mark McDaniel, PhD, professor of psychology, Washington University in St. Louis.

A Simple Trick to Help You Remember

In a study of 57 adults (average age 72), participants were told to push a computer's "F1" key once while performing a series of cognitive and perceptual tasks. One group also was asked to touch the top of their heads when they pressed the key.

Result: Those who had touched their heads were much more likely to remember having hit the F1 key.

Theory: It's easier to recall having completed a habitual task if it is accompanied by some kind of motor task, such as touching your head or crossing your arms.

If you have trouble remembering whether you've completed a daily activity (such as taking pills): Try making a specific motion each time you perform the task.

Mark McDaniel, PhD, professor of psychology at Washington University, St. Louis.

Want to Boost Short-Term Memory? Watch a Funny Video

Gurinder Singh Bains, MD, PhD, assistant professor and primary research coordinator, Loma Linda University School of Allied Health Professions, Loma Linda, California. His study was published in *Alternative Therapies*.

You forget that thing that someone told you...this morning. You misplace your keys. You walk into the kitchen to do something...but once you get there, you forget what it is.

What you're experiencing is a decline in short-term memory. It starts to go down as early as your 40s...and it's perfectly normal. (Forgetting where you live or what your keys are for, that's a different story.)

But wouldn't it be great if there were something simple and easy that you could do to improve it?

There is. In fact it's so simple, it's funny.

HOW RED SKELTON ENHANCES BRAIN POWER

Watching a humorous video for 20 minutes may be all it takes to improve your ability to remember things you've just heard or read, found researchers at Loma Linda University in California. They showed 20 older men and women (average age 70) either a video of Red Skelton (the former clown who had a popular TV comedy show in the 1950s, '60s and early '70s)...or a montage from *America's Funniest Home Videos*.

None of the participants had any cognitive impairment. However, half of them (10) had diabetes, which is known to contribute to short-term memory loss. An additional 10 participants, who did not have diabetes nor cognitive impairment and were of the same age, were the control group. They did not watch the videos but instead were asked to sit silently in a quiet room.

Before and after watching funny videos...or sitting in silence...the participants took three components of a short-term-memory test. First, a researcher read aloud 15 words, and participants were then asked to say from memory as many as they could remember...a test of learning. The test was repeated five times. The same test was then given with a different list, and then participants were asked to remember what had been on the first list...a test of recall. Finally, participants were given a piece of paper with 50 words on it and asked to circle words that had been on the first list...a test of visual recognition. Finally, a little saliva was swabbed at five different points, including before and after—you'll see why in a moment.

Result? Laughter worked. After watching the humorous videos, the healthy adults did 39% better on the learning test, 44% better on the recall test and 13% better on the visual recognition test. Those with diabetes also saw significant improvements—a 33% boost in learning, a 48% jump in recall and a 17% gain in visual recognition. Sitting silently also seemed to benefit the control group but not nearly as much. Their gains were 24%, 20% and 8%, respectively.

How can a little mirth improve memory? That's where the saliva comes in.

THE STRESS CONNECTION

Saliva contains cortisol, a stress hormone. All of the participants who watched the funny videos experienced a significant decrease in salivary cortisol levels. Stress, as the researchers already knew, suppresses the function of the brain's hippocampus, where short-term memory is pulled together. (Over time, chronic stress can even damage...and shrink...the hippocampus.) Feeling less stress and producing fewer stress hormones, the researchers speculate, is what led to better learning and memory in the video watchers.

This wonderfully simple experiment suggests a wonderfully simple way that we could all boost our short-term memory—watch humorous videos. *There are literally thousands that are easily found online...but here are three good (and free) ones...*

• **The hilarious well-known scene from the *I Love Lucy* TV show**—when Lucy and Ethel get jobs at a candy factory.

• **Comedienne Carol Burnett's spoof on *Gone With the Wind*.**

• ***Frasier*, from the TV comedy series Frasier, sings "Buttons and Bows."**

If you want to stretch out the experience, try these funny full-length movies—*Blazing Saddles* (1974), *Airplane!* (1980), *Raising Arizona* (1987), *A Fish Called Wanda* (1988), *Liar Liar* (1997), *There's Something About Mary* (1998), *Little Miss Sunshine* (2006), *Death at a Funeral* (2007) and *Bridesmaids* (2011). For more choices, go to Bottomlineinc.com/classic-comedies-to-make-you-laugh-out-loud

Of course, you don't have to watch a video to relax and laugh. Although it wasn't studied, it's a reasonable speculation that anything that lowers stress levels may enhance short-term memory. While this is the first research to show memory improvement, other research has shown that humor and laughter stimulate the immune system, make pain more tolerable, improve mood and even reduce markers of inflammation. That's fun with benefits.

Kirtan Kriya Meditation Boosts Mood and Memory

Andrew B. Newberg, MD, director of research at the Myrna Brind Center of Integrative Medicine at Thomas Jefferson University Hospital and Medical College, Philadelphia, and coauthor of *How God Changes Your Brain: Breakthrough Findings from a Leading Neuroscientist.* He is coauthor of a study published in *The Journal of Alternative and Complementary Medicine.*

We all shudder at the prospect of losing our memories and brain power as we get older. Those fears are well-founded. Among Americans age 65 and older, 13% show symptoms of Alzheimer's disease, such as memory loss, confusion, speech problems and personality changes...and an additional 10% to 20% have mild cognitive impairment, which can progress to Alzheimer's disease.

Sadly, such problems often are accompanied by depression, anxiety and other mood disorders that can further aggravate cognitive decline and erode quality of life.

What if you could think better and feel better, despite getting older, by investing just 12 minutes a day?

You might be tempted to jump at the chance. But actually, you wouldn't even have to jump—you'd get to sit.

The technique involves no drugs...requires no formal training...has no negative side effects...is easily done at home...and costs absolutely nothing.

Here's the secret...

REPEAT AFTER ME

The form of meditation called kirtan kriya (pronounced KEER-tun KREE-uh) involves repeating a mantra consisting of four syllables—Saa Taa Naa Maa—while doing a specific hand motion.

Don't laugh—because this really works!

The proof comes from a recent study involving seniors who already had memory loss from mild cognitive impairment or mild-to-moderate Alzheimer's disease. At the start and end of the study, all participants answered questions about their emotional states and underwent tests of their cognitive skills. They also had brain scans to measure cerebral blood flow in various areas of the brain linked to concentration, attention, decision-making, speech and emotions.

One group of participants (the control group) was asked to listen to classical music for 12 minutes per day for eight weeks. The other group was taught kirtan kriya meditation and asked to perform it at home for 12 minutes daily for eight weeks.

Results: Among the kirtan kriya meditators, researchers found significant improvement in the areas of tension and fatigue, and lesser but still notable improvement in depression, anger and confusion...whereas among the music group, scores worsened in all these areas. The meditation group also showed improvement in cognitive function—and interestingly, these effects were accompanied by corresponding changes in cerebral blood flow. In contrast, among the music group, there were no significant changes in cognitive function or cerebral blood flow.

More research is needed to confirm these findings and shed light on just how this form of meditation helps with age-related memory loss and mood problems. But in the meantime, there's certainly no harm in giving it a try to see if it helps you.

HOW TO DO KIRTAN KRIYA

Sit with your eyes closed. You will be using the tip of the thumb of each hand to touch the tip of each finger in sequence. As you say Saa, touch the thumb to the index finger...as you say Taa, touch the middle finger...as you say Naa, touch the ring finger...as you say Maa, touch the pinky finger. Repeat the mantra in your normal voice for two minutes...in a whisper for two minutes...silently in your head for four minutes...in a whisper again for two minutes...and in your normal voice again for two minutes.

Are you musical? Instead of speaking (or thinking) the four syllables in a monotone, you can try chanting them in a singsong fashion, hitting the note A (on Saa)...then G (on Taa)... then F (on Naa)...and then G again (on Maa).

Speak Out for a Better Memory

Speak out loud to improve memory when studying. Reading words aloud makes them easier to remember. Identify which information is most important for you to remember, and read only that material out loud.

Colin MacLeod, PhD, professor, department of psychology, University of Waterloo, Waterloo, Ontario, Canada, and leader of a study of more than 200 people, published in *Journal of Experimental Psychology: Learning, Memory, and Cognition.*

Do You Doodle?

Doodling improves memory. In a recent study, people who doodled while listening to a boring phone message remembered 29% more about the message than those who didn't doodle.

Jackie Andrade, PhD, professor, School of Psychology, Plymouth University, UK, and leader of a study published in *Applied Cognitive Psychology.*

Does Chewing Gum Boost Memory?

Michail D. Kozlov, PhD, department of psychology, University of Tuebingen, Germany. Formerly a PhD candidate at Cardiff University, UK.

Remember those studies about how chewing gum might improve your brain power? The idea was that, somehow, chomping and cogitating at the same time helped your short-term memory so that you could be better at remembering the name of someone you just met, remembering the knitting instructions you just read, remembering what you were supposed to pick up at the grocery store and the like.

Researchers from Cardiff University in the United Kingdom were never quite convinced by those studies. They wondered why chewing gum while trying to think would be such a good idea when many other studies have shown that multitasking is a bad idea—it makes us more distracted and less efficient.

So they performed their own study to try and settle the matter.

Should we stock up on Wrigley's or Trident before tackling a task that involves our short-term memory?

This recent study proposes an interesting answer...

THE DISTRACTION OF CHEWING

Michail Kozlov, who was the lead researcher and a PhD candidate at the university, described the experiments that he and his colleagues conducted.

In one experiment, subjects were shown a sequence of seven letters in a random order—each letter flashed briefly on a computer screen, one at a time. Afterward, all seven letters appeared on the screen together, and students were asked to place them in the order that they'd been shown. (That's called testing for "order.") In another experiment, students were shown eight different single-digit numbers that each flashed briefly on a computer screen in random order. Then they were shown seven of the eight single-digit numbers and were asked to name which number was missing. (That's called testing for "identity.")

When students performed the tasks while chewing gum, their recall was, overall, 5% worse on both "order" and "identity" tasks, compared with when they performed the tasks without chewing gum.

For good measure, the researchers tested both "natural" and "vigorous" gum chewing—with the same result for both.

"The findings clearly warrant a reevaluation of the assertion that chewing gum benefits short-term memory," Kozlov said. "Instead, we found that chewing has the opposite effect—a negative impact on short-term memory."

THE CHEWING GUM WARS

Now, you may be wondering, how can similar studies lead to such dissimilar findings?

And how can we be sure that these recent findings trump others from the past?

Kozlov said that the experiments that were done in prior studies tested only "identity," not "order"—and that "order" is important because it's what's really needed in everyday life tasks, such as sequencing numbers on a spreadsheet or even just remembering things you read, for example.

Plus, he said, short-term memory tasks should be done quickly, within seconds. The longer information is stored, he said, the more likely that long-term memory is involved. In previous research on gum, the tasks tended to last minutes rather than seconds (which is how long Kozlov's experiments took).

He said that there's no storage device in our brains for short-term information. Instead, we use other skills to keep that kind of information active—like repeating an unfamiliar phone number over and over to ourselves as we go to dial it. This kind of activity engages the brain, but if you're simultaneously doing something else, such as tapping your finger, twirling your hair or, it seems, chewing gum, then you don't have as much brain power to devote to remembering the phone number.

So if you find yourself in a situation where you need to process information immediately, then you're better off with nothing in your mouth. Save the gum-chewing for when you're not intensely focused on a task!

Surprising Memory Booster

Paul A. Newhouse, MD, director, Center for Cognitive Medicine, and professor of psychiatry and Jim Turner Professor of Cognitive Disorders, department of psychiatry, Vanderbilt University, both in Nashville.

When you think about nicotine, it's likely that negative words like "addiction" and "cigarettes" come to mind.

But what if you were told that there's a new use for nicotine that actually may be beneficial to the brain...and that it might not be so dangerous?

A recent study shows that the substance may help improve memory in certain people.

WHEN YOUR MIND SLIPS AWAY

There are some people who have severe memory loss, such as people suffering from Alzheimer's or other forms of dementia, but far more people experience a less severe form of memory loss called mild cognitive impairment (MCI).

MCI is more than just everyday forgetfulness—it's the stage between normal forgetfulness and the onset of dementia (though not everyone with MCI will develop dementia). MCI might include, for example, having trouble with everyday problem solving (such as balancing a checkbook), forgetting recent conversations or occasionally struggling with hobbies you once enjoyed because you can't remember the steps.

There are no drugs that are proven to help MCI, but a researcher at Vanderbilt University's Center for Cognitive Medicine in Nashville recently made an interesting find: The nicotine in the patches that are currently used to help people quit smoking seem to help improve memory in people with MCI.

ONE STIMULATING SUBSTANCE

The researchers enrolled 67 seniors (average age 76), all of whom were current nonsmokers with MCI. They were given a series of memory and cognitive tests. Then half of them started wearing nicotine patches (one 15-milligram patch for 16 hours each day) for six months, while the other half wore placebo patches. The study was "double blind," so neither the participants nor the researchers working directly with them knew which patches contained nicotine.

When the subjects were given memory tests again after six months, the patients receiving nicotine showed improvements in memory on several tests, while the placebo group did not show improvements on any tests (and sometimes showed declines). For example, on one particular long-term memory test, the nicotine-patch group improved by 46%, while the placebo group declined by 26%.

The researchers aren't sure whether the memory improvements seen in the nicotine group lasted longer than six months—and if so, for how long—because the subjects weren't followed for more than six months, but future studies will attempt to answer that question. The study was published in *Neurology*. Paul A. Newhouse, MD, director of the center and the lead author, explained why nicotine may have had this effect…

THE POWER OF THE PATCH

Dr. Newhouse noted that nicotine stimulates parts of the brain that act as receptors of acetylcholine, a neurotransmitter that is linked to attention, which is important for learning and memory. In Alzheimer's patients and in those with advanced dementia, there tend to be fewer receptors, but in patients with MCI there are more, so the researchers thought it might work…and it appears to.

Now what are the risks, you may be wondering? From what Dr. Newhouse found in this study (and from what other studies about the effects of the patches have shown), there aren't many. None of the participants developed an addiction to nicotine, including those who were former smokers, although it is possible that long-term use of nicotine patches could lead to addiction. A few had mild nausea and dizziness at first—much like you would when smoking for the first time. The only noticeable side effect was weight loss, which isn't a surprise as nicotine is an appetite suppressant. It's also possible that users could require higher and higher doses of the nicotine for it to continue to be effective, which would increase risk for side effects. The 15-mg dosage might seem high (a cigarette contains roughly 1 mg of nicotine), but with the patch, the nicotine is delivered at a slow, steady rate throughout the day, and lesser amounts are absorbed through the skin than through smoking. And there's no known cancer risk with the patches.

Nicotine patches are available over-the-counter, but Dr. Newhouse stresses that you shouldn't start using them just because you think that you're forgetful. Why? For one, larger studies need to be done to prove whether the nicotine is as helpful as this initial study makes it seem—Dr. Newhouse calls the early results "encouraging," but that doesn't make them definitive. Two, if you aren't suffering from MCI, putting on a nicotine patch can actually lead to too much stimulation in your brain and make it hard to concentrate. And three, you shouldn't self-diagnose your cognitive function—because you might be dealing with something more serious than you realize. "Consult a physician or get evaluated at a memory clinic before trying a nicotine patch or any form of treatment," said Dr. Newhouse. In the end, this will be interesting research to watch. It might just be that, though smoking is bad for you, a nicotine patch could do some good.

Phone a Friend, Boost Brain Power

Chatting for 10 minutes a day benefits your brain as much as doing the daily crossword puzzle.

Recent finding: Social interaction—such as talking on the phone and getting together with friends—boosts memory and mental performance as effectively as more traditional kinds of mental exercise, such as word and number puzzles.

Oscar Ybarra, PhD, psychologist, University of Michigan Institute for Social Research, Ann Arbor, and lead author of a study of 3,610 people, published in *Personality and Social Psychology Bulletin*.

Never Forget to Take Your Meds Again

Cynthia Russell, PhD, RN, professor at the University of Missouri Sinclair School of Nursing in Columbia. She runs a research program focused on interventions to improve health behaviors in patients with chronic kidney disease. Her recent article on improving medication adherence through a personal systems approach was published in *Nursing Clinics of North America*.

Traditionally, doctors have tried to educate and motivate patients about the importance of taking their medications, but with little effect. Now, though, a new way of dealing with the problem—called a personal systems approach—is showing great prom-

ise. "The idea is to teach people how to use their own routines and environment to ensure that their medications are there at the times they need to take them. With this approach, patients don't need to worry about forgetting because the medications are automatically built into their daily lives," said Cynthia Russell, PhD, RN, a professor at the University of Missouri Sinclair School of Nursing who has studied medication adherence.

For a personalized approach that makes it easy to remember your meds…

•**Think through your routines.** What is a typical weekday like for you? How about a weekend day? In a log, write down as much as you can about these routines—what time you get up…where and when you eat each meal…the door through which you leave the house…what you do before dinner…how you prepare for bed. Also consider what happens when a routine goes awry. You may realize that you often forget to take your pill with your morning orange juice because when you're running late, you rush off to work without the juice—or the pill. Analyze weekly and monthly routines, too. For instance, if you spend one weekend per month out of state, take notes on that as well.

•**Compare your routines to your medication schedule and identify easy matches.** Look for things that you do consistently. If you need to take a pill on an empty stomach, your log should help you spot a convenient opportunity—perhaps right after brushing your teeth in the master bathroom each morning. If a drug must be taken with food, stick with the meal that you eat most consistently (for example, if you often skip breakfast, take your meds with lunch). Clearly, the more medications you take, the trickier this can be, so ask your doctor which drugs can be taken together for simplicity's sake and which must be spaced apart. "Then look for solutions that don't rely on motivation or memory. Once the change is started, you shouldn't have to try to remember," Dr. Russell said.

•**Find the solution that is right for you.** Dr. Russell described several methods that worked for her patients. One woman who often left the house in a hurry started keeping her morning pills in her car. Another patient was always at her desk at her 8 pm medication time, so she stashed her pills next to her computer. A woman who never forgot to give her dog his twice-daily meds began storing her own drugs next to the dog's—after marking the bottles so they didn't get mixed up!

Recruit a helper if that person is involved in your medication routine. If another household member needs to take a pill at the same time of day as you, ask him or her to join you—so you can support each other's personal medication routines.

High-tech helpers: Program the calendar on your computer to issue medication reminders...set the alarm on your cell phone to ring at the appropriate time each day...or try a smartphone app.

Examples: RxmindMe and Medisafe Pill Reminder & Medication Tracker. Both are free.

•**Keep track of your progress.** In Dr. Russell's research, patients use a special pill bottle with an electronic cap that records the date and time every time it is opened. She explained, "We print out the data and go over it monthly to determine whether a patient's changes have helped her reach her goals." (Your doctor can obtain this product, the Medication Event Monitoring System from Aardex, to use with you, Dr. Russell said.)

Low-tech option: Keep a notebook next to your medicine bottle and log the date and time you take your pills. After two weeks, check your records to see how you did. If you missed any doses, reevaluate your routine.

Success story: When one woman tried this personal systems approach, she discovered the root of her problem. She kept her diabetes pills in the medicine chest in her upstairs bathroom—but she didn't even go upstairs when she got home from work, instead going straight to the kitchen to prepare dinner. Moving her pills from the bathroom to the kitchen cabinet where she kept her dinner plates made all the difference. For backup, she asked her husband to always inquire about her meds as soon as they sat down to eat. As a result, her blood glucose levels improved significantly. She even posted her latest lab report on her refrigerator to remind her of how well she's doing...and to inspire her to keep at it.

Four Easy Tricks to Remember Names Better

Scott Hagwood, author of *Memory Power* and four-time National Memory Champion. He is based in Fayetteville, North Carolina.

Imagine this—you're at a party when someone greets you by name with a hearty handshake, but you suddenly draw a blank and can't for the life of you remember his name.

How embarrassing!

We've all been in situations like that before, but we don't have to be in them again.

Your ability to remember is not necessarily something you're born with—you can train yourself to become better.

Here are my four favorite mental exercises that will train your brain to remember names more easily—and, better yet, they're all so simple!

WHEN YOU MEET SOMEONE NEW

Try at least one of the following tricks every time you meet a new person.

•**Alliterate to learn.** It's amazing how much memory power you can get by using alliteration, the stringing together of words that start with the same sound. To do this, when you first learn someone's name, think of a characteristic that describes this person and that starts with the first letter of the person's first name. For example, you might think to yourself, Hannah wears high heels...Tom is tall... or Donna loves drama.

•**Rhyme to remember.** Rhyming is also a powerful memory booster. So in your mind, rhyme a new person's first name with an associative characteristic. For instance, Anna eats a banana...Max plays the sax...Jim likes to swim. (This won't work for every person, of course, but it's worth trying whenever possible.)

• **Link new acquaintances with old ones.** Say you were just introduced to someone named George who seems to be a bit of a joker. Can you think of someone else you know well who is also named George and who has a similarly playful personality? If so, make a point of linking these two people in your mind ("the two jokers") so that the next time you see this new person, an image of the old George will pop into your mind—along with the name George. (Or maybe your old George has no sense of humor at all, so you can remember this "new George" as his complete opposite.)

• **Repeat the new name.** To firmly imprint a new name on your mind, repeat it both out loud and to yourself several times. Make a point of saying something such as "Great to meet you, Jason" at the beginning of the conversation and "Hope to see you again soon, Jason" at the end of the conversation.

WHEN YOU MEET SOMEONE AGAIN

When someone you've already met reappears and his name slips your mind…what do you do? First, think of the above tricks that you used to remember this person's name in the first place. Does he have some characteristic that you notice that starts with the first letter of his name? Does he enjoy doing something that rhymes with his first name? Is he exactly like—or the complete opposite of—someone who you know who shares the same name?

If none of those methods works, don't panic. When you're in a group, be attentive, because someone else might say the name. Or just keep talking to the person without guessing at his name, because sometimes your subconscious works while you're talking, and after a few minutes, the name might come to you. If all else fails, accept defeat and politely say, "I remember talking to you before, but I've met so many people. Can you please give me your name again?" It won't be held against you!

CHAPTER 11

Sleep Well for a Healthy Brain

How Sleep Sweeps Toxins from Your Brain

It's tempting to shortchange ourselves on sleep. There's so much that needs to get done while we're awake, and science has never given us a good explanation for why we sleep away one-third of our lives...until now.

Using state-of-the-art imaging technology, researchers have made a startling discovery about the purpose of sleep. It turns out that, as our bodies rest, our brains are busy sweeping away a certain type of toxic detritus that collects during the day—the same type of detritus that's linked to Alzheimer's disease and other neurodegenerative disorders. This cleanup process involves changes in the actual cellular structure of the brain—changes we can liken, oddly enough, to a busy movie theater!

Here's the latest advice on how to keep your brain in top form, plus lots of tips on how to sleep better...

CLEANING A CROWDED SPACE

To understand this research, it helps to think of a movie theater. When a film is showing and the theater is packed, candy wrappers and popcorn and other garbage all fall to the floor. Moviegoers are making a mess, but it would be impossible to clean up while the people are still in their seats. The theater patrons wouldn't be able to concentrate on the movie...and there wouldn't be enough room for cleaners to maneuver.

Later, though, after the movie, the people clear out and the seats fold up, and there is much more room. It's easier to get to the floor beneath to sweep away all the crud that the people left behind.

Researchers from the University of Rochester Medical Center discovered that brains are like movie theaters. When we're awake, our brains are very active, guiding all our func-

---

Maiken Nedergaard, MD, professor of neurosurgery, codirector, Center for Translational Neuromedicine, University of Rochester Medical Center, Rochester, New York. Her research was published in *Science*.

tions. As part of that process, our brains discard toxic proteins (such as the beta amyloid that's linked to Alzheimer's) and other by-products—and there's little opportunity to clean up that debris. However, as the detritus builds up, our brains can't function as well.

Cool revelation: When we sleep, our brain cells literally shrink—similar to how theater seats fold up—thus enlarging the spaces around the cells. This allows brain fluids to flow more freely, doing their job of picking up the garbage that accumulated during the day and carrying it away.

HOW THIS DISCOVERY WAS MADE

In most of the human body, the lymphatic system is responsible for collecting and disposing of waste. But the lymphatic system doesn't make it past the protective blood-brain barrier that closely guards what enters the brain. Instead, cerebrospinal fluid circulates through the brain, picking up the interstitial fluid (fluid between the cells) along with the discarded proteins. This exchange of fluid was named the glymphatic system by the same Rochester researchers after they discovered the intricate network.

For the recent study, the researchers used a technique called two-photon imaging and different colored dyes to measure the rate of cerebrospinal fluid flowing through the brains of mice (the mouse brain is remarkably similar to the human brain) when the animals were awake…when they were sleeping naturally… and when they were under general anesthesia.

What the researchers found: The glymphatic system was nearly 10 times more active when the mice were asleep or anesthetized than when they were awake…and the sleeping brains removed significantly more beta amyloid and other debris. This occurred because, when the mice were asleep or anesthetized, their brain cells contracted by more than 60%, creating more space between the cells.

We already know that sufficient sleep helps us think more clearly, do better on tests, make smarter food choices and perhaps keep blood sugar under control. Though it's too early to say that getting enough sleep helps prevent Alzheimer's and other neurodegenerative dis-

eases, the recent study findings suggest that it might—giving us yet one more reason not to shortchange our slumber time.

Get more sleep: To give your brain the rest it needs, continue reading the articles in this chapter.

Lack of Sleep Shrinks Your Brain

Study by researchers at University of Oslo, Norway, titled "Poor sleep quality is associated with increased cortical atrophy in community-dwelling adults," published in *Neurology*.

As kids we wanted no part of it. As adults we often can't get enough of it. And some of us are even proud that we "don't need" much of it. Sleep. No matter what our age or feelings about sleep, the benefits have been proven in study after study. If you don't sleep enough, even if you don't think you are tired the next day, you won't function at full capacity and you'll be more prone to making mistakes and losing focus. But now, we have learned that the penalty for not getting enough restful sleep is much worse than that.

Not getting enough sleep can literally shrink key parts of your brain.

BRAIN LOSS IS REAL

This powerful study, analyzed the brains and sleeping habits of 147 adults who ranged in age from 20 to 84. As part of the study, researchers took two MRI scans of the participants' brains three-and-a-half years apart. The participants also filled out sleep-quality questionnaires that measured how long and how well they slept over a one-month period. "Poor sleep" generally means that a person takes a long time to fall asleep and/or wakes up frequently during the night and/or doesn't get enough deep sleep.

After analyzing all the data, the researchers found that poor sleep was associated with reduced volume in the right frontal lobe of the brain. Among other things, the frontal lobe is responsible for problem-solving, making choices and memory. Poor sleep was also associated with deterioration of parts of the temporal and parietal lobes. The temporal lobe helps us sense sights and sounds but also regulates our personality, moods and behavior. The parietal lobe helps us interpret sensory information, including touch and visual perspective.

THE SLEEP (AND AGE) CONNECTION

Sleep gives the brain the chance to repair itself in a way similar to how a "defrag" application removes noise and waste from a computer so that it runs more efficiently. But this process seems to naturally become less efficient as we age. Numerous studies have borne this out, and the study on sleep and changes to brain structure did show that changes were more conspicuous in participants who were older than 60. This led the study researchers to question whether poor sleep leads to brain changes (shrinkage and deterioration)...or, in contrast, age-related brain changes lead to poor sleep.

Sleep problems and age-related brain changes might go together as a vicious cycle. Other studies have linked poor sleep with poor cognition and an increased risk of Alzheimer's disease. But whether lack of sleep ages the brain or an aging brain thwarts sleep, there is only one side of that equation that you can profoundly alter.

This is why it is vitally important that you do everything you can to keep your brain fit. And that includes getting a restful night's sleep. *The National Sleep Foundation provides these tips...*

• **Stay on schedule.** To the extent you can, stick to the same bedtime and wakeup time to train your body to keep with a healthful sleep-wake cycle.

• **Get ready.** Relax before you go to sleep. In particular, turn off your electronic devices, such as your computer and television, about an hour before bed and let quiet time replace distraction time.

• **Skip the cat nap.** Just as snacking can ruin your appetite for mealtime, napping can leave you sleepless at night, so make an effort to limit daytime naps and, as mentioned above, reinforce a sleep- and wake-time schedule.

• **Don't force the issue.** If you can't sleep, don't force it. Get up, read a book, have a cup of soothing chamomile or passion flower tea and try again later.

• **Pass on the nightcap.** Don't drink alcohol close to bedtime. Although an alcoholic drink can help lull you to sleep, it can adversely affect how well you sleep, and you will often find yourself waking up feeling restless and dehydrated a few hours later.

Disturbed Sleep Linked to Alzheimer's

Scientists monitored sleep patterns of 100 cognitively normal adults (ages 45 to 80) for two weeks and measured levels of amyloid plaque (a biomarker for early Alzheimer's disease) in their cerebrospinal fluid.

Result: Those who spent less than 85% of their in-bed time sleeping were more likely to have amyloid plaque.

Theory: Disrupted sleep could contribute to the development of Alzheimer's, possibly due to the way brain activity affects amyloid levels.

Yo-El Ju, MD, assistant professor of neurology, Washington University School of Medicine, St. Louis.

Better Sleep, Better Memory

Do you have an accurate memory? It may depend on how well you slept the night before.

Recent research: People who are sleep-deprived are more likely to develop false memories, a finding that could call into question the reliability of crime eyewitnesses.

Psychological Science.

More Bad News for Poor Sleepers

Older people who sleep poorly are more likely to have damaged blood vessels in the brain, warns Andrew Lim, MD.

Recent study: Special sensors were used to detect nighttime awakenings in older people. Those with the greater number of arousals were 27% more likely to have hardened blood vessels and 31% more likely to have oxygen-starved tissue in the brain. These factors increase the risk for stroke and cognitive impairment.

Andrew Lim, MD, assistant professor of neurology at University of Toronto, Canada.

Don't Use Just Any Old Pillow

William J. Lauretti, DC, an associate professor in the department of chiropractic clinical sciences at the New York Chiropractic College in Seneca Falls, New York, and spokesperson for the American Chiropractic Association in Arlington, Virginia. He is author of numerous journal articles and textbook chapters on neck and back pain.

Do you wake up stiff and achy? Don't be so quick to blame it on your age or arthritis—it just might be due to what you're sleeping on…

MORE THAN AN AFTERTHOUGHT

Plenty of people agonize about buying a mattress—you can easily spend $1,000 or more, and there are all those features to choose from (such as pillow toppers and coil counts).

The truth is, there's no unbiased research showing that any of these features will reduce pain. The best mattress for you is simply the one that feels best for you.

The features offered in pillows, however, do matter. That's why pillows should never be selected as an afterthought. *How to select a pillow based on where you need support and how you sleep…*

PILLOWS FOR NECK PAIN

I usually advise people to sleep on their sides because it's a neutral position that's easy on the back, shoulders and knees.* But side-sleeping leaves a large gap between the downward-facing shoulder and the head. A too-thin pillow will allow your head to dip down, which puts a lot of stress on the neck.

Best pillow for side-sleepers: One that's thick enough to fill the space between your ear and the mattress. It will support your neck and head and keep them in line with your spine. A firm foam pillow is ideal because the weight of your head won't compress it very much while you sleep.

Good products: BackJoy Comfort, $59.99, BackJoy.com/sleep. Or you could try a water pillow so you can customize your pillow height. Chiroflow Premium Water Pillow, $46.17, Amazon.com.

Best pillow for back- and stomach-sleepers: A feather pillow. You can shape a feather pillow and make it thicker under the neck for better support and thinner under the head so that it remains flat.

Good product: 700-Fill-Power Sateen White Goose Down Pillow, $199, LLBean.com.

If you like the feel of a feather pillow but are allergic, try the Grand Down All Season Down Alternative Standard Pillow Set, $41.99, Amazon.com.

Another option for neck pain is a thin conventional pillow with a "neck bone" support pillow placed under the neck.

Good product: Original Bones NeckBone Chiropractic Pillow, $14.99, Amazon.com.

You can also try a specialized pillow that is thicker at the ends, with a slight cavity in the middle and built-in neck support. These pillows help keep the head at the right height while supporting the neck. In addition, they provide flexibility for people who like to change from back-sleeping (when they would use the thinner middle part of the pillow) to side-sleeping (when the thicker end would be appropriate).

*We all have a preferred sleep position, but certain positions are better for various types of pain than others. I have found that patients can adopt a new sleep position if it helps their pain.

Good product: Core Products Core 200 Tri-Core Pillow Standard Support, $39.00, Amazon.com.

PILLOWS FOR BACK PAIN

For back pain, the usual advice is to sleep on your back on a superfirm mattress. Back-sleeping does give good support, but many people aren't comfortable in this position, and it tends to increase snoring.

I have found that back pain patients tend to do better when they sleep on their sides. It keeps the spine straight and is generally less stressful than stomach- or back-sleeping.

Stomach-sleeping tends to produce a forward curve in the low back, jamming the joints together and causing pain. Back-sleeping can be better, but if the mattress is too soft, it causes a forward curve in the low back. And if the mattress is too firm, it flattens the low back, which can lead to tight muscles.

Best pillow pick: When sleeping on your back, use a feather pillow that's "fluffed" to provide more lift under the neck, and flattened out a bit under the head. When sleeping on your side, use a fairly thick and firm foam pillow to support the head and fill the gap between the head and bottom shoulder. See feather pillow and foam pillow recommendations mentioned earlier.

PILLOWS FOR SHOULDER PAIN

It's a challenge to find a comfortable position when you have shoulder arthritis or a history of shoulder injuries. If you sleep on your stomach, you would have to keep your head turned all night, which could make shoulder pain worse. Of course, sleeping on the "bad" shoulder can be painful as well, but lying with the bad side up is also tricky because the shoulder isn't supported by a pillow or the mattress.

Best pillow pick: A large body pillow. While on your side, hug the pillow to your chest and rest your top-side arm (with your painful shoulder) on top of it. It will support the shoulder and keep it from "folding" while you sleep.

Good product: Pegasus Home Fashions Body Pillow, $30.45, Amazon.com.

PILLOWS FOR KNEE PAIN

Back-sleeping is ideal when your knees hurt, but as mentioned earlier, few people can comfortably sleep on their backs. And stomach-sleeping is a problem because it overextends the knees. Side-sleeping is less stressful to the knees, but this position can be uncomfortable when the bones of the knees press together.

Best pillow pick: While sleeping on your side, placing a pillow between your knees will prevent them from rubbing against each other and keep your upper hip at a comfortable angle.

Good product: Remedy Contoured Memory Foam Leg Pillow, $12.68, Amazon.com.

You can also put a body pillow between your knees.

HELPFUL RESOURCE

For reviews of additional types of pillows, go to SleepLiketheDead.com/pillow-reviews.html.

How to Buy a Mattress (and Still Sleep at Night)

Ronald Czarnecki, a former manager of multiple mattress stores in the Pacific Northwest. He is author of *Shop for Sleep and Survive the Bite: How to Shop for a Mattress and Save Money in the Cold White Sea of Deception.*

Mattresses might be soft to sleep on, but they are notoriously hard to buy. Various stores sell very similar mattresses under different names, thwarting attempts to compare prices. Salespeople often steer shoppers toward ultra-expensive products. And manufacturers highlight features that consumers can't easily evaluate. As a result, many shoppers pay hundreds of dollars more than necessary—or end up sleeping for years on mattresses that they hate.

Beware of these traps…

TRAP #1: **It's very difficult to compare mattress prices from store to store.** With the exception of certain specialty mattresses, each retailer typically uses product names and numbers that you won't find anywhere else. This is true even when the mattresses are virtually identical, aside from cosmetic changes involving fabric colors and quilting patterns.

What to do: When you find a mattress that feels comfortable (see end of article for evaluating comfort), jot down every available piece of information about what's inside the mattress. Include the coil count and coil wire gauge… dimensions including the height…firmness (based on your judgment of where it falls on a one-to-10 firmness scale with one the firmest)…materials used…how the sleep surface is described…and what position the list price occupies compared with other mattresses at the store from the same manufacturer. When you visit other mattress retailers, examine mattresses that fall in the same general position in the manufacturer's price scale until you find one that matches up very closely. Start there and compare coil counts, firmness and other characteristics of various models until you find one that seems to match. Lie on this mattress, if possible, to confirm that it feels about the same as the one you tried earlier.

Tell the salesperson that you found the corresponding mattress at the other store, and ask if he/she can beat the other store's price. If the second store has the lower price, you could return to the earlier store and try the same tactic. Most mattress stores and many furniture stores will negotiate. Their list prices tend to be double their cost, so it's perfectly reasonable to try to negotiate a price 20% to 40% off list price (which could mean a savings of $400 off a $1,000 mattress). Department stores often won't negotiate, but they sometimes will honor their price-match guarantee if the customer shows that a mattress at another store is essentially identical despite different names. And the department store might offer a better deal on shipping and better return options if you're not satisfied, both important considerations.

Reasonable price: You should be able to find a good queen-size mattress for $700 to $1,000—for guest rooms, $500 to $800.

TRAP #2: **"Pillow top" softness may not last.** So-called pillow-top mattresses feel great when you lie on them at the store. They have thick, soft layers of fiber and/or foam above the mattress springs. Trouble is, these thick layers soon will develop deep, annoying body indentations. The heavier you and/or your partner, the faster this will happen.

If you love the soft pillow-top feel, opt for a "plush top" instead. These have perhaps two to three inches of foam and fiber, rather than the four to six inches of a pillow top—and they will be less likely to develop deep body indentations. Plush tops also tend to be $100 to $300 less expensive than pillow tops.

Helpful: If there are two separate "tape edges"—ropelike lines—running around the mattress above and below the foam layers, it is called a pillow top.

TRAP #3: **Warranties and satisfaction guarantees are less impressive than they seem.** If you voice concern about whether a mattress is right for you, the salesperson might assure you that there's no need to worry because the store offers a satisfaction guarantee.

Quiz the salesperson about this guarantee. Can you get cash back or only exchange the mattress for a different one—and how much time do you have to return it? Is there a restocking fee for returns? What about a pick-up charge or additional shipping charge for the replacement mattress? And if you purchase a mattress during a sale, will you be able to exchange it for one of similar list price or only for a lesser one with a list price similar to the sale price you initially paid?

Caution: Most manufacturers' mattress warranties cover only major defects. They won't permit you to return the mattress because you don't find it comfortable. Mattresses generally should be replaced every eight to 10 years.

Update: Online mattress retailers, such as Casper, Leesa, Purple, and Tuft and Needle, offer "satisfaction guaranteed" return policies. Each policy varies by company.

TRAP #4: **New foundations often are unnecessary.** If you buy a mattress, expect the salesperson to push you to buy the matching foundation (what used to be called a box spring) as well. You might be told that this foundation will extend the life of your mattress or make it more comfortable or that not buying it will void the mattress warranty. None of this is likely to be true.

Unlike old-fashioned mattresses, many modern mattresses do not require you to flip them over from time to time, and these no-flip mattresses don't require springs beneath them at all. Today's "box springs" really are just simple wood-and-wire frames covered in fabric. These foundations cost retailers very little, yet they're often sold for hundreds of dollars.

If your old foundation has no obvious problems such as sagging or cracking and is the same size as the new mattress, you can continue to use it. If you have an old spring-type box that flexes when you push down on it, you don't want to use it with a new "no-flip" single-sided mattress.

If you have a platform bed or a bed with slats that are spaced no more than two inches apart, you can skip the box spring entirely—assuming that the resulting mattress height is not too low. If you do need a new foundation, purchase the one that's matched (brand-wise) to your new mattress. Don't feel that you need to match the fabrics. A lower-priced foundation of the correct size should be fine if you're buying a single-sided mattress.

TRAP #5: **A higher coil count doesn't necessarily mean higher quality.** For spring mattresses, mattress salespeople often stress high coil count—more springs per square inch—as they steer shoppers toward high-end models. It's true that having more coils is better than having fewer coils, all else being equal, but all else is not equal when it comes to coils. Coils might be made from different materials or in different ways.

Example: A mattress with independent coils—coils each made from a separate piece of wire—is likely to do a better job of conforming to the contours of your spine than a mattress with coils made from continuous strands of wire, even if the coil count isn't as high. Independent coils also do a much better job of isolating movement, a big plus for those who share a bed.

TRAP #6: **Delivery and removal charges.** Ask about delivery charges before you agree to buy a mattress. Some retailers provide free delivery, but others see it as a way to slip one last sneaky fee into the deal.

Also ask whether removal of the old mattress is included in delivery—there's sometimes an additional charge for this. Include any delivery and pick-up fees when you compare prices at different stores.

TRAP #7: **An expensive specialty mattress can have drawbacks.** Solid foam and dual-zone, air-filled mattresses look great in ads and can feel great when you lie on them—but there might be issues that the salesperson won't mention. *For instance...*

• **Memory foam mattresses such as those made by Tempur-Pedic** do a wonderful job of conforming to the contours of the body and providing support—but they also make some sleepers feel too hot.

• **If you want foam but are a warm sleeper,** consider a natural latex foam mattress, which sleeps cooler. Some synthetic foam mattresses have gel embedded in them to keep sleepers cooler, but these mattresses are extremely heavy and difficult to move.

• **Dual-zone, air-filled mattresses such as Sleep Number by Select Comfort** provide separate firmness controls for each side of the bed. But humidity and perspiration tend to build up around the internal air bladders of even the best-made air-filled mattresses. Mildew and mold can spread if the bladders are not cleaned frequently using liquid detergent.

These mattresses can be opened up for cleaning and for ventilation—but make sure that the mattress is completely dry before closing it up.

More from Ronald Czarnecki...

How to Test a Mattress

Lie on a mattress for at least 10 to 15 minutes in the showroom to make sure that it feels comfortable—and that it properly supports your spine.

Doctors used to recommend firm mattresses for back health, but they've since concluded that firm mattresses actually provide poor spine support. Backs do best in beds that allow the spine to be straight and supported as you sleep. When you lie on your side on a too firm mattress, your shoulders and hips don't sink in far enough for your spine to stay straight…and when you lie on your back, your hips don't sink in far enough for the mattress to support your lower back. A medium-firm mattress is the best choice for the vast majority of sleepers.

The mattress industry uses terms like "firm," "medium-firm," "plush," and "pillow-soft." It may be more helpful to use a one-to-10 firmness scale with one as the firmest and four-to-six as medium. Ask the salesperson where each mattress falls on this firmness scale so that you can learn what firmness number you like best. Then you can specify this number when comparing other mattresses.

Exception to the medium-firmness rule: Side-sleepers prone to hip or shoulder discomfort might do better on a soft mattress.

Helpful: Bring someone along on your shopping trip to make sure that your spine is straight as you lie on your side…and to confirm that there's no gap between your lower back and the mattress when you lie on your back.

For Better Sleep: Some Like It Chilly—Getting Your ZZZs Can Be Much Easier With One of These 6 New Products…

Joseph M. Ojile, MD, a clinical professor of medicine at St. Louis University School of Medicine. Dr. Ojile is also founder and CEO of Clayton Sleep Institute and president of the Clayton Sleep Research Foundation, ClaytonSleep. com, in St. Louis. Dr. Ojile serves on the board of directors of the National Sleep Foundation.

Manufacturers have recently introduced mattresses and other sleep products that are designed to keep the bed a few degrees—or, in some cases, many degrees—cooler than room temperature. If you and your partner cannot agree on the ideal temperature, you might want to look at products that control each side of the bed separately.

Important: Some temperature-controlled sleep products are quite expensive, and there's no conclusive scientific evidence that they'll improve the quality of your sleep. But they may be a good choice for people who can't cool or heat the room as much as they would like—especially if they are about to buy a new mattress.

Remember: Most mattresses should be replaced about every seven to 10 years—or if they begin to show signs of wear (sags or lumps) and/or you regularly awaken with stiffness and aches.

Helpful sleep products—listed from least to most expensive…

• **Iso-Cool memory foam pillow.** If you're not ready to replace your mattress but would like to try a product designed to improve your sleep quality, this pillow may be a good option. It adapts to your body's temperature with microscopic beads that absorb or release heat as needed. The 300-thread-count cover is hypoallergenic.

Cost: $42 and up. Amazon.com

• **ChiliPad.** This temperature-controlled mattress pad may be the next best thing to getting a new mattress. The pad, from Chili Technology, circulates water at temperatures ranging from 46°F to 118°F. You can adjust the water temperature in one-degree increments. If you get the dual-control model, you adjust each side of the bed separately.

Cost: $449 and up. ChiliTechnology.com

• **Sealy Optimum.** The well-known mattress maker has designed a new line for sleepers who are always migrating from one part of the bed to another in their all-night search for a cool spot.

People who use first-generation memory foam mattresses often complain that they get too hot. Newer mattresses, made with what Sealy calls OptiCool gel memory foam, draw heat away from the body, and the multilayer structure is designed to absorb motion, for firm, comfortable support.

Cost: $1,699 and up. Sealy.com

• **ComforPedic AirCool Memory Foam.** The material that's used in this mattress, called TrueTemp gel, is encapsulated inside tiny beads. The gel absorbs heat and carries it away from the mattress surface. When you move to a new spot, the area that was heated by your body quickly cools again.

Cost: $1,299 and up. Beautyrest.com/beds/comforpedic

• **BluTek.** This line of mattresses is designed to circulate air. It's almost like adding a fan to the mattress—the more the air circulates, the cooler the mattress will be.

The mattress is filled with pinholes that allow trapped heat inside to escape. It also has a permeable fabric along the edges that allows air to move sideways. According to the manufacturer, the mattress cools off much more quickly than standard mattresses do.

Cost: $1,499 and up. Kingsdown.com

• **YúMé.** Made by Mattress Firm, this climate-controlled mattress uses the same Gentherm heating/cooling technology that has been used for years in car seats. It draws in room air, heats/cools it to your preference and circulates it through the mattress. The dual wireless temperature controls provide 11 settings. The fan that circulates air is quiet enough that it will not disturb your sleep.

Cost: $1,700 and up. MattressFirm.com

Best Sleep-Easy Machines

Michael J. Breus, PhD, a clinical psychologist, a diplomate of the American Board of Sleep Medicine and a fellow of the American Academy of Sleep Medicine. He is author of *The Sleep Doctor's Diet Plan*. TheSleep Doctor.com

---

Sleep deprivation not only makes you feel miserable the next day, it's also dangerous. When you don't get enough Zs, your reaction time slows significantly and your emotional state turns fragile. You're also at greater risk for diabetes and heart disease.

People who suffer from sleep problems often try sleeping pills and lots of other approaches. But one of the most commonly overlooked issues is sound quality in the bedroom. Some sounds, such as snoring from a partner, are simply annoying, while irregular noises, such as a barking dog or sirens, keep your body on high alert, making restorative sleep virtually impossible.

To improve the sound quality in your bedroom, consider trying one of these great "white-noise" machines. *Both are available from multiple online sources…*

• **Dohm NSF.** Marpac makes high-quality sound machines that are sturdy, reliable and, not surprisingly, hugely popular.

The Dohm NSF is also the official "sound conditioner" of the National Sleep Foundation.

The machine's plastic casing houses a small fan that creates a rush of white noise, effectively masking noises that disrupt sleep. The Dohm runs on low to high speeds.

Cost: $49.99.

• **SOUND+SLEEP.** From Adaptive Sound Technologies, the SOUND+SLEEP machine has many different options such as "meadow" and "waterfall" that mimic nature sounds. It also offers white noise—and pink and brown noise that cover different frequencies on the sound spectrum. The standout feature of the unit is its adaptive mode button, which senses the ambient sounds in the room so that the machine can automatically adjust to mask any increased noise.

Cost: $99.95.

For a Better Night's Sleep, Paint Your Bedroom This Color

People who slept in blue rooms got more sleep—an average of seven hours and 52 minutes a night—than people who slept in rooms of any other color.

Possible reason: The color blue is associated with calmness and is thought to help reduce blood pressure and heart rate.

Study of 2,000 bedrooms in the UK by Travelodge, Parsippany, New Jersey. Travelodge.com

Is Your Bedroom Dark Enough?

Meir H. Kryger, MD, the former director of sleep medicine research and education at Gaylord Sleep Medicine of Gaylord Hospital in Wallingford, Connecticut. He is author of *A Woman's Guide to Sleep Disorders*, and has been researching and treating women's sleep problems for nearly 30 years.

Excess light at night inhibits melatonin production, which can wreak havoc with your sleep/wake cycle. This can be particularly problematic for women, given that they are already twice as likely as men to suffer from insomnia.

What's more: Melatonin also plays a role in regulating blood pressure and blood glucose levels—making it even more important to keep your bedroom sufficiently dark.

How dark is dark enough? You should not be able to see details in your room at night even after your eyes habituate to the darkness, Dr. Kryger said. *If your room is too bright…*

• **Get light-blocking window blinds or shades,** if necessary, to keep out streetlights and other ambient light…or at least wear a sleep mask.

• **Keep the hall light off.** If other household members are still awake when you go to bed, shut your door.

• **Replace your illuminated alarm clock.** Choose one with a built-in feature that automatically dims the clock face at night or that illuminates only when you press a button. You might even try getting rid of your alarm clock! While this seems like a shocking proposal to those who fear that they'll sleep in until noon, Dr. Kryger said that most people do not actually need an alarm clock because they wake up before it goes off.

• **Turn off the tube.** If you or your partner cannot get to sleep unless the television is on, there's help. A psychologist trained in cognitive behavioral therapy can retrain a person to fall asleep without the television.

Alternative: Invest in a television with a built-in timer that turns itself off and program it to do so at a time after which you would typically be asleep.

• **Check for other sources of light.** Lie in your bed and look around. Is light coming from a computer, house phone, cell phone, cable box, alarm keypad or any other device? Unplug it, block its glow or move the device to another room. If you need a night-light to find your way to the bathroom safely, be sure to use one that is very dim (try an energy-efficient LED night-light) and place it where its slight illumination will not disturb your slumber.

Fall Asleep Faster… Without Drugs

John Hibbs, ND, senior clinical faculty member at Bastyr University in Kenmore, Washington, and family practitioner at Bastyr Center for Natural Health, in Seattle.

If you often toss and turn for 30 to 60 minutes or more before finally falling asleep, you may be tempted to use prescription sleeping pills.

The problem is, these make it even harder to reconnect with your normal sleep cycle, robbing you of the most restorative type of sleep.

Try natural strategies that support normal sleep patterns…

• **Go to bed earlier.** This may seem counterintuitive, as if you would only lie awake even longer than you already do. But for many people, the body's biochemically preprogrammed bedtime falls between 9:00 pm and 10:00 pm. If you stay up until midnight, your body may secrete stress hormones to cope with the demands of being awake when it wants to be asleep—and this interferes with your body clock.

Best: Move up your bedtime by an hour... give yourself several weeks to adjust...then advance your bedtime again until you're regularly hitting the hay before 10:00 pm.

• **Exercise at the right time.** Don't try to exhaust yourself with strenuous workouts, especially in the evening—this raises adrenaline levels and makes sleep more elusive.

Instead: Exercise for at least 30 minutes every morning. This reduces the stress hormone cortisol, helping to reset your biochemical clock.

• **Get wet.** Hydrotherapy—especially close to bedtime—calms the nervous system by acting on sensory receptors in the skin. Typically it is most effective to take a half-hour bath in water that's the same temperature as the skin. However, some people respond better to a hot bath...others feel more relaxed after a "contrast shower," first using hot water, then cold.

• **Adopt a pro-sleep diet.** Eliminate all stimulant foods (caffeine, sweets, monosodium glutamate) from your diet. Magnesium calms the nervous system, so eat more magnesium-rich foods (pumpkin seeds, salmon, spinach)...and/or take 200 mg to 300 mg of supplemental magnesium twice daily. Do not skip meals—when hungry, the body secretes stress hormones that can interfere with sleep. Avoid eating too close to bedtime—a full stomach distracts the body from normal sleep physiology.

• **Try nutraceuticals.** Certain supplements help balance brain chemicals.

Recommended: At bedtime, take 500 milligrams (mg) to 1,000 mg of gamma-aminobutyric acid (GABA), a calming brain chemical. Another option is to take a bedtime dose of 50 mg to 100 mg of 5-hydroxytryptophan (5-HTP), a natural compound that relaxes by balancing levels of the brain chemical serotonin. GABA and 5-HTP can be used separately or together for as long as needed. Both are sold in health-food stores and rarely have side effects at these doses.

Shut Down Before Bed

Tablet users may be losing sleep. The light from backlit electronic devices, including the iPad, iPhone, Kindle Fire and certain Nooks, disrupts the body's circadian clock and reduces rapid eye movement (REM) sleep. These devices emit short-wavelength enriched light, known as blue light, that suppresses melatonin in the body—the hormone that helps start the sleep process.

Best for nighttime readers: A printed book.

Two-week sleep-lab study by researchers at Brigham and Women's Hospital, Boston, published in *Proceedings of the National Academy of Sciences.*

Better Sleep Habits

A late bedtime is actually better than a full night of sleep with interruptions.

Recent study: Adults who had a delayed bedtime experienced only a 12% reduction in positive mood versus 31% in those who were awakened several times during the night.

Explanation: The interrupted sleepers had less slow-wave sleep, the type that leaves you feeling restored and rested.

Patrick H. Finan, PhD, assistant professor of psychiatry and behavioral sciences, The Johns Hopkins University School of Medicine, Baltimore.

Can't Sleep? Surprising Causes of Insomnia

Andrew L. Rubman, ND, founder and medical director, Southbury Clinic for Traditional Medicines, Southbury, Connecticut. SouthburyClinic.com

Every night, millions of Americans have trouble falling asleep or staying asleep. Quite often this is caused by stress, anxiety, caffeine or overstimulation before bed.

But there is another common cause that few people even know to consider—a nutritional deficiency of one kind or another. If you have such a deficiency, once it is identified you can easily correct it—and start enjoying peaceful slumber once again.

This is a far superior approach to prescription sleeping pills, which not only fail to address the underlying reason for sleeplessness but often are also addictive and have side effects such as disorientation and next-day fatigue.

One example: Kathryn was usually bubbly and energetic. She suddenly started dragging at work, even nodding off during meetings. At night she would awake with unpleasant and uncontrollable urges to move her legs. The surprising cause turned out to be related to Kathryn's new vegetarian diet, which she had started several months before—without meat, her diet no longer included the iron she needed. As a result, she had developed restless legs syndrome, which makes sleeping a real challenge.

The simple solution: Her doctor prescribed iron supplements and began monitoring her levels. Now Kathryn sleeps like a baby and is once again bursting with energy at the office.

NUTRITIONAL DEFICIENCIES INTERFERE WITH SLEEP

Iron and restless leg syndrome is just one of the hidden dietary deficiencies affecting sleep. Nutrition guru Andrew L. Rubman, ND, offered more insight on potentially sleep-disturbing dietary deficiencies and how to address them. If you suffer from insomnia, he recommends consulting a doctor who is knowledgeable about nutritional biochemistry to assess your nutrient levels and offer diet advice and/or supplements to support your body's natural sleep processes.

Dr. Rubman said that the following nutrients are strongly related to sleep…

CALCIUM—NATURE'S SEDATIVE

When you run short on calcium, you are apt to toss and turn and experience frequent awakenings in the night. This mineral has a natural calming effect on the nervous system.

It works by helping your body convert tryptophan—an essential amino acid found in foods such as turkey and eggs—into the neurotransmitter serotonin, which modulates mood and sleep. Serotonin, in turn, is converted into melatonin, a hormone that helps regulate the sleep cycle.

Dr. Rubman suggests: It's always better to get the nutrients you need from food rather than supplements. Milk and dairy products are the most common dietary sources of calcium, but Dr. Rubman notes that many people have trouble digesting cow's milk, especially as they grow older. Excellent nondairy sources of calcium are leafy green vegetables such as kale and collard greens, canned sardines, sesame seeds and almonds. The Recommended Dietary Allowance (RDA) for adults over age 18 is 1,000 to 1,200 mg/day. For those not getting enough from dietary sources, Dr. Rubman often prescribes the calcium-magnesium supplement Butyrex from T.E. Neesby. Take it half an hour before going to bed.

RELIEVE LEG CRAMPS WITH MAGNESIUM

Nighttime leg cramps, often due to a magnesium deficiency, are a common cause of sleeplessness. Magnesium helps your body's cells absorb and use calcium, so this mineral pair works hand in hand to relax muscles, relieve painful cramps or spasms and bring on restful slumber.

Dr. Rubman suggests: Leafy green vegetables are the best source of dietary magnesium, followed by artichokes, nuts, legumes, seeds, whole grains (especially buckwheat, cornmeal and whole wheat) and soy products. The Butyrex Dr. Rubman prescribes for calcium deficiency contains magnesium, so it helps solve this problem too. (The RDA for magnesium for adults is 400 mg/day for men and 310 mg/day for women.)

VITAMIN B-12 FOR SEROTONIN PRODUCTION

Vitamin B-12 supports the production of neurotransmitters that affect brain function and sleep, helping to metabolize calcium and magnesium and working with them to convert tryptophan into the neurotransmitter se-rotonin. Insufficient B-12 may be a factor if you have trouble falling or staying asleep.

Dr. Rubman suggests: Foods rich in vita-min B-12 include liver and other organ meats, eggs, fish and, to a lesser degree, leafy green vegetables. For B-12 deficiency, Dr. Rubman sometimes prescribes B-12 tablets taken sub-lingually (dissolved under the tongue) one hour before bedtime—but notes that it's im-portant to take a multivitamin that contains B vitamins twice daily as well, since it helps your body use the B-12 efficiently.

Note: Most B multivitamins contain B-12 but only a minimal dose, Dr. Rubman said, so further supplementation is usually necessary.

VITAMIN D MODULATES CIRCADIAN RHYTHMS

Again with the vitamin D! We can't hear enough about the importance of this vital nu-trient, it seems—and indeed, vitamin D turns out to be essential to support your body's up-take and usage of calcium and magnesium. Its role in sleep involves modulating your circa-dian rhythm (the sleep/wake cycle that regu-lates your 24-hour biological clock).

Dr. Rubman suggests: Pointing out that most Americans have less than optimal levels of vitamin D, Dr. Rubman said he commonly prescribes daily supplements of D-3, the form most efficiently used by the body. He noted that 10 to 20 minutes of sunshine daily helps your body manufacture vitamin D, and foods such as fish and fortified milk are rich in this nutrient.

HERBS—SOME HELP, SOME INTERFERE WITH SLEEP

Although they do not specifically address nutritional deficiencies, Dr. Rubman also rec-ommends relaxing herbal supplements such as chamomile, hops or valerian to gently nudge you toward sleep. Try them in teas, capsules or tinctures from reputable manu-facturers such as Eclectic (EclecticHerb.com), taken half an hour before retiring.

Though many people swear by melatonin, Dr. Rubman said that there is not enough sci-entific evidence yet to demonstrate that this popular sleep supplement works efficiently

and without long-term ill effects. He does not prescribe it.

It's also important to be aware that a num-ber of supplements are stimulating and may cause sleep irregularities in some individuals.

The biggest stimulators: Ginseng, ginkgo, St. John's wort, alpha lipoic acid and SAM-e. If you take any of these, do so early in the day, take the lowest dose that seems effective for you or discuss alternatives with your phy-sician. These are all best used under profes-sional guidance.

A SOOTHING BEDTIME SNACK

Dr. Rubman said that his favorite sleep in-ducer is to head upstairs each evening with a soothing bedtime beverage—either a cup of herbal tea with honey or a glass of warm milk (though not everyone's digestive system easily tolerates milk). He generally advises against late-night snacking, which can disturb sleep, but if you must have something keep it light. A high-protein, low-glycemic snack, such as a banana with peanut butter or half a turkey sandwich on whole-grain bread, can help encourage serotonin production...and sweet dreams.

It's 3 am and You're Awake...Again!

Michael Breus, PhD, a Scottsdale, Arizona–based clinical psychologist who is board-certified in clinical sleep disorders. He appears regularly on national tele-vision shows, including *The Doctors* and *The Dr. Oz Show*, and is a coauthor, with Debra F. Bruce, PhD, of *The Sleep Doctor's Diet Plan: Lose Weight Through Better Sleep.* TheSleepDoctor.com

I n the world of sleep disorders, having dif-ficulty staying asleep is just as troubling as having difficulty falling asleep.

Both sleep problems rob us of the con-sistent, high-quality rest that helps protect against high blood pressure, obesity, diabetes, stroke and depression.

Plenty of people who have nighttime awak-enings turn to a prescription sleep aid, such as *zolpidem* (Ambien). But these pills are only a temporary fix and can cause prolonged drowsiness the next day or, in rare cases, sleepwalking or sleep-eating within hours of taking them.

A better option: Cognitive behavioral therapy for insomnia, known as CBT-I, is now recommended as a first-line treatment for chronic sleep problems.* With CBT-I, you work with a specially trained therapist (typically for six to eight sessions) to identify, challenge and change the patterns of thinking that keep you awake at night. A 2015 study found CBT-I, which is typically covered by health insurance, to be more helpful than *diazepam* (Valium), commonly used as a sleep aid, in treating insomnia. (See page 345 for more information.)

But if you are not quite ready to commit to a course of CBT-I—or even if you do try it—there are some simple but effective strategies you can use at home to help you stay asleep and get the deep rest you need.

Best approaches to avoid nighttime awakenings…

•**Get more omega-3 fatty acids.** While the research is still preliminary, a new study published in *Sleep Medicine* found that the more omega-3–rich fatty fish adults ate, the better their sleep quality.

My advice: Eat fatty fish…and to ensure adequate levels of omega-3s, consider taking a fish oil supplement (one to two 1,000-mg capsules daily).**

•**Avoid "blue light" at night.** Exposure to blue light—the kind emitted by smartphones, computers, tablets and LED TVs—disrupts sleep patterns by blocking the release of the sleep hormone melatonin. Even if you do fall asleep fairly easily, blue light exposure may come back to haunt you in the form of a middle-of-the-night wake-up.

If you can't force yourself to power down your electronics within two hours of bedtime, try positioning handheld devices farther away from your eyes than usual.

*To find a CBT-I therapist, consult the Society of Behavioral Sleep Medicine, BehavioralSleep.org. You can also try the free CBT-i Coach app, available at iTunes or Google Play.

**Consult your doctor if you take medication.

In addition, consider various apps that filter blue light on your smartphone or tablet. Some operating systems are automatically programmed with this feature—Apple's iOS 9.3 offers Night Shift, for example. Using your device's geolocation and clock, the colors of your display are automatically shifted to the warmer end of the spectrum (which is less disruptive to sleep) around sundown. Free apps for Android devices include Night Shift: Blue Light Filter and Twilight.

•**Use special lightbulbs.** If you wake up in the middle of the night and make a trip to the bathroom, the glare of the bathroom light tells your brain "It's morning!"

What helps: Use low-blue lightbulbs in your bathroom and bedroom that don't block the release of melatonin. A variety are available from Lighting Science (LSGC.com). Or look online for night-lights designed to emit low levels of blue light.

IF YOU DO WAKE UP

Even if you follow the steps described above, you may still have occasional nighttime awakenings with trouble falling back asleep (meaning you are awake for at least 25 minutes).

Experiment with the following strategies to see what works best for you…

•**Resist the urge to check e-mail or do anything else on your phone.** Even short exposures to blue light are enough to suppress melatonin. Mentally stimulating activities, such as loud TV, are also best avoided. (However, a TV at low volume with the setting adjusted to dim the screen can be a great distractor for an active mind at night.)

My advice: Choose a relaxing activity like reading, listening to soothing music or knitting. If you read, use a book light or a bedside-table lamp that has one of the special bulbs mentioned earlier.

•**Don't look at the clock.** If you do, you'll start doing the mental math of how many hours you have left until you need to wake up. This will cause anxiety that will spike your levels of cortisol and adrenaline, sleep-disrupting hormones that make you feel wide awake!

My advice: Turn your clock around, and try counting backward from 300 by threes to distract yourself and promote drowsiness.

Also helpful: Try the "4-7-8 method"—inhale for four seconds...hold your breath for seven...and exhale slowly for eight. Breathe in this manner for up to 15 to 20 minutes or until you fall asleep. Inhaling and holding in air increases oxygen in the body, which means your body doesn't have to expend as much energy. The slow exhale helps you unwind and mimics the slow breathing that takes place during sleep, which will help you fall asleep.

•**Turn on some pink noise.** The well-known "white noise"—used to mask conversations and potentially startling sounds—is comprised of all frequencies detectable by the human ear. Pink noise, on the other hand, has a lower, softer frequency. Pink noise is generally considered more relaxing and has a steady sound like gentle rain.

Sleep experts believe that our brains respond better to the lower spectrum of pink noise than to the fuller spectrum of white noise. The result is a more peaceful and sleep-conducive feeling.

My advice: Search for a free app that contains pink noise, and listen to it with earphones on your smartphone, laptop or tablet if you wake up in the middle of the night. Just be sure to glance only briefly at the screen when turning on the device, and turn off the screen light while listening. You can set the pink noise to play for a set amount of time, such as 30 minutes. As an alternative, you can purchase a pink-noise generator online.

Salmon and Spinach for a Sleepytime Dinner

Try salmon and spinach salad for dinner at 7 pm—omega-3s in the fish help you relax, and magnesium in spinach can calm your nerves. For dessert at 7:30, eat tart cherries—they contain the sleep hormone melatonin—or drink tart cherry juice. For a bedtime snack at 9 pm, make warm milk part of a soothing ritual—it is the routine, not the tryptophan in the milk, that is calming.

Health. Health.com

Foods That Sabotage Sleep

Bonnie Taub-Dix, RDN, CDN, a registered dietitian and director and owner of BTD Nutrition Consultants, LLC, on Long Island and in New York City. She is author of *Read It Before You Eat It.* BonnieTaubDix.com

You know that an evening coffee can leave you tossing and turning into the wee hours. *But other foods hurt sleep, too...*

•**Premium ice cream.** Brace yourself for a restless night if you indulge in Häagen-Dazs or Ben & Jerry's late at night. The richness of these wonderful treats comes mainly from fat—16 to 17 grams of fat in half a cup of vanilla, and who eats just half a cup?

Your body digests fat more slowly than it digests proteins or carbohydrates. When you eat a high-fat food within an hour or two of bedtime, your digestion will still be "active" when you lie down—and that can disturb sleep.

Also, the combination of stomach acid, stomach contractions and a horizontal position increases the risk for reflux, the upsurge of digestive juices into the esophagus that causes heartburn—which can disturb sleep.

•**Chocolate.** Some types of chocolate can jolt you awake almost as much as a cup of coffee. Dark chocolate, in particular, has shocking amounts of caffeine.

Example: Half a bar of Dagoba Eclipse Extra Dark has 41 milligrams of caffeine, close to what you'd get in a shot of mild espresso.

Chocolate also contains theobromine, another stimulant, which is never a good choice near bedtime.

•**Beans.** Beans are one of the healthiest foods. But a helping or two of beans—or broccoli, cauliflower, cabbage or other gas-producing foods—close to bedtime can make your night, well, a little noisier than usual. No one sleeps well when suffering from gas pains. You can reduce the "backtalk" by drinking a mug of chamomile or peppermint tea at bedtime. They're carminative herbs that aid digestion and help prevent gas.

• **Spicy foods.** Spicy foods temporarily speed up your metabolism. They are associated with taking longer to fall asleep and with more time spent awake at night. This may be caused by the capsaicin found in chili peppers, which affects body temperature and disrupts sleep. Also, in some people, spicy foods can lead to sleep-disturbing gas, stomach cramps and heartburn.

Sleeping Pills Are Just Plain Dangerous

Robert Langer, MD, MPH, principal scientist and medical director, Jackson Hole Center for Preventive Medicine, Wyoming.

It's bad enough that people are so desperate for sleep that they resort to taking any of a long list of pharmaceuticals in an effort to help them get a good night's rest. Even worse is that these theoretical helpers come with a long list of associated dangers, including addiction.

Well guess what? The list of dangers just got longer.

Research, conducted by physicians at the Scripps Clinic Viterbi Family Sleep Center in San Diego and Jackson Hole Center for Preventive Medicine (JHCPM) in Wyoming, has shown that use of sleeping pills has been associated with an increased risk for cancer and death.

The most troubling part is that this study found that it's not just daily users who are at risk—those who use them less than twice a month may even be at risk.

IT TAKES A WHILE FOR SIDE EFFECTS TO SURFACE

Robert Langer, MD, MPH, principal scientist and medical director at JHCPM, explained more about these frightening findings. He said that most studies on the safety of sleeping pills last only six months or less. "That's not enough time to examine the risk for many serious health consequences, such as cancer or death," said Dr. Langer. "Our research is more long-term, and we didn't just look at whether or not people were taking sleeping pills. We also looked at which type they were using and how often they were taking the pills."

The researchers looked at the electronic medical records of the population served by the Geisinger Health System (GHS) in Pennsylvania, the largest rural integrated health system in the US. Subjects (mean age 54 years) were 10,529 male and female patients who received prescriptions of sleeping pills as sleep aids (on-label), and 23,676 matched controls with no prescriptions of sleeping pills. They were followed for an average of 2.5 years.

The researchers found that the more sleeping pills that subjects took, the greater their risk for death from all causes and, shockingly, even people who were taking them only sporadically were at higher risk for death. *For example, compared with those who did not take sleeping pills, people who took…*

• **One to 18 sleeping pills a year were 3.6 times more likely to die within the 2.5-year follow-up period.**

• **19 to 132 sleeping pills a year were 4.4 times more likely to die.**

• **133 or more pills a year were 5.3 times more likely to die.**

These results did not differ whether the subjects were using older sleeping pills, such as *temazepam* (Restoril), or newer ones, such as *zolpidem* (Ambien), *eszopiclone* (Lunesta) and *zaleplon* (Sonata), which are marketed as being shorter-acting and safer.

Researchers also found an increased risk for all major cancers among moderate and heavy users of any sleeping pill. There was a 20% increased risk among any users who took 19 to 132 pills a year and a 35% increased risk among any users who took more than 132 pills a year.

It's important to note that none of these results prove cause and effect, but they certainly reveal an unsettling association.

UNDERSTANDING THE CONNECTION

Could the results simply be due to the fact that patients who take sleeping pills are usually in worse health—for example, perhaps they don't eat well or exercise as much as they should or maybe they're more stressed? Dr. Langer says no. "We controlled for every possible variation, matching subjects and controls by age, gender and health history, yet the results remained the same."

So why the increased risk for death and cancer? The authors did not have adequate information to assess possible mechanisms. However, based on prior studies, potential mechanisms include increases in sleep apnea, accidents related to sleep walking/driving, aspiration pneumonia and depression of respiratory function.

NOW WHAT?

This is a finding of major consequence, because nine million American adults took a prescription sleeping pill in 2013, according to a recent Centers for Disease Control and Prevention study. But the complicating factor is that sleeping pills do provide health benefits. In other words, not taking a sleeping pill and potentially not getting enough sleep comes with its own set of risks—for instance, insomnia can raise the risk for heart disease, stroke, diabetes, obesity, depression and other serious health conditions. So if you're taking sleeping pills, what do you do?

First, consult your prescribing physician, said Dr. Langer. "Don't stop cold turkey, because that can cause withdrawal symptoms and agitation, as well as sleepless nights. Figure out a plan with your doctor about how to taper off," he said. And then ask your doctor about safer alternatives, such as melatonin or manipulating light exposure, he said. You can also try cognitive behavioral therapy from an informed primary care doctor, behavioral therapist or sleep medicine physician, he added.

To Sleep Better, Make Your Own Placebo

Article titled *"The Placebo Effect: History, Biology, and Ethics,"* by Patrick Lemoine, MD, professor of psychiatry and director of clinical studies, University of Claude Bernard of Lyon, France, published in *Medscape*.

Ted. J. Kaptchuk, director, Program in Placebo Studies, Beth Israel Deaconess Medical Center, Boston.

Wouldn't it be great if you could just take a "sugar pill" to get to sleep? Maybe you can. Recent research has shown that placebos—sugar or other non-active material given to patients in place of actual drugs—make good sleep medicine. About half of the effectiveness of prescription sleep medications comes from the placebo effect, research shows. The "real" drugs, meanwhile, may leave us groggy, memory-impaired and more accident-prone—and can lead to a drug dependency. They are widely overprescribed, especially amongst the elderly.

But if you know you're just taking a sugar pill, is it really a placebo? Don't you need to believe you're really taking a sleeping pill for the placebo effect to work?

One French doctor has devised a clever method that lets his patients use the power of the placebo to wean themselves from reliance on prescription or over-the-counter sleeping pills. *Here's how you can do it yourself...*

THE POWER OF PLACEBOS

First, a little background. The term placebo (Latin for "I shall please") has been used to refer to medicine for more than two centuries (Thomas Jefferson wrote about them), but most physicians believed these inert pills exerted no real physiological action—they simply allowed patients to fool themselves into feeling better.

Now we know better. The belief that you are taking medicine can unleash powerful, positive physical changes in your body. "A host of studies have shown that treatment with placebos elicits an array of physiological responses," says Harvard Medical School professor Ted J. Kaptchuk, who directs the Program in Placebo Studies at Beth Israel

Deaconess Medical Center in Boston. "These include stimulating neurotransmitters such as the body's own opioids, cannabinoids, dopamine and serotonin, all of which can alleviate pain, depression, anxiety and fatigue. We have an entire pharmacy of substances within us—and placebos help trigger their action."

YOUR RECIPE FOR ZZZS?

Patrick Lemoine, MD, a professor of psychiatry at the University of Claude Bernard of Lyon in France, finds that many of his patients have trouble letting go entirely even if they have cut back. For them he uses homemade placebos to wean his patients off prescription pills. "It's a bit like when a child learns to swim and refuses to let go of a floating device the instructor has gradually deflated," he writes.

His weaning technique entails transferring prescription sleep medication into empty capsules and doing the same with sugar, then mixing the drug capsules and sugar capsules together so that on any given night, you won't know whether you're taking a real or fake pill.

Below is a plan based on his recommendations for patients who are used to taking a sleeping pill every night.

Make sure to first ask your pharmacist whether your prescription sleeping tablets can be safely crushed and ingested in capsules...

• **First, gather your materials.** Buy a bag of at least 150 empty capsules—choose the opaque sort over the clear—at your drugstore or online. Next, you'll need sugar, or, if you'd rather not take in even a tiny amount of sugar, you can substitute cornstarch. Finally, you'll need something with which to crush your sleeping pills—a mortar-and-pestle or, if you prefer, a capsule-filling kit (easily found online).

• **Next, count out 30 empty capsules.** Insert one finely crushed sleeping pill into each of 25 of the capsules. Now put about the same amount granulated sugar or whatever placebo material you have chosen into each of the remaining five capsules.

• **Put all of the capsules in a jar or empty pill bottle, and shake gently to mix them around.**

• **For the next month, take one capsule from this bottle each night.** On any given night, you won't know whether you've taken the sleeping drug or a placebo. But you will know that on any given night, there's a very good chance that you are taking the sleeping drug, because 25 out of the 30 capsules contain the drug.

• **The second month, fill 20 capsules with the sleep aid and 10 with the placebo.**

• **The third month, make it even-steven—15 drug-filled caps, 15 placebo-filled caps.**

• **For the fourth month, it's 10 drugs/20 placebos.**

• **For the fifth month, five drugs/25 placebos.**

• **For the last month, one drug/29 placebos.**

By the end of the process, if all goes well, you'll be sleeping like a baby with almost no help from drugs. You may want to wean yourself from sleep drugs in just a few months rather than the full six, and that's fine. What's described above is not a scientifically proven method, but just one doctor's approach that works for some of his patients, so feel free to adapt the approach as you see fit.

For example, there's no reason to start taking a pill every night if you're in the habit of taking sleeping pills only when you feel that you need them. In that case, mix up a batch of sleeping pills plus some number of placebos beforehand, and take one pill when you feel that you need a little help. And if you have trouble giving up the idea that you might be taking a sleeping pill, you could go back to the 5/25 or even the 1/29 formula. You'll still be taking a lot fewer sleeping pills. (*Note:* If you're traveling, especially if you're flying, leave these pills at home. You won't be able to show that they are prescription medicines if you are asked.)

Another approach: Try a half dose of your standard sleeping pills, either cut in half (check with your pharmacist to see if yours can be cut in half safely) or mixed in with placebos as above. You can also use the placebo effect to make other types of prescriptions work better.

Finally, it's also possible that taking a placebo might work for you even if you know it's a placebo. "We've done several studies using 'open label' or 'honest' placebos (where the person taking them knew they were ingesting an inactive substance) with very good results," says Professor Kaptchuk.

In the end, learning to harness the power of placebos to get better sleep is really about activating your own abilities—and there are many paths you can take.

Flower Sleep Remedy

Not sleeping well? Try lavender. When a bottle of lavender oil was left open within three feet of the bedsides of adults who were hospitalized, they slept significantly better and had lower overnight blood pressure.

Why: The soothing scent of lavender calms the nervous system.

To improve anyone's sleep: Use lavender oil in an aromatherapy diffuser at bedtime, or put a few drops on a cotton ball, and tuck it into your pillowcase.

Karen Davis, PhD, professor, department of health policy and management, The Johns Hopkins Hospital, Baltimore.

Gentle Ways to Get Better Sleep

Jamison Starbuck, ND, a naturopathic physician in family practice and a guest lecturer at the University of Montana, both in Missoula. She is a past president of the American Association of Naturopathic Physicians and a contributing editor to *The Alternative Advisor: The Complete Guide to Natural Therapies and Alternative Treatments.*

When you're really wrestling with insomnia, it's tempting to go to your doctor and ask for one of the sleep medications we see advertised on TV—Ambien or Lunesta—or an older tranquilizing drug such as Valium. While short-term use of one of these drugs might make sense for a person who feels his/her overall health is being threatened by insomnia, I generally advise against this approach. Sure, these drugs may temporarily allow you to sleep, but they don't cure insomnia. *My advice...*

• **Do some detective work.** Thinking about your own sleep issues and making some written notes can be a big help. When do you typically go to bed? How often do you have insomnia? Do you have trouble falling asleep or wake in the middle of the night? Also, look at when your problem started to determine whether it coincided with any health issues, use of new medications or habits, such as working late hours, that could lead to insomnia.

• **Get your doctor involved.** Discuss your notes with your doctor. Chronic pain, hormonal changes (including those related to hyperthyroidism and menopause) and serious illness, such as cancer and heart or lung disease, can cause insomnia. If any of these conditions is to blame, getting proper treatment may well take care of the insomnia, too.

After you've consulted your doctor, try these gentle methods...*

• **Avoid high-protein dinners.** Protein is often hard to digest. Eating a lot at dinner can lead to gastrointestinal distress that may result in insomnia. Instead, eat foods that are easy to digest (such as soup and salad) for dinner, and have larger, protein-rich meals midday.

Also helpful: Take a 2,000-mg omega-3 supplement with your evening meal. When taken before bedtime, these healthful fats can have a calming effect on the brain, promoting sleep.

• **Try Calms Forté.** This homeopathic preparation is effective and extremely safe.

Typical dose: One tablet under the tongue at bedtime and whenever you wake up in the middle of the night (up to six tablets per 24-hour period). Calms Forté, made by Hylands, is available at natural groceries and pharmacies.

*Check with your doctor before trying supplements, especially if you take medication and/or have a chronic medical condition.

•**Add skullcap.** If the steps above don't give you relief, you may want to also try this potent herb to relax the "busy brain" experience that often keeps people awake. I recommend using skullcap in tincture form—30 to 60 drops (one-sixteenth to one-eighth teaspoon) in a cup of chamomile or spearmint tea at bedtime.

Note: Skullcap can make some people too sleepy. If you are sensitive to medication, try just 10 drops of skullcap at bedtime—or simply drink chamomile or mint tea as a sedative.

•**Use melatonin with care.** If you'd rather try this popular sleep aid, do so thoughtfully. Melatonin is a hormone. Taking too much can trigger irritability. Melatonin supplements may also raise women's estrogen levels, increasing overall inflammation in the body. I recommend taking no more than 3 mg of melatonin in a 24-hour period and often start my patients on a daily dose of only 1 mg. Take melatonin 30 minutes before bedtime.

Nose Trick Puts You to Sleep

Do you have difficulty falling asleep? Look to your nose! The left nostril is connected to the right hemisphere of the brain. Breathing through the left nostril can activate the parasympathetic nervous system, which counteracts stress and helps calm you and put you into a sleep mode. *Here's the way to put that nostril to work to bring on the sleep you need...*

Lie on your right side, which will help open your left nostril, then use the thumb or index finger of your right hand to close the right nostril. Take long, deep breaths through your left nostril for a few minutes...and you will feel much more relaxed and closer to sleep.

Joan Wilen and Lydia Wilen are folk-remedy experts based in New York City. They are authors of *Bottom Line's Treasury of Home Remedies & Natural Cures* and *Bottom Line's Household Magic.*

Pill-Free Cure for Insomnia

YAWN! Not getting enough sleep is exhausting. Most people have trouble sleeping every once in awhile. If you just can't catch those Zs and you hate the groggy morning-after feeling you get from sleeping pills, try this acupressure trick. Just before you go to bed, press the center of the bottoms of your heels with your thumbs. The easiest way to do this is to lie on your back (on a carpeted floor is best) and bend your knees, using your right hand on your left foot and left hand on your right. Press as hard as you can without cramping your hands. Keep pressing for at least two minutes—up to four minutes is even better. You should feel yourself starting to really relax, with tension leaving your body. Ease into bed for blissful zzzzzzzs.

Joan Wilen and Lydia Wilen are folk-remedy experts based in New York City. They are authors of *Bottom Line's Treasury of Home Remedies & Natural Cures* and *Bottom Line's Household Magic.*

Natural Cures Tailored to Your Sleep Problem

Laurie Steelsmith, ND, LAc, a licensed naturopathic physician and acupuncturist in private practice in Honolulu and author of *Natural Choices for Women's Health.* DrSteelsmith.com

Let's say you have trouble sleeping. You want to avoid prescription and even over-the-counter sleep drugs, which can be habit-forming and have bad side effects. You're leaning toward a safer, natural alternative...possibly melatonin.

You're wondering, *What's the best sleep supplement?*

But that's the wrong question.

The right question is, *What's the best supplement to help me with my specific sleep problem?*

There are lots of herbs and supplements to choose from that can help with sleep problems. Some work better for certain situations than others. In fact, melatonin, the most popular sleep supplement, is usually not the best choice (see next page).

There are also lifestyle changes that may help with each specific situation. For most people, these lifestyle changes—and, if needed, specific herbs and supplements tailored to particular situations—can help restore good sleep.

One caveat: If you have a chronic medical condition or take any kind of medication, check with your doctor before taking supplements.

IF YOU HAVE TROUBLE FALLING ASLEEP

This is usually due to a busy mind, anxious thoughts and high levels of the stress hormone cortisol in the evening, when it should be low.

Before taking supplements, do this for a week: Try a calming bath to unwind at night, or relaxation therapy such as meditation or listening to a guided imagery recording. Lower the lights, quiet the house, turn off all electronics. If you're still experiencing insomnia after a week, try taking one of the following supplements to help you drop more easily into sleep…and make sure you continue with the lifestyle changes.

•**Phosphatidylserine.** This supplement, usually derived from cabbage or soy, decreases cortisol at night. Phosphatidylserine can help optimize your reaction to stress and support the proper release of cortisol. A product called Seriphos that contains 90 mg of phosphatidylserine. Start with one pill an hour or two before bedtime taken with a small high-protein snack (such as a cracker with almond butter) for better absorption and to prevent stomach upset. If you tolerate it well and you need more support, take two pills. You can take up to two pills before bed and two in the middle of the night if you're waking up. Side effects are rare—occasionally, you might feel a little sleepy the next day, and very rarely, a paradoxical feeling of being more awake at bedtime. Avoid phosphatidylserine if you have kidney problems.

•**Valerian root and GABA.** Valerian root (an herb) and GABA (gamma-aminobutyric acid, an amino acid supplement) help to calm the nervous system. They both bind to GABA receptors in the brain and can be taken alone or together. The standard dose of valerian root is 300 mg to 500 mg of a standardized extract of 0.5% essential oils taken one hour before bedtime. The standard dose of GABA is 250 mg to 1,000 mg taken one hour before bed. Start with GABA first to see if you get the desired effect. Start with 250 mg at night, and increase the dose to up to 1,000 mg if necessary. (GABA can cause serious cardiovascular side effects and nightmares in very large doses—10,000 mg—and should be avoided entirely by pregnant and lactating women.)

Valerian root is safe and effective for most people, but side effects can occur, such as headaches, insomnia, excitability and a feeling of uneasiness. If falling asleep is still a huge effort, take both at the same time. It's safe to take valerian root (up to 500 mg at night) and GABA (250 mg to 500 mg at night) for up to three months—while working on the underlying causes of your insomnia.

IF YOU HAVE TROUBLE STAYING ASLEEP

Nighttime wakening can be one of the most difficult-to-treat sleep conditions.

One lifestyle tip: Make sure you're eating adequate calories for dinner. Skipping dinner causes your blood sugar level to drop, which increases cortisol in your body and can wake you up. Eating a solid, healthful dinner that contains all three macronutrients—protein, fat and carbohydrate—can mitigate this.

•**5-HTP.** Another common culprit is too little serotonin. This neurotransmitter makes us feel happier, calmer and more balanced and plays an important role in sleep. To boost serotonin, try 5-HTP. This supplement is the active form of tryptophan, an amino acid that your body needs to make serotonin. It's often used to help people who are depressed, a condition that can be characterized by low serotonin levels. But your levels can be lower than ideal even if you aren't experiencing depression—and if so 5-HTP supplements can help you stay asleep. Start with 100 mg taken at least one hour before bed, and gradually increase to 300 mg if you need it. At these doses, side effects are rare—but don't take this supplement if you are taking a prescription antidepressant (such as an SSRI) that also increases serotonin levels.

IF MENOPAUSAL SYMPTOMS ARE WAKING YOU UP…

Women who are in the menopausal transition (perimenopause) often have sleep problems due to hormonal fluctuations.

First step: Get your hormone levels assessed to see if your estrogen is too high and progesterone too low, or if both hormones are low. If progesterone is low, chaste tree berry (see below) can balance levels, but sometimes bioidentical hormones can help, too. Start with bioidentical progesterone, and if that isn't enough, try an estrogen cream to apply to the vagina or vulva.

•**Chaste tree berry.** For women in perimenopause, this herb can help to naturally increase waning progesterone levels. Progesterone is a calming hormone and can help even out a woman's fluctuating hormonal levels through its action on the pituitary gland. It has been shown to help support healthy ovulation, which is essential for supporting progesterone levels, even during perimenopause. Try Asensia, a chaste tree berry-containing product that also contains other ingredients, including L-arginine and green tea extract, which in combination help the chaste tree berry be better utilized by your body. It is very safe to user.

•**Especially for night sweats.** Asensia can help in women who are waning in progesterone, and Seriphos works great for insomnia associated with night sweats.

•**Got to pee?** Try to get up and do your business without turning on the lights or peeking at the clock. But if every night you're being wakened about the same time, you could try taking a drop of a homeopathic sleep remedy such as Quietude by Boiron. It contains homeopathic doses of hyoscyamus niger, nux moschata, passiflora incarnata and stramonium. The tablets can be placed under the tongue and allowed to dissolve while you drift off to sleep.

IF YOU HAVE JET LAG OR WORK THE NIGHT SHIFT

If you've crossed a few time zones or regularly work through the night, you know that it throws off your circadian rhythm, making it hard to get back into a regular sleep pattern. Expose yourself to sunlight, especially morning sunlight, when you can, which will help regulate your internal clock. *A few specific tips…*

•**For jet lag,** before your trip, wake up and go to sleep earlier several days before a trip heading east…go to sleep later for a westward trip…and when you get to your destination, make yourself get up in the morning and work out.

•**For shift work,** you'll sleep better and be more awake on the job if you stick to the same sleep and wake schedule every day, even on days you're not working.

If these approaches don't work for you, consider…

•**Melatonin.** A lot of people think they should pop melatonin whenever they have trouble sleeping, but it's really only best for resetting a body clock that has been thrown off by shifting time zones or shift work. A typical dose is 3 mg under the tongue to be taken within one hour of when you want to fall asleep. For jet lag, you can use it for a few nights to settle into a new time zone…or it can be used longer by people who have night shifts. It's often used long term for men and women who change their day/night sleep cycle frequently—such as doctors and nurses. Side effects can include headache, short-term depression, daytime sleepiness, dizziness, cramps and irritability. Some people are very sensitive to melatonin, and even a typical 3-mg dose may be too much for them. Start with a 1-mg dose and slowly increase to 3 mg if you tolerate it well. This is not recommended for children or young women who want to get pregnant. Because melatonin levels tend to naturally drop as people get older, melatonin is best for people older than 50.

NOURISH YOUR CALM

All these strategies can help you feel rested and restored, but to truly improve sleep, you need to take stock of how your energies are being spent—and adjust your lifestyle so that you nourish a calm nervous system. This alone will do wonders for people who are having trouble sleeping.

After all, you can't expect to be mentally overstimulated all day and then have your mind turn off at night like a switch. Exercise is also key—it discharges stress and tension, and encourages sound sleep. Get regular physical exercise but avoid exercising in the three hours before bedtime, when it could rev you up.

Finally…as a last resort, it's ok to occasionally take prescription sleep aides. There is a time and place for them especially for those who have intractable insomnia. Some need these only occasionally, but others stay on these long term.

Recommended: Benadryl, which allows a person to wake up, rather than others such as Ambien, which could put a person into a trancelike state where he/she doesn't remember what he has done if he gets up in the middle of the night.

Sleep Better with Cognitive Behavioral Therapy for Insomnia

Donn Posner, PhD, CBSM (Certified in Behavioral Sleep Medicine), psychologist, Palo Alto VA Medical Center, Palo Alto, California. A clinical associate professor of psychiatry and human behavior at The Warren Alpert Medical School of Brown University, Providence, he also is a coauthor of *Cognitive Behavioral Treatment of Insomnia: A Session-by-Session Guide*.

D o you lie awake night after night, struggling to catch the sleep that eludes you…then feel exhausted and miserable during the day? Don't just suffer stoically—insomnia is serious! It increases the risk for high blood pressure, obesity, diabetes, anxiety and substance abuse. What's more, although insomnia often is considered a sign of depression, recent research reveals that the insomnia can come first and double a person's risk of developing depression.

Sleeping pills may seem like a quick fix, but don't be too hasty in taking that route. Though these drugs do help some people, they also can have bad side effects…and according to one study, long-term use is associated with increased risk for early death.

There's a much better option that can get you the deep, blissful sleep you need. It's completely safe and drug-free, and because it addresses the underlying causes of insomnia (unlike medication), its benefits persist even long after treatment ends. It's called cognitive behavioral therapy for insomnia (CBT-I), and just a few sessions can go a long way to restore normal sleep patterns. CBT-I has been shown to relieve insomnia for a wide variety of people, including older adults and those who suffer from chronic pain, fibromyalgia, cardiovascular disease, mood disorders and other health problems. It can even help people who have been taking sleeping pills for years. *Here's what you should know about CBT-I…*

IS THIS SLEEP SOLUTION RIGHT FOR YOU?

A few restless nights should not be considered insomnia (important to know so that you don't feel overly stressed about an occasional bad night!).

True chronic insomnia means difficulty initiating or maintaining sleep, despite adequate opportunity to sleep, that occurs at least three times a week and lasts for at least three months. How long can it take you to fall asleep before it's a problem? Most experts in the field consider 30 minutes of lying awake, either before first falling asleep or after having woken up in the middle of the night, as the cut-off. In addition, insomnia leads to some daytime consequences—for instance, fatigue, memory problems, difficulty concentrating, poor work performance or even anxiety about being unable to fall sleep. Insomnia is not just a nighttime disorder…it's a 24-hour disorder.

If you think that your sleep pattern fits the above description of insomnia, talk to your doctor—a medical problem could be interfering with your slumber, and you may find that sleep comes more easily once that underlying condition is addressed. If your insomnia persists, however, you should strongly consider trying CBT-I.

WHAT TO EXPECT DURING TREATMENT

The first step with CBT-I is for you to find a sleep specialist who offers it. To do this, ask your doctor for a referral to a qualified professional with expertise in CBT-I...or find a practitioner through the Society of Behavioral Sleep Medicine (BehavioralSleep.org) or contact the nearest certified sleep center and say that you're interested in CBT-I.

Once you choose a sleep specialist, you can expect to undergo a thorough evaluation of all areas of functioning to determine all the factors that are contributing to your sleep problems. Genetic makeup, internal rhythm, social life, home life and work life are all evaluated...and you are instructed to keep a sleep diary to help pinpoint problematic patterns. Your therapist also tries to determine whether an emotional issue or even another sleep disorder precipitated your insomnia. When the evaluation is complete, the therapist creates an individualized treatment plan, typically consisting of four to six weekly one-hour sessions.

Then the real work begins. As the name implies, CBT-I involves both behavioral and cognitive elements. *Though therapy is tailored to each patient, a typical protocol includes the following...*

•**Sleep restriction.** You may be instructed to stop napping...stay active in the evening to avoid dozing off in front of the TV...go to bed later than you usually do...and get out of bed at precisely the same time every morning regardless of how well you slept. Your sleep therapist also may restrict the amount of time you spend in bed, for instance, by allowing you only 30 minutes more than your actual sleeping time—so if you usually get just five hours of sleep, you'll be told to spend no more than five and a half hours in bed. Only as your "sleep efficiency" improves do you start going to bed earlier and staying in bed longer. The idea is for you to be very sleepy at bedtime... which makes it much easier to fall asleep.

•**Stimulus control.** You are cautioned against using your bed at any time of day for anything other than sleeping or sex. That means no lounging on the bed to read, watch TV, talk on the phone or surf the Internet. For times when you do go to bed and do not fall asleep (or fall back to sleep) within 15 to 20 minutes, you are told to get up and go do something in another room, returning to bed only when you feel sleepy again—and repeating this instruction as many times as necessary.

•**The rationale**—when a person habitually struggles to fall asleep, he/she "works" at what should be a natural process...and he becomes conditioned to associate the bed with anxiety, frustration and effort. In contrast, by getting out of bed whenever he cannot sleep, he gives up that struggle. If he applies this rule consistently, over time the bed becomes a trigger for sleep rather than for wakefulness. That association between bed and sleep is further reinforced when he avoids using the bed at all while awake. The only exception is sex. If we asked people to give up the bed as a place for sex, they wouldn't comply anyway. But more importantly, during sex you presumably are not trying to sleep, so it doesn't present the same problem as, say, reading in bed with the intention of getting to sleep. It is really sleep effort above all that we try to eliminate.

•**Sleep hygiene.** Typically patients are advised to avoid caffeine after noon...and to avoid exercise, alcohol, heavy meals and nicotine within two hours of bedtime. Your sleep therapist also reviews your bedroom environment to make sure it is dark and cool enough to be conducive to sleep. (Many people keep their bedrooms too warm for good sleep.)

•**Anxiety abatement.** The therapist teaches you how to deal with the anxiety you may feel before heading to bed. For instance, you may often think, *I'll be a wreck if I don't get to sleep*...or *I can't stand lying awake like this!* As you learn to counteract that "catastrophic thinking" with rational thoughts—*I can function OK even if I don't sleep for eight hours*...or *Insomnia is unpleasant but hardly unbearable*—your anxiety lessens and sleep comes more easily. You also may be shown relaxation techniques to practice during the day and at bedtime. And you learn to avoid staring compulsively at the clock, which only makes you fret more as you calculate how much sleep you're losing. If you need an alarm clock, you may be told to use one without illumination… or to place the clock under your bed where you can't keep checking it.

Commitment is key: Too many people try one or two of the techniques for a few nights, and then if they don't immediately start sleeping better, they get frustrated and give up. There is nothing magic that will work tonight. It takes dedication and commitment to make CBT-I work because you have to rebuild your innate sleep drive and realign your body's natural rhythms before you'll be able to sleep well. Be forewarned—during treatment, sleep problems often get worse before they get better… but that's a sign that the protocol is working. It can take a week or two to start seeing real progress. Given that most people with chronic insomnia have had the problem for years, a couple weeks of work should be a good trade.

Covering the costs: The Affordable Care Act now requires insurance companies to cover behavioral health treatments, but benefits vary depending on the state you live in, your insurance plan and your sleep therapist's professional degree. The price for a course of CBT-I treatment averages about $460 for up to six sessions. It's also worth noting that you may end up saving money in the long run. A recent study showed that older adults with insomnia spent an average of $1,100 more on health care over a six-month period compared with those who did not have insomnia—and that, after completing as few as three sessions of CBT-I, participants' total health-care costs dropped significantly.

So even if you have to pay out of pocket, you may want to consider CBT-I an investment in yourself. Chances are good that it will end up saving you anxiety, aggravation and money…promoting optimal health overall.

"Voodoo" Cure for Insomnia

Pina LoGiudice, ND, LAc, clinical director of Inner Source Health and Acupuncture, a center for integrative naturopathic care in New York City. She also is a contributing author of *Textbook of Natural Medicine* and a member of the adjunct faculty of the Natural Gourmet Institute for Food and Health in New York City, and has appeared on various TV shows, including *The Dr. Oz Show.* InnerSourceHealth.com

Getting stuck all over with needles may seem the stuff of voodoo nightmares—but in fact, if you suffer from insomnia, it may be just the fix for your sleepless nights. OK, don't volunteer to be a voodoo doll, though it may seem that way to you if you've never tried acupuncture. But do set aside your squeamishness and give it some consideration.

There's a growing amount of real science behind it. For instance, a meta-analysis of 46 randomized trials found that acupuncture does ease insomnia. And a study published in *Asian Journal of Psychiatry* found that acupuncture may be as effective as the sedative drug *zolpidem* (Ambien) in alleviating sleeplessness, particularly for women and older patients.

Big advantage: Acupuncture has no serious adverse effects—unlike sleeping pills, which can lead to breathing problems, pounding heartbeat, chest pain, blurred vision and addiction.

Studies aside, you might still wonder how well acupuncture works for real insomniacs in the real world. New York City naturopathic physician and licensed acupuncturist Pina LoGiudice, ND, LAc, said, "I can confirm that acupuncture has helped many of my patients sleep. I use it on its own for mild insomnia…for chronic cases, I use it in combination with other natural modalities to address underlying conditions that can interfere with sleep."

How it works: From the perspective of Western medicine, acupuncture helps regulate various hormones and neurotransmitters—including melatonin, serotonin, endorphins and many others—that play major roles in sleep regulation, according to a recent study from

Emory University School of Medicine. In traditional Chinese medicine, the theory is that various symptoms develop when a patient's qi (vital energy) gets blocked...and acupuncture removes these blockages by stimulating specific acupoints that correspond to different parts of the body. As Dr. LoGiudice explained, "Acupuncture helps strengthen the body's ability to heal itself. When tension and pain are removed, you eliminate much of what is causing the insomnia."

What to expect: While the course of treatment is tailored to an individual's needs, typically a patient receives 10 to 20 hypoallergenic needles at a time in a treatment session that lasts about 30 to 45 minutes. Placement of the needles depends on where the qi is blocked and on any underlying health problems that may be contributing to poor sleep. Discomfort is minimal—the needles are extremely thin and only go through the first layer of skin.

Insomnia patients typically go for treatment once per week for six to 12 weeks, then follow up once or twice a year for maintenance, Dr. LoGiudice said. How soon can patients expect results? "Some feel a difference as soon as the third treatment, while others may take up to 12 sessions. If we are not seeing results by the eighth session, I start thinking about adding nutrients or herbs to the treatment plan," she said.

To find a qualified acupuncturist: Visit the website of the American Association of Acupuncture and Oriental Medicine at AAAOM online.org and click on "Patients." Dr. LoGiudice noted that acupuncture generally is safe for everyone...there are no side effects except for rare cases of slight bruising...and some health insurance policies now cover acupuncture—all facts that may help you sleep better as you consider this treatment option.

Sleep Soundly: Safe, Natural Insomnia Solution

Rubin Naiman, PhD, psychologist specializing in sleep and dream medicine and clinical assistant professor of medicine at the University of Arizona's Center for Integrative Medicine. He is author of the book *Healing Night* and coauthor with Dr. Andrew Weil, of the audiobook *Healthy Sleep*.

A good night's sleep...there's nothing more restorative—or elusive...for the 64% of Americans who report regularly having trouble sleeping. A disconcertingly high percentage of the sleepless (nearly 20%) solve the problem by taking sleeping pills. But sleeping pills can be dangerously addictive, physically and/or emotionally—and swallowing a pill when you want to go to sleep doesn't address the root cause of the problem. What, exactly, is keeping you up at night?

SLOW DOWN...

According to Rubin Naiman, PhD, a psychologist and clinical assistant professor of medicine at the University of Arizona's Center for Integrative Medicine, most of our sleep problems have to do not with our bodies, per se, but with our habits. The modern American lifestyle—replete with highly refined foods and caffeine-laden beverages, excessive exposure to artificial light in the evening, and "adrenaline-producing" nighttime activities, such as working until bedtime, watching TV or surfing the Web—leaves us overstimulated in the evening just when our bodies are designed to slow down...and, importantly, to literally cool down as well.

Studies show that a cooler core body temperature—and warmer hands and feet—make you sleepy. "Cooling the body allows the mind and the heart to get quiet," says Dr. Naiman. He believes that this cooling process contributes to the release of melatonin, the hormone that helps to regulate the body's circadian rhythm of sleeping and waking.

DEEP GREEN SLEEP

Dr. Naiman has developed an integrative approach to sleep that defines healthy sleep as an interaction between a person and his/

her sleep environment. He calls this approach Deep Green Sleep. "My goal was to explore all of the subtleties in a person's life that may be disrupting sleep. This takes into account your physiology, emotions, personal experiences, sleeping and waking patterns and your attitudes about sleep and the sleeping environment." This approach is unique because it values "the subjective and personal experience of sleep," he says—in contrast with conventional sleep treatment, which tends to rely on "computer printouts of sleep studies—otherwise known as 'treating the chart.'"

It's important to realize that lifestyle habits and attitudes are hard to change, so Dr. Naiman cautioned that it often can take weeks, even months, to achieve his Deep Green Sleep. The good news is that the results are lasting and may even enhance your waking life.

Here are his suggestions on how you can ease into the night…

• **Live a healthful waking life.** "The secret of a good night's sleep is a good day's waking," said Dr. Naiman. This includes getting regular exercise (but not within three hours of bedtime) and eating a balanced, nutritious diet.

• **Cool down in the evening.** It's important to help your mind and body cool down, starting several hours before bedtime, by doing the following…

  • Avoid foods and drinks that sharply spike energy, such as highly refined carbohydrates and anything with caffeine, at least eight hours before bedtime.

  • Limit alcohol in the evening—it interferes with sleep by suppressing melatonin. It also interferes with dreaming and disrupts circadian rhythms.

  • Avoid nighttime screen-based activities within an hour of bedtime. You may think that watching TV or surfing the Web are relaxing things to do, but in reality these activities are highly stimulating. They engage your brain and expose you to relatively bright light with a strong blue wavelength that "mimics daylight and suppresses melatonin," said Dr. Naiman.

  • Create a sound sleeping environment. It is also important that where you sleep be stimulation-free and conducive to rest.

IN YOUR BEDROOM

• **Be sure that you have a comfortable mattress, pillow and bedding.** It's amazing how many people fail to address this basic need—often because their mattress has become worn out slowly, over time, and they haven't noticed.

• **Remove anything unessential from your bedside table that may tempt you to stay awake,** such as the TV remove control or stimulating books.

• **When you are ready to call it a night, turn everything off**—radio, TV and, of course, the light.

• **Keep the room cool (68°F or lower).**

• **Let go of waking.** Each day, allow your mind and body to surrender to sleep by engaging in quieting and relaxing activities starting about an hour before bedtime, such as…

  • Gentle yoga

  • Meditation

  • Rhythmic breathing

  • Reading poetry or other nonstimulating material

  • Journaling

  • Taking a hot bath

Also: Sex seems to help most people relax and can facilitate sleep, in part because climaxing triggers a powerful relaxation response, Dr. Naiman said.

• **Consider supplementing with melatonin.** If sleep is still elusive after trying these Deep Green Sleep tips, Dr. Naiman often suggests a melatonin supplement. Dr. Naiman believes that this is better than sleeping pills since melatonin is "the body's own natural chemical messenger of night." "Melatonin does not directly cause sleep, but triggers a cascade of events that result in natural sleep and dreams," he said, adding that it is nonaddictive, inexpensive and generally safe. Not all doctors agree however, so it is important to check with your doctor first.

If you're interested in learning more about Dr. Naiman's Deep Green Sleep program, you can visit his website (TheSleepAdvisor.com) and take a free quiz that helps identify your particular sleep challenges. But, since it is computer-based, make sure you do it several hours before bedtime!

The 15-Minute Secret to Sleeping Better (Boost Energy and Mood, Too)

Michael Terman, PhD, director of the Center for Light Treatment and Biological Rhythms at Columbia University Medical Center, New York City. He is founder and president of the Center for Environmental Therapeutics (CET), New York City. A leading authority on the circadian clock and the role that light plays in regulating it, Dr. Terman is coauthor of *Chronotherapy: Resetting Your Inner Clock to Boost Mood, Alertness, and Quality Sleep.*

Many of us have trouble sleeping and experience times during the day when our energy or mood lags. This can be more pronounced in the fall and winter when the days are shorter and darker.

The good news is that you don't have to turn to medication to fix these problems. The way to restful sleep, increased energy and a better mood may be as easy as exposing yourself to the right amount of light at the right time of day. *Here, how to do it…*

HOW LIGHT AFFECTS US

Many of us spend most of our days indoors. Even if our homes or offices seem to get a lot of natural light through windows, a light meter held in the room would show that the amount of light indoors registers much lower than just outside the window. In the evening, when our inner clock needs to wind down, we are inundated by artificial light from lamps, computer monitors and television screens. In our bedrooms at night, a night-light, streetlights, bathroom light, etc., can disturb sleep timing and quality.

BRIGHT-LIGHT THERAPY

By changing the amount and patterns of your daily light exposure, remarkable changes in your mood, energy and sleep can occur within days.

What to do: Buy a fluorescent light box that provides 10,000 lux of illumination (lux measures the light level reaching your eyes from the source). That is the equivalent of the amount of light that you would get while walking on the beach on a clear morning about 40 minutes after sunrise. The lamp should have a screen that filters out ultraviolet (UV) rays, which can be harmful to the eyes and skin. It should give off only white light, not colored light, which has been hyped to be especially potent but is visually disturbing and no better than white. To be sure of a big enough field of illumination, the screen area should be about 200 square inches (for example, 12 inches x 16 inches) or larger.

A good brand that meets all of the requirements is the DL930 Day-Light Classic by UpLift Technologies. It costs about $150. Many insurance companies will fully or partially cover the cost of a light box if you provide a physician's letter. Adjust the light box so that the light comes from above your line of sight and you feel comfortable and are not squinting. You should be positioned 12 to 13 inches from the screen. You can get the benefits of the light while talking on the phone, using your computer or enjoying breakfast. You sit facing forward, focused on the work surface, while the light shines down at your head from in front.

While side effects from light therapy are rare and relatively minor, they can occur. If you experience eyestrain, headache, queasiness or agitation after beginning light therapy, reduce the light dose by sitting farther away from the light box or shorten the duration of exposure.

SLEEP PROBLEMS

When do you prefer to go to sleep, and when do you like to wake up? Your answer indicates your chronotype, your individual inner clock. To determine your chronotype, take the chronotherapy quiz at CET.org. Click on "Education," then "Resource Centers" and then "Your Circadian Rhythm Type (Auto MEQ)."

The quiz will tell you the amount and timing of light therapy that will work best for you, but here are general recommendations…

• **You fall asleep too early.** You find it hard to stay awake at night and typically wake up very early in the morning.

Prescription for light therapy: Use a bright-light therapy box for 15 to 30 minutes about an hour before you typically get sleepy.

Other helpful strategies for staying awake and pushing your sleep cycle forward…

•Make lunch your major meal of the day, then eat only a light dinner.

•Avoid napping, especially in the afternoon and evening. Instead, distract yourself from your fatigue by moving around and doing stretches.

•Turn up room lights during the evening.

•**You fall asleep too late.** You try to get to bed at a decent hour but can't fall asleep. Then you have trouble waking up for work or school.

Prescription for light therapy: Use a light box for 15 to 30 minutes within 10 minutes after your natural wake-up time. If this time is later than your work schedule allows, begin light therapy on a long weekend. Then begin shifting your wake-up time and light-therapy schedule earlier—in 15-minute increments—as soon as you feel comfortable waking up at the new time.

More strategies for shifting your inner clock earlier include…

•Finish dinner at least three hours before bedtime. Avoid alcohol after dinner.

•Minimize napping, especially in the second half of the day. Try to get outdoors, keep moving and do some stretches instead.

•Keep your bedroom dark until you wake up. Early morning light seeping in through the windows actually can worsen a late-sleep pattern.

•**You sleep fitfully.**

Prescription for light therapy: Take light therapy—or spend time in the sun—in the middle of the day. Enhancing midday light exposure often improves sleep quality at night.

Other strategies to help you sleep through the night include…

•Do not drink alcohol after dinner.

•Keep your bedroom dark.

If you tend to wake up at night to use the bathroom, install amber-colored night-lights in the bathroom and hallway instead of turning on bright lights, which can disrupt your sleep.

•**You are unable to fall back to sleep after waking in the middle of the night.** There could be many causes for this type of sleep problem, such as anxiety, depression and physical illness, so it is best to consult a doctor. However, using light therapy in the evening to push sleep onset later (see "fall asleep too early") may help some people sleep through the night.

ENERGY AND MOOD

You can use bright-light therapy at any time during the day to increase your energy and alertness. Some people can quickly recharge with a brief session of light therapy (as little as 10 minutes) when they first feel an energy slump.

Caution: See a doctor if you are chronically lethargic—this can be a sign of depression, a medical sleep disorder (such as apnea) or other illness.

If you're feeling sad or mildly depressed, the light-therapy regimen is the same as the prescription for falling asleep too late.

Caution: It can be difficult for an individual to know the difference between mild depression and moderate or severe depression. If you are suffering from moderate or severe depression, a physician will need to monitor your progress with light therapy and consider other treatment options. To help determine where you fall on the depression spectrum, go to CET.org.

Mindfulness Brings on the ZZZs

Mindfulness meditation can help sleep. People over age 55 with sleep problems who were taught a standardized, structured course of meditation reported significantly better sleep quality. You can learn this meditation through programs such as Mindful

Awareness Practices or Mindfulness-Based Stress Reduction.

David S. Black, PhD, MPH, assistant professor of preventive medicine at Keck School of Medicine, University of Southern California, Los Angeles, and leader of a study published in *JAMA Internal Medicine*.

To Get to Sleep Fast, Do These 6 Easy Yoga Moves

Loren Fishman, MD, assistant clinical professor of rehabilitation and regenerative medicine, Columbia Medical School, New York City, medical director, Manhattan Physical Medicine and Rehabilitation, and author of several books on yoga for health, including the upcoming book, *Healing Yoga: Proven Postures to Treat Twenty Common Ailments—from Backache to Bone Loss, Shoulder Pain to Bunions, and More.*

Losing a good night's sleep is a bummer, isn't it? You walk around in a groggy fog the next day and run the risk of getting snippy with coworkers, friends and loved ones because sleep deprivation has made you grumpy. So many factors in modern daily life can make it tough for us to fall asleep, stay asleep and rest peacefully. Gentle stretching and certain breathing techniques, such as long deep breathing, are good to do right before bedtime. So it is great to learn that the trick to de-stress and set the stage for a good night's sleep, recommended by Loren Fishman, MD, assistant clinical professor of rehabilitation and regenerative medicine at Columbia Medical School in New York City, is a quick set of simple yoga poses.

"Yoga is a powerful tool to relieve stress and help your body relax and prepare for sleep," Dr. Fishman said. "By stretching muscles, yoga poses trigger mechanisms in the body that send powerful relaxing signals to the brain. When performed daily, yoga can make us into better sleepers."

Dr. Fishman instructs his patients to do the following yoga routine nightly at bedtime. Poses can even be done while in bed. Otherwise, do them on a cushioned surface on the floor. A plush blanket or towel will do if you don't have carpeting or a yoga mat.

•**Seated forward bend.** This will give a great stretch to your legs and back muscles. To prepare for the forward bend, sit with your legs straight in front of you. First, stretch one leg and then the other by extending from the hip through the heel to elongate the leg. Then 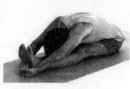 relax your legs and stretch your arms straight upward to feel your torso and back extend long and lean. Now you are ready to bend forward from the hips and reach out with your hands to grasp your ankles or feet (or as far down your legs as you comfortably can—you should be stretching, but not straining). Let gentle, deep breaths help you relax into the stretch. Hold this pose for one to three minutes.

•**Revolved abdomen pose.** This pose massages the abdominal organs, gives a nice stretch to the lower back and muscles across the rib cage and opens the chest so you can breathe more deeply. To do it, lie on your back, bend your knees to your chest and stretch your arms out to your sides. With bent knees pressed together, inhale. Then, while ex- 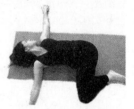 haling, twist from your hips to lower your legs to the right while turning your face to the left. Again, give yourself a nice stretch, but do not strain or force yourself to go deeper into the pose than you comfortably can. Hold the pose for five breaths, then bring your knees and head back to center. Repeat the pose on the opposite side by dropping your knees to the left while turning your head to the right. Hold the pose for five breaths.

•**Reclining big toe pose.** This is a leg lift that gives a good stretch to the muscles all down the back of the leg. Unless you are very limber, you will need a prop to help you get the most stretch. The prop can be a long belt, 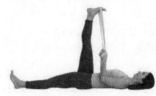 scarf, cord or necktie that you can brace against the arch or ball of your foot and use as a lever to stretch your leg until your foot faces the ceiling. To do this posture, lie on your back, take a deep breath, and, while gently exhaling, bend your right knee to your chest and loop the prop around the arch or ball of the right foot, holding the ends of the prop in both hands. Inhale while straightening your knee so that your right heel is turned toward the ceiling. Guide the prop to comfortably increase the stretch. Hold this pose for a minute or two and then repeat with the other leg.

• **Child's pose.** This restorative yoga pose helps get more blood flowing in the head and can be so deeply relax-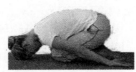ing that when you roll out of it, you may just nod off to sleep like a baby. Begin by kneeling so that you are sitting on your heels, and take a nice, deep, relaxing breath. Bend forward while exhaling and place your forehead on the floor (or on your bed if that's where you are doing the exercise). Place your arms at your sides so that the hands, palms turned up, are near your feet. As you breathe, especially focus on relaxing your back and shoulders. Hold this pose for five to seven long, slow deep breaths.

• **"Stop-action" breathing.** This is an easy and deeply relaxing breathing technique that strengthens the respiratory system. While lying down on your back in bed, exhale completely through the nose. Then inhale a little bit of air—just enough for a count of two or three seconds. Hold that little bit of breath for two or three seconds and, without exhaling, take another two or three seconds of breath, hold, and keep on taking those little sips of air, inhaling and pausing, until your lungs are full as if you've just taken only one big breath instead of a series of small ones. Hold for a second or two. Then slowly exhale in the same manner, exhaling a little bit for two or three seconds, pausing with breath held for two or three seconds and continuing like this until you've completely exhaled air from the lungs. Do four or five rounds of this breathing technique, taking a normal breath between each round of the stop-action breaths.

• **Corpse pose.** If you're not in your bed yet, it's time to crawl into it and get into this pose—you're going to be asleep soon! Lie on your back with your legs stretched out and your arms comfortably at your sides, palms turned up. Slowly inhale and exhale through the nose, feeling your abdomen expand and contract. While you do so, start mentally scanning your body, beginning at your toes and working your way up to the top of your head, assessing whether you are holding tension anywhere. Mentally release muscular tension as you go, allowing your body, inch by inch, to comfortably sink into the surface it is lying on. You may fall asleep in the process or you might simply hold the pose for five breaths and then slowly transition into your favorite sleeping posture to fall asleep.

Fall Asleep Faster

Michael Terman, PhD, head of the Center for Light Treatment and Biological Rhythms at Columbia University Medical Center in New York City. He is founder and president of the New York City–based Center for Environmental Therapeutics. A leading authority on the circadian clock and the role that light plays in regulating it, Dr. Terman is coauthor, with Ian McMahan, PhD, of *Chronotherapy: Resetting Your Inner Clock to Boost Mood, Alertness and Quality Sleep.*

I f you can't fall asleep at a reasonable hour, you might tell yourself that you are a "night owl" or just suffer from insomnia. But turning to sleeping pills, as many insomnia sufferers do, can be a big mistake. These medications may not improve your situation and could even make it worse if you have a type of sleep disorder known as delayed sleep phase disorder (DSPD)—a condition that affects about 10% of people who complain of chronic insomnia.

Even worse: Your situation can be exacerbated by the shorter days and later sunrises of winter.

Could you have DSPD? How to find out—and what to do about it…

WHY CAN'T YOU
GET TO SLEEP?

People who have DSPD find it hard to fall asleep before 2 am or sometimes even later. With this disorder, the sufferer's circadian rhythm, or internal sleep clock, is shifted later at night and, as a result, he/she awakens later in the morning. If you have DSPD, you might, for example, naturally fall asleep at 2 am and feel ready to get up about 10 am.

The problem is, most people need to get up at around 7 am or so to get to work or start their daily activities. If you drag yourself out of bed in order to meet a typical daily schedule, you will then have to deal with the fatigue, grogginess and irritability that can occur when you do not get enough sleep.

While most cases of DSPD are due to a circadian rhythm disorder, symptoms of insomnia also could be due to other causes, such as depression, anxiety disorders, neurological impairments (including dementia) or even certain drugs such as the beta-blockers commonly used for high blood pressure.

Important: Talk to your doctor about your sleep symptoms so that he/she can confirm that they are due to problems with your circadian rhythm. You may be advised to consult a sleep specialist.* If you are diagnosed with DSPD, chronotherapy, which aims to reset your body's biological rhythms, usually improves symptoms within a week.

A SECRET THAT
REALLY WORKS

Your body's inner clock expects sleep to begin at a certain time, which varies from person to person. About two hours before that time, the clock signals the pineal gland, a small, pinecone-shaped gland located near the center of the brain, to begin releasing small amounts of the "sleep hormone" melatonin. For the average sleeper, melatonin levels start to rise about 9 pm to prepare the body to fall asleep around 11 pm. The melatonin itself is not putting you to sleep the way sleeping pills do—rather it is

*To find a sleep specialist, consult the American Academy of Sleep Medicine, AASMnet.org.

signaling the sleep centers in the brain, via the inner clock, that nighttime is beginning.

While using a melatonin supplement, sold over-the-counter in drugstores, might seem like an obvious aid to help you fall asleep earlier, most people take it right before sleep, which overwhelms the body with excessive levels of the hormone. This can lead to side effects such as difficulty awakening, fatigue and even a feeling of sadness the next day.

However, melatonin can be used very successfully to synchronize one's circadian rhythms and shift the body clock earlier so that the urge to sleep occurs earlier. The secret is to take tiny amounts of the hormone—no more than what the pineal gland releases naturally. The other crucial point is to take the melatonin well before the inner clock typically signals the pineal gland to release melatonin.

Important study: At the Center for Light Treatment and Biological Rhythms at Columbia University Medical Center in New York City, researchers developed and tested a controlled-release melatonin tablet that allows a fine stream of melatonin to be absorbed over hours. In research volunteers, the microdose tablet (0.2 mg) produced blood levels of melatonin that were in the same range as those produced naturally by the pineal gland.

What's more, the melatonin from the tablet was washed out of the blood by the morning, mimicking the body's normal removal of pineal melatonin. In contrast, when the volunteers took a higher-dose tablet, melatonin was still lingering in the blood the next day, which can counteract the desired effect and actually shift the inner clock even later.

What to do: Until the microdose tablet is commercially available, DSPD sufferers can try using a 1-mg tablet cut into quarters with a pill cutter—one-quarter of the tablet should be taken six hours before your "natural bedtime" (driven by your natural circadian sleep–wake cycle).

Caution: A 1-mg tablet cut into quarters is not a precise dose, and some people may experience grogginess in the early evening.

To determine your natural bedtime: Take the quiz at CET.org, the website of the Center for Environmental Therapeutics (CET), a nonprofit organization that educates the public and professionals on sleep disorders. Click on: "Education"…"Resource Centers"…"Your Circadian Rhythm Type." Once you determine your natural bedtime, count back six hours and take the melatonin tablet at that time.

DON'T FORGET TO DIM THE LIGHTS

Exposure to bright indoor or outdoor lights suppresses melatonin levels. *What to do…*

•**Use low-level "soft white" bulbs**—they are easy on the eyes and produce minimal glare.

•**Dim computer and TV screens to the lowest comfortable level at least two hours before bedtime.**

•**Wear "blue-blocking" protective glasses if you must be in bright light after taking your evening melatonin.** The filter on the lenses screens out the blue rays from computer and TV screens and bright lights. Unlike sunglasses, blue-blocking glasses enhance night vision. These glasses (on the CET website for about $80) can fit over prescription glasses.

Once you start taking melatonin and dimming the lights in the evening, DSPD should improve within one week (some people improve the first night). Be sure not to get into bed until you start feeling sleepy, which will likely be earlier than usual. If you get into bed before the urge to sleep kicks in, you can worsen insomnia. As your sleep-onset time becomes earlier, be sure to gradually move up the time you take the melatonin so that it continues to be six hours before you are ready for sleep.

If you stop chronotherapy and return to a later sleep pattern, the problem should subside when you resume the melatonin regimen. Some people will need to take melatonin indefinitely—this is fine.

Don't Let Your Bed Partner Ruin Your Sleep—Simple Solutions for the Most Common Problems

Jeffry H. Larson, PhD, licensed marriage and family therapist for more than 25 years and a professor of marriage and family therapy at the College of Family, Home and Social Sciences at Brigham Young University in Provo, Utah. He is author of *Should We Stay Together? A Scientifically Proven Method for Evaluating Your Relationship and Improving Its Chances for Long-Term Success.*

Sooner or later, one in every four American couples ends up sleeping in separate beds. Maybe it's your spouse's tossing and turning or TV watching in bed. Whatever the reason, it may seem easier just to turn that spare bedroom into a nighttime sanctuary of your own. But is that arrangement healthy?

New thinking: Even with the challenges that can come with sharing a bed, the net effect is usually positive for your health. While the exact mechanism is unknown, scientists believe that sleeping with a bed partner curbs levels of the stress hormone cortisol and inflammation-promoting proteins known as cytokines…while boosting levels of the so-called "love" hormone oxytocin.

Sleeping in the same bed also cultivates feelings of intimacy and security, which can strengthen a relationship and promote better sleep—factors linked to living a longer life. *Here, six common challenges and how to overcome them…*

•**You like to keep the room dark, while your partner prefers it light.** Sleep experts recommend keeping the room dark to help stimulate the production of the naturally occurring sleep hormone melatonin.

My advice: Room-darkening shades or light-blocking curtains help create the darkness we need for a good night's rest. But if your partner insists on having some light in the room, consider placing a dim night-light near his/her side of the bed. The person who prefers darkness may want to wear a sleep mask.

• **You're always cold, but your bed partner is too warm.** Sleep experts agree that a cooler room is generally more conducive to sleep and complements the natural temperature drop that occurs in the body when you go to sleep.

My advice: Optimal room temperature for the best sleep varies from person to person—most insomnia experts recommend a range of 60°F to 68°F. To help achieve your personal comfort level, use separate blankets so you can easily cover yourself or remove the blanket during the night without disturbing your bed partner. If you like to use an electric blanket during the winter, choose one with separate temperature controls.

• **You're a night owl, but your partner is a lark.** If the two bed partners prefer different bedtimes, this can cause both of them to lose sleep and can be a major contributor to marital strife. In a study involving 150 couples, which I conducted with several colleagues at Brigham Young University, the University of Nebraska–Lincoln and Montana State University, those who had mismatched body clocks argued more, spent less time doing shared activities and had slightly less sex.

The first step in trying to resolve conflicting bedtimes is to understand that one's circadian rhythm, the internal body clock that regulates sleep and wakefulness as well as other biological processes, dictates whether you are a natural early riser or a night owl. One's particular circadian rhythm is determined by genetics but can be influenced by sunlight, time zone changes and work schedules. Bedtime tendencies also can be socially learned.

My advice: Have a conversation with your partner. Avoid blaming the other party for having a different sleep schedule—we can't control our circadian rhythms or such factors as work schedules. Then, like everything else in a partnership, you'll need to compromise.

For instance, say your partner likes to go to bed at 10 pm and get up at 6 am, while you're rarely in bed before 1 am and sleep until 10 am. As a compromise, you might agree to get in bed with your partner at 9:30 pm to talk, snuggle, relax, read together, etc. Then, when your partner is ready to go to sleep, you can

get up and continue with your night. Alternatively, you and your partner could agree to go to bed at the same time two or three nights a week. A night owl could also lie in bed and listen to music or an audiobook with headphones while his partner sleeps.

• **Your bed partner wants to watch TV, but you want peace and quiet.** Watching TV—or looking at any illuminated screen, such as a laptop or smartphone—promotes wakefulness and can interfere with sleep. So it's not really something anyone should do just before lights out. However, if one partner wants to watch TV or use a laptop before bed, he should do it in another room.

• **Your partner thrashes all night long.** Some individuals are naturally restless sleepers, tossing and turning throughout the night. Others may have restless legs syndrome (RLS) and/or periodic limb movement disorder (PLMD)—two related but distinct conditions.

RLS causes unpleasant sensations, such as tingling and burning, in the legs and an overwhelming urge to move them when the sufferer is sitting or attempting to sleep. PLMD causes involuntary movements and jerking of the limbs during sleep—the legs are most often affected but arm movements also can occur.

With RLS, the sufferer is aware of the problem. Individuals with PLMD, on the other hand, frequently are not aware that they move so much.

My advice: To help ease symptoms, you may want to try natural strategies such as taking warm baths, walking regularly and/or using magnesium supplements, which also promote sleep. But be sure to check with a doctor. If you have RLS or PLMD, it could signal an underlying health condition, such as iron deficiency.

If symptoms persist, you may want to talk to your doctor about medications such as *ropinirole* (Requip) and *pramipexole* (Mirapex), which can help relieve symptoms. Side effects may include nausea and drowsiness.

• **Your partner snores a lot—and loudly.** This is not only a nuisance, it also makes it hard for you to sleep.

My advice: In some cases, running a fan, listening to music through earbuds or using a white-noise machine can help.

If the snoring occurs almost every night, however, your partner may need to see an otolaryngologist (ear, nose and throat doctor) to determine whether there's an underlying medical condition.

Loud snoring that is accompanied by periods in which the person's breathing stops for a few seconds and then resumes may indicate sleep apnea, a serious—but treatable—disorder usually caused by a blocked or narrowed airway.

The New Anti-Snoring Workout

Murray Grossan, MD, a board-certified otolaryngologist at Tower Ear, Nose & Throat at Cedars-Sinai Medical Center in Los Angeles. He is also author of *The Whole Person Tinnitus Relief Program* (DrGrossanTinnitus. com) and founder of Hydro Med Inc. Dr. Grossan's Hydro Pulse nasal-sinus irrigator was named *Time* magazine's "Invention of the Year" in 2000.

Snoring can be a nightmare—both for the sufferer and his/her bed partner. But until recently, the treatments have been limited. A snorer might be told to lose weight, for example, wear a mouth guard or a mask (part of a continuous positive airway pressure, or CPAP, system) that delivers a steady stream of air at night…change his sleeping position… or, in severe cases, get surgery.

Recent development: In a 2015 study of 39 men who snored or had mild obstructive sleep apnea (OSA), a common cause of snoring, scientists found that performing mouth and tongue exercises reduced the frequency and intensity of snoring by up to 59%—a reduction on par with other therapies, including mouth guards or surgery.

And while snoring may seem like more of an annoyance than a health problem, that is simply not true. Snoring has been linked to medical conditions, including heart attack, stroke and glaucoma. *How mouth and tongue exercises can help…*

SIT-UPS FOR YOUR THROAT

If your bed partner has complained of your snoring or you have unexplained daytime sleepiness, consider trying the following exercises.

About half of my patients improve enough after doing these exercises (think of them as "throat sit-ups") for five minutes three times a day for six weeks to avoid surgery or other inconvenient therapies such as wearing a mouth guard or using CPAP. They also awaken feeling more refreshed and reduce their odds of developing OSA.

Here are the main exercises included in the recent study mentioned above (led by Geraldo Lorenzi-Filho, MD, PhD)—along with some slight variations that I have found to be effective for my patients. The tongue positions for these exercises strengthen your tongue muscle and the sides of your throat. However, my variations give these muscles a more rigorous strength-training workout.

- **Tongue Push.**

What to do: Push the tip of your tongue forcefully behind your upper front teeth and move it all the way back along the roof of your mouth (palate) 20 times.

My variation: Say the vowel sounds "A, E, I, O, U" while doing the exercise.

- **Flat Tongue Press.**

What to do: Suck your tongue up against the roof of your mouth, pressing the entire tongue against your palate 20 times.

My variation: Repeat "A, E, I, O, U" while doing the exercise.

- **Say "Ahhh."**

What to do: Focus on raising the back of the roof of the mouth and uvula (the fleshy appendage in the throat that's responsible for the rattling sound made by snorers) 20 times.

My variation: Say the vowel "A" (or "Ahhh") while doing the exercise.

THESE THERAPIES HELP, TOO

Colds, allergies and sinus infections can cause nasal congestion and/or postnasal drip—two common conditions that can make your throat swell, increasing your risk for snoring. *What helps...*

•**Nasal lavage** (using a saline solution to irrigate and cleanse the nasal cavity) helps clear nasal congestion and postnasal drip. Subjects in the study mentioned above performed nasal lavage three times a day. Based on my clinical experience, once a day does the job.

A product that I created called The Hydro Pulse Sinus System ($89.99, HydroMedOnline. com) works well. It includes a special throat attachment that directs pulsating irrigation to the tonsils and throat to ease swelling. But you could also use a neti pot (*typical cost*: $10)—just be sure to keep it clean and sanitized between uses and use distilled or sterile water to prevent a sinus infection. Or you can buy sterile squeeze bottles filled with nasal saline.

•**Nose taping.** With age, the tip of one's nose naturally begins to droop some. This can obstruct the nasal valve, which impedes breathing and contributes to snoring.

Try this simple test: Use your finger to press the tip of your nose up. If breathing feels easier when you do this, try taping your nose up before bedtime.

What to do: Cut a three-inch strip of one-half-inch medical grade tape. Place it under the nose at the center, without blocking the airway. Gently lift the nose as you run the tape up the midline of the nose to the area between the eyes. The taping should be comfortable and is for use during sleep.

Important: Commercial nasal strips, such as Breathe Right, spread the sides of the nose apart. Taping up the nose, as described above, also does this, with the additional advantage of opening the nasal valve.

Saline Spray Solution for Snoring

Murray Grossan, MD, a board-certified otolaryngologist and head and neck surgeon with Tower Ear, Nose & Throat at Cedars-Sinai Medical Center in Los Angeles, and author of *Free Yourself from Sinus and Allergy Problems—Permanently*. Grossan.com

D oes your partner complain that your snoring keeps him awake at night...or do his raucous snores rob you of needed rest? Snorers' partners really do suffer—for instance, if we wind up sleep-deprived, our risk for accidents rises.

To the rescue: Simple saline.

Sometimes snoring signals sleep apnea, a breathing disorder that should be checked by a doctor. But in many cases, snoring is simply the result of nasal congestion, according to otolaryngologist Murray Grossan, MD, author of *Free Yourself from Sinus and Allergy Problems—Permanently*. Allergies or an infection such as a cold can trigger swelling of the inner lining of the nose, which causes a vibration of the soft palate that creates the snoring sound. Using a saline nasal spray at bedtime moisturizes the nasal passages and reduces inflammation, in turn helping to quiet the snores. But commercial saline sprays often contain preservatives that some people are sensitive to, so they can actually increase congestion. That's why Dr. Grossan recommended using a homemade solution instead.

What to do: You need one-quarter teaspoon of salt—preferably kosher or canning salt, which are free of the anti-drying agents some people are sensitive to. Stir the salt into one-half cup of water (for safety, use distilled or boiled water) until it dissolves. Pour the mixture into an empty nasal spray bottle (I found one online for $1.50 plus shipping at http://bit.ly/J1W4TN). Each night at bedtime, spray two or three squirts into each nostril. Use or discard homemade saline within five days.

Option: Take a quick hot shower after using the spray, Dr. Grossan suggested. The steam will further moisturize nasal passages...

increasing the odds for blissfully quiet, snore-free slumber.

Don't Ignore Sleep Apnea

Ralph Downey III, PhD, adjunct associate clinical professor of medicine and past chief, sleep medicine, Loma Linda University Medical Center, Loma Linda University Children's Hospital.

D octors have long known that obstructive sleep apnea (repeated interruptions in breathing during sleep) can harm the overall health of men and women who suffer from the condition.

Now: Recent research shows that sleep apnea is even more dangerous than experts had previously realized, increasing the sufferer's risk for heart attack, stroke, diabetes and fatal car crashes.

What you need to know…

NO ROOM TO BREATHE

Sleep apnea occurs about twice as often in men as in women, but it is overlooked more often in women. An estimated 70% of people with sleep apnea are overweight. Fat deposited around the neck (men with sleep apnea often wear a size 17 or larger collar, while women with the disorder often have a neck circumference of 16 inches or more) compresses the upper airway, reducing air flow and causing the passage to narrow or close. Your brain senses this inability to breathe and briefly awakens you so that you can reopen the airway.

The exact cause of obstructive sleep apnea in people of normal weight is unknown, but it may involve various anatomical characteristics, such as having a narrow throat and upper airway.

RED FLAG 1: **About half of all people who snore loudly have sleep apnea.** One telling sign is a gasping, choking kind of snore, during which the sleeper seems to stop breathing. (If you live alone and don't know whether you snore, ask your doctor about recording yourself while you are sleeping to check for snoring and other signs of sleep apnea.)

RED FLAG 2: **Daytime sleepiness is the other most common symptom.** Less common symptoms include headache, sore throat and/or dry mouth in the morning, sexual dysfunction and memory problems.

DANGERS OF SLEEP APNEA

New scientific evidence shows that sleep apnea increases risk for…

•**Cardiovascular disease.** Sleep apnea's repeated episodes of interrupted breathing—and the accompanying drop in oxygen levels—takes a toll on the heart and arteries.

Recent finding: Heart attack risk in sleep apnea sufferers is 30% higher than normal over a four- to five-year period, and stroke risk is twice as high in people with sleep apnea.

•**Diabetes.** Sleep apnea (regardless of the sufferer's weight) is linked to increased insulin resistance—a potentially dangerous condition in which the body is resistant to the effects of insulin.

Recent finding: A Yale study of 593 patients found that over a six-year period, people diagnosed with sleep apnea were more than two-and-a-half times more likely to develop diabetes than those without the sleep disorder.

•**Accidents.** Sleep apnea dramatically increases the risk for a deadly mishap due to sleepiness and impaired alertness.

Recent finding: A study of 1,600 people, presented at an American Thoracic Society meeting, found that the 800 sleep apnea sufferers were twice as likely to have a car crash over a three-year period. Surprisingly, those who were unaware of being sleepy were just as likely to crash as those who were aware of being sleepy.

DO YOU HAVE SLEEP APNEA?

If you think you may have sleep apnea, see a specialist at an accredited sleep center, where a thorough medical history will be taken and you may be asked to undergo a sleep study. This involves spending the night in a sleep laboratory where your breathing, oxygen level, movements and brain wave activity are measured while you sleep.

BEST TREATMENT OPTIONS

The treatment typically prescribed first for sleep apnea is continuous positive airway pressure (CPAP). A stream of air is pumped onto the back of the throat during sleep to keep the airway open. The air is supplied through a mask, most often worn over the nose, which is connected by tubing to a small box that contains a fan.

In recent years, a larger variety of masks have become available, and fan units have become smaller and nearly silent. A number of adjustments may be needed, which may require trying several different devices and more than one visit to a sleep lab.

Other treatments for sleep apnea are usually prescribed to make CPAP more effective, or for people with milder degrees of the disorder who have tried CPAP but were unable or unwilling to use it.

These treatments include…

• **Mouthpieces.** Generally fitted by a dentist and worn at night, these oral appliances adjust the lower jaw and tongue to help keep the airway open.

• **Surgery.** This may be recommended for people who have an anatomical abnormality that narrows the airway and for whom CPAP doesn't work. The most common operation for sleep apnea is uvulopalatopharyngoplasty (UPPP), in which excess tissue is removed from the back of the throat. It works about 50% of the time.

HELPING YOURSELF

Several measures can make sleep apnea treatment more effective and, in some cases, eliminate the condition altogether. *What to do…*

• **Lose weight, if you are overweight.** For every 10% of body weight lost, the number of apnea episodes drops by 25%.

• **Change your sleep position.** Sleeping on your side—rather than on your back—typically means fewer apnea episodes. Sleeping on your stomach is even better. Some obese people who have sleep apnea do best if they sleep while sitting up.

• **Avoid alcohol.** It relaxes the muscles around the airway, aggravating sleep apnea.

• **Use medication carefully.** Sleep medications can worsen sleep apnea by making it harder for your body to rouse itself when breathing stops. If you have sleep apnea, make sure a doctor oversees your use of sleep medications (including over-the-counter drugs).

Hidden Brain Dangers of Sleep Apnea…Especially for Women

Paul M. Macey, PhD, assistant professor in residence, associate dean for information technology and innovation, School of Nursing, University of California, Los Angeles. His study was published in *PLoS ONE*.

You probably know that obstructive sleep apnea causes people to gasp, snort and snore as their sleep is interrupted by repeated stops and starts in their breathing. And you know that these mini-suffocations, which can occur dozens of times each hour, increase the risk for all kinds of serious health problems.

But you probably don't know that sleep apnea causes permanent changes to the structure of the brain and how the brain controls blood pressure. These changes create a vicious cycle that leaves apnea patients starved for oxygen not only at night, but also during the day—particularly at times when their bodies are most in need of oxygen!

Though sleep apnea often is thought of as a "man's problem," women develop it, too… and women are at especially high risk for the dangerous nervous system changes, a recent study reveals. *Male or female, if you (or a loved one) have or may have sleep apnea, you need to know about this research…*

AUTONOMIC GLITCH

Participants in the recent study included male and female patients who recently had been diagnosed with sleep apnea and were not receiving treatment, plus some healthy "controls" (people without sleep apnea who served as a basis of comparison).

The point of the experiment was to see how people's bodies respond to various physical "challenges" that use different nervous system pathways to signal increased cardiovascular demand. These challenges mimic day-to-day activities, such as straining, lifting and touching something cold. Normally such challenges, like many everyday activities, cause heart rate to speed up. This is a protective response of the autonomic regulatory system (the part of the central nervous system that regulates heart rate, blood pressure, breathing, etc. without you having to think about it), sending extra blood and oxygen to cells that are in greater need.

The challenges in the experiment included a hand-grip task (squeezing an inflatable bag with one hand as hard as possible for 16 seconds)…keeping a foot in icy water for one minute…and breathing out hard with the mouth closed and nose pinched shut (similar to what happens when a person is straining over a bowel movement).

Results: For all three challenges, compared with the healthy controls, the sleep apnea patients showed an impaired response—meaning that they had heart rate increases that were less pronounced and slower to kick in.

Also, in comparing male sleep apnea patients with female sleep apnea patients, the researchers found that the degree of impairment was worse in women. Take the bag-squeezing test, for example. The heart rate of women with apnea increased just 3.3% and returned to normal very quickly, whereas in healthy women, heart rate increased 5.8% and remained elevated significantly longer. For men, however, the differences between those with and without apnea were much less pronounced. Heart rate increased 7.4% in apnea patients, compared with 8.6% in healthy men…and there was only a small difference in how long it remained elevated in the two male groups.

Why such an impaired response is dangerous: An impaired response means that tissues, including sensitive brain cells, are being starved of oxygen because blood flow is inad-equate. Obviously, sleep apnea patients are oxygen-deprived whenever they stop breathing during sleep—but this study shows that people with sleep apnea also often are deprived of oxygen when they are awake and during daily physical tasks, when oxygen is needed most. That's because their nervous systems don't do a good job of increasing heart rate as needed to meet demands at times when the body is physiologically challenged.

What's more, this impaired response creates a vicious cycle—impaired blood flow leads to structural changes in the brain and cardiovascular system, which leads to further impaired blood flow—and so on. The worse this gets, the greater the risk may be for heart disease, high blood pressure and other chronic illnesses associated with autonomic dysfunction, the study researchers noted. While both male and female sleep apnea patients are at risk, the dangers for women may be particularly high, given their greater magnitude of autonomic response impairment and the fact that they are less likely to be properly diagnosed in the first place.

Self-defense for women and men: Sleep apnea affects an estimated 28 million adults in the US, more than 80% of whom do not realize that they have the disorder. If you have been told that you snore, gasp or grunt as you sleep, or if you often feel groggy during the day even after a full night's rest, ask your doctor about being tested for sleep apnea. Early detection and treatment can help protect against damage to the brain, cardiovascular system and other organs…and allow you to sleep better and feel better, too.

Sleep Device Bonus

When a person with sleep apnea begins treatment with a continuous positive airway pressure (CPAP) device, which forces air into the lungs during sleep, the person's resistance to insulin (a hallmark of diabetes) improves dramatically.

If you have sleep apnea: Treatment with a CPAP device may not only improve your sleep but also help lower diabetes risk.

Imran H. Iftikhar, MD, assistant professor of internal medicine, University of South Carolina, Columbia.

How to Finally Fix Your Sleep Apnea

Michael Breus, PhD, a sleep specialist in private practice in Scottsdale, Arizona, and author of *Good Night: The Sleep Doctor's 4-Week Program to Better Sleep and Better Health*. He is a Diplomate of the American Board of Sleep Medicine and a Fellow of the American Academy of Sleep Medicine.

I f you've got obstructive sleep apnea (OSA)—that well-known sleep disorder marked by snoring and gasping—you've no doubt been told that it's a serious condition. It can lead to high blood pressure, heart disease and stroke, along with severe fatigue and night after night of disrupted sleep.

In case that all sounds pretty frightening, don't lose hope. OSA can be virtually eliminated with a nondrug treatment. The problem is, about half of all patients stop using the treatment within the first year. Some last only a few nights.

Why do so many people give up on a treatment that works so well? Because they hate it!

However, there are ways to make "CPAP"—the nickname of this treatment—much more tolerable so that you can finally get the pleasant sleep you need and deserve.

Here's how to make CPAP a much better experience…

TREATMENT THAT WORKS

The gold standard treatment for sleep apnea is continuous positive airway pressure (CPAP). With this therapy, a machine about the size of a shoe box delivers a constant flow of air that opens your airways and improves your breathing.

Unfortunately, CPAP machine users are tethered to the machine all night, and some of these machines are noisy. You also have to wear a mask over your mouth and/or nose, which makes some people claustrophobic. And the flow of air can cause uncomfortable mouth/nose dryness and eye irritation.

Startling study: Only 46% of patients prescribed CPAP used the devices for more than four hours a night on 70% of all nights—the threshold for effective treatment.

Because proper use of CPAP can reduce health risks associated with sleep apnea to close to zero, this is not a treatment that you want to give up if you have this condition.

MAKING PEACE WITH CPAP

If you're prescribed CPAP therapy, you may want to start out with a basic machine just to see how well you respond. Ask your respiratory therapist about renting a machine to try it out first. This device might do a good job of improving your symptoms, and the purchase price is usually $500 or less, compared with pricier, more sophisticated units (see below).

But what if you find the machine to be so uncomfortable that you stop using it? You have a lot of options. A sleep specialist or respiratory therapist can help you sort them out. CPAP machines are usually covered by insurance. *Where to start…*

•**Different masks.** A full-face style that covers the mouth and nose provides a good fit and is more likely than other masks to stay put during the night. A total face mask extends all the way from the forehead to the chin. But you'll look like Darth Vader and might, ironically, feel like you're suffocating.

You may prefer a nasal "pillow," an under-the-nose mask with nostril tubes that's less obtrusive and won't obscure your vision if you like to read before falling asleep.

A nasal mask that fits only over the nose is yet another choice. It's more likely than the nasal pillow to stay in place. Many people find this more comfortable than a full-face configuration. Prices for the masks described above generally range from $40 to $200 (in addition to the cost of a CPAP machine).

•**A "ramp" feature.** Most CPAP machines, starting at around $500, have a feature that gradually ramps up air pressure so that the full force won't be felt right away. The machine can be programmed to automatically raise pressure every five minutes or so until the prescribed amount is reached—and you have fallen asleep.

•**Heated humidification.** This is now a standard feature on many units. Everyone who uses CPAP occasionally suffers from nose or mouth dryness. The humidity added by certain machines reduces this effect and makes you more comfortable. You need to fill and clean a water tank with these models. They are available at all price levels, from less than $500 to more than $1,500.

Also helpful: A squirt of saline solution into each nostril before you put on any CPAP mask. Doing this will help prevent dryness and nighttime congestion.

•**Bilevel PAP.** Unlike the continuous pressure in some machines, bilevel PAP (also known as BiPAP) units match the airflow to your breathing. They increase pressure during inhalations—when apneas (breathing cessations) usually occur—and decrease it when you exhale. Research has shown that people with bilevel PAP machines are more likely to keep using them than those with non-bilevel PAP units. Prices start at about $600.

•**AutoPAP.** These machines are a bit different from bilevel PAP machines because they automatically change air pressure on a breath-by-breath basis. When you sleep on your back, for example, you will naturally tend to have more apneas. The machine will detect breathing changes and make the necessary adjustments in air pressure. Prices start at around $400.

"NO MORE CPAP!"

Some people never get comfortable using CPAP of any kind. For these individuals—especially if they have milder OSA—other options include…

•**Oral appliance.** This custom-made mouthpiece helps keep the airway open and is especially effective for people who sleep on their backs. The $1,800 to $2,000 cost may be covered by insurance.

•**Nasal valves.** When you go to bed, you apply a small, Band-Aid–like strip over each nasal opening. The strips have nasal plugs with small valves. The valves open when you inhale, then partially close when you breathe out. This creates expiratory positive airway pressure that helps keep the airways open.

Example: Provent Sleep Apnea Therapy. This FDA-approved sleep apnea treatment requires a prescription and costs about $60 a month, which might not be covered by insurance. It may not be suitable for people with chronic health conditions such as heart disease.

•**Winx Sleep Therapy System.** This consists of a small, flexible mouthpiece and a plastic line that connects to a console. This system creates oral airway pressure, similar to CPAP units. But it doesn't require a mask and is more tolerable for some people. It costs about $700. Some insurers may cover it. It should not be used by anyone with a severe respiratory disorder, loose teeth or periodontal disease.

Better Sleep Apnea Alternative

A customized oral appliance that moves the jawbone slightly forward during sleep helps keep the airway open and may work better for some adults who cannot tolerate a continuous positive airway pressure (CPAP) mask and machine.

Recent finding: Nearly 100 adults with mild-to-moderate sleep apnea who wore this type of mouth guard nightly showed improvement in sleep apnea and snoring.

If you've been diagnosed with sleep apnea: Ask your doctor whether an oral appliance would be appropriate. If so, a dentist can custom-fit one. Most devices cost about $2,000 and may be covered by insurance.

Karl Franklin, MD, senior lecturer, Umea University, Sweden.

CPAP Heals Brain Damage Caused by Sleep Apnea

Study titled "White Matter Integrity in Obstructive Sleep Apnea Before and After Treatment," published in *Sleep*.

If you suffer from obstructive sleep apnea, you may be among the very many people who would rather endure it and its health consequences, such as heart disease, than use a noisy and uncomfortable continuous positive airway pressure (CPAP) machine while you sleep. About 25% of people with sleep apnea refuse to use CPAP. And of those who do use it, only 30% to 60% use their machines enough to be considered adherent (that is, cooperative about therapy) by their doctors. And adherent, as far as CPAP goes, is use for at least four hours a night for at least seven out of every 10 nights.

But now, the time for "blowing off" your CPAP machine has truly passed, because the results of a recent study show something chilling: People who don't consistently use their CPAP machines are damaging their brains. That's right—if you don't use CPAP enough, it could be costing you your ability to think and your memory.

Here's why that happens...and how you can recover your lost brain function...

DIRE EFFECT OF SLEEP APNEA

The study was small but well-designed. It included 32 men who were in the prime of life (average age 43). Seventeen of them had severe sleep apnea but had never used CPAP...and 15 were healthy men who acted as controls. The researchers used MRI scans to study participants' brains and, in particular, their white matter, which is the part of the brain that conducts nerve impulses and basically allows the different parts of the brain to communicate with each other. The men also took neuropsychological tests to evaluate their attention, reasoning, reaction times and long- and short-term memory.

The results, to put it mildly, were not good for the patients with sleep apnea. Neuropsychological tests taken before CPAP treatment began showed that the men with sleep apnea were simply not as sharp as the other men. Their thinking and reasoning were significantly slower and less accurate than the controls, and their short- and long-term memories were not as good. And the brain scans showed that the patients' white matter was not intact—in other words, neural connections weren't, in fact, connecting as efficiently as they should.

They had decided to delay treatment of their sleep apnea—and now their brains were disintegrating. But there was good news, too.

REGAIN YOUR BRAIN

Saving grace: In tracking the men's functioning over time, researchers discovered that CPAP can reverse the damage to the brain's white matter caused by sleep apnea. In fact, new white-matter connectedness began to be seen after only three months of regular CPAP use. After 12 months of use, a near complete reversal of white-matter damage in all of the affected parts of the brain was seen. This improvement in brain structure was reflected with improvement in memory, attention and other cognitive functions. In fact, scores on a series of neurocognitive tests matched nearly all the scores of the healthy controls. In short, CPAP virtually reversed brain damage caused by untreated sleep apnea.

In an earlier study, the same researchers found the same sort of results when they looked at how CPAP affected the brain's gray matter. Gray matter controls muscle function and the senses.

Bottom line: If left untreated, sleep apnea can wreck your brain. CPAP therapy is very effective and can save your brain—but only if you use it. Alternatives such as an implantable device and wearable devices that force you to change sleep positions when you roll over onto your back (which can set off sleep apnea) are alternatives that do not work as well as CPAP but are better than no treatment at all. Also, new CPAP designs that are more comfortable and quieter are becoming available. Your doctor can also adjust the CPAP machine that you already have to make sure it fits comfortably. So, no more excuses...save your heart and your brain by doing what you can to manage your sleep apnea.

$50 Fix Reduces Sleep Apnea by 36%

Stefania Redolfi, MD, university researcher, Respiratory Medicine Department, University of Brescia, Italy.

Would you rather wear a strange-looking and uncomfortable mask while you sleep…or tight stockings during the day?

The obvious answer is "um, neither"…but it is entirely possible that people who have a certain type of chronic obstructive sleep apnea may be presented with exactly this choice, based on recent European research. A study published in the American Thoracic Society's *American Journal of Respiratory and Critical Care Medicine* reports that wearing compression stockings can reduce sleep apnea episodes significantly for one-third of the people whose apnea is caused by chronic venous insufficiency—a pretty dramatic difference for such an easy treatment. Since it was a small, brief and preliminary study focused on just this one cause of obstructive sleep apnea, it's entirely possible that longer treatment may yield even more impressive results that are helpful to even more patients.

OUT FROM BEHIND THE MASK

If you have ever seen a continuous positive airway pressure (CPAP) mask, but—even though the designers have done their best and there now are quite a few different models to choose from—there's not a single one that is truly comfortable. They are bulky and uncomfortable on the face and force many wearers to sleep in positions they'd rather not sleep in. Many people who need them refuse to wear them. That's why the news that there is a safe, easy-to-use and inexpensive treatment option for a good portion of people with sleep apnea is quite welcome!

Stefania Redolfi, MD, of the University of Brescia in Italy, lead researcher of this practical and surprisingly promising study, explained that chronic venous insufficiency is a vascular problem in which veins (primarily in the legs) can't efficiently pump blood back to the heart. Fluid builds up in the legs during the day and then shifts at night to the neck, bloating tissue there. This causes the person to experience the partial collapse of the pharynx in between breaths during sleep—and so begins the loud, unpleasant "gasp and snore" pattern that characterizes obstructive sleep apnea in these patients.

What does wearing tight stockings during the day have to do with insufficient oxygen at night? It is actually quite ingenious. "Wearing compression stockings during the day helps to reduce the daytime fluid accumulation in the legs," Dr. Redolfi explained, "which in turn reduces the amount of fluid flowing into the neck at night." Absent the pressure created by that fluid, the respiratory system does not narrow as much and, for many people, this intervention is enough to allow them to get adequate oxygen into their lungs by breathing—and sleeping—normally. This is a wonderful thing, because sleep apnea and the constantly interrupted sleep that goes with it can severely undermine a person's health.

WHAT THE RIGHT SOCKS CAN DO

The study was small, involving 12 patients—half randomly assigned to wear compression stockings during the day (putting them on as soon as they awakened and taking them off only after getting into bed for the night) for a week, while the other half served as the control, with the two groups switching places after the first week. Subjects spent their nights at a sleep center, where their physiological signs (including brain waves, respiration and eye movements) were measured continuously. Researchers also measured each person's overnight changes in leg fluid volume and neck circumference at the start of the study and at the end of both the compression-stocking and control periods.

Dr. Redolfi said that the researchers expected the compression stockings would help—but they were somewhat surprised by the degree to which they helped! *Wearing the stockings resulted in…*

• **An average of a 62% reduction in overnight leg fluid volume change,** as compared with when subjects did not wear the stockings.

• **A 60% reduction in neck circumference increase** (used as a proxy measurement to estimate fluid shift into the neck).

• **A 36% reduction in the number of apnea episodes.**

EFFECTIVE AND INEXPENSIVE

This is a very basic intervention that has the potential to make a big difference for patients who are struggling with obstructive sleep apnea. The stockings cost less than $50 and, though they aren't exactly cute or comfortable, Dr. Redolfi said that all the study participants preferred them to the CPAP mask. As simple as it sounds, though, she said that people with sleep apnea shouldn't try this on their own—she said it is important to have a sleep study done to measure whether the stockings are making a difference and if so, how much. Talk to your doctor about this. Dr. Redolfi plans further research to ascertain whether wearing the stockings for longer than a week shows more significant results…to learn whether other measures, such as using diuretics or exercises to reduce fluid volume, are useful… and also to examine whether wearing compression stockings can help people with sleep apnea due to other causes, such as obesity.

Alternative Treatment for Sleep Apnea

Inspire Therapy is a new type of pacemaker implanted in the chest that delivers electrical impulses to the nerve that controls the tongue and improves function of the upper airway. In recent tests, it was found to reduce nightly sleep apnea severity by 68%. Inspire Therapy was approved by the FDA in 2014.

Ryan J. Soose, MD, assistant professor of otolaryngology at University of Pittsburgh Medical Center. He is author of a study published in The New England Journal of Medicine.

The Buzz About Positional Therapy for Sleep Apnea

Lawrence J. Epstein, MD, program director of the Sleep Medicine Fellowship Program and associate physician, division of sleep and circadian disorders, departments of medicine and neurology at Brigham & Women's Hospital, and instructor in medicine at Harvard Medical School, all in Boston. Dr. Epstein also is past president of the American Academy of Sleep Medicine.

It happened again—a night's sleep was wrecked by the gasping for air, snoring and snorting caused by obstructive sleep apnea (OSA). The symptoms strike whenever you roll over onto your back, and even though you know a CPAP machine would fix the problem, you just can't get yourself to use one. You might even have a machine gathering dust in a corner of your bedroom.

No worries. If lying on your back really is what sets off your OSA, there is, in fact, a new way to avoid symptoms and get some shut-eye.

DON'T LET SLEEP APNEA GET YOU FLAT ON YOUR BACK

Half of people with OSA generally have symptoms only when they are sleeping on their backs. This is called positional OSA. Until recently, CPAP was the main and doctor-preferred treatment for positional OSA even though simply not sleeping on your back prevents symptoms, too. Studies have shown that, although not quite as effective as CPAP, positional therapy—which offers a variety of techniques to keep a sleeper off his or her back—is adequate to control OSA symptoms in people who won't or can't use a CPAP machine.

Until now, positional therapy has been pretty basic, involving use of low-tech objects such as tennis balls, body pillows or foam belts that discourage or prevent a person from rolling onto his back during sleep. Now, a new approach, called vibro-tactile positional therapy, uses vibration to prevent a person from sleeping on his back. And the device, called Night Shift, does not restrict movement like the older options do.

NO LOST SLEEP

Night Shift is a relatively thin neck collar with a sensor that vibrates when you roll onto your back. The intensity of the vibration increases until you change your sleep position.

Surprisingly, this vibrating gadget will not disrupt sleep and keep you up as much as your OSA will, says Lawrence J. Epstein, MD, an expert in sleep medicine and positional therapy from Harvard Medical School and past president of the American Academy of Sleep Medicine. Although you might be briefly roused to roll over, you usually won't completely awaken, he said. You simply will shift position and fall right back into deeper sleep.

The device also electronically monitors how often you roll onto your back, how long you stay in that position before shifting and how much you snore or have breathing problems during sleep, explained Dr. Epstein. "This information can be downloaded onto a computer and sent to your doctor to determine how effective the device is for you," he said.

According to a small published study sponsored by Advanced Brain Monitoring, Inc. (the makers of Night Shift) and conducted by the inventors of the device, Night Shift reduced sleep apnea by more than half in 83% of the study participants who used the device nightly for four weeks. This had a greatly improved effect on snoring, daytime depression and sleepiness and, most importantly, getting enough oxygen during sleep. At some point though, a larger, independent study will need to confirm Night Shift's effectiveness and also compare it to CPAP. But the bottom line is that using any technique that will help prevent OSA is better than nothing. OSA is a risk factor for cardiovascular problems, such as irregular heartbeat, high blood pressure and heart attack, and eye problems, such as glaucoma—so it is vital to do what you can to prevent it.

HOW TO GET THE DEVICE

Night Shift is available by prescription only, so if you want to try it, speak with your doctor. Dr. Epstein advised that it may be worth your while to see a board-certified sleep specialist rather than your primary care physician to get a prescription for the device. Unlike a primary care doctor, a sleep specialist (a physician with training and board certification in sleep medicine) can ensure that positional therapy is right for you. Such a doctor will also best use the product's technology to closely monitor your response to treatment.

Although Night Shift is not yet widely covered by insurance, at $349, it's about one-third of the price of a CPAP machine.

What You Need to Know About Exploding Head Syndrome

Brian Sharpless, PhD, associate professor of psychopathology at Argosy University Northern Virginia in Arlington.

Imagine lapsing into a peaceful sleep. The transition from wakefulness to slumber will be hardly noticeable but surely inevitable— after all, the night is so quiet, the bedsheets cozy and your bedroom just the right temperature. Consciousness has just about faded to dreamy sleep when suddenly…BOOOOOM!!! An explosion jerks you awake! You jump up in a panic, expecting to be in the midst of a catastrophe, but nothing has changed. Nothing at all. So there you are in bed in the dark and quiet of night wondering what in heck just happened.

Exploding head syndrome (EHS) is a sleep disorder that more people probably experience than experts have imagined, and it can happen once and never again…rarely…or monthly, weekly or even nightly.

Even though medical books say it's rare, Brian Sharpless, PhD, associate professor of psychopathology at Argosy University Northern Virginia in Arlington, has done research on EHS, and here explains what it is...

IS IT DANGEROUS?

EHS generally happens not in the middle of sleep, but either as you're drifting off to sleep or while in the early stages of naturally waking. The hallmark of EHS is hearing a sudden, very loud sound—literally as loud as an explosion—but it doesn't always sound like an explosion. Besides explosions, people describe EHS sounds as slamming doors, gunshots, clashing cymbals, electrical zapping or a loud clunking or popping noise. About 10% of people who have EHS also perceive light flashes or some form of "visual static," or they may feel an electrical sensation flow from their torsos to their heads just before the loud noise strikes.

Despite the disorder's name and the fright it puts into people who experience it, it is not a sign of a physical disease. But if you do have such an experience and have significant head pain when you wake up, this is a clear indication that you're not experiencing EHS but a headache syndrome or possibly something more serious that should be checked out by a doctor.

THE CAUSE IS MYSTERIOUS

Scientists aren't exactly sure what causes EHS, but ordinary stress and emotional tension or just feeling out of sorts on a particular day might set if off. More severe psychological stressors that need to be addressed with a mental health-care professional might be behind EHS in people who experience it very frequently, such as several times a week—or night. Biologically, a glitch or something out of sync might be happening in the reticular formation, the part of the brain that monitors movement, balance, visual and auditory activity and is basically responsible for shutting you "off" so that you can go to sleep.

A lot of things have to happen in your brain and body before you fall asleep. It's kind of like shutting down a computer, and there is a lot of room for things to go wrong Although the reticular formation is responsible for shutting everything down for sleep, our best guess about what happens in EHS—and

there is some disagreement on this among researchers—is that instead of shutting down, the auditory neurons fire all at once. That's why an explosive or otherwise startling noise is "heard" even though no loud noise actually happened around you.

EHS was first described in 1876—yet now, 138 years later, we still don't know how common it is. From reviewing the few scientific reports that have been published, researchers have hypothesized that 10% to 50% of the population will have an EHS episode at least once. Meanwhile, medical books on sleep disorders have traditionally claimed that EHS is rare and that it generally targets people who are age 50 and older. My own research shows that neither of these points is true and has documented EHS in adults of all ages, including college students.

DEALING WITH EXPLODING HEAD SYNDROME

Remember, there's no indication that EHS will harm you, and it is not a sign of disease. At best, it might make an interesting topic for conversation at the next day's breakfast. At worst, it can delay your sleep and lead to troubled sleep if it happens frequently...especially if you're wracked with worry because you don't understand what it is or why it's happening.

There is no standard treatment for people who experience EHS on a regular basis (whether "regular" is a few times a year or a few times a month or week), but a low-dose magnesium supplement taken before bedtime may help. Magnesium is a natural calcium channel blocker, and calcium channel blocker drugs (used to reduce blood pressure and also for migraine relief) have been shown to relieve EHS in case studies of people who had episodes of EHS several times per night.

Besides prescription calcium channel blockers such as *flunarizine* and *nifedipine* (Procardia), the antidepressant *clomipramine* (Anafranil) also has been successfully used to stop EHS in people who have very frequent episodes. My advice for people who do experience EHS frequently is, again, to be reassured that you aren't going crazy or experiencing anything life threatening. Because very frequent EHS episodes may be related to more serious stress-related psychological issues, people who do have very frequent episodes should consider seeing a behavioral sleep medicine specialist (usually a doctor trained in neurology and psychiatry who specializes in sleep disorders), a psychiatrist or a psychologist to deal with the stress and, thereby, alleviate EHS.

Sleep Paralysis—How to Stop This Waking Nightmare

Brian Sharpless, PhD, associate professor of psychopathology at Argosy University Northern Virginia in Arlington. He is author of *Sleep Paralysis: Historical, Psychological, and Medical Perspectives.*

Have you ever had the truly horrific experience of waking up in your own bed and realizing that you are paralyzed? You may have simply found yourself overwhelmed with an eerie sense of foreboding or panic or else experienced a more classic scenario, which goes something like this…

You know that there is an intruder in the room and then the intruder attacks—pressing on and restraining you, suffocating you. You try to scream but you can't utter a sound or move. And the intruder is not even a human being! It's a demon, an outer-space alien or some other monstrous creature! Yet, however surreal this experience is, you are certain, at least for the first few moments in, that you are awake. You may struggle against the paralysis to wake yourself up out of what you realize is a very vivid nightmare. Then, in the midst of the horror and panic, you actually do wake to find yourself quite safe and sound.

About 8% of the general population will experience this phenomenon, called sleep paralysis, at least once, and some will experience it periodically—even several times a week. Some victims also truly believe that sleep paralysis episodes aren't mere nightmares but veritable supernatural or alien attacks. But if you have such recurrent nightmares or know someone

who does, be assured that you are not being attacked and you're not going crazy. And if you ever have such a nightmare for the very first time, this article could help you recognize what is happening and get a handle on it.

NOT THE BOGEYMAN

Sleep paralysis historically has been attributed to supernatural bugaboos—demons, witches and ghosts and, in modern times, space aliens. But rather than being a supernatural or space-age horror, sleep paralysis is a REM-sleep glitch in which certain aspects of REM sleep continue after you have, in part, emerged from sleep. In this state, you are both awake and asleep, dreaming and hallucinating, explained Brian Sharpless, PhD, associate professor of psychopathology at Argosy University Northern Virginia in Arlington. You are paralyzed because the brain chemistry that keeps your body immobile so that it won't act out dreams is still in full force. Other signature aspects of sleep paralysis—intense fear or panic and the creepy sense of being watched or attacked, restrained or suffocated by a gruesome intruder—also can be chalked up to neurochemical interactions in the brain.

DEFUSING A WAKING NIGHTMARE

Although sleep paralysis has been discussed by physicians since at least the time of ancient Rome, there's no clear-cut treatment for it. Findings from a recent study by Dr. Sharpless, however, may help people with periodic sleep paralysis get relief.

Because sleep paralysis is common in college students (occurring at least once in nearly 30% of them), Dr. Sharpless, who is a coauthor of *Sleep Paralysis: Historical, Psychological, and Medical Perspectives*, conducted his study in this population group. The study, in part, investigated how people try to disrupt or prevent sleep paralysis episodes and how successful their tactics are.

A total of 156 participants with sleep paralysis were included in the study. They were identified out of a much larger group of would-be participants using an evaluation called the Fearful Isolated Sleep Paralysis Interview, which assesses the frequency of sleep paralysis episodes, the level of fear and distress they evoke and hallucinations that occur during episodes. The Fearful Isolated Sleep Paralysis Interview also includes questions that help doctors identify whether a medical condition, such as narcolepsy, or a psychiatric problem, such as post-traumatic stress disorder, is causing the sleep paralysis and even if drug use is the culprit. (None of the study participants fell into these categories.) The participants also were questioned about whether and how they disrupted or prevented their sleep paralysis episodes.

THE RESULTS

Although most participants (70%) who had had sleep paralysis said they had tried to disrupt episodes by using various tactics to force themselves awake, only half of them felt that they had been successful. The most common tactic was to try to move, which worked for some and not for others but may be worth a try. Dr. Sharpless suggests that, rather than struggling to move arms or legs, attempt to simply twitch a finger or toe during a sleep paralysis episode. This might be enough to jog yourself out of the episode and into fully waking consciousness.

One of the less used but more successful tactics was to simply stay calm, not give into participating in the narrative of the dream, and remind yourself that the experience is just a dream. Not participating in the nightmare can have the result of simply waking up out of it.

Of course, it would be better to prevent sleep paralysis from occurring at all! Among the study participants with periodic sleep paralysis who had tried ways to prevent it, most (nearly 80%) felt they were generally successful at keeping episodes at bay. *Based on feedback from these folks and previous research by himself and others, Dr. Sharpless offered these suggestions for discouraging sleep paralysis episodes…*

•**Avoid alcohol and coffee several hours before bedtime.** These substances affect the types of sleep you have and may make you more likely to have an episode of sleep paralysis when you wake.

•**Avoid sleeping on your back or stomach.** Studies show that these postures are more likely to encourage the feeling of suffocation and chest pressure during a sleep paralysis episode.

•**Keep a regular sleep schedule and maintain a routine that encourages healthy sleep.** This means going to bed at the same time every evening and turning off the cares of the day as well as the computer, television and other overstimulating diversions at least a half hour before you turn in.

•**Avoid becoming overtired before deciding to hit the sack and also avoid oversleeping.**

•**Practice progressive relaxation before going to sleep and whenever you can throughout the day.**

•**Get exercise on most days.** It can help you sleep more soundly at night.

WHEN TO GET HELP

Although sleep paralysis more commonly occurs in people with narcolepsy or epilepsy and in people with stress and anxiety disorders—or simply in people under stress—it can also occur in average, healthy people. If sleep paralysis is occurring frequently and causing emotional distress and/or daytime fatigue, Dr. Sharpless recommends that you consult a psychologist or psychiatrist who specializes in the treatment of sleep disorders.

PART 3

Your Brain at Full Speed

CHAPTER 12

How Your Brain Can Heal Your Body

Use Your Brain to Ease Your Pain Without Pills

More people are disabled by chronic pain than by diabetes, heart disease and cancer put together. An estimated 27% of US women (and 29% of men) suffer from debilitating pain, yet the problem remains vastly undertreated. Pain medications do not always bring sufficient relief—plus they can lead to side effects and/or addiction.

The good news: Like everything in your body, pain is affected by the workings of your mind. No matter what the cause of your pain, you can harness the power of your brain to reduce your suffering. *Here's how...*

Your limbic system, the most primitive part of your brain, controls your involuntary nervous system and emotions. Pain activates the limbic system, triggering the fight-or-flight response. As stress hormones are released, your heart beats faster, blood pressure soars, muscles tense...and various emotions are sparked, including anxiety, panic, anger and sadness. Normally, these responses are temporary—but with chronic pain, the stress of these intense reactions creates a downward spiral.

Example: The pain of chronic arthritis provokes a continuous release of stress hormones, leading to headaches and insomnia that exacerbate discomfort. As your body weakens, it produces fewer mood-boosting endorphins. Soon you're too tired and despondent to socialize, and the resulting isolation only makes you feel worse.

Helpful: If you learn to cultivate a sense of distance from your pain, you can mute the limbic system's response, reducing physical

James N. Dillard, MD, DC, CAc, board-certified physician, doctor of chiropractic and certified medical acupuncturist who pioneered the integrative model in pain medicine. He is author of *The Chronic Pain Solution: Your Personal Path to Pain Relief.* Dr. Dillard now maintains private practices in New York City and East Hampton, New York. DrDillard.com.

pain signals and easing the accompanying emotional suffering.

At least twice a day, go somewhere quiet and safe where you won't be disturbed…sit or lie in whatever position is most comfortable… and practice one or more of the techniques below for five to 15 minutes.

CALMING BREATH

Pain can take your breath away, triggering a pattern of shallow breathing that increases muscle tension and deprives cells of oxygen. Deep breathing—especially when combined with a meditative focus—helps by relaxing muscles, stimulating endorphins and reducing emotional distress.

Remember: For both of the deep-breathing techniques below, inhale slowly through your nose and then exhale slowly through your mouth. Clear your mind, and focus only on your breath. If other thoughts intrude, let them float away and refocus on your breath.

• **Flare-control breath.** This is particularly effective for pain flare-ups. As you inhale, notice your lungs filling with the vitality of your breath. Imagine your breath flowing to the area of your pain, bringing healing energy to this spot. As you exhale, imagine the pain flowing out of your body along with your breath.

• **Purifying breath.** This is especially helpful for easing troubling emotions that accompany pain. Picture your body surrounded by pure, white light.

Inhaling: Imagine this light being drawn into your lungs and then spreading until your whole body glows with healing light.

Exhaling: Picture a dark essence—representing fear, anger and sorrow—being expelled with your breath, leaving your body pain-free and your mind at ease.

HEALING IMAGERY

The guided imagery method quiets the nervous system by convincing your mind that it does not feel pain. *Close your eyes and imagine either of these…*

• **A place of peace.** Picture yourself in an ideal setting of your choosing—a favorite vacation spot, a mountaintop, a lush garden, a tranquil lake. Immerse yourself in this scene by imagining what you see (majestic trees, an azure sky)…feel (a soft breeze, the warm sun)…smell (a campfire, fresh lilacs)…hear (singing birds, rustling leaves)…and taste (the salty sea, a perfect strawberry). The more details you can conjure up, the more effective the imagery is.

• **Soothing hues.** Take a few deep breaths, then focus on your pain. Note its location and intensity…describe its qualities (aching, throbbing, burning). Think of a color that represents pain (black, purple, hot pink), and imagine that your painful area is suffused with that color. Now choose a healing hue (such as white, silver or pale blue), and imagine that it has the power to dissolve your pain. Visualize the healing color pouring onto the painful area and spreading out wider and wider, until the painful color completely disappears. In your mind's eye, let that healing color continue to pour out for as long as you want—you have an unlimited supply.

PAIN-RELIEVING ACUPRESSURE

Like acupuncture, acupressure is based on a principle of traditional Chinese medicine—that chi (energy) flows throughout the body along invisible channels called meridians, and that pain occurs when the chi becomes blocked or unbalanced. In terms of conventional Western medicine, the firm pressure applied during acupressure is thought to distract the nervous system, halting pain messages from traveling up the spinal cord to the brain.

The following techniques are particularly good for head, neck and shoulder pain, but they also ease the tension that pain elsewhere in the body can trigger in the neck area. Do each technique for several minutes per side.

• **Catwalk.** With your right hand, feel along the top of your left shoulder for any tender, tight or tense spot…then massage that area by "walking" your index, middle and ring fingers along it (like a cat kneading with its paws). Do this repeatedly and quickly—each finger press should last only about half a second. Repeat on the other side.

• **Thumb press.** Place your right hand behind your head, palm facing you and thumb pointing downward. With the pad of your thumb, press firmly into the base of your skull, working all the way across the right side and paying extra attention to any tight or tender spots. Repeat on the other side.

SOOTHING AROMATHERAPY

Certain scents can invigorate you when pain saps your energy…or calm you when pain leaves you tense or anxious. Aromatherapy also distracts your attention from pain and may relax muscles. Add a few drops of essential oil to a hot bath or sprinkle a few drops on a handkerchief that you hold near your nose (do not apply essential oil directly to skin).

Or: Smooth a scented lotion into your skin, especially on painful areas.

• **Invigorating scents.** Try cedar…eucalyptus…or peppermint (this one also eases the nausea that can accompany pain).

• **Calming scents.** Try bergamot…geranium…lavender…rose…or sandalwood.

Unraveling the Mystery of Pain

Gary Kaplan, DO, founder and medical director of the Kaplan Center for Integrative Medicine in McLean, Virginia. He is also clinical associate professor of family medicine at Georgetown University School of Medicine in Washington, DC. Dr. Kaplan, who is board-certified in both family medicine and pain medicine, is author of *Total Recovery: Solving the Mystery of Chronic Pain and Depression.* KaplanClinic.com

Anyone who lives with unexplained chronic pain knows that it can be depressing. In fact, of the more than 47 million American adults who suffer from chronic pain—often with no identifiable cause—at least two-thirds also have depression.

It's no coincidence, according to Gary Kaplan, DO, a pain expert who believes that the two disorders may be an important symptom of the same underlying condition—inflammation in specific cells of the brain. *Dr. Kaplan explained his theory…*

• **What actually causes chronic pain?** There are many possible causes, including joint or nerve damage and cancer. However, if a doctor cannot identify the origin of chronic pain or pain persists beyond the point of expected healing, inflammation in the brain could be the cause.

• **What role does brain inflammation play in causing pain?** The brain contains different kinds of cells, among them microglia, which make up about 10% of brain cells. These cells act as the immune system of the central nervous system. If threats (see below) make it into the brain, microglia go into attack mode—they become upregulated—to destroy the threat.

While upregulated, microglia secrete inflammatory chemicals to create swelling that helps to protect the healthy brain cells. Even in relatively tiny amounts, inflammatory chemicals make us feel sick, even though the body is fighting illness. Signs of inflammation include fever, fatigue, headaches and pain virtually anywhere in the body.

• **What causes microglia to become upregulated?** Infections (such as meningitis or Lyme)…toxins (including heavy metals, mold or excessive alcohol)…loss of oxygen to the brain, which occurs in sleep apnea…autoimmune disorders such as celiac disease… physical traumas…surgery…and chronic use of narcotics. In addition, emotional traumas— experienced due to long periods of stress, a physical assault or a car accident, for instance—can turn on the microglia. That explains why a person who grew up in an emotionally or physically abusive household is more likely to suffer chronic pain as an adult—an association that has been shown in numerous studies.

With enough repetitive assaults, the microglia can become so hyperreactive that they constantly spew inflammatory chemicals. Constant inflammation in the brain can result in not only chronic pain but also depression, anxiety disorders and other health issues.

• **Why does chronic pain affect only certain people?** Each of us has a different level of resilience (due to genetics and environmental factors such as emotional nurturing). Some people can take a huge number of physical or mental blows and remain healthy...others can be physically affected by just a few assaults.

• **So how do we "turn off" the microglia that are making us sick?** That's still being researched. In my practice, however, we try to address each of the factors provoking the inflammation in the brain.

My advice for people who are suffering from unexplained chronic pain...

1. Create a time line of life and health. On one sheet of paper, write down the major traumas of your life—physical and emotional—along with the dates (or approximate dates) they happened. On another sheet, write down the dates your pain, depression or illnesses began. By comparing the two, you should be able to see a correlation between them.

2. Consider psychotherapy. If you recognize a pattern in your time line, some of your pain could be due to unresolved feelings about the traumas. Unresolved guilt, shame, resentment and anger inflame neurons in the central nervous system. But resolving these issues can reduce or reverse inflammation.

MRIs of patients who have post-traumatic stress disorder (PTSD) have shown that with cognitive behavioral therapy or eye movement desensitization and reprocessing—in which certain eye movements and discussion of the trauma are combined—neuron function can return to normal.

3. Avoid NSAIDs. Occasional use of non-steroidal anti-inflammatory drugs (NSAIDs), such as Aleve or Motrin, is fine, but frequent use (three or more times a week) can, over time, lead to chronic intestinal inflammation, which can spread to other organs, including the brain.

4. Ask about medication. I sometimes prescribe low-dose (1.25 mg to 4.5 mg) *naltrexone* (a medication that is used to treat addiction), which can return microglia to a noninflammatory state. Other drugs that may help include *minocycline,* an antibiotic, or an angiotensin receptor blocker, a medication that relaxes blood vessels. If you have chronic pain, ask your doctor about these.

EXTINGUISH YOUR INFLAMMATION CYCLE

Certain lifestyle factors can promote pain-causing inflammation. *What helps...*

• **Test your diet.** For six weeks, avoid all foods with wheat, soy, milk and milk products (foods that often trigger allergies or sensitivities that promote inflammation). Eat only fresh fruits, vegetables, brown rice, fish, chicken and eggs—these foods, in general, are the least likely to cause inflammation.

After six weeks, add back one category of food—such as dairy—per week. Note whether these foods have a negative effect on your energy, mood or level of pain. If so, eliminate that food from your diet entirely.

• **Try meditation.** Research shows that meditation builds new neuronal tissue and helps create a natural resilience to future trauma. Your meditation doesn't have to be a formal program—you can start by simply sitting quietly in a room for 20 minutes each day, allowing your body to gradually relax while you focus on your breathing. Aerobic exercise and adequate sleep also help control inflammation.

Beat Disease with These Powerful Mental Techniques

Ellen Langer, PhD, professor of psychology, Harvard University, Cambridge, Massachusetts, and head of the Langer Mindfulness Institute at Harvard. She is author of *Mindfulness...The Power of Mindful Learning...On Becoming an Artist: Reinventing Yourself Through Mindful Creativity...Counterclockwise: Mindful Health and the Power of Possibility.* LangerMindfulnessInstitute.com

D id you know that you can turn back the clock and regain the vigor of your youth by putting yourself in a "time capsule" for a few days? Sounds crazy, but it's actually fun, festive and easy to do.

THE MIND-BODY CONNECTION

Our culture operates on the assumption that the mind and body are separate. What we're learning is that you can't separate them…the mind and body are one. And prioritizing the mind-body connection is fast becoming the best approach to not only physical health, but all-around well-being.

Take, for instance, my time-machine study on ageless aging—a program you can easily do with a group of friends in your age bracket. The study involved a group of 80-year-olds who were basically put in a time machine for a week. Yes—a time machine. They were first tested on vision and hearing, grip strength, memory and dexterity before being taken to a monastery that was decorated to replicate life in 1959. The décor included photos of their younger selves. The participants wore 1950s fashions during their stay, and entertainment consisted of TV shows, movies, books, newspapers and music of the 1950s. The participants also were instructed to discuss sports and events that occurred during that era in the present tense. Most importantly, the participants were told to not reminisce about the old days, but, instead, to think of themselves as actually being younger.

Five days later, the participants did, in fact, look younger and their scores on grip strength, dexterity, memory and even eyesight had improved. These results showed that thinking you're in your prime (even if you are way past it) can trigger the body to become healthier.

THINK YOURSELF WELL

Here's more on how you can become a healthier and younger you…

• **Believe you're in control of your health.** But you really have to believe.

Real-life results: A group of college students hoping to enter the military were divided into two subgroups. All participants had 20/20 vision or better. One group was given flight suits to wear and told to think of themselves as Air Force pilots doing flight simulation exercises while they used flight simulators. The other group was just seated at the flight simulators and told that the simulator was broken and that they should just pretend to fly the plane. After the exercise, the participants' were given vision tests. The eyesight of the group members who believed they were actu-

ally enacting a flight simulation—a skill that requires precise vision—was 40% better than those in the group that was just pretending.

• **Transform the mundane into a vital health routine.** For example, recognize that any kind of physical activity—not just sweating through a Zumba workout—can be a calorie-burning exercise. Be like a group of maids who were told that cleaning is good exercise. They lost weight and had improved body mass indices and hip-to-waist ratios compared with maids who weren't told this. When questioned, those other maids said that they didn't think of housecleaning as exercise. They didn't lose any weight at all.

• **Describe your health in the most positive terms possible.** Although doing so won't necessarily miraculously cure you of whatever you've got, it can make living with a chronic disease or health risk a lot easier by relieving pain and stress. For example, don't be like a group of breast-cancer survivors who said they were "in remission." They were less functional, in more pain and in poorer health than another group who thought of themselves as "cured."

• **Act how you want to feel.** Surely, you have had experiences when you've "thought yourself well"—or "made yourself sick."

This "don't try this at home" experiment makes a strong point: Healthy volunteers were given tissues and asked to act as if they had a cold while watching a film of people coughing and sneezing. Forty percent of the volunteers reported cold symptoms afterward, and blood tests taken at that time showed that all of those reporting symptoms had high levels of IgA antibody, which means that their bodies were launching an immune response against a cold they were imagining that they had!

Practice thinking of yourself as healthy, vibrant, young and resilient, and engage your imagination to cause change in accordance with will.

Stop Chronic Back Pain Without Surgery

David Hanscom, MD, board-certified orthopedic spine surgeon, Swedish Neuroscience Specialists, Seattle. He is the author of *Back In Control: A Spine Surgeon's Roadmap Out of Chronic Pain*. BackinControl.com

It hurts just to read the latest statistics on back pain. Every year, Americans spend an estimated $86 billion on back pain treatments, including pain pills, injections and surgery. And although about 800,000 surgical procedures are performed each year for back pain, in about 75% of those cases, the surgery doesn't help.

That's why David Hanscom, MD, an orthopedic spine surgeon at Swedish Neuroscience Specialists in Seattle, does something that few surgeons would dream of—he talks most of his patients out of having surgery. Instead, he recommends a new six-step approach to treating chronic back pain that he finds far more effective than surgery for most people.

AN OLD PROBLEM

Expensive yet ineffectual spine surgeries are currently a hot topic—but even decades ago, questions were being asked about whether too many were being performed. For example, back in 1989, *Iowa Orthopaedic Journal* published "Are We Performing Too Much Spinal Surgery?"...and the 2001 American Academy of Pain Medicine annual meeting presented the session "Failed Back Syndrome: The Disturbing Statistics." Research continues to raise questions about the associated dangers, including a recent Stanford University study that linked spinal fusion surgery with a higher risk for stroke.

Dr. Hanscom acknowledged that overzealous surgeons and hospitals looking to maximize profits play a role in how many spine surgeries are performed. However, he said, it's also important to realize that many surgeons are loath to turn away desperate patients who are begging for help. "These patients can't work, they can't sleep, they're miserable—so they're willing to try anything, even if there's no guarantee that surgery will get rid of their pain," he said.

WHY SURGERY USUALLY WON'T HELP

The main reason why spine surgery so often doesn't work, Dr. Hanscom said, is that an operation can relieve back pain only if there is a structural abnormality, such as a ruptured disk or pinched nerve. But the vast majority of chronic, severe back problems don't fall into that category. Instead, the back pain is nonspecific, rooted in inflammation in the body's soft tissues (ligaments, tendons, fascia, muscles). "These types of problems cannot be seen on imaging tests—and if you can't see it, the best surgeon in the world won't be able to fix it," said Dr. Hanscom.

So when the problem is a soft-tissue issue, whether or not the patient undergoes surgery, his pain is likely to go on and on. Understandably, this leads to a lot of frustration (because nothing is helping) and fatigue (because pain is exhausting). A vicious cycle is created—pain leads to frustration and fatigue, and frustration and fatigue exacerbate pain.

The longer the pain continues, the worse the situation gets. "Long-lasting pain creates neurologic pathways that outlast the root cause," Dr. Hanscom explained. "Once these pain pathways are formed and remembered, the cycle is established and the pain becomes chronic. So even after the soft-tissue problems are gone, the pain often isn't. The only way to fix this type of chronic pain is to tackle the central nervous system's response to pain."

TAKING CONTROL

Dr. Hanscom knows firsthand whereof he speaks. His book *Back In Control: A Spine Surgeon's Roadmap Out of Chronic Pain* describes his own battle with chronic pain—from tennis elbow, migraine headaches, burning feet syndrome and more—and the surprising strategy that he used to overcome it. Based on his personal and professional experience, he has developed a program—called Defined, Organized, Comprehensive Care (DOCC)—that he uses in treating his own patients and in training other surgeons. Its premise is that pain is a perception...and that understanding it gives you greater power to gain control over it. "Freedom from pain is not only possible, with the right tools it is probable," he said.

Basically, the DOCC approach works by calming down the nervous system and allowing it to heal while also laying down new neurological pathways so the nervous system isn't trapped in the endless loop of pain signals. Dr. Hanscom explained, "It's not that you simply learn to live with the pain. Instead, your brain stops responding to the pain—so you literally do not feel it." *The DOCC program involves six basic steps…*

•**Sleep.** Getting at least eight hours of sleep per night is a cornerstone of the program. "If sleep issues aren't addressed, nothing else will work," Dr. Hanscom said. For people who have trouble sleeping due to their pain, prescription sleep medications are an option.

•**Stress management.** Chronic stress creates a cascade of biological events that exacerbate inflammation and sleeplessness, which in turn perpetuate chronic pain. Managing stress requires a two-pronged approach—making time for activities that build up your energy reserves (exercise, hobbies, socializing, spending time alone)…and learning to deal more effectively with aspects of your life that drain your energy (things that make you anxious, angry or unhappy).

•**Pain medication.** If you (or your doctor) have been leery of using pain medication for fear of its potential side effects, it is worth reconsidering this issue. Taking pain medication to achieve short-term relief while you work to resolve your chronic pain problem can help you halt that vicious cycle through which pain begets more pain, Dr. Hanscom said.

•**Physical therapy.** Rehabilitation of soft tissues soothes inflammation and facilitates true healing.

•**Goal setting.** Creating a detailed picture of what you are trying to achieve and devising a plan to work toward that goal helps you decrease anxiety, frustration and depression. This, in turn, calms the central nervous system and eases physical pain.

•**Retraining the brain.** The DOCC program moves people from being reactive to being creative in their lives. Meditation, visualization and creative play are among the primary tools Dr. Hanscom recommends. Particularly helpful is writing, he said.

Example: Write down a situation that bothers you (for instance, "My spouse is always late and it stresses me out"). Then, on paper, examine your thought processes about this situation (such as, "When she's late, I imagine that she's been in a terrible accident…or that she just doesn't care enough about me to be on time"). Next, look for errors in your thinking ("It's highly unlikely that she's had an accident…and she shows me in many ways every day that she loves me"). Finally, write about more rational ways in which to view the situation ("She's just not good at budgeting her time. I'll ask her to meet me 15 minutes earlier than necessary so that, by the time she arrives, we'll be right on schedule"). Even though the problem or problems you write about might not seem to be related to your back pain, the writing exercises essentially help reprogram your nervous system to undo the old pain pathways, allowing your brain to lay down new, positive, pain-free neural pathways.

For more information on how to conquer your chronic back pain and take control of your life, visit BackinControl.com.

Boost Memory, Ease Anxiety, Erase Pain… with Your Brain Waves

Paul G. Swingle, PhD, RPsych, registered psychologist board-certified in biofeedback and neurotherapy and author of *Biofeedback for the Brain*. Formerly a professor of psychology at the University of Ottawa in Canada, he currently is in private practice in Vancouver, British Columbia. SwingleClinic.com

Imagine finding relief from medical or psychological problems by changing the way your brain works. You can—with neurofeedback, a type of biofeedback in which you learn to control brain wave activity. As brain function improves, symptoms associated with inefficient brain function also improve. Even physical pain is eased, because pain management has a psychological component—and there are no drug side effects to worry about.

How it works: The brain produces electrical signals in the form of waves that correspond to specific mental states (see "Which Brain Waves Do What" at the end of this article). Neurofeedback boosts your ability to produce particular brain waves that have specific desired effects. The process is painless and noninvasive.

You don't even have to be ill or in pain to reap the advantages. Many healthy executives, musicians and athletes use neurofeedback to sharpen the mind, ease stage fright or just perform at their peak.

USEFUL TO YOU?

To explore whether neurofeedback can help you, consult a neurotherapist—a specially trained psychologist, psychiatrist, naturopathic doctor, medical doctor, chiropractor or other health-care professional.

Recommended: Choose one who is certified in neurofeedback by the Biofeedback Certification International Alliance (720-502-5829, BCIA.org).

At your initial diagnostic meeting, the neurotherapist uses an electroencephalogram (EEG) machine to map your brain wave activity. For relatively straightforward problems, such as depression or sleep disorders, or in cases where the goal is simply to maximize cognitive performance, several electrodes (sensors) are dabbed with conductive gel and attached to specific spots on your head. For complex problems, such as traumatic brain injury or epilepsy, you wear a close-fitting cap with 19 sensors.

These sensors, connected with wires to a computer, measure electrical impulses produced by your brain. The practitioner reads these impulses while your eyes are open, while your eyes are shut and while you are reading—because some abnormalities are apparent only under certain circumstances.

Example: With one form of attention deficit disorder, brain waves look normal when the mind is not challenged—but when given a task, such as reading, the brain produces a wave that is not conducive to concentrating.

Your brain map is compared with internationally recognized reference data showing which brain patterns are normal under which circumstances. This identifies areas of the brain that are functioning abnormally or suboptimally. These areas are then targeted for treatment.

DURING A TREATMENT SESSION

A typical treatment session lasts about 50 minutes. The practitioner places an electrode at the spot where your brain needs to become more or less active when producing a specific frequency. The electrode is connected to a computer that gives you feedback. When you succeed in altering your brain waves to the target frequency, the computer produces a special sound or visual cue.

At first, achieving this is a matter of trial and error—more the result of passively observing the mental and physical states that seem to work rather than actively trying to think or do something specific. For instance, if you're trying to create alpha waves to ease anxiety, you may notice that the tone sounded when you closed your eyes and pictured a ship sailing into the horizon but not when you imagined yourself in a meadow. With practice, your brain learns to regulate these brain waves.

Which Brain Waves Do What

Common brain wave frequencies (in hertz), the mental states they are normally associated with and the consequences of excess or deficiency...

Type of Wave	Normal State	Too Much Leads to...	Too Little Leads to...
Delta: 0-3 hz	Asleep	Mental fog, pain	Poor sleep
Theta: 4-7 hz	Drowsy	Poor memory	Inability to relax
Alpha: 8-13 hz	Relaxed	Insomnia	Mental chatter
Beta: 14-30 hz	Alert	Anxiety	Distraction

The severity of the problem determines the length of treatment. Some people have 10 to 30 weekly sessions...others come three times a week for up to 100 sessions. A follow-up session assures that the brain wave change is stable. Some people get "tune-ups"—many older clients come four times a year to adjust the frequencies associated with mental focus. Cost varies but typically runs about $100 per session. Insurance sometimes covers treatment.

Recommended: Neurofeedback is a complementary therapy, best used in conjunction with psychotherapy, physical therapy, nutritional counseling, medical care or other treatment.

For instance: Neurofeedback can ease cravings for alcohol or drugs—but a person with a substance use disorder also needs counseling to learn how to create a new social environment that does not include drinking or drugs.

Important: Inform your medical doctor and other health-care providers before beginning neurofeedback (as you should with any new treatment) to make sure that none of your therapies conflict.

NEUROFEEDBACK HELPS

- **Age-related cognitive decline**
- **Alcohol and drug cravings**
- **Anxiety**
- **Attention disorders** (such as ADD and ADHD)
- **Brain damage from head injury**
- **Depression**
- **Epilepsy, seizures**
- **Fibromyalgia**
- **Migraine**
- **Post-traumatic stress**
- **Sleep problems**
- **Stroke effects**

Brain Retraining Eases Tinnitus

Steven Lamm, MD, practicing internist, clinical faculty, NYU School of Medicine, New York City. He is a panel physician for the New York State Athletic Commission and is coauthor of *The Hardness Factor: How to Achieve Your Best Health and Sexual Fitness at Any Age.*

Anyone who has experienced tinnitus—an uncontrolled ringing or roaring noise in the ears—knows how maddening it can be. All the more so because there really is no treatment to stop it. Doctors typically offer patients an array of remedies that may or may not help, including tranquilizers, antidepressants and mechanical devices that attempt to mask the plaguing noises. But thus far there is nothing that has worked well and consistently. Fortunately there's a new way to train the brain to ignore the nerve signals that simulate ringing, according to a recent study.

The research, conducted by scientists at the University of Texas at Dallas, examined a way to reprogram the brain so that it no longer "hears" the tones that have become so intensely disturbing. Using a form of treatment called vagus nerve stimulation (VNS), already in use to help patients with treatment-resistant epilepsy or depression, the scientists first induced tinnitus in rats (how they did this is way too complicated to go into here, but believe me, they did it—and confirmed it by the rats' failure to respond to a gap in the background noise) and then set out to see if they could correct it. They delivered painless electrical pulses to the vagus nerve, which leads to the auditory cortex in the brain. The rats were exposed to tones with frequencies just above and below the range of the tinnitus sounds.

Results: The rats now responded appropriately to the gap in the background noise (they recognized the silence)—and scans of their brains three weeks after the therapy showed what the researchers expected to see, that tinnitus had been stopped in all of them.

HOW GREAT IS THIS?

Steven Lamm, MD, a member of the clinical faculty at NYU School of Medicine, says that tinnitus is "probably one of the most annoying, irritating and exasperating complaints that a patient can have. It's like an alarm clock that can't be turned off." According to Dr. Lamm this research demonstrates that the nerve activity of the brain is capable of modification. "Tinnitus involves an abnormality of the brain circuitry," he said. "If you reshuffle the circuitry, you may be able to eliminate the unwanted noise."

ON THE HORIZON

VNS treatment could be an improvement over current tinnitus therapies because it may offer a possible end to the condition without any significant side effects—unlike antidepressants and tranquilizers—say the study's authors.

Research on this therapy in humans is ongoing. People with tinnitus will participate in clinical trials much like those that worked with the rats. They will have electrodes attached to their vagus nerves in an outpatient procedure and then, every day over a period of three weeks, they will visit the clinic to listen to a range of tones and receive electrical impulses to the vagus nerve. The hope is that researchers will for the first time be able to "reset" the brain's circuitry to actually eliminate tinnitus for these people. We don't know whether the treatment will result in any collateral problems—such as, perhaps, the inability to hear certain actual tones. But given the fact that about 10% of adults are plagued by tinnitus, this treatment could be nothing less than a godsend...an end to the ringing alarm clock in your head that refuses to turn off.

Hypnosis: It's Not Hooey! 6 Medical Problems It's Been Proven to Help

Marc I. Oster, PsyD, a psychologist and professor of cognitive behavioral therapy at the Illinois School of Professional Psychology at Argosy University in Schaumburg, Illinois. He is a fellow and past president of the American Society of Clinical Hypnosis and the recipient of the Milton H. Erickson Award for Scientific Excellence in Writing on Clinical Hypnosis. MarcOster. Homestead.com

Don't confuse medical hypnosis with the flamboyant stage shows that feature a swinging watch, a performer in a glittery jacket and volunteers from the audience, all quacking like ducks.

Hypnosis-enhanced therapy is a legitimate treatment for various medical problems—and unlike many treatments, it is noninvasive and totally safe.

Here's what hypnosis really helps...

IRRITABLE BOWEL SYNDROME

IBS is a mysterious, often debilitating condition that causes cramps and intermittent episodes of diarrhea, pain and constipation. Medications to treat it aren't very effective.

Several well-designed studies of hypnotherapy for IBS have shown that IBS patients who were treated with hypnosis had "substantial, long-term improvement" of gastrointestinal symptoms, along with less anxiety and depression. It's possible that hypnosis alters how the central nervous system responds to intestinal signals. It also diverts people's attention from their intestinal sensations and causes them to perceive less discomfort.

PAIN RELIEF

Hypnosis doesn't necessarily reduce pain, but it does alter how people react to it. Studies have shown, for example, that hypnotized dental patients have a higher pain threshold. They also have less anxiety, which reduces sensitivity to pain.

One study, which looked at patients with burn injuries, used virtual-reality technology to induce hypnosis. Patients wore a fiber-optic helmet that immersed them in a make-believe environment. As they descended into a snowy, three-dimensional canyon, an audiotape with a clinician's voice prepared them for what they would experience during the treatment of the burn.

Result: They had a decrease in both pain and anxiety—and their need for potent painkillers was reduced by half.

HELP QUITTING SMOKING

About 65% to 70% of smokers who are treated with medical hypnosis quit successfully, according to research. That's much better than the quit rate from going cold turkey (about 20%) or using stop-smoking drugs including nicotine therapy (35% to 40%).

Hypnosis isn't a miracle cure for smoking or other addictions. Anyone who takes the time to schedule appointments with a therapist already is highly motivated. The success rate would be lower for those who remain on the fence about quitting. That said, hypnosis still is more effective than standard treatments.

BETTER CANCER CARE

The radiation therapy that's used to treat some cancers often causes fatigue as a side effect. Researchers at Mount Sinai Hospital, New York City, found that cancer patients who underwent hypnosis during a common kind of counseling called cognitive-behavioral therapy experienced less fatigue than participants in a control group.

The study, published in *Journal of Clinical Oncology*, showed that after six months, the average patient treated with hypnosis had less fatigue than 95% of those who weren't hypnotized.

LESS SURGICAL PAIN

Another study of cancer patients found that those who had a single, 15-minute hypnosis session prior to their surgery required less sedation and experienced less nausea, pain and fatigue than those in a nonhypnosis group.

Mount Sinai researchers analyzed 20 studies on hypnosis and surgery, and they found that in 89% of cases, hypnotized surgical patients had less pain, used less pain medication and recovered faster.

CHRONIC FATIGUE

A six-month study at Beth Israel Deaconess Medical Center, Boston, showed that 73% of participants who had chronic fatigue syndrome reported increased energy, more restful periods of sleep and better concentration at work. This is far better than the national average of 23% of people who improve with other types of therapy.

HOW YOU CAN TRY HYPNOSIS

Because of its long association with parlor tricks, hypnosis still is a subject of confusion.

A few facts: You don't go into a trance during hypnosis...you are more in control of yourself than usual, not less...and you won't do anything that you don't want to do.

A specially trained therapist will use guided imagery to focus and direct your imagination. It is the same technique sometimes used during meditation.

Example: While you relax, the therapist will encourage you to breathe slowly and deeply...to imagine a soothing scene (such as walking in the woods)...and to keep your mind focused on just that one thing. This is known as the induction phase. Your brain activity slows, but you still are focused and alert.

At this point, medical hypnosis diverges from traditional meditation. While you are in a relaxed state, the therapist will guide your thinking toward particular issues.

Suppose that you have arthritis and that your arm always hurts. The therapist might describe a scene in which you're walking to a lake...submerging yourself in icy water...and feeling your arm go pleasantly numb. The positive effects can last for minutes to hours to forever.

Research has shown that people who are mentally and physically relaxed are more receptive to taking in new ideas and feeling in new ways.

To find a hypnotist who can help you, look for a licensed health-care professional who offers hypnosis as only one part of his/her practice. Someone who only does hypnosis may not have the understanding of health-care issues to properly diagnose and treat you. The websites for the American Society of Clinical

383

Hypnosis (ASCH.net) and the Society for Clinical & Experimental Hypnosis (SCEH.us) have referral pages that can help you find an expert in your area.

Expect to complete between four and 10 sessions. The cost per session is about the same as you would pay for other types of counseling.

Example: Depending on where you live, you might pay about $150 for a session with a psychologist. You will pay less if you see a social worker, nurse or mental-health counselor.

Most insurance companies do not cover hypnosis per se, but they may cover therapy that includes hypnosis. Medicare covers "hypnotherapy" for certain conditions.

Grow a Happy Brain

Richard O'Connor, PhD, psychotherapist in private practice, Canaan, Connecticut, and New York City. He is former executive director of the Northwest Center for Family Service and Mental Health and author of *Undoing Depression: What Therapy Doesn't Teach You and Medication Can't Give You.* UndoingDepression.com

---

About three-quarters of patients who are treated for depression take one or more antidepressant medications. In fact, about 10% of all Americans are taking these drugs.

Antidepressants, including Prozac and other selective serotonin reuptake inhibitors (SSRIs), can help patients with severe depression, but they are not effective for most patients with mild-to-moderate depression. A recent report in *The Journal of the American Medical Association* concluded that some of the most widely prescribed antidepressants are no more effective than placebos for these patients.

Also, these drugs commonly cause sexual problems, weight gain and other side effects, including an inability to feel empathy for others. These side effects might be acceptable for someone who is incapacitated with depression, but the risk-benefit ratio isn't acceptable for the types of depression that can be treated with other methods. *Here's how to relieve depression without taking medications…*

Important: Never stop taking an antidepressant without your doctor's approval, and be sure to taper off slowly.

GROW A HAPPY BRAIN

It has been discovered in recent years that chronic depression causes significant brain-damage. Patients produce less dopamine, one of the neurotransmitters that affects the ability to feel pleasure. The hippocampus, one part of the brain associated with emotions, can shrink by up to 20%. Cells lose endorphin (the pleasure hormone) receptor sites, which further inhibits pleasurable feelings.

Good news: Much of this damage can be reversed with positive emotions—by trying the strategies in this article and continuing to use the ones that work for you. Just as the areas of the brain associated with hand coordination get larger when a musician practices his/her instrument, people with depression can increase the areas of the brain associated with positive emotions.

KEEP TRACK

Sudden mood changes can be a hallmark of depression. The dramatic ups and downs that some patients experience are triggered by unfelt feelings. Because of their past experiences (such as childhood trauma), they have learned to mute their feelings—experiencing them is too painful.

Example: You might go to bed feeling fine, then wake up in the throes of depression. You are reacting to something, but because you don't know what that something is, you feel buffeted by forces beyond your control.

Solution: A mood journal. Every day, keep track of what's happening when you experience any type of mood change. Write down what you're feeling, what you were doing when you first noticed the feeling and what you were thinking about or remembering at the time.

This is a powerful tool to help you circumvent your defense mechanisms. You will start to recognize more of your feelings and understand why you're having them. This won't make the emotional pain disappear (you might even feel more upset when you first start doing this), but you will start to recognize emotional causes and effects. This knowledge will lead to solutions as well as a greater sense of control.

DO SOMETHING

Patients with severe depression can be almost catatonic—just getting out of bed or taking a shower can seem impossible. With milder forms of depression, procrastination is one of the biggest hurdles. Starting something is risky. There might be failure. There will be frustrations and setbacks. Self-esteem may be threatened. Doing nothing can feel like a safer alternative even though the lack of accomplishment will make the depression worse.

People don't accomplish things because they are naturally productive and energetic. They become productive and energetic by doing things.

Solution: Every day, make yourself do something that gives you a sense of accomplishment. You might make a commitment to work in the yard or fix a garden fence. You might decide to write a few lines of a poem.

It doesn't matter what the activity is, as long as you do something. People who set goals and deadlines (I'm going to write for 10 minutes tomorrow at 10 am) and follow through almost always notice an improvement in mood. Once they experience that uplift, they are more likely to keep trying new things.

GET OFF THE ROLLER COASTER

Depression is accompanied by thought patterns that are rife with distorted perceptions and faulty logic.

Example: A healthy individual who gets a flat tire will focus on the immediate problem—Darn, I have a flat tire. I'll have to get it fixed.

Someone with depression will imagine the worst possible scenario. All of my tires must be going bad. I don't have the money to replace them all. I might have to get another job....

They get so worked up that they forget they are dealing with a simple problem. Instead, the imaginary scenario dominates their thinking.

Solution: Take yourself off the mental rollercoaster. When you start imagining the worst, think Stop. Ask yourself how likely any of these dire outcomes really is. Once people understand that they're prone to making exaggerated—and erroneous—generalizations, they find it easier to mentally step back and focus on the real problem. Oh, it's just a flat tire. It feels like a huge problem, but it's not.

WATCH YOUR MIND

Studies have found that people who practice mindful meditation—noting the thoughts that run through their minds without letting those thoughts upset them—have increased activity in the prefrontal part of the brain. This is where positive emotions are processed and negative emotions are controlled.

Mindfulness means watching your mind at work. You are aware of yourself and your thoughts, but you are detached from the emotional components. People who practice mindfulness become more thoughtful about their emotions and are less likely to react to them.

This is critical for people with depression. They tend to ruminate too much. They worry about things that haven't happened and attach too much importance to things that don't matter.

Solution: Daily meditation. Find a quiet place where you won't be interrupted for 20 or 30 minutes. Get comfortable, close your eyes and start to breathe slowly and deeply. Focus only on your breathing. As thoughts or feelings drift in and out of your mind, acknowledge them, then let them float off, like bubbles in a pool of water. Whenever you get distracted, return your mind to your breathing.

Don't expect to experience bliss—that's not the purpose. It's more like exercise for the brain. People who do this daily find that they're generally calmer and more resilient against stress. They learn to detach from their emotions long enough to think about what those feelings really mean and how important (or unimportant) they are.

WALK IT OFF

Studies of depressed adults show that those who exercise three times a week improve just as much in the short-term as those who take antidepressants. People who continue to exercise are more likely to avoid future depressive episodes than those who rely solely on medication.

Exercise appears to stimulate the growth of new brain cells, the opposite of what happens with depression. It stimulates the production of endorphins. It also promotes feelings of accomplishment and physical well-being.

Solution: Walk briskly three or more times a week. You will probably notice significant improvement in mood within the first week. Those who exercise harder or more often tend to report the greatest improvement.

The Power of a Personal Mantra

Ronald A. Alexander, PhD, a clinical psychotherapist and executive director of the OpenMind Training Institute in Santa Monica, California. He is author of *Wise Mind, Open Mind: Finding Purpose & Meaning in Times of Crisis, Loss & Change* and created the audio CD *Mindful Meditations for Creative Transformation.* RonaldAlexander.com

---

If you can't keep your mind and body still long enough to reap the benefits of healing meditation, a mantra can make all the difference.

The concept of a mantra (which means *sacred message* in Sanskrit) was developed thousands of years ago by yogis to enhance meditation and promote enlightenment.

How does that translate to today's frenetic world? Consistent users report that mantras can change your state of mind, mood, thought processes and even physiology. Research shows that mantras may help you calm down…reduce stress…moderate emotional responses…focus attention…set priorities…sleep more soundly… and improve overall quality of life.

Several simple sounds can bring stillness to the mind, including Ohm, Ra…Ma…and Sa. Or you can select a phrase that has personal relevance and use this unique mantra during meditation.

Modern twist: Today's mantras often meld principles of Eastern meditation, such as Buddhist mindfulness (being fully aware of the present moment, without judgment), with contemporary Western psychotherapy techniques that aim to replace unwholesome self-criticisms with positive thoughts. The idea is to choose a mantra that is meaningful to you… gently dispels sorrows about the past and worries about the future…and/or reinforces a desirable emotional state, such as tranquility, acceptance or mental clarity.

Developing your mantra repertoire: First, consider the specific change you desire. For instance, suppose an inner voice keeps telling you that you're unworthy, incompetent or unlovable. *To find a mantra that can redirect your thoughts…*

• **Identify the unwholesome self-judgment and challenge its validity.** Ask yourself, Is it really true that I am unworthy? Chances are that the answer is no.

• **Determine the healing opposite of unworthiness, and turn that into a mantra—** for instance, "I am worthy."

• **Compose two additional mantras expressing the same idea,** such as "I deserve to be happy" and "I am learning to value myself." We often struggle with deep negative thoughts, beliefs and feelings…so it helps to have a repertoire of three mantras that instill and reinforce a more wholesome core message.

• **Choose a particular place in your body** (such as your heart, forehead or belly) in which to "ground" your affirmation by placing your hand on that spot or imagining your breath going there as you repeat your mantra. This physical action helps you focus on the positive resources that exist in your physical body.

Sample mantras: Depending on your situation and goals, select mantras that have significance for you, such as, "The healing bright light resides within me"…"I am at peace now"…"I am strong"…"Love surrounds me"…"I relax and breathe"…"I attract healthy relationships"…"Today is my day"…"Success is mine"…"My creativity is flowing."

When to use your mantra: Meditate by repeating one of your chosen mantras, silently or aloud, for at least five minutes three times daily—when you wake up in the morning…at mid-afternoon, when biorhythms naturally produce an energy lag…and at sunset or just before bed.

Alternative: Meditate for a minimum of 20 minutes once or twice daily, using part of this time to focus on your mantra.

Also repeat your mantra whenever you feel stressed or sad or otherwise struggle as you go about your day. It will help you identify the uncomfortable emotion…acknowledge it for a moment…and then release it as you embrace a more positive and joyful feeling.

Easy 20-Minute Way to Prevent Heart Disease

Norman E. Rosenthal, MD, a clinical professor of psychiatry at Georgetown University School of Medicine in Washington, DC. He is author of *Transcendence: Healing and Transformation Through Transcendental Meditation*. NormanRosenthal.com

Wouldn't it be great if there were a simple way to lower blood pressure, reverse heart disease and sharpen your brain? There is! It's called transcendental meditation, or TM for short.

Many people think of TM as a vestige of the 1960s, a vaguely religious practice that was popularized when the Beatles went to India to study with Maharishi Mahesh Yogi.

TM is not a religious practice. It does not involve immersing yourself in a particular belief system. It's a mental technique that changes brain wave patterns and alters, in beneficial ways, physiological processes, such as blood pressure, heart rate and hormone levels.

Bonus: TM is easier to do than many other forms of meditation and relaxation therapy. And beginners exhibit the same brain wave changes as long-time practitioners, sometimes within just a few weeks after starting TM.

WHAT IT INVOLVES

Various relaxation techniques require you to sit with your eyes closed, focus on your breathing and/or visualize a particular scene. TM requires the repetition of a mantra, a meaningless word that you mentally focus on.

There's nothing mystical about the mantra. It's simply a tool for quieting the mind and "transcending" stressful thoughts, worries and concerns.

Most people who practice TM do so twice a day for 20 minutes each time. During a session, the breathing slows and the brain (as measured on an EEG) produces a preponderance of alpha waves, slow frequency signals (eight to 12 cycles per second) that indicate deep relaxation. There's also an increase in brain wave coherence, in which activity in different parts of the brain is roughly synchronized.

TM has been studied more than most other forms of meditation and relaxation—and, in some cases, appears to have more pronounced health effects. Researchers have published approximately 340 peer-reviewed articles on TM, many of which appeared in respected medical journals. *Important benefits…*

LOWERS BLOOD PRESSURE

A University of Kentucky meta-analysis that looked at data from 711 participants found that those who practiced TM averaged a five-point reduction in systolic pressure (top number) and three points in diastolic (bottom number). This might sound like a modest benefit, but it's enough to potentially reduce the incidence of cardiovascular disease by 15% to 20%.

Scientists speculate that TM lowers blood pressure by reducing the body's output of hormones, such as epinephrine, that accompany and stimulate the natural stress response. People with hypertension who meditate twice a day for more than three months require, on average, 23% less blood pressure medication.

Other nondrug treatments for hypertension, including biofeedback, progressive relaxation and stress-management training, don't have these same effects.

REVERSES HEART DISEASE

Researchers divided participants with hypertension into two groups. Those in one group were given health education (the control group), while those in the second group practiced TM for six to nine months. The thickness of the intima (inner lining) of the carotid artery was measured at the beginning and end of the study.

Result: The intima thickened slightly in the control group, indicating that cardiovascular disease had progressed. In the TM group, the thickness of the intima decreased. This study, published in *Stroke*, indicates that TM actually can reverse cardiovascular disease.

It's not known why TM has this effect. We suspect that it's more effective in patients with early-stage disease. In those with advanced atherosclerosis, which is accompanied by calcification of plaques (fatty deposits) in the coronary arteries, TM might slow disease progression but is unlikely to remove plaque that has already accumulated.

REDUCES PAIN

I sometimes recommend TM for patients who suffer from chronic-pain conditions, such as arthritis. We know that pain tends to be more severe in patients with high levels of anxiety and stress—and TM is very effective at reducing stress.

In one study, participants dipped their fingers into painfully hot water, then rated the pain. Those who practiced TM rated their pain exactly the same as those who didn't use TM, but they were less bothered by it. Interestingly, participants who practiced TM for just five months achieved the same results as those who had meditated for decades.

SHARPENS YOUR BRAIN

When people meditate, the coherence of alpha brain waves throughout the brain is accompanied by slightly faster beta waves in the prefrontal region of the brain, behind the forehead. The alpha waves produce relaxation, while the beta waves increase focus and decision-making.

Brain studies of top-level managers show that they have higher levels of both alpha and beta coherence than lower-level workers. A similar thing occurs in elite athletes.

Practice helps: Some of the physiological changes produced by TM occur immediately, but people who keep doing it for several months tend to have better results, probably because of increased synaptic connections (connections between brain cells). The brain may literally rewire itself, with practice.

HOW TO START

During a TM session, you'll achieve a state of restful alertness, during which your thoughts are clear but without the distractions of the internal noise that we live with. How people achieve this is highly individual. I like to relax in a comfortable chair in a quiet room. I dim the lights, turn off the telephones and start repeating my mantra. A friend of mine who has practiced TM for 40 years can enjoy a brief session in the back of a taxi.

You might find it tricky to keep mentally repeating the mantra. You might be distracted by physical sensations, outside sounds, etc. All of this is natural and expected. At some point during the session, you'll feel mentally silent. You will be present in the moment but removed from it.

Important: TM is easy to practice but difficult to learn on your own. People start with one-on-one sessions with an instructor. In general, each teaching session lasts about 90 minutes. Your instructor will assign a mantra and give instructions for using it. Sometimes people wonder why they can't pick their own mantras. One reason is that it is a tradition not to. Another is that someone who chooses his/her own mantra might do so because of underlying meanings or associations. A mantra from a teacher won't have this baggage.

You will work with the instructor once a day for four consecutive days. After that, you might return once every month to make sure that your technique is working. The website TM.org can provide referrals to instructors in your area.

CHAPTER 13

Brain Tricks for a Better Life

How to Have an "Einstein Brain"—Here Are His Tricks—You Can Use Them, Too!

Albert Einstein was a genius, but sheer intelligence was not all that he had. The man who cracked secrets of the universe also knew the secret of using his own brain for maximum effect. But unlike Einstein, most people fail to actively use the brain in order to heighten its powers.

The first step to changing this is to recognize the various parts of the brain and how each functions…

• **Brain stem.** Sometimes referred to as the "reptilian brain," the brain stem generates instinctive drives for survival and reproduction. The fight-or-flight response to threat comes from the reptilian brain, as does stress and lust.

• **Limbic system.** Situated on top of the brain stem, the limbic system filters the instinctive drives of the reptilian brain through a network of past experiences, producing emotions such as fear, desire and jealousy.

• **Frontal cortex.** Located behind the forehead, the frontal cortex is known as the "thinking brain." It allows us to plan, create and find meaning and purpose in life.

A 10-SECOND EXERCISE

Much of the time, one part of the brain dominates. Uncontrolled rage, ravenous hunger or the health-eroding grind of stress takes over when the reptilian brain is in charge. If the limbic system is leading the way, we're filled with confidence or self-doubt, longing or delight. When the frontal cortex dominates, we plan and judge, seek knowledge and weigh costs against benefits.

Rudolph E. Tanzi, PhD, Joseph P. and Rose F. Kennedy Professor of Neurology at Harvard Medical School and director of the Genetics and Aging Research Unit at Massachusetts General Hospital, both in Boston. He is coauthor, with Deepak Chopra, MD, of *Super Brain*.

The brain actually is at its best when all three parts work together.

Examples: You're falling into the grip of reptilian drives when you become furious after receiving unfair criticism from your spouse. Or perhaps you've had two slices of pizza but a powerful craving for a third is about to take over. *To restore balance to your brain functions, think of the acronym STOP…*

• **Stop what you're doing.**

Take three deep breaths, then force yourself to "feel" a smile all through your body.

• **Observe yourself.** How do you feel now? Paying attention to your whole body takes you out of purely reptilian mode, bringing the limbic circuit and frontal cortex into the game. Think about what you're doing—and the consequences for your health and well-being.

• **Proceed with full awareness of yourself and those around you.** This simple 10-second process allows you to take charge of your brain.

WATCH OUT FOR THE "LOOPS"

Whatever has happened in your life has left its traces in your memory, regardless of whether you have conscious access to these thoughts.

The patterns, or "feedback loops," created by intricate connections within the brain are what shape the attitudes, beliefs, fears and desires we bring to new experiences. The limbic system takes over, and that's why if you were criticized regularly by parents for coming home with poor grades, a situation where you will be judged today is likely to activate old feelings of inadequacy and arouse fear and anxiety. You may see work demands as a trial, not a challenge. Or you may not try a new type of exercise for fear of failure.

Surprisingly, even positive feedback loops have a downside. When something feels good, you want to do it again and again. Unchecked, the limbic reward circuit can cause overindulgence that leads to health problems or even addiction.

What to do: Become aware of feedback loops—both positive and negative. Ask your-

self where the feeling is coming from and how past associations are shaping present feelings.

Simply observing and recognizing the source of these unproductive feelings will give your brain the new input it needs to begin changing the self-defeating circuits and start "rewiring" it with healthier connections and associations.

LET YOUR THOUGHTS RUN WILD

Einstein opened up his mind to all possibilities, which allowed his brain to form new neural connections that dramatically boosted his mental capacities.

You can do the same thing. When faced with a task or situation in which previous solutions have been unsatisfactory, the logical frontal cortex is likely to take over in an attempt to "figure out" an answer.

What to do: Instead of approaching such situations with logic alone, let your brain activity run wild—allow associations that might seem far-fetched, nonsensical or even outlandish to pop up. Step back and observe what emerges without judgment or fear of being foolish.

Then put your thinking brain to work in sifting through the creative work that the other part of your brain has done. You may very well discover interesting ideas, solutions to vexing problems and refreshing approaches.

How to Break a Bad Habit for Good—Hint: Willpower Won't Work

Charles Duhigg, an investigative journalist for *The New York Times,* New York City. He is author of the best-seller *The Power of Habit: Why We Do What We Do in Life and Business.* CharlesDuhigg.com

Almost all of us have bad habits that we have tried to break but can't. That's because we have relied on willpower. Willpower can be effective, but it's like a muscle that grows fatigued after a while, and we tend to slip back into old patterns.

I spent the past few years uncovering new scientific research on the neurology and psychology of habits. *The findings indicate a much more effective way to break bad habits...*

THE HABIT LOOP

Habits are neurological shortcuts that we use to save mental effort and get through life more efficiently. But the dependence on automatic routines—MIT researchers say more than 40% of our daily actions are habits—has a downside. Our brains go on autopilot, and we reach for a cigarette, bite our nails or turn on the TV without thinking.

Habits like these may seem complicated, but they all can be broken down into three components...

•**Cue,** which triggers an urge or a craving that we need to satisfy and causes a habitual behavior to unfold (for example, you feel sluggish and want to perk up).

•**Routine** or actual behavior you want to change (you reach for a can of cola).

•**Reward,** the deep-seated desire satisfied by your behavior (the soda's sugar, caffeine and fizziness energize you).

Over time, these three components become so intertwined and encoded in the structures of our brains that they form an intense loop of craving and anticipation of the associated reward.

STEP 1: ANALYZE THE LOOP

Awareness of the mechanisms of your own particular habit can make it easier to change...

•**Identify the routine.** It's the most obvious and visible part of the loop.

Example: Every day, I would get up from my desk at The New York Times building, wander to the cafeteria and eat a cookie while I chatted with whomever was there. I am a disciplined person, so it was frustrating and embarrassing that this daily habit had caused me to gain several pounds over the course of a year despite my efforts to resist. I would even put notes on my computer that read "No More Cookies." But most days, I gave in.

•**Isolate the cue.** Scientists have determined that almost all habitual cues fit into one

of five categories. Ask yourself the following questions when you feel an urge that sets off a behavior pattern—What time is it?...Where am I?...Who else is around?...What was I just doing?...What emotion am I feeling? One or more of the answers is your cue. It took me several days of self-observation to discover the trigger for my cookie binge. It would happen every day between 3 pm and 4 pm. I wasn't hungry or stressed out at the time, but I did feel isolated after working alone in my office for many hours.

•**Figure out the actual reward.** Because I wasn't eating cookies to stem my hunger, some other powerful craving was being satisfied. You can pinpoint the craving with some experimentation using alternate rewards.

Example: One day when I felt the urge to go to the cafeteria and get a cookie, I walked briskly around the block without eating anything. The next day, I brought a cookie from home and ate it at my desk. The day after, I had an apple and a cup of coffee with people at the cafeteria. After each experiment, I waited 15 minutes. If I still felt the urge to go to the cafeteria for a cookie, I assumed that the habit wasn't motivated by that particular reward. I soon realized what I was craving was the distraction and relief that came from socializing. Only after gossiping with colleagues in the cafeteria was I able to get back to work without further urges.

STEP 2: ADJUST THE ROUTINE

Trying to ignore my craving and suppress my behavior took what seemed like bottomless reserves of willpower. Studies suggested that I would have much more success if I tinkered with the routine, simply modifying it to be less destructive. That's the secret to gaining leverage—cues and rewards are primal needs that are difficult to deny, but routines are quite malleable and often can be replaced. Every afternoon when I felt the urge to have a cookie, I would visit the office of a friend and chat with him for at least 10 minutes.

STEP 3: GIVE IT TIME

My new behavior pattern, which I tracked on paper each day, still required effort and willpower. I often felt like slipping back into the old routine, and in fact, I did have setbacks, especially when I was under a lot of stress or out of my usual environment. But resisting the cookie was more manageable than applying blind discipline and writing notes to myself. Habits are an accretive process—each time you perform a modified loop, there is a thickening of neural pathways in the brain and the new behavior gets marginally easier. After about a month, I suddenly realized that I had a powerful craving to chat with a friend in the afternoon—but I no longer felt the urge to eat cookies.

Other helpful findings…

• **Begin with minor, easy-to-change habits.** A series of small wins makes you believe that you can cope with deeply entrenched cravings in a different way.

• **Get involved with others trying to break the same habit.** Becoming part of a like-minded social group provides more than just inspiration and a measure of accountability. Their experience is helpful in analyzing your cues and rewards and in suggesting alternative routines and behaviors.

CREATING GOOD HABITS

Trying to start a positive, new habit, such as exercising more or eating better, presents a different kind of challenge. Instead of analyzing and altering an existing loop, you have to establish one from scratch. *What works…*

• **Focus on "keystone" habits.** There are certain good habits that seem to echo through one's life and make it easier to change other habits. For instance, people who exercise regularly start eating better, stop using their credit cards quite so much, procrastinate less and have more patience with colleagues and family. Other keystone habits include a healthful, consistent sleep routine…maintaining good track of your finances…and keeping your living space organized.

• **Use a concrete and consistent cue.** Studies show that if you are hungry when you get home at the end of the day and there is nothing readily available to eat for dinner, you are much more likely to eat poorly. Just a simple cue like leaving vegetables out on the counter—even if you don't eat them—results in healthier eating.

Make sure that the reward you choose is something you really crave. For instance, you want to get in better shape. When you first start jogging or going to the gym, the rewards (such as losing weight or gaining more energy) may not happen quickly enough to keep you motivated or to turn the behavior into an automatic habit. You may need to trick your brain the first few weeks by rewarding yourself with something more lavish and immediate after you exercise, such as a piece of chocolate or a soak in a hot tub.

The Power (and Fun!) of Lucid Dreaming

Jayne Gackenbach, PhD, a professor of psychology at Grant MacEwan University in Edmonton, Alberta, Canada. She has done extensive research and writing on lucid dreaming and is coauthor of *Control Your Dreams*.

Imagine that you're standing on a mountaintop when an angry pit bull charges up and clamps its jaws around your hiking boot. You are terrified…but then you exclaim, "You're no real threat," and fearlessly grab the dog by the scruff of the neck and bring it up to eye level—at which point it licks your face like a friendly puppy.

This is a dream, but not the usual type of dream we all have several times a night. Instead, the scenario above illustrates a lucid dream, one that differs in an essential way from a regular dream or nightmare—because the lucid dreamer realizes that he or she is dreaming while the dream is occurring. And rather than being helpless to control the action, the lucid dreamer can actively work to influence the elements of the dream.

Though lucid dreaming sometimes occurs spontaneously, it is a skill you can develop—and doing so has valuable benefits, according to Jayne Gackenbach, PhD, a psychology professor and dream researcher at Grant MacEwan University in Edmonton, Alberta, Canada. While a regular dream might provide inspiration or insight, a lucid dream can deliberately focus that process, helping you to…

• **Face down nightmares,** diminishing their power to terrify—for instance, by letting you purposely turn that ferocious dream hound into a harmless pup.

• **Creatively solve real-life problems.** Lucid dreamers often actively look for and find in their dreams the answers to specific questions that eluded them when awake—about, say, how to improve their athletic performance or fix an error in a project they are working on. One reason this can happen is that, during dreaming, the mind handles many basic tasks involved in learning, memory and information processing.

• **Resolve psychological conflicts.**

Examples: If you're not sure whether you want to quit your job, you can rehearse your resignation in a lucid dream and see how it makes you feel. This might give you a more insightful result than simply imagining resigning while you are awake because dream images are so much more vivid than waking mental imagery. If you're struggling with grief, a lucid dream can provide an opportunity to feel as if you are saying the things you wish you had said to a loved one who has passed away…thus bringing a sense of closure.

• **Reduce anxiety and promote inner calm,** just as the stress-relieving technique of guided imagery does—because lucid dreaming is a particularly vivid form of imagery.

Have fun experiencing unlikely or impossible things, such as meeting a movie star, making love with an old flame or breathing underwater like a mermaid.

Dr. Gackenbach noted several ways to encourage lucid dreaming. She credited many ideas to psychophysiologist Stephen LaBerge, PhD, a pioneer in the field of lucid dreaming research, with whom she coedited the classic book *Conscious Mind, Sleeping Brain.*

To hone your lucid dreaming skills…

• **Get enough sleep.** Approximately every 90 minutes during sleep, you complete a cycle that includes light sleep, deep sleep and the rapid eye movement (REM) stage. While each 90-minute cycle includes each of these stages, the duration of the various stages changes through the night. The REM stage—which tends to produce dreams that are emotionally evocative and easiest to recall—lasts only about five minutes at the beginning of the night…but by early morning, REM may last half an hour or so. Therefore, if you don't have time for sufficient sleep, you cut off the longest dream stage. How much sleep is enough? According to the National Sleep Foundation, the average adult needs seven to nine hours of sleep per night.

• **Before you fall asleep, briefly focus on your goal for your lucid dream,** such as solving a particular problem or making an important decision—this increases the likelihood that you'll dream about that issue. If feelings that were stirred up during the day get in your way, write about those feelings in a journal to "clear your emotional slate," Dr. Gackenbach suggested—then you'll be better able to focus on your goal.

• **As soon as you wake up, try to recall your dreams.** Instead of jumping out of bed, lie quietly with your eyes closed and think about what you dreamed…or immediately write down your dreams in a journal. If no dream images come to mind, try to remember the mood or emotions of your dream.

Purpose: Developing dream recall skills helps you identify recurring features or patterns in your dreams, which prepares you for the technique below.

• **Learn to recognize your personal "dreamsigns."** Dr. LaBerge coined this term to refer to things that occur in dreams that are incongruent with waking life, such as flying like a bird…or objects or people that often recur in your dreams, such as zebras or a particular friend from childhood. Once you identify your dreamsigns, you are more likely to be able to say to yourself—while you are still asleep—"Oh, this must be a dream because I am seeing zebras." At that point, you have brought lucidity to your dream state!

When you realize that you are having a lucid dream, stay calm and focused. Dr. Gackenbach said that she used to get so excited upon recognizing that she was in the midst of a lucid dream that she would wake up.

Helpful: In his book *Exploring the World of Lucid Dreaming*, Dr. LaBerge suggests that you can prevent a premature awakening by stretching out the arms of your dream body and spinning like a top—perhaps because even imaginary spinning activates a mechanism in the inner ear believed to be associated with REM. Then you can continue with your lucid dream, deliberately directing the action in a way that brings you pleasure or lets you look for insights or answers to real-life problems.

Caution: Purposely exploring lucid dreaming is safe for most people. However, Dr. Gackenbach cautioned against it for anyone with schizophrenia, psychosis or a history of hallucinogenic drug use. For such people, lucid dreaming may contribute to confusion as to whether it is the dream world or the waking world that is real.

Solve Any Problem in Three Simple Steps

Ken Watanabe, author of the best-selling *Problem Solving 101: A Simple Book for Smart People.* He is founder and CEO of Delta Studio, an education, entertainment and media company in Tokyo. Formerly, he was a consultant at McKinsey & Co.

More than 10 years ago, Ken Watanabe, a Harvard MBA who worked at one of the world's leading consulting firms, walked away from a lucrative career to write a children's book. He was alarmed that school-age kids in his native Japan were good at memorizing large amounts of information but not very effective at applying it to real-life situations. He wanted to teach them in a fun way to broaden and organize their approach to problem-solving and become more proactive in shaping the world.

But something unexpected happened. Watanabe's 110-page book became a phenomenon among adults in Japan...and the country's best-selling business book of the year. Since then, it's been published in countries around the world, including the US.

Here are Ken Watanabe's secrets to problem-solving...

THE THREE STEPS

Good problem-solving isn't an innate talent. It comes from a way of thinking using a set of techniques that you can practice and improve upon. Most people rely too much on their instincts when they try to solve a problem, especially when they feel flustered or overwhelmed. They tend to grasp at the first or second solution that pops into their heads, even if it doesn't seem completely adequate.

I developed a simple, structured approach that works for addressing almost any kind of problem, big or small. In fact, I've used the same approach helping my Fortune 500 company clients as I do trying to fix the pepper shaker in my kitchen.

STEP 1: **Identify your problem and the root difficulties causing it.** People tend to think about their situations in such vague, universal terms that they get overwhelmed.

Example: You feel stressed and unhappy because you never have enough money each month. Stress and unhappiness are symptoms, not underlying problems that you can take action to remedy. You have to analyze more deeply. Is the actual problem that you're not earning enough money? Or is it that you're spending too much each month? To identify problems, I find it helpful to think of myself as a doctor trying to cure a patient. I list potential causes for a problem, arrive at a hypothesis for the most likely cause and focus on addressing that cause.

STEP 2: **Come up with multiple solutions.** List as many as you can, no matter how improbable. This often leads you to creative and unexpected solutions. Even if you think a particular solution may be the right one, get into the habit of challenging this conclusion. Ask yourself, What are the shortcomings of this solution? Is there a better way?

STEP 3: **Prioritize your actions and implement a plan.** After you select a solution, you need to follow through on it and be prepared to modify it—or replace it—until the problem is resolved.

MY FAVORITE TOOLS

I find that jotting down my thoughts and creating graphic representations of them are essential to breaking down problems into manageable parts and making sure that I explore every possible avenue…

• **The Logic Tree.** This is useful for clarifying your problem and its root causes.

How it works: Write your problem in a box on the left side of a piece of paper. Ask "Why?" you have that problem. For each answer, draw an arrow to the right, and put it in a box. Now ask "Why?" for each of the answers in the boxes. Keep repeating the process until you have identified all of the possible root causes of the problem.

The Logic Tree also can help you brainstorm a variety of solutions to a problem after you've identified the root cause.

Example: Say that you have determined from the first Logic Tree that the root cause of your money problems is that you don't track your spending well enough. Start a new Logic Tree for possible solutions. In a new box on the left side of a piece of paper, write "I need to track my money more carefully." Then ask "How?" Follow the same format as the first Logic Tree, answering every "How" until applicable solutions are determined.

• **Pros and cons box.** This is useful for evaluating which competing solutions are the best ones. The box allows you to line up and compare the benefits and drawbacks of possible solutions at a glance.

How it works: Draw three columns. Label the first "Possible Solutions," the second "Pros" and the third "Cons." List each solution, and fill in its corresponding pros and cons. You can further refine the process by marking each pro and con entry using a star system. Three stars is very attractive or very unattractive depending on whether it's in your pro or con list, two stars is moderately attractive/unattractive, one star is marginally attractive/unattractive.

• **Count the stars.** If they are in the pro column, more stars is good. If they are in the con column, more stars is bad.

MY PEPPER SHAKER PROBLEM

I had an expensive new pepper shaker that I had to shake and shake over my food just to get enough pepper out. It was a small problem, but one that annoyed me almost every day. I thought about throwing it out and buying a new pepper shaker, but that seemed like a waste. I decided to find out whether thinking through the problem in a structured way would allow me to find a more satisfying solution. A pepper shaker, of course, is trivial in the scheme of things, but the process used to solve the pepper shaker problem can solve any problem.

In this case, identifying the problem was easy—I wasn't getting enough pepper from my pepper shaker.

Possible root causes…

• **I need too much pepper on my food.** I rejected this because I really like pepper on my food and didn't want to change my preferences. My tastes were not the issue.

• **I wasn't shaking the shaker long enough or hard enough.** I dismissed this cause, too, because I felt that giving one or two vigorous shakes should be sufficient.

• **The small openings on the top of the pepper shaker were too small.** Yes, this seemed like the most reasonable cause. I decided to pursue this line of thought and develop solutions.

Possible solutions…

• **Buy a new pepper shaker with larger openings.** I had already rejected the idea of buying a new one.

• **Increase the amount of pepper that was coming out of the shaker.** Yes, this seemed promising, but how to do it?

I had to continue generating more refined solutions.

Possible refined solutions…

• **Increase the number of holes in the shaker by poking more of them.** I didn't want to do this, because it would ruin the look of my nice pepper shaker.

- **Make each existing hole bigger.** No, again for the same reason.
- **Use more finely ground pepper.** Yes, that seemed like the smartest, most practical idea.

I then put the solution into action. I called the store to check whether it carried finely ground pepper—it did. I stopped by the store on the way home from work.

Unleash the Power of Your Brain to Lose Weight Once and for All

Rudolph E. Tanzi, PhD, the Joseph P. and Rose F. Kennedy Professor of Neurology at Harvard University and director of the Genetics and Aging Research Unit at Massachusetts General Hospital, both in Boston. He is coauthor, with Deepak Chopra, MD, of *Super Brain: Unleashing the Explosive Power of Your Mind to Maximize Health, Happiness, and Spiritual Well-Being.*

Think about all of the changes that you make when you're trying to lose weight. You change your food choices, serving sizes and daily calories. The pounds come off—only to come back on again.

Reason: You haven't made the most important change of all—to your brain. There could be an imbalance in the brain's circuitry. The areas that trigger impulsive behavior have been strengthened from years of bad habits, while the areas that control rational decision-making have been weakened.

Everyone knows the weight-loss basics. The challenge is to restore mental balance so that you automatically make healthier choices. *What to do…*

LOOK AT YOUR FEELINGS

When you wish to eat, ask yourself whether you really are hungry. Pay attention to your stomach. Is it full or empty? Ask yourself, Do I really need food right now?

People often eat for reasons that have nothing to do with hunger. We eat when we're upset, frustrated, bored, etc. The act of eating is a distraction from uncomfortable feelings and a coping mechanism that makes the feelings less intense.

Studies have shown that mood strongly affects food choices. One study published in *American Demographics* found that people gravitate toward ice cream and cookies when they're sad…potato chips when they're bored… and pizza or steak when they're happy.

My advice: Before you eat anything, seriously ask yourself why you want it. If you haven't eaten for several hours, you're probably just hungry. But if you're craving a snack even though you ate recently, you're probably dealing with emotional hunger. Ask yourself, How am I feeling about the world today?…What's my mood?…What do I really need at this particular moment?…Does my stomach feel empty?

When you eat only when you're hungry and you don't use food for an emotional fix, you've achieved homeostasis, a type of mind-body balance in which you desire only what you need.

Imagine a single cell floating in a petri dish. It doesn't think about food. It takes in nutrients when it needs them and stops when it has had enough. It is in a perfect state of homeostasis.

You can achieve the same harmony by being self-aware, or mindful.

What to do: Suppose that you come home from work and already are anticipating the taste of chocolate. Don't go straight to the pantry. Instead, run through the mindful list. If you determine that you are experiencing only emotional hunger, take three very deep breaths and smile. This simple exercise can make the craving go away. It also works if you've already started eating and don't want to overeat.

DON'T RESIST

It's human nature to crave what you can't have, so forcing yourself to resist may not be the answer. Whatever you resist persists. So if you've gone through your mindful eating list and still feel like eating, don't fight the feeling.

Even if you know that you tend to eat more on those days when nothing's going right, it's better to lose the battle than to lose the war.

Instead of resisting, try to reshape your brain. Focus on awareness, not resistance.

Example: You're standing in front of the refrigerator, staring at a slice of pecan pie. You go through your mindful checklist and realize that you're not really hungry, but it's been a lousy day and that pecan pie sure will make you feel better. Go ahead and eat it, but be mindful of why you are eating it. This will train your brain about when and how you wish to eat.

Maintaining a healthy weight is a lifelong endeavor. You can't spend your entire life fighting urges. What you can do is gradually become more aware of your feelings…know when you're weak…and learn not to depend on food to get you through. Along the way, you will train your brain to eat healthier.

EAT MUCH MORE SLOWLY

Many people race through meals. By the time they realize that they are full and the appropriate message is sent to the brain, they've already consumed hundreds of extra calories—and later feel bloated and uncomfortable.

In a recent study, researchers found that people who ate quickly consumed 55% more food per minute than those who ate slowly. In the study, people who ate slowly consumed two ounces of food per minute. Those who ate a little more quickly consumed 2.5 ounces per minute…and those who really gobbled their food consumed 3.1 ounces per minute.

Hunger and eating involve a balancing act between two hormones. While you're eating, the hormone that stimulates appetite, ghrelin, starts to decline. At the same time, the hormone that suppresses appetite, leptin, starts to rise. The hormones work together to control how much you eat. But they take time to work. If you're a fast eater, they can't keep up—and you wind up consuming more calories than your body needs.

My advice: Eat slowly and mindfully. Enjoy each bite of food. Notice the smell, texture and taste. Don't take another bite until you've thoroughly chewed the previous bite.

Ideally, you should take at least 20 minutes to eat a meal. That's about how long it takes for the hormones to send the appropriate signals to the brain.

Try This Memory Trick to Get Motivated to Exercise

Mathew Biondolillo, PhD, and David Pillemer, EdD, Dr. Samuel E. Paul Professor of Developmental Psychology, department of psychology, University of New Hampshire, Durham. Their study was published in *Memory*.

Remember the fun you had when biking off to a special place with your best friend when you were a kid? Or how about the fabulous time you had playing volleyball or soccer at the family picnic? What about the anniversary party where you "cut a rug"?

On the other hand, can you stand to recall the stress and embarrassment of dropping a winning catch in a childhood ball game…or the hell you went through running an obstacle course during basic training?

Researchers studied whether vividly remembering exercising could motivate people to actually exercise. They recruited 186 volunteers, divided them into three groups and had them fill out questionnaires that assessed how they felt about exercise and quizzed them on their exercise habits. Then, depending on their group assignment, the volunteers were asked to describe a positive exercise-related memory (Group 1) or a negative exercise-related memory (Group 2) or were not queried at all about memories (Group 3). Groups 1 and 2 were instructed to be as detailed and specific as possible about their memories and were asked questions intended to really get them to relive the recalled events. *Specifically, they were asked…*

• **To gauge how vivid their memories were and how intense the positive (or negative) feelings in them were.**

• **Whether the recalled events were typical experiences for them,** how they felt while recalling the memories and whether looking back at the memories made them feel self-sufficient or competent.

Eight days after completing the questionnaire and memory-recall exercise, the volunteers were asked to describe their exercise activity for the previous week and also mention whether the memories they had drummed up had helped motivate them.

THE MYSTERY OF MOTIVATION

The folks in the positive-memory group exercised the most—they exercised 17% more intensely than the negative-memory group and 47% more intensely than the no-memory group, which in itself is an interesting look at how the simple act of recalling positive efforts can motivate us to repeat, in some form, those efforts.

But what's especially interesting is that even people in the negative-memory group exercised more than people in the no-memory group. In fact, volunteers who had been asked to relive painful exercise memories in excruciating detail went right out and exercised 26% more intensely than the group that had not recalled any memories.

Since none of the volunteers reported consciously using a memory that had been thought up the week before as motivation to exercise, something more subtle must have been going on in the volunteers' minds. Recalling either a positive or negative memory about exercise may have prompted feelings—even on a subconscious level—about self-worth and encouragement or desire for self-improvement that translated into motivation to exercise.

Hypnotists and hypnotherapists, however, know that when people remember and visualize a practiced activity in detail (be it playing tennis or the trombone or giving a speech), they not only are more likely to do the activity, they're more likely to do it just as well as if they had been physically practicing it.

The takeaway? If, for whatever reason, you aren't naturally inclined to be physically active—which is vital for good health—you now have a shockingly simple and effective way to change that. You can take a tip from this study and give yourself some quiet time a few days a week to vividly recall a memory—the better, the more motivating—of a time when you

were very physically active. Really immerse yourself in the memory. Relive it. What did the event feel like when it was happening, and how do you feel looking back on it? Then let the mysteries of the mind do their magic.

Retrain Your Brain and Break Free from the Patterns That Are Holding You Back

Rebecca Gladding, MD, former staff psychiatrist with the Veterans Administration California Healthcare System. She recently served as a clinical instructor and medical director of the UCLA Adult Inpatient Eating Disorders Program. She is coauthor of You Are Not Your Brain: The 4-Step Solution for Changing Bad Habits, Ending Unhealthy Thinking, and Taking Control of Your Life.

Habits are hard to break because of the way the brain is wired. Each time you repeat a harmful behavior—overeating, overspending, procrastinating or something else—the brain circuits involved in that action become stronger. The brain associates the action with the situation that gave rise to it, such as being under stress. Over time, the brain becomes hardwired to choose that behavior automatically any time a similar situation arises.

Example: If you reach for a sugary snack whenever you are worried about a project at work, after a while, you may crave sugar the moment that you start feeling anxious about anything anywhere.

That's the bad news.

The good news: You can rewire your brain to choose constructive habits…

STEP 1: RELABEL

Negative habits are triggered by deceptive brain messages—thoughts, beliefs and impulses that run counter to your positive, healthy intentions. These thoughts and urges are accompanied by unpleasant emotions or physical sensations such as anger, sadness, anxiety or fatigue. Because the discomfort is so intense, you are driven to get rid of it as fast as you can, usually by indulging in an unhealthy habit. This brings temporary relief but in reality makes the situation worse—each time you give in, you further strengthen the brain pathways that connect the thought or urge with the bad habit.

Relabeling means recognizing your impulses and negative thoughts as deceptive brain messages and calling them what they are. It means simply noting to yourself what is happening, such as, *I am having a craving even though I just ate 30 minutes ago* or *My boss just yelled at me, and because of that, now I need some chocolate.* The more you are aware of these habits, the more opportunities you have to stop acting on them.

Becoming aware of these messages can be challenging at first. *To develop your ability to relabel…*

●**Practice making mental notes.** Any time you feel "off" or uneasy in some way, notice what is going on in your body or mind, and pick a simple word or phrase to describe it. For example, if you notice that you are thinking about a conversation with a friend that went awry—when you really need to be working—say to yourself, *Mind wandering.* If you are having physical symptoms, such as heart pounding, shakiness, feeling a pit in your stomach, note this as anxiety. The key is to snap yourself back into awareness—which is the first step toward doing something about the situation in a healthy, productive way.

●**Focus on your breathing.** One way to enhance your ability to notice what's happening in a moment-to-moment way is by focusing on your breath. For five minutes, sit in a quiet place, close your eyes and simply pay attention to your breath as you inhale and exhale. What you will find as you try to do this is that your brain is constantly running, thinking about plans for later in the week or stressing about what you have to do today. Whenever you realize that you have become lost in thought in these ways, say to yourself, *Thinking* or *Planning* or *Wandering,* then gently turn your focus back to your breathing.

Do this focused breathing exercise once a day, and gradually extend the length of time to 20 or 30 minutes.

STEP 2: REFRAME

As you become aware of deceptive brain messages, you can begin changing your perception of their importance. You do this by reframing—challenging your default response.

Reframing does not mean denying the existence of a thought or impulse or judging yourself for having it. Instead, you look at the thought from a new perspective and diminish its importance so that you do not automatically react in your habitual way.

Example: I feel upset right now, but that doesn't mean I have to have a cigarette (or that I am a bad person because I am craving one).

To change your perspective…

●**Use distancing phrases.** When you notice a deceptive brain message, say to yourself, *That's not me, it's just my brain…*or *Oh, that's just mental chatter…*or *I'm having a bad brain day.*

●**Look for thinking errors.** We often make inaccurate assumptions about difficult situations and painful feelings. To uncover these erroneous, unhelpful thoughts, ask yourself nonjudgmental questions, such as, *What is it about this situation that is upsetting me? What am I telling myself about what is happening? What are some other interpretations?*

Common thinking errors include…

All-or-nothing thinking: Seeing situations and people in extremes, such as perfect or hopeless, all good or all bad.

Worst-case thinking: Assuming that something terrible inevitably is going to happen.

Discounting the positive: Ignoring your good qualities and failing to notice or take seriously other people's positive reactions toward you.

●**Be compassionate with yourself.** Write down the deceptive brain message—the thought, sensation or impulse—that is bothering you. Then ask yourself what a kindhearted friend would advise or think.

●**Use the 15-minute rule.** When you experience an especially powerful impulse, try to wait 15 minutes before you act. Then if you still cannot resist the urge, slowly and mindfully engage in the activity that your deceptive brain message is insisting upon.

Important: Do not try to talk yourself out of an uncomfortable feeling. Simply examine it. You are training yourself to be less frightened of discomfort, to learn that it will pass and that it is not such a big deal.

STEP 3: REFOCUS

Once you have relabeled and reframed a deceptive brain message, you may find it surprisingly easy to actively shift your attention to a healthy, constructive activity—even as your deceptive thoughts are urging you to act in your old, habitual way. By refocusing repeatedly, you weaken the brain circuits associated with your cravings and retrain your brain to choose healthier responses when you are stressed or sad.

The best refocusing activities are ones that engage and interest you. If they require strategy or learning something new, they will be even more effective, but any wholesome activity that you enjoy is fine.

Examples: Do a crossword puzzle…read… exercise…call a friend…play with a pet…sing a song…pursue a hobby…cook a healthy recipe.

If you are at work, refocus on a task that you can accomplish quickly or that is less demanding.

What makes this step powerful is that you allow uncomfortable sensations and impulses to be present…but then you act constructively anyway. You are learning that the messages do not have to dominate your attention or control your actions. You are training your brain to create new associations between thoughts and healthy actions. This takes patience.

STEP 4: REVALUE

The final step is really about gaining perspective and the strength to believe in yourself. Each person gets there at his/her own pace, and when you do, you can look at the deceptive brain message and unhelpful impulses and simply say to yourself, *This is nothing more than the feeling of a deceptive brain message. I do not have to act on it, and it does not define me.* The more you are able to relabel, reframe and refocus, the more empowered you will be to dismiss those deceptive brain messages and move on with your life in a positive direction—one that you define. That's the essence of revalue and the goal of the four steps.

Jack Canfield's Seven Principles of Success and Happiness

Jack Canfield, motivational speaker and cocreator of the *Chicken Soup for the Soul*® series, which has sold more than 80 million books. He is CEO of Chicken Soup for the Soul Enterprises, a publishing and training company in Santa Barbara, California. JackCanfield.com

J ack Canfield has made the study of success in one's personal and professional lives his own life's work. He has interviewed hundreds of successful people, read more than 3,000 books on success and given thousands of lectures on the topic. *Here Canfield reveals the principles of success that are most often overlooked…*

• **Develop four new good habits each year.** Most of everything we do is based on ritual. We eat at certain restaurants…wear certain clothes…brush our teeth in a certain way… and watch certain TV shows simply because that is what we have always done. These are our habits, and we perform them without really thinking.

The trouble with habits is that they preserve the status quo, making dramatic improvement unlikely. If we want more out of life, we must be willing to evaluate and replace some of our rituals with more productive ones.

Example: Instead of spending the hour after dinner watching TV, go for a brisk walk… study a second language…read a book…or make the extra sales calls that you need to advance your career.

It takes a minimum of 25 days for the brain to build the neural links required to make a new behavior a habit. I suggest practicing a new habit for three months to ensure that it sinks in. Once it becomes second nature, add another new habit. At three months per habit, there's time to add four each year. In five years, you will have 20 new habits that will help fuel your success.

• **Practice appreciation.** Studies of employee motivation inevitably find that feeling appreciated is the single greatest motivator in the workplace, even ahead of higher wages. Yet many people fail to put the power of appreciation to full use in their business and personal lives.

When you show people that you appreciate them, you not only make them feel better, you make yourself more successful. People are more likely to help you achieve your goals if they believe that you appreciate their efforts. There's no downside—appreciation costs nothing, and no one has ever complained about being overappreciated.

Helpful: I used to carry in my pocket an index card with 10 circles on it. Every time I let someone know that I appreciated him/her, I filled in one of the circles. If at the end of the day I hadn't filled in all 10, I sent out appreciative e-mails. After a few months, showing appreciation became second nature for me, and I no longer had to carry the cards. I haven't had anyone leave my nine-employee company in more than five years. I attribute a big part of that loyalty to everyone feeling appreciated.

• **Solicit and respect feedback.** Rather than guess how you're doing, ask. Periodically ask employees, employers, customers and loved ones to rate your performance on a scale of one to 10. If the answer is anything less than 10, ask, "What would it take to make it a 10?"

If you follow this strategy, you're encouraging people to help you become great. The main reason that people don't solicit feedback is because they're afraid of what they might hear—but the information we can obtain is worth facing such fears.

Not all feedback is accurate, but watch for patterns and never get angry at the source, even if you disagree.

• **Keep all of your agreements.** When you break an agreement, the person you let down loses faith in you and is less likely to want to work with you in the future. Even more important, you lose some faith in yourself. It's all but impossible to become a success if you don't have faith in yourself.

To avoid breaking agreements, teach yourself to say no to things that you would rather not do. Then you won't have to back out later. Write down everything you agree to do on your calendar as soon as a commitment is made—you would be surprised by how many people don't do this.

If you must break an agreement, let the other parties involved know as soon as possible, and do everything in your power to fix any problems that the broken agreement creates for them.

• **Exceed expectations.** Don't ask yourself, *How can I get a little more out of this situation?* Instead, ask, *How can I give a little more to those around me?* Sacrificing usually isn't a sacrifice—it's a path to success. If you consistently go the extra mile for clients, colleagues, employers, family and friends, you'll earn their loyalty for life.

Example: When UPS went on strike, David Morris, the owner of Dillanos, a small, Seattle-based coffee roasting company, rented a truck and drove 2,320 miles to deliver an order to a small client in Southern California. That client, It's a Grind Coffee House, is now a large franchise with 50 stores and an additional 100 planned. It is Dillanos's largest customer and has remained loyal to Dillanos because of the extra effort Morris put in years ago.

• **Reject rejection.** Rejection does not prevent success—fear of rejection does. What stops a man from asking an attractive woman out on a date? What stops an inexperienced salesman from asking the most successful salesman at his firm for advice? They're afraid of rejection—afraid that if they ask, the answer might be no. But there's absolutely no rational reason to fear rejection.

Example: You ask a successful person to give you career advice, and he says no. You didn't have his advice before you asked, and you don't have his advice after. You're no worse off than when you began, so why be afraid of asking?

If you want to be a success, you must treat rejection as an illusion—a negative response conjured up by your mind that really doesn't exist.

- **Eliminate small obstacles.** Make a list of the problems that you would like to remove from your life—include even minor things, such as a lamp that doesn't work right. Schedule a day or two to fix as many of these problems as you can, starting with the easiest to solve.

In this way, you'll get into the habit of thinking, *I know what I want, I know how to get it.* Once you're in this mindset, you'll stop resigning yourself to your current situation and start making larger positive changes as well.

The Amazing Power of Affirmations

Louise L. Hay, one of the founders of the self-help movement. She is author of numerous books, including *You Can Heal Your Life*, which has sold more than 50 million copies. She is founder and head of Hay House, Inc., a self-help publishing company, Carlsbad, California, whose best-selling authors include Wayne Dyer and Joan Borysenko. LouiseHay.com

Affirmations are statements that reflect our views of who we are and what we want. They can be positive or negative. They influence our feelings and thoughts—and what actually happens in our lives.

Example: I grew up in an abusive family. As a child, I believed that it was natural for men to beat women. As I went though life, I always attracted men who abused me. It wasn't until I learned about self-esteem and self-worth that I let go of that pattern of thinking. As a result, I started to attract men who valued and respected me.

Positive affirmations don't miraculously create a new reality—but they do open the mental channels that can allow good things to happen. People who are happy and self-confident welcome good things into their lives. They attract positive people. They create their own opportunities. *Here's how…*

- **Turn a negative into a positive.** Statements such as, "I don't want to be fat," "I don't like this relationship" or "I don't want to be unhappy"

are actually negative affirmations. Dwelling on things that we don't want merely creates more mental space for those things to thrive.

When delivered as positive affirmations, the statements above become "I am slender," "I have a wonderful new relationship" and "I am happy."

- **Train yourself.** Most of us have trained ourselves to be self-critical. We can just as easily train ourselves to be accepting.

Exercise: For the next month, say a few hundred times a day, "I approve of myself." Repeat it out loud or to yourself when you're in the shower, walking to the mailbox, etc.

At first, you'll probably notice that repeating this mantra brings up opposite feelings. You'll find yourself thinking, *I don't believe it* or *Saying this makes me feel silly.*

These are resistance thoughts. Let them pass through your mind. They have no power unless you choose to believe them. Counter them with the original mantra, *I approve of myself.* Your thinking will start to change.

- **Look in the mirror every morning and say, "I really love you."** Do this—and use your name. The universe loves gratitude and appreciation. Appreciating yourself means appreciating the universe.

Imagine that you give someone a gift. If that person is grateful and appreciative, you want to give him/her more presents. But if he is negative about it and says something like, "I don't like the color," you won't want to be so generous again.

When you love yourself, you're thanking the universe for the wonderful gift that is you—and more gifts will come your way.

- **Say "thank you."** I say "thank you" to the universe at least a dozen times a day—when I see the beauty of a tree, a breathtaking sunset, etc. The more grateful you are for the good things in your life, the more life gives you to appreciate.

If you want a joyous life, you must think joyous thoughts.

Example: Some people notice that it's raining and say, "What a lousy day." It's not a lousy day. It's merely a wet day. There are lots of good things to do on rainy days. Why greet it with despair?

• **Eliminate "should" thinking.** Many people force themselves to do things that they dislike, because someone (often a parent) said they should do them—go to a certain school, become a lawyer, marry a particular person, etc.

Better: Replace "should" with "could." The word "could" means that you have choices… that you can follow your own judgment and listen to your instincts.

Exercise: Write the phrase "I should" at the top of a piece of paper, followed by five or six ways to finish the sentence.

Examples: "I should be thin"…"I should be smarter"…"I should have more money now." You'll probably find that most of the items reflect your own fears and imagined limitations.

Now, instead of writing "I should," substitute it with, "If I really wanted to, I could…"

Examples: "If I really wanted to, I could be thin"…"If I really wanted to, I could be smarter"…"If I really wanted to, I could have more money now."

• **Tell yourself it's easy.** Several times a day, tell yourself how easy it is to do something. "It's easy to have good friends"…"It's easy to find a job I love"…"It's easy to bring good into my life."

This type of affirmation is one of the simplest—and most powerful. We tend to think that things are much more difficult than they really are. The fear of difficulty is really the fear of trying, which keeps us from moving forward.

• **Learn from failure.** The fear of failure can be paralyzing. How many times have you been too afraid to try something new?

We encourage children when they're learning to walk. Every tiny step is a success! Yet we're not so kind to ourselves. We tell ourselves that we're clumsy or stupid…that our initial, halting steps are a failure.

Not true. Every experience that we have is a learning experience. We get better with practice…discover new strengths…and find opportunities.

Exercise: Several times a day, use "success affirmations." Say things such as, "Everything I touch is a success"…"I am blessed beyond my fondest dreams"…and "Golden opportunities are everywhere for me."

Much of life is a rehearsal, a time to make mistakes, try new approaches and learn how to make things better. Everything brings us closer to success.

• **Forgive others and yourself.** We give away our power when we harbor anger toward people and events from the past. Maybe you had an unhappy childhood…an abusive spouse…a job that didn't work out. Let it all go.

Dwelling on old hurts never makes people happy. Worse, it hampers the ability to enjoy the future because you stop believing that you—and only you—can make things better.

Forgiving doesn't mean forgetting or condoning bad behavior. The goal is to free yourself from negativity.

Exercise: Sit with your eyes closed and say, "The person I need to forgive is so-and-so, and I forgive him/her." Repeat it over and over for five to 10 minutes. Then turn your attention inward and take a minute or two to forgive yourself for things you've done.

Repeat this exercise at least once a week. Do it for every injustice or hurt that you still feel. You'll come to realize that the past doesn't control your present…and that you have the inner strength to make yourself happy.

Teach Your Brain to Be More Organized

Margaret Moore, MBA, CEO, Wellcoaches Corporation, codirector, Institute of Coaching, McLean Hospital (Harvard Medical School-affiliated), Belmont, Massachusetts, and Paul G. Hammerness, MD, assistant professor, psychiatry, Harvard Medical School, and specialist in psychiatry, Boston Children's Hospital, both in Boston. Ms. Moore and Dr. Hammerness are coauthors of *Organize Your Mind, Organize Your Life*.

Many self-help books and seminars include advice like "buy a bunch of baskets to sort your mail," "use an electronic calendar," "color-code your e-mails" and "multitask so things don't pile up."

However, a recent book on the subject—*Organize Your Mind, Organize Your Life*—has a surprise inside.

The authors refute pretty much all the organization advice that we've ever heard. They claim that to get more organized, we need to start by organizing our brains—in other words, a frenzied and scattered mind is what truly leads to a messy life.

The coauthors of the book, Margaret Moore, MBA, an executive wellness coach and codirector of the Institute of Coaching at McLean Hospital—a pioneering hospital in terms of instituting psychological interventions—in Belmont, Massachusetts, and Paul Hammerness, MD, assistant professor of psychiatry at Harvard Medical School in Boston, who has spent a lot of time researching attention-deficit/hyperactivity disorder (ADHD) and how the brain gets distracted, explained how they translated complex brain science into easy-to-follow, powerful tactics that may help people regain control over their lives…

THREE SIMPLE STEPS
TO BETTER ORGANIZATION

What do the authors mean by "organized?" Let's face it, if you want to get things done, you do have to have a calendar, a place for your mail, etc.! But while those things can be helpful, they're all useless if your brain itself isn't focused. For example, you can schedule all sorts of tasks on your calendar, but if you can't learn how to manage your attention span, then you won't finish any of the tasks. *So here's how to control your ability to concentrate…*

STEP 1: **Calm the brain.** You can't properly focus when you're overwhelmed, anxious, sad or frustrated by, say, work or family issues, said Dr. Hammerness. The solution to this is taking a "brain break"—instead of dwelling on the stress and becoming paralyzed by thoughts of your sick mother, for instance, or the fact that you didn't get a raise last year, spend two minutes doing something totally different that will distract you from thinking those thoughts. This could include exercise

(such as a brisk walk, a stair climb or anything that gets your blood pumping)…closing your eyes and breathing deeply…listening to calming music…calling a friend (short conversation, please!)…or gazing at and appreciating a photo or flower on your desk. This brain break will cleanse your mental palate and put you in a more positive state of mind, giving you a fighting chance to refocus on the task at hand, said Dr. Hammerness.

You may have to experiment to find out what sorts of brain breaks work for you. But that's no burden—they last only two minutes each.

STEP 2: **Sustain your attention.** Lots of organization gurus recommend "chunking" tasks into short bursts as a way to feel less intimidated by large projects. But five or 10 minutes on a complicated task such as writing a business report or planning an event often doesn't cut it, because large projects require creative problem-solving and extensive, adventurous explorations of thought, not just fragments of attention.

Solution: Tell yourself that you'll give 30 consecutive minutes or, better yet, a full hour to your next big priority (you can even set a timer)—and then follow through. That means close your door and ignore (or shut off) the phone ringer, e-mail and text notifications, Facebook status updates, tweets, background music or TV noise, and all other potential distractions. This step takes self-discipline, but Moore says that it'll teach you mindfulness. In other words, we usually drift in and out of tasks, letting each interruption steal us away from whatever we were working on, and then we wonder where the time went. But by blocking out larger chunks of time, you'll pay more attention to the project at hand and make more of each passing minute.

STEP 3: **To stay on track, file away new ideas.** Say you're finally starting to clean out your garage one morning (a task that you've been trying to complete for months) and you think of a great recipe that you want to make for dinner that evening. Your first impulse might be to put down your trash bag so you can run to the supermarket to buy those ingredients—and you might be telling yourself, "Better do it before I forget."

That's a trap. "Many people fear that they'll forget important information if they don't act on it immediately—leading them to jump sporadically from action to action," Dr. Hammerness said. "But many people remember more than they think if they just try it."

Here's an experiment: Try trusting yourself to remember your new thoughts so that you can act on them later. Regularly getting seven to eight hours of sleep will help with that. But if, after several weeks, you find that too many of your new ideas end up slipping away, then go ahead and make a habit of writing them down.

While having some physical system for keeping track of things is critical for most people, no system will work if your brain isn't ready to engage and do its part.

How to Make Positive Thinking Work for You

Gabriele Oettingen, PhD, professor of psychology at New York University, New York City, and University of Hamburg in Germany. She is author of *Rethinking Positive Thinking: Inside the New Science of Motivation.* WOOPMyLife.org

We're often told to think positive. Whether we want to lose weight…quit smoking…negotiate a raise or promotion…achieve great wealth…or get elected president, we're assured that the key is to ignore self-doubt, banish pessimism and believe that we can do it.

But positive thinking leads to productive action only if we know how to handle it. If we don't, pie-in-the-sky daydreams and unbridled optimism are more likely to lead to stagnancy than success. For example, a recent study found that people were less likely to make a substantial donation to a charity if they first fantasized that the problem the charity addresses had been solved. Indulging in

the positive-thinking fantasy gave their minds the same positive feelings that they would have experienced if they actually had helped solve the problem, robbing them of the drive to take action.

Or consider the upcoming presidential election. Some of the candidates are relentlessly positive about what they could achieve if they are elected—an attitude that whips up crowds and attracts admirers.

The problem: The more an incoming president displays positive thinking, the worse the country seems to do. A 2014 study published in *Psychological Science* examined inaugural addresses from 1933 to 2009 and found that the more idealistic a portrait a president paints, the higher the unemployment rate and the lower the gross domestic product during the ensuing four years. That may be because an overly idealistic president might be more likely to ignore the obstacles…downplay the necessary steps to achieve the economic goals…and pursue risky ventures.

So how do you employ positive thinking as a powerful force? The key is to use it as part of the following four-step strategy, which has been shown to actually increase our odds of taking productive action and achieving a goal…

•**Identify a goal.** Choose something you would like to achieve, whether you call it a "goal" or a "wish." This could be a short-term goal—something you could accomplish today—or a long-term goal that will take much longer. Your goal should be something that you believe you can realistically accomplish but that is somewhat challenging to you. Boil your goal down to a phrase of just three to six words.

Examples: "Book a trip" or "Lose five pounds."

•**Picture the best outcome.** Now imagine what it would be like if your wish came true in the very best possible way. How would you feel? How would your life change?

Let yourself mentally experience this imagined outcome. Revel in it for a few minutes. This helps link the wish to pleasurable feelings in your mind—indulging in fantasies can feel wonderful. Your blood pressure actually might drop, enveloping you in a sense of calm and contentment.

Dreamers tend not to progress beyond this stage, but two crucial steps remain to maximize your odds of making your wish come true.

• **Picture your greatest internal obstacle.** As soon as you stop fantasizing about the best possible outcome of your wish, ask yourself, *What one thing in me is most holding me back from making this wish come true?*

The goal here is to uncover your main internal obstacle, not an external one. If you see an external force as your main hindrance, there's a good chance that the problem will seem insurmountable. If you see something within yourself as the main problem, there's a good chance you will be able to develop a solution.

Example: If your wish is to get a promotion at work, the first obstacle that comes to mind might be, *My boss is a fool who does not appreciate me.* This is not the obstacle you need to identify—a foolish boss is an external problem. Make this obstacle internal by rephrasing it as, *I feel resentment toward my boss that makes it hard for me to earn his respect.*

Your internal obstacle might be instantly obvious, or it might take time to figure out. If it proves elusive, seek it through quiet, private contemplation. Do not ask other people for their input—your odds of understanding and overcoming the obstacle are much higher if you discover it yourself. If you're not certain whether you have identified the critical internal obstacle, you probably haven't—there's usually a "That's it!" moment of revelation when you have discovered it.

Helpful: People often initially conclude that their main obstacle is, *I don't have time to pursue the goal.* These people may want to dig deeper into why they can't seem to find the time. For example, someone might realize that he/she cannot find time to pursue his wish because he devotes lots of time to helping other people pursue their wishes…and that he does this because he fears not being needed. That

fear is a major obstacle. Someone else might realize that he is not finding time for a project because he is afraid of failing.

Boil your obstacle down to three to six words, then spend some time thinking about it. Picture how this obstacle stands in your way, stopping you from reaching your goal.

This reduces the odds that your mind will be satisfied with mere fantasy and helps you do what it takes to make the wish a reality.

Once you have identified and pictured your obstacle, you might realize that you need to modify or even switch your goal because the obstacle is so formidable that you can't overcome it—or the goal is just not worth pursuing.

Example: Your wish is to get up each morning and exercise. Your obstacle is that you feel distracted by everything you have to do during the day. Perhaps it makes sense to change your initial wish to "exercise in the evenings."

• **Develop a plan to overcome your obstacle.** This plan should fit a simple if/then format—If [obstacle X occurs], then I will [take action Y].

Example: If I feel insecure when someone questions my proposal, then I will remind myself that I am just as knowledgeable on this topic as anyone.

Developing a plan in advance to overcome your internal obstacle will not just help you overcome this obstacle…it may improve your odds of overcoming any obstacle that appears. The process of obstacle identification and if/then planning described above trains the mind to look for and get past obstacles, rather than get stopped by them on a non-conscious level.

Helpful: Find a quiet moment each day to identify your goal, your best outcome, your central internal obstacle and your if/then plan. By practicing this procedure every day, you will be much more successful in understanding your wishes and attaining your goals.

The Secret to Stopping Negative Thinking: Toss Those Thoughts in the Trash

Richard E. Petty, PhD, professor and chair, department of psychology, The Ohio State University, Columbus. His study (done in collaboration with Spanish colleagues Pablo Briñol, Margarita Gascó Rivas and Javier Horcajo) was published in *Psychological Science*.

Have you tried to talk yourself out of unwanted negative thinking—those inner diatribes against your own body, likability, accomplishments or luck, for instance, or against someone or something else—but had little success? It could be because your inner pep talks lack one simple yet crucial physical element, a recent series of three fascinating experiments shows.

The missing key: A garbage can! Here's what the researchers discovered about how a trash can help halt inner trash talk…

EXPERIMENT #1: **Body blues.** Participants were given sheets of paper and instructed to spend three minutes writing down thoughts about their own bodies. Some participants were asked to write positive thoughts…others were asked to write negative thoughts. Next, within each group, half of the participants were told to reread what they had written, contemplate those thoughts, then review what they'd written for spelling and grammar errors. The other half of the participants were told to reread and contemplate their thoughts, then to rip up their papers and throw them into a garbage can. Afterward, all participants answered various body-image questionnaires that used nine-point scales to assess how much each person liked or disliked his/her own body.

Fascinating findings: When participants held onto the pieces of paper containing their written thoughts, those thoughts had a significant impact on how they felt about their bodies. In other words, participants who had been assigned to write positive remarks about their bodies rated themselves higher on the nine-point scales, while those assigned to write negative remarks rated themselves lower.

However, among participants who were told to throw out the pieces of paper containing their written thoughts, there was no difference in body-image test scores between the positive and negative groups—strongly suggesting that the act of physically discarding the written-down negative thoughts took away the power of those thoughts to damage self-image.

EXPERIMENT #2: **Diet judge.** Each participant was instructed to write either negative or positive thoughts about the Mediterranean diet after being reminded that it involves lots of fruit, vegetables, legumes and unrefined grains, with olive oil as the main fat. One group of participants was then instructed to toss their papers away…a second group was told to place their papers in their pockets or purses…a third group was told to leave their papers at their desks. Afterward, all participants were asked to rate the healthiness and desirability of the Mediterranean diet using various nine-point scales.

Intriguing results: Interestingly, the Mediterranean diet—which is generally regarded as quite healthful—was ranked most highly by people who wrote positive thoughts about it and then kept the paper in their pocket or purse…and by people who wrote negative thoughts and then discarded the paper. This suggests you can magnify the power of positive thoughts by writing them down and then protecting that paper…and that you can neutralize the power of negative thoughts to wrongly influence your judgment and attitude by writing them down and then throwing them away.

EXPERIMENT #3: **Imagination investigation.** Researchers wanted to know whether the physical act of throwing away the written thoughts was necessary or whether just imagining the act would be enough to influence subsequent attitudes. This time, participants were seated at computers and asked to type their negative thoughts about the Mediterranean diet into a document. Then one group of participants was instructed to dispose of their documents by using the mouse to drag them to the computer's recycle bin…other participants protected their documents by saving them onto storage disks…and still other participants were told to simply imagine moving their files to either the recycle bin or a storage disk. Then, as in the earlier experiment, all the participants were asked to rate the diet.

What happened next: Even though sending the typed thoughts to the recycle bin did not require physically tossing out a piece of paper, the physical act of using the mouse to perform the disposal had the same effect as throwing out a piece of paper—it reduced the impact of the participants' written thoughts on their evaluations. However, the diet evaluations of those who simply imagined moving their files to the recycle bin demonstrated that these participants were still under the influence of their written thoughts.

How remarkable it is to know that physically tossing away your negative thoughts really does toss them away!

USE THESE INSIGHTS TO YOUR ADVANTAGE

Though this study focused primarily on the effects of discarding negative thoughts, it also suggests that the phenomenon works both ways—so that by protecting positive thoughts, you can increase their power. Why not give it a try? For instance, if you have a job interview and want to portray yourself as confident, you could tuck a note into your pocket, telling yourself that you are competent and in control. When your brain is stuck on a negative thought that's interfering with your attitude or behavior, scribble it on a piece of paper—and then deliberately and mindfully toss it in the trash. Good riddance!

Bad Thoughts About Others: The Poison Inside Your Mind

Friedemann Schaub, MD, PhD, physician specializing in cardiology, molecular biologist, American Board of Hypnotherapy–certified trainer of clinical hypnotherapy, and certified master practitioner in Neuro-Linguistic Programming (NLP) and Time Line Therapy. Dr. Schaub maintains a private practice in Seattle and is author of *The Fear & Anxiety Solution*. TheFearAndAnxietySolution.com

You've heard many times how much damage you do to your self-esteem when you bash yourself with criticism: *I'm such an idiot…klutz…wimp.* But did you know that when you mentally bash other people, even in the privacy of your own mind, you're actually hurting yourself physically as well as psychologically?

It's true. *So consider whether you recognize yourself in scenarios such as these…*

• **A man driving a sports car cuts you off,** and your inner voice screams, *Hey, #)@%! Do you think you own the road?*

• **A cashier gives you the wrong change,** and you think to yourself, *What a dope. She should lose her job.*

• **When a coworker points out a mistake you made, you inwardly snarl,** *Does she really need to make a big deal of this? She's the one who blew the presentation last month. I'll get her!*

If those kinds of silent diatribes seem familiar, you are filling your mind with toxic thoughts —which is, as the saying goes, kind of like drinking poison yourself and hoping that it kills the other person. Don't drink the poison. *Here's why it hurts you…and how to stop doing it…*

OUCH, IT HURTS

When you wallow in negativity toward someone else, the person you are silently deriding goes merrily along his/her way with no clue as to what you are thinking. But inside your own body, those seething thoughts are triggering a cascade of physiological responses that, over time, take a toll on your physical health, according to Friedemann Schaub, MD, PhD, author of *The Fear & Anxiety Solution*.

"The nervous system reacts to negative emotions by releasing stress hormones, which affect the body in many different ways," said Dr. Schaub, a physician specializing in cardiology and a molecular biologist. The immediate effects include increased blood pressure, faster heartbeat and tightened muscles. Over the long term, your cholesterol rises and your immune system weakens. These changes make you more vulnerable to a host of ills, including heart disease, cancer and autoimmune disorders.

You suffer psychologically, too. "What most people don't realize is that the subconscious mind takes everything personally. So when you're cursing a clueless driver or incompetent coworker, your subconscious registers only feelings of anger and disdain. It is unable to determine whether you're upset with somebody else or yourself," Dr. Schaub said.

MENTAL JUNK FOOD

Sometimes an angry inner dialogue is an important signal that you need to take action to change the situation—for instance, by having a conversation with your teen about respect or by telling your spouse that something he/she did was hurtful. But if you often find yourself ruminating furiously about minor slights, it's a sign that your inner dialogue habits need a makeover.

Recognizing the problem is the first step toward change.

The second step: Get yourself a small notebook, Dr. Schaub suggested. Carry it with you, and write down the circumstances whenever you catch yourself indulging in inner bashing of others. After you've done this for a week or two, read over your entries and look for patterns, keeping an eye out for these four particularly damaging mental habits...

• **Passing judgment.** You're irritated because someone has done something that you believe is wrong, such as bringing too many items into the express line at the supermarket.

• **Making comparisons.** You put others down as a way to pull up your self-esteem. For instance, you think uncharitable thoughts about how fat your cousin has gotten and congratulate yourself on staying slim.

• **Deriving pleasure from another's misfortune.** The Germans have a specific word for this—schadenfreude. Something bad happens to someone else and you secretly take pleasure from it. He deserves it, you tell yourself with a grin when the coworker who got the promotion you wanted ends up being laid off.

• **Gossiping.** You enjoy talking about others, especially when they're in trouble.

Example: You learn that your neighbors are divorcing because one spouse discovered the other's huge gambling debts...and you can't wait to spread the news.

"Indulging in such unwholesome thinking is like allowing yourself to eat a giant bag of potato chips for lunch just because you're hungry—even though you know that you could find healthier and more satisfying food to fill your stomach," Dr. Schaub said. "You can imagine the detrimental impact such a mental diet can have."

REFORMING YOUR INNER DIALOGUE

You can do much better for yourself. You can choose to fill your mind with more productive and positive thoughts. To start, take your notebook again. When you catch yourself judging, comparing, taking pleasure in another's pain or gossiping, consider how you are feeling about yourself at the same moment, Dr. Schaub suggested. *You are likely to discover that you're feeling one of three ways...*

• **Insecure about your own abilities.**

• **Powerless to control the situation.**

• **Isolated, as though you don't really fit in and/or people don't like you.**

Again, look for patterns. Where do those feelings come from? Perhaps during your childhood, your parents made you feel insecure by comparing you unfavorably with a sibling. Perhaps your sense of powerlessness or isolation comes from having been bullied or ostracized as a teen. Perhaps you are just jealous of people with really nice cars.

Developing greater self-awareness about your own state of mind provides an opportunity to address those underlying issues. "Your goal is to shift away from internally commenting on what others are doing and instead focus on understanding yourself," said Dr. Schaub. "Such self-awareness doesn't have to be intense or painful. It's actually a way to expand your point of view and make life more enjoyable and fulfilling."

To accomplish that, try practicing these three steps whenever your inner bombs start exploding on someone else's unsuspecting head...

• **Acceptance.** If you know the other individual personally, consider him in the fuller context of his whole life. For instance, maybe that overweight cousin you disparage spends every day caring for his elderly mother, so he has no time for the gym. If your ire is directed toward a stranger, Dr. Schaub's suggestion is to spin your own story. That guy in the sports car who cut you off? Maybe he's rushing to the hospital because his child was injured. You can make the story simple, complicated or even funny—and it doesn't matter whether any of it is true. Its only purpose is to remind you that other people's lives are complicated in ways you can't always understand.

• **Appreciation.** Next, think positive thoughts about your situation. For example, if you are irritated because your neighbor doesn't clean up after her dog (and you are scrupulous about doing so when you walk your own dog), remind yourself to feel grateful that you live in a nice neighborhood where people want to walk their pets…and give yourself a little commendation for doing the right thing yourself.

• **Action.** This is empowering. That coworker who pointed out your mistake? Instead of plotting how to reveal her own errors to the entire department, privately thank her for alerting you to a potential problem with your project…then fix the mistake. Dr. Schaub said, "This final step brings inner resolution because it directs your thoughts away from the person you are bashing—whose actions, after all, you cannot control—and back toward solutions that you can implement yourself."

Five Ways to Think Yourself Out of Winter Depression

Kelly Rohan, PhD, professor of psychological science, The University of Vermont, Burlington. Her primary research interest is the treatment of adult mood disorders such as SAD with cognitive behavioral therapy.

Can you think your way out of winter depression?

It might seem a simplistic approach to seasonal affective disorder (SAD). But working with a therapist trained in cognitive behavioral therapy (CBT) to reframe your thoughts about winter can lead to lasting relief from SAD, according to a recent study. Over the long term, it's even more effective than bright-light therapy, which definitely helps but only as long as you keep doing it.

How does a CBT therapist work with a patient who has SAD, a form of depression that tends to strike hardest in the cold, dark winter months? What kind of thought experiments do they engage in? *The study's lead author, Kelly Rohan, PhD, a professor of psychological science at The University of Vermont in Burlington, explained her three-step process to thinking yourself out of winter depression…*

• **The first step is to take note of your negative thoughts by writing them down in a diary.**

• **Next, identify ways your thought patterns may be distorting what's really happening**—making things seem worse than they really are.

• **Finally, challenge your thoughts.** Ask yourself questions such as, What's the evidence to support this thought?…Is there any other way to look at this?…How can I reframe this thought so it's less negative and more positive—or at least neutral?

The ultimate goal? To identify and create new thoughts—ones you can really believe in—that help you feel that you have more control over your moods. *Here are five examples…*

FIVE SAD IDEAS—CHALLENGED AND REFRAMED

SAD IDEA: **Winter is such a hassle—I can't do what I want to do.**

Cognitive distortions: This blanket statement is an example of the ways our thoughts can distort what is really the case—magnification (blowing things out of proportion) and global negative labeling (overgeneralizing an observation or quality into a judgement that this is always a negative reality under all circumstances).

Challenge it! Consider what that statement actually means for you—that you need to put on more layers of clothing? That it's dark when you go out in the evening? How much of a hassle is that, really?

Reframe the thought: With these factors in mind, you might reframe this thought as, *Sure, there are inconveniences associated with winter—but I can handle them…*

SAD IDEA: **The dark, dreary days of winter make me feel depressed.**

Cognitive distortions: Filtering (taking negative details and magnifying them while ignoring positive aspects of the season) and all-or-nothing thinking (looking at things in absolute, black or white terms).

Challenge it! For starters, ask yourself how helpful this thought is. Does it make you feel better or worse? If it makes you feel worse, replace it with a more neutral but still realistic thought.

Reframe the thought: I prefer sunny days to gray days, but regardless of the weather, I can find ways to cheer myself up.

SAD IDEA: **I'm so tired during the winter that I never have the energy to exercise.**

Cognitive distortions: All-or-nothing thinking (the word "never" is a tip-off) and overgeneralization (viewing fatigue as an ever-present pattern rather than something you feel sometimes but not at every moment).

Challenge it! Recall a time when you enjoyed winter activities (such as ice-skating, skiing or sledding) or were able to push through your fatigue and be active in other ways. Then think of physical activities you'd like to try this winter. It could be as ambitious as learning how to snowshoe or as simple as a brisk daily walk. With these ideas in mind, you may be able to come up with a more positive yet still realistic thought.

Reframe the thought: It's true I'm often tired in the winter, but I can muster the energy to do physical activities that appeal to me.

SAD IDEA: **Some people look great in winter clothes, but when I put mine on, I'm sure I look fat to everyone.**

Cognitive distortions: Filtering, negative labeling and personalization (taking something personally that isn't personal at all).

Challenge it! Point out to yourself that the primary reason you change the way you dress in the winter is to stay warm—it's that simple. So while you may feel like you look better in lighter clothes, there's a benefit to feeling cozy, warm and comfortable in a soft sweater. Consider small changes you can make to feel more attractive in winter wear—a new coat if you need one and can afford it…or even just a nice new scarf. That could be all you need to feel better about your appearance.

Reframe the thought: I like the feeling of dressing for warmth and comfort, and I can do so in my own personal style.

SAD IDEA: **I always gain weight in the winter because I'm overwhelmed by cravings for comfort food, and eating them makes me happy.**

Cognitive distortions: All-or-nothing thinking, control fallacies (believing you're at the mercy of your cravings) and catastrophizing (expecting the worst—weight gain—to occur).

Challenge it! Point out to yourself that while you often crave high-calorie foods in the winter, you can find healthier ways to feel happy—perhaps by calling an old friend or doing a hobby you really enjoy. Behavioral changes are an essential part of the picture with CBT—it's not just "cognitive" therapy but cognitive "behavioral" therapy. That means that part of your solution is to change what you do, not just how you think. If you enjoy gardening in your backyard in the spring, for example, you might decide to grow herbs in a window box in the winter. Make no mistake—your behavior can definitely lift your mood.

Reframe the thought: I can find new ways to boost my mood that don't involve food.

GETTING HELP THIS WINTER

If you're prone to SAD, the best approach is to seek out a therapist who is trained in CBT so that you can figure out the thought and behavioral patterns that are bringing you down—and work together to fix them. It's not a one-size-fits-all approach. Since the use of CBT for SAD is fairly new, your best bet is to ask your primary-care physician for a referral to a good CBT therapist, or use the online finder on the website of the National Association of Cognitive-Behavioral Therapists at NACBT.org. When you make contact, explain that you want help with changing your thoughts and behaviors toward the season of your discontent—and let the therapist you choose guide you from there.

Index

413